American Academy of Pediatrics
DEDICATED TO THE HEALTH OF ALL CHILDREN™

American College of
Emergency Physicians®
ADVANCING EMERGENCY CARE

APLS

The Pediatric Emergency Medicine Resource

FIFTH EDITION

D1594931

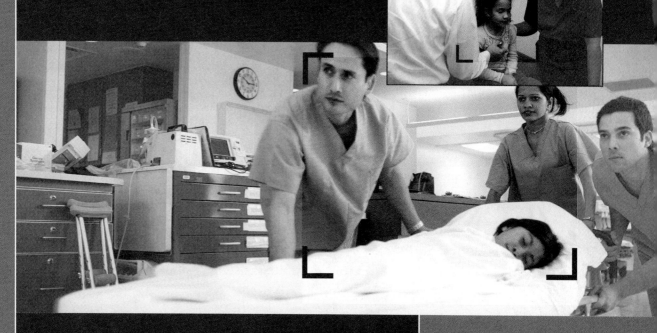

Susan Fuchs, MD, FAAP, FACEP
Editor

Loren Yamamoto, MD, MPH, MBA, FAAP, FACEP
Editor

Children are one-fourth of our population— and all of our future.

JONES & BARTLETT
LEARNING

World Headquarters
Jones & Bartlett Learning
5 Wall Street
Burlington, MA 01803
978-443-5000
info@jblearning.com
www.jblearning.com

Substantial discounts on bulk quantities of Jones & Bartlett Learning publications are available to corporations, professional associations, and other qualified organizations. For details and specific discount information, contact the special sales department at Jones & Bartlett Learning via the above contact information or send an email to specialsales@jblearning.com.

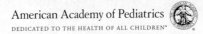

American Academy of Pediatrics
DEDICATED TO THE HEALTH OF ALL CHILDREN™

Thaddeus Anderson, Manager, Life Support Programs
Rory Hand, EdM, Life Support Simulation and Course Specialist
Rebecca Bretaña, Life Support Assistant
Melissa Marx, Manager, Life Support Programs
Wendy Simon, MA, CAE, Director, Life Support Programs
Robert Perelman, MD, Director, Department of Education

American Academy of Pediatrics
141 Northwest Point Boulevard
Post Office Box 927
Elk Grove Village, IL 60009-0927
847-434-4795
www.APLSonline.com
www.aap.org

American College of Emergency Physicians®
ADVANCING EMERGENCY CARE

Marta Foster, Director, Educational Publications
Jessica Hamilton, Publications Assistant
Thomas S. Werlinich, Associate Executive Director, Educational Products Division

American College of Emergency Physicians
1125 Executive Circle
Irving, TX 75038
Post Office Box 619911
Dallas, TX 75261-9911
800-798-1822
www.APLSonline.com
www.acep.org

Jones & Bartlett Learning books and products are available through most bookstores and online booksellers. To contact Jones & Bartlett Learning directly, call 800-832-0034, fax 978-443-8000, or visit our website, www.jblearning.com.

Production Credits
Executive Publisher: Kimberly Brophy
VP, Sales, Public Safety Group: Matthew Maniscalco
Managing Editor: Carol B. Guerrero
Senior Editorial Assistant: Amber Hodge
Editorial Assistant: Carly Lavoie
VP, Production and Design: Anne Spencer

Production Editor: Jessica deMartin
Director of Marketing: Alisha Weisman
Online Products Manager: Dawn Mahon Priest
VP, Manufacturing and Inventory Control: Therese Connell
Cover Design: Kristin E. Parker
Rights and Permissions Manager: Katherine Crighton

Photo Research Supervisor: Anna Genoese
Composition: Nicolazzo Productions
Cover Image: (patient on gurney) © Blend Images/ Alamy Images; (patient being examined) © NorthGeorgiaMedia/ShutterStock, Inc.
Printing and Binding: LSC Communications
Cover Printing: LSC Communications

The material is made available as part of the professional education programs of the American Academy of Pediatrics. No endorsement of any product or service should be inferred or is intended. Every effort has been made to ensure that contributors to the *APLS: The Pediatric Emergency Medicine Resource, Fifth Edition* materials are knowledgeable authorities in their fields. Readers are nevertheless advised that the statements and opinions expressed are provided as guidelines and should not be construed as official policy of the American Academy of Pediatrics. The recommendations in this publication and the accompanying materials do not indicate an exclusive course of treatment. Variations, taking into account individual circumstances, nature of medical oversight, and local protocols, may be appropriate. The American Academy of Pediatrics disclaims any liability or responsibility for the consequences of any actions taken in reliance on these statements or opinions.

Equipment depicted within the text and accompanying materials may vary from that utilized in your clinical practice. Learners are advised to become familiar with and review the manufacturer's directions for use of the actual therapeutic equipment utilized within his/her work place.

Neither the equipment nor procedures demonstrated in the materials represent an exclusive course of treatment. Learners are advised that differences in local protocols and equipment are likely and variations due to individual circumstances and nature of medical oversight may be appropriate.

The American College of Emergency Physicians (ACEP) makes every effort to ensure that contributors to its publications are knowledgeable subject matter experts. Readers are nevertheless advised that the statements and opinions expressed in this publication are provided as the contributors' recommendations at the time of publication and should not be construed as official College policy. ACEP recognizes the complexity of emergency medicine and makes no representation that this publication serves as an authoritative resource for the prevention, diagnosis, treatment, or intervention for any medical condition, nor should it be the basis for the definition of, or standard of care that should be practiced by all health care providers at any particular time or place. Drugs are generally referred to by generic names. In some instances, brand names are added for easier recognition. Device manufacturer information is provided according to style conventions of the American Medical Association. ACEP received no commercial support for this publication. To the fullest extent permitted by law, and without limitation, ACEP expressly disclaims all liability for errors or omissions contained within this publication, and for damages of any kind or nature, arising out of use, reference to, reliance on, or performance of such information. To contact ACEP, write to PO Box 619911, Dallas, TX 75261-9911; or call toll-free 800-798-1822 or 972-550-0911.

Some images in this book feature models. These models do not necessarily endorse, represent, or participate in the activities represented in the images. Additional illustrations and photographic credits appear on page 535, which constitutes a continuation of the copyright page.

To order this product, use ISBN: 978-1-4496-9596-5
Book alone ISBN: 978-1-4496-9595-8

Library of Congress Cataloging-in-Publication Data
APLS : the pediatric emergency medicine resource / American Academy of Pediatrics, American College of Emergency Physicians. — 5th ed.
    p. ; cm.
Pediatric emergency medicine resource
Rev. ed. of: Pediatric emergency medicine resource. 4th rev. ed. c2007.
Includes bibliographical references and index.
ISBN-13: 978-1-4496-2445-3
ISBN-10: 1-4496-2445-6
1. Pediatric emergencies. 2. CPR (First aid) for children. I. American Academy of Pediatrics. II. American College of Emergency Physicians. III. Pediatric emergency medicine resource. IV. Title: Pediatric emergency medicine resource.
[DNLM: 1. Cardiopulmonary Resuscitation. 2. Emergencies. 3. Child. 4. Infant. WS 205]
RJ370.A34 2012
618.92'0025—dc23
                                 2011025584

6048
Printed in the United States of America
20 19 18 17 16   10 9 8 7 6 5 4

Online Chapters

Contents

Contents

Contents

8 Nontraumatic Surgical Emergencies 298

9 Nontraumatic Orthopedic Emergencies 360

10 Medical Emergencies . . 392

11 Neonatal Emergencies 424

Acknowledgments

The editors would like to acknowledge the work of the Board-appointed reviewers:

Lee S. Benjamin, MD, FACEP, FAAP
Board Reviewer, American College of Emergency Physicians
Assistant Professor of Surgery and Pediatrics
Divisions of Emergency Medicine and Pediatric Emergency Medicine
Duke University School of Medicine
Durham, North Carolina

Michael J. Gerardi, MD, FAAP, FACEP
Board Reviewer, American College of Emergency Physicians
Board of Directors, American College of Emergency Physicians
Associate Professor, Emergency Medicine
Mt. Sinai School of Medicine
Director of Pediatric Emergency Medicine
Goryeb Children's Hospital
Faculty, Department of Emergency Medicine
Morristown Memorial Hospital
Morristown, New Jersey
Senior Vice President, Emergency Medical Associates
Livingston, New Jersey

Mark A. Hostetler, MD, MPH, FACEP
Board Reviewer, American College of Emergency Physicians
Associate Division Chief
Clinical Professor, Pediatrics and Emergency Medicine
University of Arizona
Pediatric Emergency Medicine
Phoenix Children's Hospital
Phoenix, Arizona

Ramon W. Johnson, MD, FAAP, FACEP
Board Reviewer, American College of Emergency Physicians
Board of Directors, American College of Emergency Physicians
Mission Hospital Regional Medical Center
Children's Hospital at Mission Viejo
Mission Viejo, California

Carden Johnston, MD, FAAP, FRCP
Board Reviewer, American Academy of Pediatrics
Emeritus Professor of Pediatrics
University of Alabama at Birmingham School of Medicine
Birmingham, Alabama

Audrey Z. Paul, MD, PhD
Board Reviewer, American College of Emergency Physicians
Assistant Fellowship Director, Pediatric Emergency Medicine
Assistant Professor, Department of Emergency Medicine
Mount Sinai School of Medicine
New York, New York

Rick Place, MD, FAAP, FACEP
Board Reviewer, American College of Emergency Physicians
Associate Clinical Professor of Emergency Medicine
George Washington University
Pediatric Medical Director
Department of Emergency Medicine
Inova Fairfax Hospital for Children
Falls Church, Virginia

Ghazala Q. Sharieff, MD, FACEP, FAAEM
Board Reviewer, American College of Emergency Physicians
Director of Pediatric Emergency Medicine
Palomar-Pomerado Health System/California Emergency Physicians
Clinical Professor
University of California, San Diego
San Diego, California

The American Academy of Pediatrics, the American College of Emergency Physicians, the lead editors, and the authors of this edition would like to thank editors, authors, contributors, and reviewers for their significant contributions to past editions. Without their efforts, this edition would not have been possible.

Contributors

The American Academy of Pediatrics, American College of Emergency Physicians, and Editors acknowledge with appreciation the contributions of the following individuals in the development of this resource.

Terry Adirim, MD, MPH, FAAP
Shady Grove Adventist Hospital
Rockville, Maryland

Mark Adler, MD
Feinberg School of Medicine, Northwestern
    University
Division of Pediatric Emergency Medicine
Children's Memorial Hospital
Chicago, Illinois

Jeffrey R. Avner, MD, FAAP
Children's Hospital at Montefiore
Albert Einstein College of Medicine
Bronx, New York

Russell E. Berger, MD
Harvard Medical Toxicology Fellow
Children's Hospital Boston
Boston, Massachusetts

Carol D. Berkowitz, MD, FAAP, FACEP
Harbor-UCLA Medical Center
Rancho Palos Verdes, California

Casey Buitenhuys, MD
Harbor-UCLA Medical Center
Torrance, California

Michele Burns Ewald, MD, FAAP
Harvard Medical Toxicology Fellowship,
    Children's Hospital Boston
Boston, Massachusetts

William A. Carey, MD, FAAP
Assistant Professor of Pediatrics
Medical Director, Neonatal Transport
Division of Neonatal Medicine
Mayo Clinic
Rochester, Minnesota

Meta L. Carroll, MD, FAAP
Assistant Professor Pediatrics
Division of Pediatric Emergency Medicine
Department of Pediatrics
Northwestern University Feinberg School of
    Medicine
Children's Memorial Hospital and Northwest
    Community Hospital
Chicago, Illinois

Lei Chen, MD, FAAP
Yale University School of Medicine
New Haven, Connecticut

Adam Cheng, MD
BC Children's Hospital
Vancouver, British Columbia

Wendy Coates, MD, FACEP
Department of Emergency Medicine
Harbor-UCLA Medical Center
Torrance, California

Chris Colby, MD, FAAP
Division of Neonatology
Mayo Clinic
Rochester, Minnesota

Cole Condra, MD, FAAP
Assistant Professor of Pediatrics
Division of Emergency Medical Services
Children's Mercy Hospitals and Clinics
University of Missouri-Kansas City
Kansas City, Missouri

Teena Cortese, PharmD
Our Lady of Lourdes Medical Center
Camden, New Jersey

Contributors

Andrew DePiero, MD, FAAP, FACEP
Assistant Professor of Pediatrics
Jefferson Medical College
Alfred I DuPont Hospital for Children
Wilmington, Delaware

Peter J. Di Rocco, MD
Medical College of Wisconsin
PEM, Children's Corporate Center
Milwaukee, Wisconsin

Ronald A. Dieckmann, MD, MPH, FACEP
Professor Emeritus of Pediatrics and
    Emergency Medicine
UCSF School of Medicine
Oakland, California

Stephanie J. Doniger, MD, RDMS, FAAP
Children's Hospital and Research Center –
    Oakland
Oakland, California

Timothy B. Erickson, MD, FACEP, FAACT, FACMT
Professor of Emergency Medicine and Medical
    Toxicology
Department of Emergency Medicine and
    Division of Medical Toxicology
University of Illinois
Chicago, Illinois

Jason W. Fischer, MD, MSc
Assistant Professor, Department of Paediatrics
University of Toronto
Director Emergency Ultrasound Program
Division of Emergency Medicine
The Hospital for Sick Children, Toronto
Toronto, Ontario

Laura Fitzmaurice, MD, FAAP, FACEP
Children's Mercy Hospitals and Clinics
University of Missouri-Kansas City
Kansas City, Missouri

George L. Foltin, MD, FAAP, FACEP
Director, Center for Pediatric Emergency
    Medicine
Associate Professor
Departments of Pediatrics and Emergency
    Medicine
NYU School of Medicine
Bellevue Hospital Center
New York, New York

Susan Fuchs, MD, FAAP, FACEP
Professor of Pediatrics
Feinberg School of Medicine
Northwestern University
Associate Director, Pediatric Emergency
    Medicine
Children's Memorial Hospital
Chicago, Illinois

Marianne Gausche-Hill, MD, FAAP, FACEP
Professor of Medicine
David Geffen School of Medicine at UCLA
Director of EMS and Pediatric Medicine
    Fellowships
Harbor-UCLA Medical Center
Department of Emergency Medicine
Torrance, California

Nicole Glaser, MD
University of California, Davis
Department of Pediatrics
Sacramento, California

Nicole Green, MD
Alfred I. DuPont Hospital for Children
Wilmington, Delaware

Phyllis L. Hendry, MD, FAAP, FACEP
University of Florida Health Science Center,
    Jacksonville
Jacksonville, Florida

Barry A. Hicks, MD, FAAP, FACS
Thomas Jefferson University and Hospitals
Philadelphia, Pennsylvania

Dee Hodge III, MD, FAAP
Washington University in St. Louis School of
    Medicine
St. Louis, Missouri

Daniel J. Isaacman, MD, FAAP
Director, Vaccines
Vaccines Clinical Research
Merck Research Laboratories

Elka Jacobson-Dickman, MD
State University of New York
Downstate Medical Center
Brooklyn, New York

**Stephen R. Karl, MD, NREMTP, FAAP,
    FACS**
Principal Investigator
South Dakota EMS for Children Project
Director, Pediatric Surgery
Avera Children's Hospital & Clinics
Sioux Falls, South Dakota

Brent R. King, MD, MMM, FAAP, FACEP
Clive, Nancy, and Pierce Runnells Distin-
    guished Professor of Emergency Medicine
Professor of Pediatrics
Chairman, Department of Emergency Medicine
Executive Vice-Dean for Clinical Affairs
The University of Texas Medical School at
    Houston
Houston, Texas

Christopher King, MD, FACEP
Associate Professor
Emergency Medicine and Pediatrics
University of Pittsburgh School of Medicine
Division of Pediatric Emergency Medi-
    cine
Pittsburgh, Pennsylvania

Steven E. Krug, MD, FAAP
Children's Memorial Hospital
Chicago, Illinois

Nathan Kuppermann, MD, MPH, FAAP
Professor, Department of Emergency Medicine
    and Pediatrics
Bo Tomas Brofeldt Endowed Chair,
    Emergency Medicine
UC Davis School of Medicine
UC Davis Medical Center
Sacramento, California

Sharon Elizabeth Mace, MD, FAAP, FACEP
Cleveland Clinic
Cleveland, OH

Michael Martin, MD
Inova Fairfax Hospital
Falls Church, Virginia

Kemedy K. McQuillen, MD, FAAP
Central Maine Medical Center
Lewiston, ME

Chris Merritt, MD, MPH
Hasbro Children's Hospital, Alpert Medical
    School of Brown University
Providence, Rhode Island

Pamela J. Okada, MD, FAAP
The University of Texas Southwestern Medical
    Center at Dallas
Dallas, Texas

Parul B. Patel, MD, MPH, FAAP
Children's Memorial Hospital
Feinberg School of Medicine, Northwestern
    University
Chicago, Illinois

Ronald I. Paul, MD, FAAP
University of Louisville
Louisville, Kentucky

Rick Place, MD, FAAP, FACEP
Associate Clinical Professor of Emergency
    Medicine
George Washington University
Pediatric Medical Director
Department of Emergency Medicine
Inova Fairfax Hospital for Children
Falls Church, Virginia

Contributors

Alfred Sacchetti, MD, FACEP
Our Lady of Lourdes Medical Center
Camden, New Jersey

John P. Santamaria, MD, FAAP
Affiliate Professor of Pediatrics
USF School of Medicine
Tampa, Florida

Steven M. Selbst, MD, FAAP
Professor of Pediatrics
Jefferson Medical College
Alfred I. DuPont Hospital for Children
Wilmington, Delaware

Ghazala Q. Sharieff, MD, FAAP, FACEP,
   FAAEM
Director of Pediatric Emergency Medicine
Palomar-Pomerado Health System/California
   Emergency Physicians
Clinical Professor
University of California, San Diego
San Diego, California

Paul E. Sirbaugh, DO, FAAP
Baylor College of Medicine / TCH
Houston, Texas

Jennifer L. Trainor, MD, FAAP
Children's Memorial Hospital
Feinberg School of Medicine, Northwestern
   University
Chicago, Illinois

Michael G. Tunik, MD, FAAP
Associate Professor
Departments of Pediatrics and Emergency
   Medicine
NYU School of Medicine
Bellevue Hospital Center
New York, New York

Debra L. Weiner, MD, PhD, FAAP
Emergency Medicine
Children's Hospital Boston
Boston, Massachusetts

Loren Yamamoto, MD, MPH, MBA, FAAP,
   FACEP
Professor of Pediatrics
University of Hawaii
Emergency Medicine Director & Vice
   Chief of Staff
John Burns School of Medicine
Honolulu, Hawaii

Working in crisis situations is demanding and requires that you be at your best. Prepare yourself with APLS, the definitive resource on pediatric emergency medicine. This resource is the core of the APLS course with features that will reinforce and expand on the essential information. These features include:

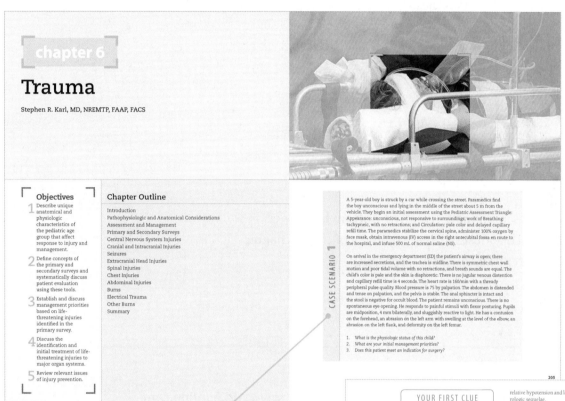

Case Scenario: Chapters contain multiple case scenarios. Case scenarios prompt readers to think about what they might do if they encountered a similar situation. A summary of assessment and management considerations for each case scenario appears at the end of the chapter.

Your First Clue: Outlines the most important signs and symptoms.

The Classics: Outlines significant diagnostic study findings.

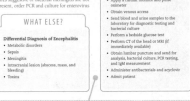

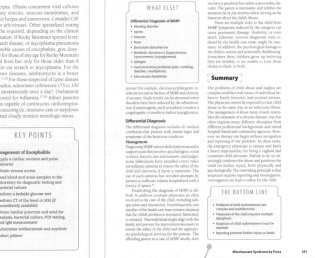

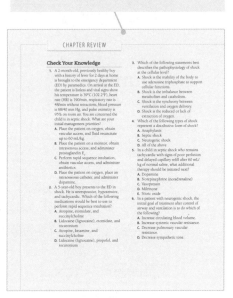

What Else?: Outlines important points of differential diagnosis.

Key Points: Outline critical management steps.

The Bottom Line: Brief summary of crucial chapter concepts.

Check Your Knowledge: End-of-chapter questions for your own self-assessment.

Instructor's ToolKit CD-ROM

978-1-4496-5179-4

Preparation is made easy with the resources found on this CD-ROM, including:

- PowerPoint® Presentations
- Lecture Outlines
- Image Bank
- Table Bank
- And much more

www.APLSonline.com

The engaging APLS technology resource provides a wealth of tools to assist in running an APLS course and to promote further learning. At the site, users will have access to:

- Background information on APLS and guidelines on how to start an APLS course.

- Additional digital content. This content is unlocked by redeeming the access code bound into the front of this textbook.

This current edition of *APLS: The Pediatric Emergency Medicine Resource* is an updated course for practitioners of pediatric acute care and emergency medicine. The content is authored by those with expert knowledge in their respective areas of study. Our shared goal is for APLS to be a highly efficient resource by conveying the most useful and important information in a concise, compact, and accessible format.

As with the last editions, the textbook serves as the core of the APLS course. In the Fifth Edition, however, supplemental materials are available in alternate electronic formats. This enhancement lightens the textbook while ensuring that content best conveyed in digital format be made highly deliverable and mobile.

Some new features of the Fifth Edition of APLS include:

- Updated and improved chapters
- A section on bedside ultrasound
- A guideline for the ED management of diabetic ketoacidosis
- Advances in procedural sedation and a recommended deep sedation protocol
- A standard set of discharge instruction forms (after-care instructions) translated into several languages, which may be used by EDs (in place of EDs creating their own translated discharge instruction forms)
- A simulation primer with fully developed cases
- Updated recommendations and algorithms from *Pediatric Advanced Life Support* (PALS)

It is our hope that you found all of the enhancements and improvements to be valuable in advancing the care of children experiencing emergencies.

Susan Fuchs, MD, FAAP, FACEP
Loren Yamamoto, MD, MPH, MBA, FAAP, FACEP
Editors
APLS: The Pediatric Emergency Medicine Resource
Fifth Edition

chapter 1

Pediatric Assessment

Ronald A. Dieckmann, MD, MPH, FACEP

Objectives

1 Describe the epidemiology of emergency pediatrics.

2 Distinguish the three components of the Pediatric Assessment Triangle.

3 List the pediatric-specific features of the primary assessment or ABCDEs for infants, children, and adolescents.

4 Differentiate between the goals and components of the primary assessment and the secondary assessment.

5 Outline the components of history taking and performing a physical examination.

Chapter Outline

Introduction
Developing a General Impression: The PAT
The Primary Assessment: The Pediatric ABCDEs
Summary of General Impression and Primary Assessment
The Secondary Assessment: History Taking and the Physical Examination
The Tertiary Assessment: Diagnostic Evaluations
Reassessment

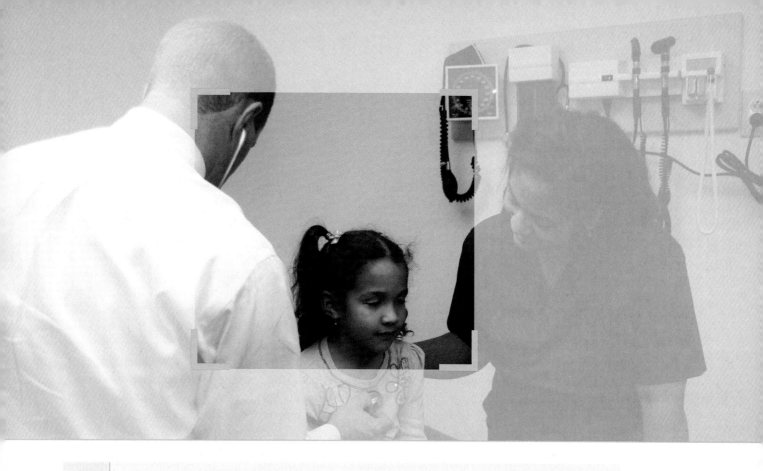

A 6-month-old boy who has had persistent vomiting for 24 hours presents to the emergency department (ED). The infant is lying still and has poor muscle tone. He is irritable if touched, and his cry is weak. There are no abnormal airway sounds, retractions, or flaring. He is pale and mottled. The respiratory rate (RR) is 45/min, heart rate is 170/min, and blood pressure is 50 by palpation. Air movement is normal, and breath sounds are clear to auscultation. The skin feels cool, and capillary refill time is 4 seconds. The brachial pulse is weak. His abdomen is distended.

1. *What are the key signs of serious illness in this infant?*
2. *How helpful are heart rate, RR, and blood pressure in evaluating cardiopulmonary function?*

Introduction

Emergency assessment of a child with an acute illness or injury requires special knowledge of normal and abnormal growth and development, as well as pediatric-specific evaluation skills. Emergency assessment of children is different from conventional physical assessment performed in nonurgent circumstances without critical time pressure and from adult emergency assessment. Conventional assessment includes a comprehensive history and a thorough anatomical head-to-toe (or toe-to-head) examination—a time-consuming approach that is not possible under emergency conditions when a highly prioritized sequence is required that integrates evaluation and critical interventions to preserve vital functions. Time-honored, adult emergency assessment often includes techniques that do not work well when evaluating acutely ill and injured children, especially preschool-aged children—in whom measurements of heart rate, RR, and blood pressure can be misleading. Adjustments to the emergency assessment based on the child's expected behavior and development will permit more subtle detection of real illness or injury.

Emergency assessment is a different process than diagnosis. Emergency assessment is a clinical evaluation, the primary goals of which are identification of abnormal anatomical and physiologic features, estimation of severity of injury or illness, and determination of urgency for emergency treatment. Diagnostic imaging and laboratory investigations are usually not essential components. Performing the rapid general impression and primary assessment allows the clinician to start general treatment to restore normal body homeostasis and physiologic function and to help prevent deterioration to respiratory or circulatory failure. The clinician might not establish a specific diagnosis after the general impression and primary assessment. Specific diagnosis is rarely necessary during resuscitation, when preserving basic airway patency, breathing, and circulation are the dominant concerns.

For patients of all ages, the emergency assessment has several specific components. The first component is the general impression, obtained from the doorway before the laying on of hands, which includes a general visual and auditory assessment of the child. This first phase or observational assessment should be accomplished using a highly efficient, prioritized, and focused approach termed the Pediatric Assessment Triangle (PAT). The next step is the primary assessment (sometimes called the initial assessment), a stepwise and prioritized approach that involves the hands-on determination of the ABCDEs (airway, breathing, circulation, disability, and exposure).

The general impression and primary assessment together are designed to detect physiologic abnormalities that can be life threatening and require immediate resuscitative actions. These assessment phases require modification to accommodate different developmental stages of childhood. Any serious physiologic abnormality that is identified must be treated before completing the next component of the sequence of the ABCDEs.

When the primary assessment is complete and after the child is stabilized, the clinician then proceeds to the secondary assessment. The secondary assessment, which is sometimes called the additional assessment, consists of taking a history and performing a physical examination structured to detect anatomical abnormalities, determine more subtle physiologic abnormalities, and identify dangerous signs and symptoms of impending problems. Secondary assessment integrates traditional, detailed history taking and head-to-toe (or toe-to-head) physical examination. This component of emergency assessment is oriented toward anatomical rather than physiologic abnormalities and emphasizes clinical diagnosis. In life-threatening or emergency conditions, secondary assessment might never be possible because the clinician has to continue aggressive resuscitation to restore vital functions.

After the secondary assessment, specific diagnostic tests are often necessary to identify the cause and severity of illness and injury. This component of patient evaluation is termed diagnostic assessment or tertiary assessment and uses laboratory and other ancillary procedures (eg, radiologic, invasive hemodynamic monitoring) to help establish specific diagnosis.

Reassessment is an important component of assessment. Reassessment includes repeated physical assessments and monitoring intended to evaluate trends of physiologic response to therapy and developing signs of distress.

Children experience a diverse array of acute illnesses and injuries, many of them unique to the vulnerable anatomical structure, immature immunologic and physiologic features, and normal exploratory behavior of youth. Fortunately, most pediatric emergencies are minor and can be readily managed with simple first aid measures at home or in school or by a primary care physician in a community office, clinic, or hospital pediatric ambulatory practice. Sometimes, pediatric illness or injury is of high acuity or life threatening or involves serious pain, and the more sophisticated medical capabilities of the ED are necessary.[1] Identifying and tracking the types of illnesses and injuries in children presenting to EDs, as well as their ages, sex, ethnicity, demographic and socioeconomic characteristics, mode or arrival, and treatment requirements, provide critical epidemiologic information for planning and managing systems for pediatric emergency care.

Epidemiology

The National Hospital Ambulatory Medical Care Survey (NHAMCS) is a national probability sample survey of visits to hospital EDs and outpatient departments of nonfederal, short-stay, and general hospitals in the United States. The survey was inaugurated in 1992 to gather, analyze, and disseminate information about the health care provided by hospital EDs and outpatient departments. In 2005, there were 115.3 million ED visits, about 39.6 visits per 100 persons. Children younger than 15 years accounted for 21.2% (24,497,000) of these visits. An additional 16.2% (18,682,000) of visits involved adolescents and young adults from 15 to 24 years old. The age group with the highest annual per capita ED visit rate was infants younger than 12 months, who made 91.3 visits per 100 infants, or approximately 3.8 million visits. Most pediatric ED patients arrived by private vehicle or were walk-ins and had either private insurance or Medicaid. The NHAMCS indicated that among children younger than 15 years, the rate of ED visits (the number of visits per 100 persons per year) was higher for males (43.0) than for females (37.6) and significantly higher for African Americans (64.7) than whites (37.7).[2,3]

Most children are seen in approximately 4,600 general and pediatric EDs throughout the United States.[4–6] These data pertain only to ED pediatric patients, who can be significantly different in their epidemiologic and demographic characteristics from children with emergency conditions cared for in private offices or clinics. Several physician surveys have found an important but significantly diminishing role for pediatricians in out-of-hospital management of many moderate to severe childhood emergencies, including meningitis, severe asthma, severe dehydration, seizures, altered mental status, anaphylaxis, and cardiopulmonary arrest.[7,8] Illnesses seem to predominate in office and clinic pediatric emergency patients, whereas injuries are far more likely in children in EDs. Other data point to a significant trend in overuse of EDs by children with many minor acute conditions easily treatable in the office or clinic.[9]

Out-of-Hospital and In-Hospital Epidemiology

In the out-of-hospital setting, 10% to 13% of ambulance runs are for infants, children, and adolescents.[10,11] Trauma represents a high number of pediatric out-of-hospital conditions, comprising approximately 54% of transported cases.[11] The most frequent mechanisms of injury among children using ambulances are motor vehicle crashes and falls. Among out-of-hospital illnesses, the most common are toxic exposures, seizures, and respiratory problems.[11] The epidemiology of out-of-hospital pediatrics is age dependent, with illnesses more common among younger children and injuries more common with increasing age. Among all patients seen in the ED, 14% arrive by ambulance. For children younger than 15 years, only 5.3% arrive by ambulance, compared with 10.3% for those 15 to 24 years and 43.1% for patients 75 years and older.[2] The epidemiology of critical illness and injury varies in different geographic locations, as does transportation and access to emergency care.

Hospitalization rates of children from EDs are markedly lower than rates for adults. One factor in pediatric hospitalization rates is the type of hospital where the ED evaluation occurred. A 2002 Canadian report on admission rates for bronchiolitis in Calgary found a 24% admission rate for children seen in pediatric EDs, compared with a 43% admission rate for those seen with similar characteristics in general EDs.[12] Admission experiences vary widely in geographic locations, and children's hospital EDs appear to care for children with different levels of illness and acuity than general EDs. Children with injuries and children and adolescents in older age groups tend to seek care at general EDs, whereas younger patients, especially infants, and children with medical illnesses often favor children's hospitals. One analysis indicated that 41% of children in a general ED had injuries, compared with only 22% at a pediatric ED.[11]

Injury Epidemiology

On the basis of mortality data, it appears that serious pediatric injuries are most frequently caused by motor vehicles, with the child being either an occupant or a pedestrian. The exception is infants for whom homicide secondary to child maltreatment is most prominent. Occupant injuries are the most common cause of death among teenagers and young adults, whereas pedestrian and bicycle-associated motor vehicle crashes are the most common cause in children. Burns, submersion injury, and violent death from homicide and suicide are also extremely important mechanisms of injury-related death in childhood.[13–15]

One study revealed that sprains, lacerations, fractures, and mild head injuries accounted for 90% of pediatric trauma in a general ED. Lacerations on the head and face accounted for 60% of all lacerations; the phalanx was the most common fracture site, followed by the radius/ulna.[2]

Illness Epidemiology

Respiratory diagnoses were the leading cause of illness-related ED visits for all age groups (0–20 years), accounting for 30% of visits.[16]

Respiratory illness is the leading reason for hospitalization of children. Asthma, pneumonia, and bronchiolitis together represent approximately one-third of pediatric hospitalizations. Seizures and gastroenteritis are also important reasons for hospitalization. Deaths from illness during the neonatal period were most frequently due to congenital malformations, disorders related to prematurity, and low birth weight.[12] Most postneonatal noninjury mortality in childhood is secondary to sudden infant death syndrome.[14] Most unexpected pediatric (<18 years) out-of-hospital cardiopulmonary arrests occur in children younger than 2 years, and most of those before the age of 1 year are due to sudden infant death syndrome. Overall, pediatric death from illness is more common than from injury, but after the age of 12 months, injury is more likely.[14]

Clinical Features of Assessment

Using an ordered sequence to emergency assessment will enforce a prioritized evaluation and management approach that will not only ensure an organized resuscitation but also help avoid missing important physiologic derangements or significant injuries. Table 1-1 outlines the entire assessment sequence, which is described in detail below. The terms used in the assessment sequence were agreed on in a national conference in 2005.[17]

TABLE 1-1 Pediatric Emergency Assessment Sequence

- General impression (Pediatric Assessment Triangle)
- Primary assessment (initial assessment)
- Secondary assessment (additional assessment)
  - History taking
  - Focused examination
  - Detailed exam (trauma)
- Diagnostic (tertiary) assessment
- Reassessment

General Impression

Emergency pediatric assessment begins with the "general impression," a visual and auditory assessment performed from the doorway. An accurate general impression is key to help identify physiologic abnormalities, determine severity and urgency for intervention, and prioritize initial treatment. Using a developmentally appropriate approach will improve the accuracy of all phases of assessment by adjusting the evaluation techniques to the expected growth and behavioral characteristics of the individual child. For injury, the assessment is sometimes straightforward because the cause or mechanism of injury is usually known, the child's main symptom is usually pain, and signs of obvious anatomical deformity often identify the problem. The child still needs careful physical evaluation for physiologic problems and for less obvious but possibly serious injuries, particularly involving the brain or abdomen. For illness, the assessment can be much trickier, especially in the infant, because onset, progression, and specific symptoms can be vague and physical signs of disease can be nonspecific.

A 21-month-old girl is brought to the ED after a 911 call. The mother explains that the child, who has severe cerebral palsy and a tracheostomy, has had copious secretions and has required more frequent suctioning and breathing treatments for 2 days. The mother is anxious and demanding immediate hospitalization for the child. The child turns blue and becomes agitated whenever you approach but is easily consoled by the mother and is interactive with the father. She follows every action of yours closely. There are no retractions or flaring. Her skin is pink if not provoked. Her RR is 50/min, and heart rate is 120/min. You are unable to obtain a blood pressure.

1. *How can the PAT be used to evaluate the severity of illness and urgency for care in a child with special health care needs?*

Developing a General Impression: The PAT

The PAT is a rapid, simple, and useful tool to assess children of all ages with all levels of illness and injury. The tool encapsulates the pediatric features of the general impression, and it works for children with either illness or injury.[18] Since the introduction of the PAT in the Advanced Pediatric Life Support and Pediatric Education for Prehospital Professionals[19] courses, this pediatric evaluation tool has become a basic assessment model in US and international life support education.[20]

The PAT is an easy way to begin the assessment of any child (**Figure 1.1**). It is based on listening and seeing and does not require a stethoscope, blood pressure cuff, cardiac monitor, or pulse oximeter. The PAT can be completed in 30 to 60 seconds. In reality, the PAT is a structured paradigm for the "across-the-room assessment"—an intuitive process for experienced pediatric providers. The components of the PAT are appearance, work of breathing, and circulation to skin. Together, the three components reflect the child's overall physiologic status or the child's general state of oxygenation, ventilation, perfusion, and brain function. It is not a diagnostic tool; the PAT is a general assessment tool that facilitates immediate physiologic evaluation in emergency circumstances that require rapid life support decisions.

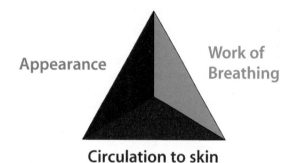

Figure 1.1 Pediatric Assessment Triangle (PAT).

Used with permission of the American Academy of Pediatrics, Pediatrics Education for Prehospital Professionals, © American Academy of Pediatrics, 2000.

Appearance

The child's general appearance is the most important thing to consider when determining whether the child is or is not sick. Appearance reflects the adequacy of ventilation, oxygenation, brain perfusion, body homeostasis, and central nervous system function.

> YOUR FIRST CLUE
>
> PAT
> - Appearance
> - Work of breathing
> - Circulation to skin

There are many physical characteristics that help define a child's appearance. Some of the most important are summarized in the "tickles" (TICLS) mnemonic: tone, interactiveness, consolability, look/gaze, and speech/cry (Table 1-2).[18] Although this is not intended as an inclusive list of all features of a distressed child, TICLS is an easy mnemonic to recall key physical characteristics of a child's appearance.

TABLE 1-2 **Characteristics of Appearance**
The "tickles" (TICLS) mnemonic
Characteristic features to look for:
• Tone
Is she moving or vigorously resisting examination? Does she have good muscle tone? Or is she limp, listless, or flaccid?
• Interactiveness
How alert is she? How readily does a person, object, or sound distract her or draw her attention? Will she reach for, grasp, and play with a toy or examination instrument, such as a penlight or tongue blade? Or is she uninterested in playing or interacting with the caregiver?
• Consolability
Can she be consoled or comforted by the caregiver? Or is her crying or agitation unrelieved by gentle reassurance?
• Look/Gaze
Does she fix her gaze on a face? Or is there a nobody-home, glassy-eyed stare?
• Speech/Cry
Is her speech or cry strong and spontaneous? Or is it weak, muffled, or hoarse?

Adapted from: Dieckmann RA, Brownstein D, Gausche-Hill M. The Pediatric Assessment Triangle: A novel approach to pediatric assessment. *Pediatr Emerg Care.* 2010:26;312–315.

Using appearance as a predictor of distress will usually detect earlier and less obvious signs of physiologic stress from illness or injury. Children with mild to moderate illness or injury can be alert on the AVPU (Alert, responsive to Verbal stimuli, responsive to Pain, Unresponsive) scale and 15 (best score) on the Glasgow Coma Scale and have an abnormal appearance.

Techniques to Assess Appearance

Assess the child's appearance from the doorway. This is step 1 in the PAT. Techniques for assessment of a conscious child's appearance include observing from a distance, allowing the child to remain in the caregiver's lap or arms, using distractions such as bright lights or toys to measure interactiveness, and kneeling down to be on eye level with the child. An immediate hands-on approach can cause agitation and crying and might confuse the assessment. Unless a child is unconscious or obviously lethargic, get as much information as possible by observing before touching the child or taking vital signs.

One example of a child with a normal appearance might be an infant with good eye contact and good color who is reaching for a tongue blade. An example of a child with a worrisome appearance might be a toddler who makes poor eye contact and is pale or mottled and listless (**Figure 1.2**).

Abnormal appearance can be due to lack of oxygen, ventilation, or brain perfusion. It can be the result of systemic problems, such as poisoning, infection, or hypoglycemia. It can also be due to acute brain injury from hemorrhage or edema or to chronic brain injury from shaken baby syndrome. Regardless of the cause, a grossly abnormal appearance establishes that the child is seriously ill or injured. In such a child, life support efforts should be started immediately to increase oxygenation, ventilation, and perfusion while the next phase of hands-on physical assessment is completed.

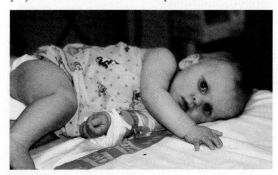

Figure 1.2 Worrisome appearance.

Although an alert, interactive child is usually not critically ill, there are some cases in which a child is critically ill or injured without having an abnormal appearance. Toxicologic or traumatic emergencies are good examples as follows:

• A child with a dangerous intoxication, such as from acetaminophen (paracetamol), iron, or cyclic antidepressants, might not show symptoms immediately after ingestion. Despite normal appearance, the child can develop deadly complications in the coming minutes or hours.

- A child with blunt trauma might be able to maintain adequate core perfusion despite internal bleeding by increasing cardiac output and systemic vascular resistance and might appear normal. When these compensatory mechanisms fail, the child might show rapid progression to decompensated shock.

Age differences are associated with important developmental differences in psychomotor and social skills. Normal or expected appearance and behavior vary by age group. Children of all ages engage their environment. For newborns, this occurs by energetic sucking and crying. For older infants, it occurs through smiling or tracking a light; for toddlers, it is by exploring and touching their surroundings; and for adolescents, it is by talking. Knowledge of normal childhood development should guide the approach to children and will result in more accurate judgments about appearances. Table 1-3 summarizes important behavioral characteristics of children of different developmental ages and provides developmentally appropriate assessment techniques.

Although appearance reflects real illness or injury, it does not always show the cause of injury or illness. Appearance is the screening portion of the PAT. The other elements of the PAT—work of breathing and circulation to skin—provide more specific information about the type of physiologic derangement. They help to show the likely cause of system dysfunction while also providing additional clues about severity.

Work of Breathing

Work of breathing is a more accurate indicator of oxygenation and ventilation than RR or chest sounds on auscultation—the traditional measures of breathing in adults. Work of breathing reflects the child's attempt to compensate for abnormalities in oxygenation and ventilation. Assessing work of breathing requires listening carefully for audible abnormal airway sounds and looking for signs of increased breathing ef-

fort. It is another hands-off evaluation method. Table 1-4 summarizes the key characteristics of work of breathing.

Abnormal Audible Airway Sounds

Examples of abnormal airway sounds that can be heard without a stethoscope are snoring, muffled or hoarse speech, stridor, grunting, and wheezing. Abnormal airway sounds provide excellent anatomical and physiologic information about breathing effort and type and anatomical location of the breathing problem. They also help determine the severity of the problem.

Snoring, muffled or hoarse speech, and stridor suggest upper airway obstruction. The location in the upper airway where the obstruction exists determines the quality of the abnormal sounds. Snoring occurs if the oropharynx or hypopharynx is partially obstructed by the tongue and soft tissues. A gurgling sound suggests the presence of blood, secretions, or foreign body in the oropharynx or hypopharynx. Muffled or hoarse speech is abnormal vocalization or expiratory sounds that occur when the child attempts to talk. Obstruction at or slightly above the level of the vocal cords or larynx produces these alterations in speech. Stridor is an inspiratory, high-pitched sound produced by obstruction at the level of the larynx or lower in the trachea and bronchi.

Obstruction of upper airway passages occurs in a variety of illnesses and injuries. Snoring or gurgling can be heard in a postictal child with posterior displacement of the tongue or in a child with a large tongue hematoma. Muffled or hoarse speech, or a "hot potato" voice, is common in the setting of peritonsillar abscess. Abnormal speech can also reflect a laryngeal fracture after blunt neck trauma. Stridor is most often from viral laryngotracheobronchitis (croup); foreign-body aspiration is another cause in younger children.

Grunting is an instinctive mechanism to keep alveoli open for maximal gas exchange. Grunting involves exhaling against a partially closed glottis. It is a marker of alveolar lung disease or injury. This short, low-pitched sound is best heard at the end of the exhalation. Grunting is often present in children with moderate to severe hypoxia, and it reflects poor gas exchange

TABLE 1-3 Behavioral Characteristics and Special Assessment Techniques

Developmental Age	Behavioral Characteristics	Special Assessment Techniques
Neonate	Primitive reflexes only	Immediately assess airway, breathing, heart rate, and color. Because the neonate has no interactive behavior yet, focus assessment of appearance on muscle tone, spontaneous motor activity, and quality of cry.
Infant <2 months old	Physiologic responses No separation anxiety	Obtain the pregnancy and delivery history because manifestations of intrapartum or perinatal disease often manifest in this age. Signs of serious illness might be nonspecific, so a history of fussiness, feeding difficulty, or poor sleeping can be a significant symptom of sepsis, metabolic abnormality, or a central nervous system problem. An episode of choking, apnea, loss of tone, or change in skin color might represent an apparent life-threatening event. Examine with the patient in any position.
2–6 months old	Social skills (smiles, tracks) Motor skills (rolls over, sits, reaches) Vocalization	As infants develop a wider range of behaviors and become more interactive with the environment, TICLS as a measure of appearance becomes a more reliable indicator of disease and injury. Examine with the patient in any position and use distraction. Use calm, lilting speech to soothe and engage child.
6–12 months old	Socially interactive Stranger/separation anxiety Sits without support Plays, babbles	Leave child on caregiver's lap. Anticipate stranger anxiety. Sit or squat at child's level. Offer toys and distractions (tongue blade, penlight). Examine from toe to head.
Toddler	Fearless curiosity Strong opinions, illogical Egocentrism Stranger/separation anxiety Wide verbal variability	Approach gently and observe from the doorway. Leave the child on the caregiver's lap and get down to the child's level. Enlist the caregiver's assistance. Use distraction. Talk to the child about herself. Use endless praise and reassurance. Explain procedures simply. Examine from toe to head.

TABLE 1-3, Behavioral Characteristics and Special Assessment Techniques, cont'd

Developmental Age	Behavioral Characteristics	Special Assessment Techniques
Preschooler	Magical, illogical thinkers Misconceptions about illness and injury but logical Fears of mutilation, loss of control, death, darkness, and being alone Good language skills	Speak directly to the child. Choose words carefully and clarify misconceptions. Use dolls or puppets for explanation. Allow the child to handle equipment and ask for help. Set limits on behavior. Use games and distractions. Praise cooperation and avoid ridicule. Examine head to toe.
School-aged child	Talkative, analytical Understand cause and effect Want involvement in care Fears of separation, loss of control, pain, and physical disability	Speak directly to child and provide simple explanations. Anticipate questions and fears. Explain procedures and never lie. Respect privacy. Do not negotiate but provide options. Involve the child in the treatment.
Adolescent	Mobile, experimental, illogical Understand cause and effect Expressive Fears of loss of independence, loss of control, body image	Explain everything. Encourage questions. Show respect and speak directly to child. Be honest and nonjudgmental. Honor modesty and confidentiality. Do not succumb to provocation. Ask friends for assistance.
Child with special health care needs	Developmental age can be quite different than chronological age Child might represent mix of physical and emotional abnormalities	Use understandable language and techniques. Do not assume the child is mentally impaired. Use information from caregiver and physician when possible.

Adapted from: Dieckmann R, ed. *Pediatric Education for Prehospital Professionals*. 2nd ed. Sudbury, MA: Jones & Bartlett Publishers, American Academy of Pediatrics; 2006:32–50.

because of fluid in the lower airways and air sacs. Some of the conditions that cause hypoxia and grunting are pneumonia, pulmonary contusion, and pulmonary edema.

Wheezing is the movement of air across partially blocked small airways. It is caused by lower airway obstruction, usually because of bronchoconstriction and edema from asthma or bronchiolitis. In the early phases of lower airway obstruction, wheezing is present during exhalation only and can be heard only by auscultation. As the obstruction increases and breathing requires more work, wheezing occurs during both inhalation and exhalation. With more obstruction, wheezing is audible without a stethoscope.

Finally, if respiratory failure develops, work of breathing can diminish and the wheezing might not be heard at all. The most common cause of wheezing in childhood is asthma, although bronchiolitis, allergic reaction, and foreign objects in the lower airway are also possible causes, especially in infants and toddlers.

Visual Signs

There are several useful visual signs of increased work of breathing. These signs reflect increased breathing effort by the child to improve oxygenation and ventilation. Examples of visual signs that represent instinctive actions to compensate for hypoxic stress are abnormal positioning, retractions, nasal flaring, and tachypnea.

TABLE 1-4	Characteristics of Work of Breathing
Characteristic	Features to Look for
Abnormal airway sounds	Snoring, muffled or hoarse speech; stridor; grunting; wheezing
Abnormal positioning	Sniffing position, tripoding, refusal to lie down
Retractions	Supraclavicular, intercostal, or substernal retractions of the chest wall; head bobbing in infants
Flaring	Nasal flaring

Dieckmann R, ed. *Pediatric Education for Prehospital Professionals.* 2nd ed. Sudbury, MA: Jones & Bartlett Publishers, American Academy of Pediatrics; 2006:10. Reprinted with permission.

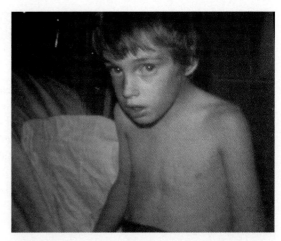

Figure 1.3 The sniffing position is an abnormal position and reflects upper airway obstruction.

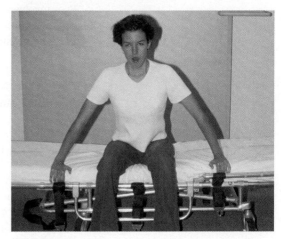

Figure 1.4 The abnormal tripod position indicates the patient's attempts to maximize accessory muscle use.

Abnormal positioning is immediately evident from the doorway. There are several types of posture that indicate compensatory efforts to increase airflow. A child who is in the "sniffing" position is trying to line up the axes of the airways to open the airway and increase airflow. This position is usually the result of severe upper airway obstruction (**Figure 1.3**) from such conditions as retropharyngeal abscess, foreign-body aspiration, or (rarely) epiglottitis. The child who refuses to lie down or who leans forward on outstretched arms (tripod position) is trying to use accessory muscles to improve breathing (**Figure 1.4**). This sign is observed in children with severe bronchoconstriction from asthma or bronchiolitis. The sniffing position and the tripod position are abnormal and indicate increased work of breathing and severe respiratory distress.

Retractions are common physical signs of increased work of breathing. They represent use of accessory muscles to help breathing. Retractions are easily missed unless the clinician looks for them specifically after the child is properly exposed. Retractions are a more useful measure of work of breathing in children than in adults.

This is because a child's chest wall is less muscular and thinner, and the inward excursion of skin and soft tissue between the ribs is visually more apparent. Retractions are a sign that the child is recruiting extra muscle power to try to expand the chest more fully and move more air into the lungs. They can be in the supraclavicular area (above the clavicle), the intercostal area (between the ribs), or the substernal area (under the sternum), as illustrated in **Figure 1.5**.

The amount and location of retractions reflect the severity and degree of hypoxia. A child with mild retractions in only one anatomical area, such as the intercostal area, is obviously not working as hard and does not have as severe a hypoxic insult as a child with deep retractions in more anatomical areas. When a child exhausts compensatory mechanisms and

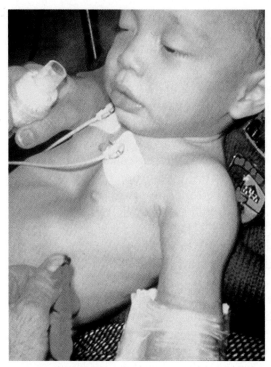

Figure 1.5 Retractions indicate increased work of breathing and can occur in the supraclavicular, intercostal, and substernal areas.

approaches respiratory failure, retractions can paradoxically decrease. This is an ominous trend and signals impending respiratory arrest. Assisted ventilation is imperative.

One form of accessory muscle use in infants is head bobbing—the use of neck muscles to improve breathing during severe hypoxia. The child extends the neck while inhaling, then allows the head to fall forward while exhaling. This visual sign suggests moderate to severe hypoxia.

Tachypnea is another visual clue to increased work of breathing, but it can be deceptive. The specific, counted RR must be age adjusted for interpretation. The range of normal RRs in children is wide and is subject to great variability in emergency settings where pain, cold, and anxiety can cause mild to moderate tachypnea in the absence of hypoxia. In addition, tachypnea can reflect a physiologic response to metabolic acidosis and might not represent a primary respiratory abnormality at all. Respiratory rates that are too fast (>60/min) or too slow (<12–20/min) might not be adequate to maintain minute ventilation (MV). Remember, MV is equal to RR times tidal volume (TV), or MV = RR × TV. Rates that are too slow will decrease MV,

because TV cannot be increased to compensate, and rates that are too fast result in a marked decrease in TV and therefore MV.

Nasal flaring is another form of accessory muscle use that reflects significantly increased work of breathing (**Figure 1.6**). Flaring is the exaggerated opening of the nostrils during labored breathing and indicates moderate to severe hypoxia. Inspect the face specifically to detect flaring because it is easily missed.

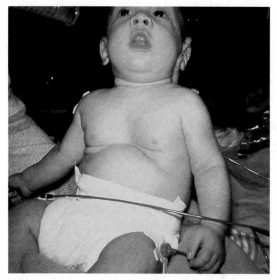

Figure 1.6 Nasal flaring indicates increased work of breathing and moderate to severe hypoxia.

Techniques to Assess Work of Breathing

Step 2 in the PAT is assessing work of breathing. The initial step is to listen carefully from a distance for abnormal audible airway sounds, then look for key visual signs. Abnormal sounds should be listened for from the doorway. Then it should be noted whether the child has abnormal positioning, especially the sniffing posture or tripoding. Next, the caregiver should uncover the chest of the child for direct inspection or have the child undress on the caregiver's lap. The quality and location of the intercostal, supraclavicular, and substernal retractions should be determined and whether there is head bobbing in infants should be noted. After examination for retractions, whether the RR is grossly increased should be noted. Inspect for nasal flaring should be performed last.

Children can have increased work of breathing because of abnormalities anywhere in their airways, air sacs, pleurae, or chest walls. Assessing these auditory and visual characteristics together helps to define the type of problem and the degree of distress. The type of abnormal airway sound gives an important clue to the anatomical location of the illness or injury process, whereas the number and type of visual signs of increased work of breathing help in determining the degree of physiologic stress.

Combining assessment of appearance and work of breathing can also help establish the severity of the child's illness or injury. If a child readily compensates for hypoxic stress by increasing work of breathing, the brain is perfused with relatively normal levels of oxygen and carbon dioxide (CO_2), so appearance is relatively normal. A child with normal appearance and increased work of breathing is in respiratory distress—a compensated physiologic state that describes most cases of respiratory illnesses and injuries of childhood. However, if increased work of breathing does not compensate for the hypoxic stress, the brain is perfused with blood with decreased oxygen content. If further decompensation occurs and breathing becomes increasingly inadequate, the brain experiences both decreased oxygen and increased CO_2. Hypoxia causes restlessness and agitation, and hypercapnia causes lethargy and diminished responsiveness. Hence, the patient's appearance in states of acute hypoxia and hypercapnia is distinctly abnormal. The combination of abnormal appearance and increased work of breathing indicates an uncompensated physiologic state that is termed respiratory failure. Finally, the combination of abnormal appearance and abnormally decreased work of breathing implies impending respiratory arrest.

Circulation to Skin

The goal of rapid circulatory assessment is to determine the adequacy of cardiac output and the perfusion of vital organs. Heart rate, blood pressure, and cardiac auscultation—key indicators of circulatory function in adults—are not helpful in forming an accurate general impression in a child and, like RR, can be deferred to the ABCDEs, hands-on phase of the primary assessment. The child's appearance is one indicator of perfusion because inadequate perfusion of the brain will cause abnormal behavior. However, abnormal appearance can be caused by many conditions other than decreased perfusion. For this reason, other signs of perfusion must be added to the appearance evaluation to assess the child's circulatory condition.

An important sign of perfusion in children is circulation to skin. When cardiac output is too low, the body compensates by increasing heart rate and by shutting down circulation to nonessential anatomical areas, such as the skin and mucous membranes, to preserve blood supply to the most vital organs (brain, heart, and kidneys). Therefore, in most children who have inadequate core perfusion, circulation to skin is significantly diminished by intense neuromotor regulation. Hence, visual signs reflect the overall status of core circulation. Pallor, mottling, and cyanosis are visual indicators of reduced circulation to skin and mucous membranes. Table 1-5 summarizes these characteristics.

Pallor is usually the first sign of poor skin or mucous membrane perfusion. It can also be a sign of anemia or hypoxia. Mottling is caused by constriction of blood vessels to the skin and is another sign of poor perfusion (**Figure 1.7**).

Cyanosis is a blue discoloration of the skin and mucous membranes. Do not confuse acrocyanosis—blue hands and feet in a newborn or infant younger than 2 months—with true cyanosis. Acrocyanosis is a normal finding when a young infant is cold, and it reflects vasomotor instability rather than hypoxia or shock (**Figure 1.8**). True cyanosis is a late finding of

Signs of Increased Work of Breathing
- Abnormal airway positioning
- Retractions
- Nasal flaring
- Head bobbing
- Stridor
- Wheezing
- Grunting

TABLE 1-5 Characteristics of Circulation to Skin	
Characteristic	**Features**
Pallor	White or pale skin or mucous membrane coloration from inadequate blood flow
Mottling	Patchy skin discoloration due to vasoconstriction
Cyanosis	Bluish discoloration of skin and mucous membranes

Dieckmann R, ed. *Pediatric Education for Prehospital Professionals.* 2nd ed. Sudbury, MA: Jones & Bartlett Publishers, American Academy of Pediatrics; 2006:13. Reprinted with permission.

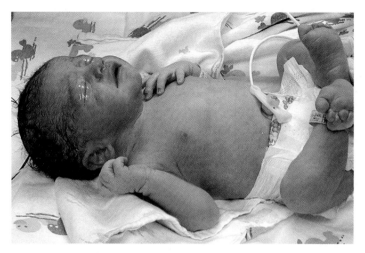

Figure 1.8 Acrocyanosis.

Kattwinkel J, ed. *Textbook of Neonatal Resuscitation.* 5th ed. Elk Grove Village, IL: American Academy of Pediatrics and American Heart Association; 2006:A-4. Reprinted with permission.

respiratory failure or shock. A hypoxic child is likely to show other physical abnormalities long before turning blue, including abnormal appearance and increased work of breathing. A child in shock will also have pallor or mottling. Never wait for cyanosis to begin supplemental oxygen. Acute cyanosis is always a critical sign of either hypoxia and/or ischemia that requires immediate intervention with breathing support.

Abnormal circulation to skin in combination with normal appearance can suggest compensated shock. The abnormal appearance in compensated shock can be subtle, and some children seem remarkably alert. However, if the circulatory stress continues and compensatory mechanisms fail to compensate, the brain

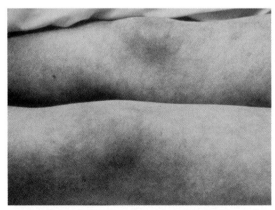

Figure 1.7 Mottling is the result of constriction of blood vessels to the skin and can indicate poor perfusion.

receives inadequate blood supply and appearance becomes abnormal. Poor motor tone, lack of interactiveness, restlessness, and listlessness are important indicators of physiologic disorders. When observed in a child with abnormal circulation to skin, especially with a history of volume loss or blunt injury, these characteristics suggest perfusion failure or decompensated shock.

Another clue for the presence of shock is tachypnea without signs of increased work of breathing; this is called effortless tachypnea and represents the child's attempt to blow off extra CO_2 to correct the metabolic acidosis generated by poor perfusion.

Techniques to Assess Circulation to Skin

Step 3 in the PAT is evaluating circulation to skin. Be sure the child is exposed enough for visual inspection but not cold. Cold can cause false skin signs. In other words, the cold child can have normal core perfusion but abnormal circulation to skin. Cold circulating air temperature is the most common reason for misinterpretation of skin signs.

Inspect the skin and mucous membranes for pallor, mottling, and cyanosis. Look at the face, chest, abdomen, and extremities. Then, inspect the lips for cyanosis. In dark-skinned children, circulation to skin is sometimes more difficult to assess. The lips and mucous membranes in the mouth might be the best places to look.

Using the PAT to Evaluate Severity and Illness or Injury

Combining the three components of the PAT can answer three critical questions: What is the most likely physiologic abnormality? How severe is the child's illness or injury? How fast do I have to intervene, and what type of general and specific treatment should I give?

The PAT has two important advantages. First, it quickly gives the clinician critical information about the child's physiologic status before touching or agitating the child. This is important because it can be difficult to identify abnormal appearance, increased work of breathing, or decreased circulation to skin when a child is agitated and crying. Second, the PAT helps set priorities for the rest of the hands-on primary assessment. The PAT takes only seconds to complete, it identifies the need for lifesaving interventions, and it blends into the next phase of hands-on physical assessment.

For example, if a child is interactive and pink but has a few intercostal retractions, the general impression would be respiratory distress. In this PAT configuration, the child should be approached slowly and in a developmentally appropriate manner to complete the primary assessment, including a careful hands-on ABCDE evaluation. On the other hand, if the child is limp with unlabored rapid breathing and pale or mottled skin, the PAT suggests decompensated shock. In this case, the primary assessment should be performed rapidly and resuscitation started based on the ABCDEs. A child who has abnormal appearance but normal work of breathing and normal circulation to skin could have an important and potentially dangerous combination of PAT characteristics, suggesting a primary brain dysfunction or a major metabolic or systemic problem, such as postictal state, subdural hemorrhage, brain concussion, intoxication, hypoglycemia, or sepsis. Table 1-6 provides a summary of different PAT configurations with the general impression or physiologic state and potential emergency causes.

CASE SCENARIO 3

A 7-year-old boy is hit by a car in front of his home. He was thrown 1.5 m (5 ft) and had a brief loss of consciousness. The father decided to take him to the physician's office when he noted the boy becoming sleepy.

In the office, the boy opens his eyes with a loud verbal stimulus but will not speak or interact. There are no abnormal airway sounds, but intercostal retractions and flaring are present. His skin is pale. Respiratory rate is 50/min, heart rate is 145/min, and blood pressure is 90 by palpation. The chest is clear with decreased tidal volume. The skin feels cool; capillary refill time is 4 seconds, and brachial pulse is present. Pupils are equal and reactive. He has a large frontal hematoma.

1. *Does this child's assessment suggest serious injury?*
2. *What actions are required by the physician in the office?*
3. *How should this child be transported to the ED?*

The Primary Assessment: The Pediatric ABCDEs

The primary assessment is an ordered, hands-on, physical evaluation of the ABCDEs. It provides a prioritized sequence of life support interventions to reverse organ failure. As in adults, there is a specific order for treating life-threatening problems as they are identified, before moving to the next step. ABCDE assessment includes the following components:

- Airway
- Breathing
- Circulation
- Disability
- Exposure

TABLE 1-6 PAT Configurations and Emergency Causes

Appearance	Work of Breathing	Circulation to Skin	Possible Systemic Causes of Altered Physiologic State	Examples of Causes
Abnormal	Normal	Normal	Primary brain dysfunction Systemic problems	Shaken baby Brain injury Sepsis Hypoglycemia Intoxication
Normal	Abnormal	Normal	Respiratory distress	Mild asthma Bronchiolitis Croup Community-acquired pneumonia Foreign-body aspiration
Abnormal	Abnormal	Normal	Respiratory failure	Severe asthma Pulmonary contusion Penetrating chest trauma
Normal	Normal	Abnormal	Compensated shock	Diarrhea External blood loss
Abnormal	Normal	Abnormal	Decompensated shock	Severe gastroenteritis Major burn Major blunt injury Penetrating abdominal injury
Abnormal	Abnormal	Abnormal	Cardiopulmonary failure	Cardiopulmonary arrest

Adapted from: Dieckmann R, ed. *Pediatric Education for Prehospital Professionals*. 2nd ed. Sudbury, MA: Jones & Bartlett Publishers, American Academy of Pediatrics; 2006:2–31.

Using Length as the Index for Drug Dosing and Equipment Sizing

During a critical emergency, performing the appropriate interventions to support the ABCDEs requires accurate equipment sizing and drug dosing. The child's age and estimated weight are unreliable predictors of equipment sizes and drug doses and are more likely to result in medical error.[21] Length is the ideal index because this size characteristic is the best predictor of equipment sizes. Length predicts lean mass, the most precise basis for drug dosing. Most resuscitation drugs have a small volume of distribution, which is associated with lean weight not real weight.[22] Length-based equipment sizing and drug dosing can be accomplished with either a colorized resuscitation tape or with a simple tape measure and a computerized decision support program. The colorized tape or decision support tool uses the 50th percentile weight for any measured length—an index known to be safe for pediatric equipment sizing and drug dosing.

Airway

The PAT will usually identify the presence of airway obstruction. However, the loudness of the stridor or wheezing is not necessarily related to the amount of airway obstruction. For example, asthmatic children in severe distress might have little or no wheezing. Similarly, a child with an upper airway foreign body below the vocal cords could have minimal stridor.

Abnormal airway sounds tell whether there is any amount of upper or lower airway obstruction.

Techniques to Assess and Manage the Airway

If the airway is not open, manual airway-opening maneuvers, such as the head tilt–chin lift, or in the trauma patient, the jaw-thrust maneuver, should be performed. A neutral neck position should be maintained. Suction should be frequently performed. Whether the airway is maintainable or not maintainable with manual techniques and suction should be determined. If the infant or child has a clinical history or signs suggesting cervical spine injury, spinal stabilization should be maintained while performing airway maneuvers.

If positioning and suctioning do not establish a patent airway, airway obstruction should be considered. Age-specific obstructed airway techniques (back blows [back slaps] and chest thrusts for children <1 year of age; abdominal thrusts [Heimlich maneuver] for children ≥ 1 year of age) should be performed, then direct laryngoscopy with Magill forceps should be considered. If airway obstruction continues, alternative airway access procedures should be performed using needle or surgical cricothyrotomy, depending on the child's age, physician skill level, and available equipment (see Online Chapter 26, Critical Procedures).

If the airway is open, chest rise with breathing should be looked for. If gurgling is present, carefully suction because this means there is mucus, blood, or a foreign body in the mouth or airway.

Breathing

Respiratory Rate

The RR per minute should be determined by counting the number of chest rises in 30 seconds, then doubling that number. However, the RR should be interpreted carefully. Healthy infants might show periodic breathing or stopping and starting breathing for less than 20 seconds. Therefore, counting for only 10 to 15 seconds can result in a RR that is too low.

Respiratory rates can be difficult to interpret. Rapid RRs can simply reflect high temperature, anxiety, pain, or excitement. As an example, for every degree in temperature elevation, the RR will increase by 2 to 5/min. A rapid RR without an increased work of breathing (effortless tachypnea) can also occur due to metabolic acidosis as the child attempts to blow off extra CO_2 to correct the acidosis. Normal rates, on the other hand, can occur in a child who has been breathing rapidly with increased work of breathing for some time and is now becoming fatigued. Finally, the RR should be interpreted based on what is normal for age. Table 1-7 lists the ranges of normal RRs for age.

TABLE 1-7 **Normal Respiratory Rates for Age**	
Age	Respiratory Rate/min
Infant	30–60
Toddler	24–40
Preschooler	22–34
School-aged child	18–30
Adolescent	12–16

Dieckmann R, ed. *Pediatric Education for Prehospital Professionals*. 2nd ed. Sudbury, MA: Jones & Bartlett Publishers, American Academy of Pediatrics; 2006:15.

Recording serial RRs can be especially useful, and because trend is sometimes more accurate than the first documented rate, a sustained increase or decrease in RR is often significant. The RR should be used in conjunction with other information about breathing.

Pay close attention to extremes of RR. A very rapid RR (>60/min for any age), especially with abnormal appearance or marked retractions, indicates respiratory distress and possibly respiratory failure. An abnormally slow RR is always worrisome because it might mean respiratory failure. Red flags are RRs of less than 20/min for children younger than 6 years and of less than 12/min for children 6 to <15 years. A normal RR alone never determines that breathing is adequate. The RR must be interpreted with appearance, work of breathing, and air movement.

Auscultation

A stethoscope should be used to listen over the midaxillary line to hear abnormal lung sounds in inhalation and exhalation, such as crackles and wheezing (**Figure 1.9**). Inspiratory crackles indicate alveolar disease. Expiratory wheezing indicates lower airway obstruction. Air movement and effectiveness of work of breathing should also be evaluated. A child with increased work of breathing and poor air movement might be in impending respiratory failure.

Table 1-8 lists abnormal breath sounds, their causes, and common examples of associated disease processes.

Oxygen Saturation

After the RR has been determined and auscultation performed, the child's oxygen saturation level should be measured. Pulse oximetry is an excellent tool to use in assessing a child's breathing (**Figure 1.10A**). **Figure 1.10B** illustrates the technique of placing a pulse oximetry probe on a young child. There are various anatomical

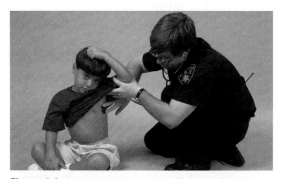

Figure 1.9 A stethoscope should be used to listen over the midaxillary line to hear abnormal lung sounds.

locations for application of sensors, including fingers, toes, nose, and ear lobe.

A pulse oximetry reading above 94% saturation indicates that oxygenation is probably adequate. A reading below 90% in a child with 100% mask oxygen could be an indication for assisted ventilation. *The possibility of respiratory distress in a child with a reading above 94% should not be underestimated.* A child in respiratory distress or early respiratory failure might be able to maintain oxygenation by increasing work of breathing and RR. This child might not appear to be ill by pulse oximetry findings alone. Interpret oxygen saturation together with work of breathing. Table 1-9 summarizes circumstances in which pulse oximetry can be deceptive and underestimate the level of gas exchange abnormality.

Measurement of CO_2

Measurement of CO_2 is becoming increasingly available as a monitoring method in selected children. This monitoring method can identify respiratory depression earlier than pulse oximetry and can help prevent development of hypoxia.[23] The common techniques include capnometry, capnography, and end-tidal CO_2 detection. Capnometry suggests measurement or analysis of CO_2 production alone, without graphic waveform records (**Figure 1.11**). The devices usually provide a continuous, digitalized quantitative measurement. Digitalized colorimetric devices

TABLE 1-8 Interpretation of Breath Sounds		
Sound	Cause	Examples
Stridor	Upper airway obstruction	Croup, foreign-body aspiration, retropharyngeal abscess
Wheezing	Lower airway obstruction	Asthma, foreign body, bronchiolitis
Expiratory grunting	Inadequate oxygenation	Pulmonary contusion, pneumonia, drowning
Inspiratory crackles	Fluid, mucus, or blood in the airway	Pneumonia, pulmonary contusion
Absent breath sounds despite increased work of breathing	Complete airway obstruction (upper or lower airway), physical barrier to transmission of breath sounds	Foreign body, severe asthma, hemothorax, pneumothorax, pleural fluid, or pneumonia

Dieckmann R, ed. *Pediatric Education for Prehospital Professionals.* 2nd ed. Sudbury, MA: Jones & Bartlett Publishers, American Academy of Pediatrics; 2006:16.

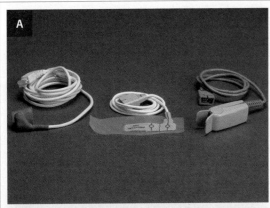

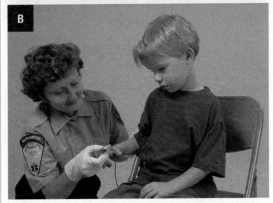

Figure 1.10 A. Various pulse oximeter probes wrap around or clip onto a digit or earlobe. B. Pulse oximetry is an excellent tool for assessing the effectiveness of breathing.

TABLE 1-9 Conditions Associated With Deceptive Pulse Oximetry	
Condition	Effect on Arterial Oxygen Saturation
Inadequate signal • Poor perfusion • Patient movement • Wrong probe	Abnormally low
Tachypnea	Abnormally high
Methemoglobinemia	Abnormally high
Cyanotic congenital heart disease	Abnormally low
Carboxyhemoglobin	Abnormally high

will have either a transcutaneous probe or an infrared sensor in a nasal adaptor or attached to a tracheal tube. Capnometry and capnography can be used on nonintubated and intubated children. Digital capnometers provide real-time measurements of exhaled CO_2 levels through the entire respiratory cycle and will display a digital readout of the inspired and end-tidal CO_2 concentrations, as well as the RR. Infrared sensors can be positioned either in the mainstream tubing or as a side stream of the oxygen delivery system.[24]

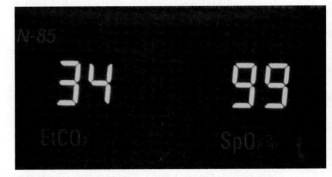

Figure 1.11 Capnometry.

A second option in intubated patients is a qualitative, colorimetric end-tidal CO_2 measurement. Colorimetric detectors are inexpensive detection devices attached to a tracheal tube; they read only the highest CO_2 concentrations at the end of expiration. They use a filter paper that changes color on contact with CO_2. Color readings include purple (<4 mm Hg of CO_2), tan (4–15 mm Hg of CO_2), and yellow (>15 mm Hg of CO_2) (**Figure 1.12**).[25] The filter paper begins as purple and should change to yellow with the exhalation phase as CO_2 contacts the filter paper. Lack of change of color from purple indicates either esophageal placement of the endotracheal tube or that the patient is not perfusing, as is the case in cardiopulmonary arrest. Tan represents either retained CO_2 in the stomach or states of poor perfusion with tracheal placement of the tube.

Measurement of CO_2 has variable value in respiratory assessment but in selected cases allows better detection of potentially life-threatening problems than clinical judgment alone.[23] It is extremely useful when the child has respiratory distress and is being treated in a monitored setting. The most important use of digital capnometry and capnography is its noninvasive ability to provide an instantaneous measurement of the level of CO_2 in the arterial blood.

Important applications of CO_2 measurement include the following:

- Procedural sedation—during procedural sedation, apnea and respiratory depression

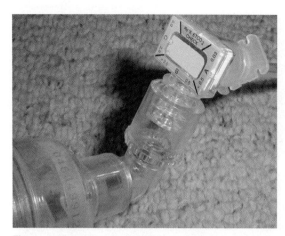

Figure 1.12 Carbon dioxide detector device.

are important untoward effects of many sedation and analgesic agents. When ventilation decreases, CO_2 concentration at the sampling site will decrease rapidly and can be instantaneously detected by capnometry or capnography. Therefore, CO_2 monitoring can serve as an apnea monitor in neonates, infants, and children and might identify respiratory depression before pulse oximetry or clinical assessment.

- Tracheal tube placement—CO_2 monitoring is probably the best way to detect esophageal intubation and displacement of a tracheal tube. Carbon dioxide values less than 4 mm Hg indicate esophageal placement in patients with a pulse. In addition to confirmation of the tracheal tube placement in the trachea, capnography can detect a total occlusion or unintentional extubation.
- Monitoring of ventilation—capnography not only is a reliable noninvasive monitor to predict Pa_{CO_2} in awake infants and children who are breathing spontaneously, but also serves as a useful device to monitor Pa_{CO_2} during mechanical ventilation of intubated children.
- Monitoring response to treatment—in severe airway obstruction from conditions such as asthma and croup, the shape of the capnogram is altered. With adequate treatment, the capnogram reverts to normal. Hence, capnography appears to be useful as a measure of response to therapy (**Figure 1.13**).

- Predicting survival in cardiopulmonary arrest—in the child in cardiopulmonary arrest, a persistent capnometry reading less than 4 mm Hg is associated with mortality. One pediatric study and several adult studies have demonstrated significant differences in capnometry readings between survivors and nonsurvivors of cardiopulmonary arrest.[26,27]
- Treatment of herniation syndrome—capnometry can be helpful in early intracranial pressure regulation in the patient with head injuries. If a child with a unilateral blown pupil and brainstem herniation responds to above-normal ventilatory rates, the capnometer reading should be noted at the time the pupil constricts and minute ventilation (MV) maintained at that level pending surgical intervention.

Techniques to Assess and Manage Breathing

If the child is in respiratory distress, oxygen should be applied using an age-appropriate technique that delivers a desired oxygen concentration. If the child is in respiratory failure based on the PAT and primary assessment, ventilation should be assisted with a bag-mask device and 100% oxygen. In selected cases, where the airway is potentially unstable, an airway adjunct, either a nasopharyngeal or oropharyngeal airway, should be inserted. Then, after appropriate preoxygenation and ventilation with the bag-mask device, tracheal intubation should be performed when intubation equipment and personnel are ready. If the child is conscious, rapid sequence intubation and neuromuscular paralysis should be used. Rarely, a child cannot receive ventilatory assistance because of severe airway obstruction from edema, foreign body, or facial or neck trauma. In such cases, either needle cricothyrotomy (in those <8 years old) or surgical cricothyrotomy (in those ≥8 years old) should be performed.

Most children requiring emergency assessment do not need immediate assisted ventilation, and hands-on assessment of breathing is possible in most cases with the child on the caregiver's lap. First, the RR should be counted and the rate interpreted for the child's age. Then,

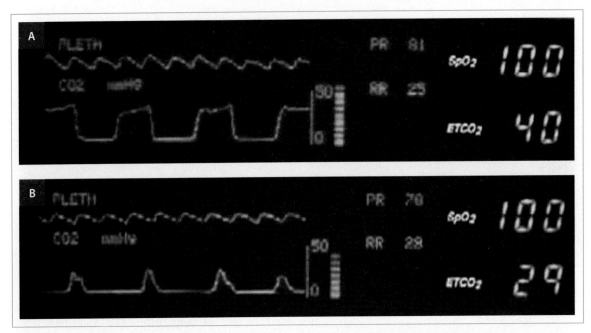

Figure 1.13 A. Capnograph monitor showing normal end-tidal carbon dioxide (CO_2) waveform. The upper waveform is the pulse oximeter signal (SpO2). The lower waveform is the end-tidal CO_2 (ETCO$_2$) reading. The expected waveform is flat and near 0 during inhalation. During exhalation, the CO_2 rises rapidly to a plateau, which then falls rapidly as exhalation ends (forming a square wave). The numerical readout of 40 indicates the CO_2 measured during the latter part of exhalation (end tidal), which should correlate with Paco$_2$ if pulmonary perfusion is good. If the ETCO$_2$ monitor is in line with an endotracheal tube, such a square wave pattern is a reliable indicator of tracheal intubation. B. Capnograph monitor showing abnormal end-tidal CO_2 wave form. The lower wave form (ETCO$_2$) does not have the expected square wave pattern and indicates an abnormal reading. The numerical readout of 29 will not correlate with Paco$_2$ because the wave form indicates a source other than normally perfused lungs. Possible causes of this abnormal wave form could be an esophageal intubation or tracheal intubation of poorly perfused lungs (eg, during less-than-optimal cardiopulmonary resuscitation).

the chest should be listened to, using a non-threatening approach that does not upset the child and prompt crying. Sometimes it is easier to have the caregiver apply the stethoscope to the chest wall. Next, oxygen saturation by pulse oximetry should be determined using a suitable probe to obtain a good waveform, and the saturation level should be interpreted in the context of work of breathing. Finally, in selected circumstances, when capnometry or capnography is available in conjunction with pulse oximetry, measurements of CO_2 should be used to further evaluate effectiveness of ventilation.

Achieving an appropriate minute volume (TV × RR) during ventilation is a key management task during assisted ventilation and requires the highest vigilance because of the tendency for clinicians to ventilate too fast and too hard in a crash situation. Hyperventilation and hypocapnia are deleterious to cardiac and brain perfusion because hypocapnia increases intrathoracic pressure, impairing venous return and cardiac

output.[28] Hyperventilation must be used cautiously in a child with traumatic brain injury because excessive hyperventilation can cause cerebral vasoconstriction, leading to brain ischemia.[29,30] In critical patients with traumatic brain injury, hyperventilation is indicated only when there are acute signs of cerebral herniation. In this clinical setting, a RR that is 5/min above the following recommended normal age-based ventilation rates should be used: 30/min for infants, 20/min for toddlers and children, and 12 to 15/min for adolescents. This assumes that the volume of each breath (TV) is provided to just achieve chest rise, and the patient has a perfusing rhythm. Whenever possible, during assisted ventilation for any purpose, a capnometer or capnograph should be used to ensure proper minute ventilation.

Circulation

The PAT provides important visual clues about circulation to skin. More information from the hands-on evaluation of heart rate, pulse quality, skin temperature, capillary refill time, and blood pressure should be added to these observations. In cases where there is potential physiologic instability, a cardiac monitor should be used.

Heart Rate

Guidelines often used to assess adult circulatory status—heart rate and blood pressure—have important limitations in children. First, normal heart rate varies with age, as noted in Table 1-10. Second, tachycardia can be an early sign of hypoxia or low perfusion, but it can also reflect less serious conditions, such as fever, anxiety, pain, and excitement. Like RR, heart rate should be interpreted within the overall history, the PAT, and entire primary assessment. A trend of increasing or decreasing heart rate can be useful and might suggest worsening hypoxia or shock or improvement after treatment. When hypoxia or shock becomes critical, heart rate falls, leading to frank bradycardia. Bradycardia (heart rate <60/min in children or <100/min in newborns) indicates critical hypoxia and/or ischemia. When the heart rate is greater than 180/min, a cardiac monitor is necessary to accurately determine heart rate.

Pulse Quality

Feel the pulse to determine the heart rate. Normally, the brachial pulse is palpable inside or medial to the biceps (**Figure 1.14**). Note the quality as either weak or strong. If the brachial pulse is strong, the child is probably not hypotensive. If a peripheral pulse cannot be felt, attempt to find a central pulse. Check the femoral pulse in infants and young children or the carotid pulse

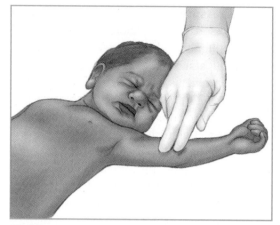

Figure 1.14 The anatomical position of the brachial pulse is medial to the biceps muscle.

in an older child or adolescent. Comparison of peripheral with central pulses (brachial in infants and carotid in older children), proximal with distal pulses, and upper limbs with lower limbs can reveal early signs of decompensated shock. Critically ill children with inadequate perfusion are able to maintain strong central pulses by shunting blood away from peripheral areas.

Skin Temperature and Capillary Refill Time

Next, do a hands-on evaluation of circulation to skin. Is the skin warm or cool? With enough perfusion, the child's skin should be warm near the wrists and ankles. With decreasing perfusion, the line of separation from cool to warm advances up the limb.

Check capillary refill time at the kneecap, foot, toes, hands, or forearm. Be sure the child is not cold from exposure because skin signs will be deceptive. Normal capillary refill time is less than 2 to 3 seconds. The value of capillary refill time is controversial. Peripheral perfusion can vary in some children, and environmental factors, such as cold room temperature, can affect capillary refill time. Also, it might be difficult to accurately count seconds under critical circumstances. The capillary refill time is just one element of the assessment of circulation. It must be evaluated in the context of the PAT and other perfusion characteristics, such as heart rate, pulse quality, and blood pressure.

Signs of circulation to the skin (skin temperature, capillary refill time, and pulse quality) are tools to assess a child's circulatory status.

TABLE 1-10 Normal Heart Rate for Age	
Age	Heart Rate/min
Infant	100–160
Toddler	90–150
Preschooler	80–140
School-aged child	70–120
Adolescent	60–100

Dieckmann R, ed. *Pediatric Education for Prehospital Professionals.* 2nd ed. Sudbury, MA: Jones & Bartlett Publishers, American Academy of Pediatrics; 2006:18.

Blood Pressure

Blood pressure determination and interpretation can be difficult in children because of lack of patient cooperation, confusion about proper cuff size, and problems remembering normal values for age. **Figure 1.15A** depicts the different sizes of blood pressure cuffs, and **Figure 1.15B** demonstrates the technique for getting a correct blood pressure in the arm or thigh. Always use a cuff with a width of two-thirds the length of the upper arm or thigh. Although technical difficulties reduce the reliability of a cuff blood pressure in patients younger than 3 years, make an attempt to determine a blood pressure in all patients.

Even if obtained accurately, blood pressure can be misleading. Although a low blood pressure definitely indicates decompensated (hypotensive) shock, a normal blood pressure frequently exists in children with compensated

TABLE 1-11 Normal Blood Pressure for Age	
Age	Minimal Systolic Blood Pressure, mm Hg
Infant	>60
Toddler	>70
Preschooler	>75
School-aged child	>80
Adolescent	>90

Dieckmann R, ed. *Pediatric Education for Prehospital Professionals.* 2nd ed. Sudbury, MA: Jones & Bartlett Publishers, American Academy of Pediatrics; 2006:19.

shock and sometimes with early decompensated shock. An easy formula for determining the lower limit of acceptable blood pressure by age is as follows: minimal systolic blood pressure = 70 + (2 × age [in years]). For example, a sick 5-year-old with a systolic blood pressure of 70 mm Hg is probably in decompensated shock. Table 1-11 gives the approximate normal systolic blood pressures for age. High blood pressure is not a common clinical problem for children but is covered in Chapter 10, Medical Emergencies.

Techniques to Assess and Manage Circulation

If a child is apneic and unresponsive based on the PAT and primary assessment, a carotid or femoral pulse (central pulse) or brachial pulse (peripheral pulse) should be checked. If no central pulse is present, chest compressions and assisted ventilation should be started using appropriate rates and techniques for the child's size. A cardiac monitor should be attached and the rhythm evaluated. Then, vascular access should be obtained with an intraosseous or an intravenous needle if a peripheral vein is visible, and drug administration should be started based on the presenting rhythm and treatment protocol.[31] Sometimes, as with ventricular fibrillation, pulseless ventricular tachycardia or unstable supraventricular tachycardia, it is necessary to perform electrical countershock before gaining vascular access.

For children who are not pulseless or in shock, the comprehensive circulatory assessment should be started by determining heart

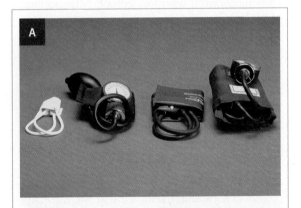
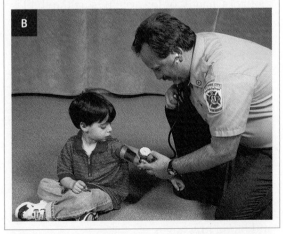

Figure 1.15 A. There are several different blood pressure cuff sizes: neonatal, infant, child, and adult. B. To obtain an accurate blood pressure reading, a cuff that is two-thirds the length of the child's upper arm should be used.

rate. A cardiac monitor should be used and a brachial pulse (peripheral pulse) or femoral pulse (central pulse) should be checked. Then, the skin at the kneecap should be examined to assess for color, temperature, and capillary refill time. Last, a blood pressure should be obtained using an appropriate-sized cuff and the measurement interpreted based on the child's age.

Identification, Categorization, and Treatment of Shock

When the assessment suggests a perfusion problem, shock type should be distinguished and the severity and urgency for treatment estimated. Then, vascular access should be obtained and drugs, fluids, and sometimes blood products administered to normalize perfusion. Vasoactive drugs might also be necessary. Table 1-12 summarizes the different forms of shock. In infants and children, shock is most often hypovolemic shock.

After the form of shock has been distinguished, the severity of shock should be characterized to help determine the type of treatment. Compensated shock refers to a physiologic state where perfusion of end organs (brain, heart, lungs, and kidneys) is preserved and the child's appearance is normal; at this level of shock severity, there might be signs of significant dehydration with tachycardia, diminished peripheral pulses, mottling or pallor, cool skin, and delayed capillary refill time. Decompensated (hypotensive) shock refers to a state of critical loss of perfusion to end organs, with altered appearance. Usually the child has hypotension or, in the absence of blood pressure measurement, loss of detectable peripheral pulses with weak central pulses. Shock, however, represents a continuum of severity so that decompensated shock can actually occur with a normal blood pressure. However, if present, hypotension always indicates decompensated shock (see Chapter 3, Shock, for treatment).

Disability

Assessment of disability or neurologic status involves quick evaluation of the two parts of the central nervous system: the cerebral cortex and the brainstem. Neurologic status (controlled by the cortex) should be assessed by looking at appearance as part of the PAT and at level of consciousness with the AVPU scale during the primary assessment (Table 1-13). The Pediatric Glasgow Coma Scale, also called the Modified Glasgow Coma Scale, is a second option if the child is a trauma patient, although the Pediatric Glasgow Coma Scale has never been well validated as a predictive instrument in children. None of these scales has undergone validation in children with altered level of consciousness not related to trauma.

TABLE 1-12 Shock Types*				
	Hypovolemic	Distributive	Cardiogenic	Obstructive
Common causes	Vomiting Diarrhea Blood loss	Sepsis Toxins Spinal cord injury Anaphylaxis	Myocarditis Supraventricular tachycardia Left to right defects	Pericardial tamponade Tension pneumothorax
Distinguishing clinical signs and symptoms	History of fluid loss Cool skin Thready pulses	Fever (Ingestion history) Major trauma	Crackles in lungs Extreme tachycardia Heart murmur	Poor heart sounds Elevated jugular venous pressure
Treatment	Crystalloid Blood products	Crystalloid Pressors	Pressors Countershock Cardiotoxic drugs	Decompression of hemopericardium or hemo-pneumothorax

*See Chapter 3, Shock, for an in-depth discussion of this topic.

TABLE 1-13 AVPU Scale

Category	Stimulus	Response Type	Reaction
Alert	Normal environment	Appropriate	Normal interaction for age
Verbal	Simple command or sound stimulus	Appropriate	Withdraws from pain
		Inappropriate	Nonspecific or confused
Painful	Pain	Appropriate	Withdraws from pain
		Inappropriate	Sound or motion without purpose or localization of pain
		Pathological	Posturing
Unresponsive	No perceptive response to any stimulus	Pathological	Not required

Dieckmann R, ed. *Pediatric Education for Prehospital Professionals.* 2nd ed. Sudbury, MA: Jones & Bartlett Publishers, American Academy of Pediatrics; 2006:22.

Always evaluate the brainstem by checking the responses of each pupil to a direct beam of light. A normal pupil constricts after a light stimulus. Pupillary response can be abnormal in the presence of drugs, ongoing seizures, hypoxia, or impending brainstem herniation. Next, evaluate motor activity. Look for symmetrical movement of the extremities, seizures, posturing, or flaccidity.

AVPU Scale

The AVPU scale (Table 1-13) is a conventional way of assessing level of consciousness in all patients with either illness or injury conditions. It categorizes motor response based on simple responses to stimuli. The patient is alert, responsive to verbal stimuli, responsive only to painful stimuli, or unresponsive.

Abnormal Appearance and the AVPU Scale

The PAT and the AVPU scale are not the same. A child with an altered level of consciousness on the AVPU scale will always have an abnormal appearance according to the PAT. Assessing appearance using the PAT might give an earlier indication of the presence of illness and injury. A child with a mild to moderate illness or injury can be alert on the AVPU scale but have an abnormal appearance.

The application of the AVPU scale is controversial. It has not been well tested for effectiveness in children. However, there is no other easy way to assess disability in children. The more complicated Pediatric Glasgow Coma Scale (or Modified Glasgow Coma Scale) for neurologic injury involves memorization and numerical scoring tasks that can be hard to accomplish in critical situations.[32,33] A study demonstrated that for pediatric blunt injury patients, inpatient mortality could be predicted using the unresponsive component of the AVPU scale and the motor response from the Glasgow Coma Scale.[34] Hence, these components of the two common rapid neurologic scoring systems are worthy of highest vigilance in assessment.

Techniques to Assess and Manage Disability

With knowledge of the child's appearance from the PAT, another specific assessment of overall central nervous system function should be performed. Either the AVPU scale or the Pediatric Glasgow Coma Scale should be used on trauma patients. On nontrauma patients, the AVPU should be used. Next, both pupils should be checked for light reaction. Then, symmetrical or abnormal motor activity should be determined.

If the disability assessment demonstrates altered level of consciousness, general life support/monitoring with oxygen, a cardiac monitor, and pulse oximetry should be started. Then vascular access should be obtained, a rapid bedside test for serum glucose should be performed, and isotonic fluid should be administered at a minimal infusion rate. Measure exhaled CO_2 if possible.

If the child has a brainstem herniation syndrome, assisted ventilation should be started at a higher than normal rate for age and CO_2 levels monitored. If pupillary constriction occurs, the ventilatory rate should be maintained at the same frequency to sustain a measured CO_2 level. Drug therapy should be started to reduce intracranial pressure. If the child begins seizing, anticonvulsant drugs should be administered.

Exposure

Proper exposure of the child is necessary for completing the emergency assessment. The PAT requires that the caregiver remove part of the child's clothing to allow careful observation of the face, chest wall, and skin. Completing the ABCDE components of the primary assessment requires further exposure, as needed, to fully evaluate physiologic function and anatomical abnormalities. Rapid heat loss, especially in a cold environment, should be avoided with infants and children.

Techniques to Assess and Manage Exposure

The child should be disrobed completely so the entire body, including the back, can be examined. If the child is alert, the physician should be sensitive to modesty by exposing one body area at a time. A warm ambient environment should be maintained, especially in infants and toddlers, by using an external heat source. The intravenous fluids should be warmed. In some patients undergoing prolonged resuscitation, a rectal probe might need to be attached to allow ongoing monitoring of core body temperature.

Use of Bedside Ultrasonography During Primary Assessment

Bedside ultrasonography in infants and children with traumatic conditions can significantly improve detection of intraperitoneal fluid, hemoperitoneum, and cardiac tamponade. If the equipment is available, during the primary assessment a focused abdominal sonography in trauma (FAST) evaluation of the heart, upper quadrants, and pelvis should be performed. FAST can detect 200 to 650 mL of free fluid or blood and takes only 3 to 5 minutes.[35] The FAST examination can provide the indication for immediate laparoscopy or laparotomy. Focused

cardiac ultrasonography can help determine the presence of pericardial fluid, diagnose cardiac tamponade, and confirm the diagnosis of pulseless electrical activity.[35] The utility of FAST and ultrasonography of the heart is highly dependent on the experience and training of the sonographer.

Another significant advantage of bedside ultrasonography is to assist in achieving vascular access.[35]

Summary of General Impression and Primary Assessment

The hands-off general impression and the hands-on primary assessment of the ABCDEs have the goal of identifying physiologic abnormalities. The PAT is the basis for the general impression. It includes characteristics of appearance, work of breathing, and circulation to skin and uses auditory and visual clues obtained from across the room. The primary assessment includes an evaluation of pediatric-specific indicators of cardiopulmonary or neurologic abnormalities and includes the hands-on physical assessment of the ABCDEs. Although vital signs can be useful in the primary assessment, they can also be misleading. They must be examined carefully and looked at together with other parts of the primary assessment. Interventions might be necessary at any point in the ABCDE sequence, and the clinician must identify and treat the higher priority physiologic problem before proceeding to the next component. If available, bedside ultrasonography should be used to perform a FAST examination of the heart, abdomen, and pelvis in all critical trauma patients. Ultrasonography will significantly improve detection of several life-threatening conditions and also assist with vascular access.

The Secondary Assessment: History Taking and the Physical Examination

After a general impression has been developed and the primary assessment completed, while immediate physiologic or major anatomical abnormalities have been addressed, a secondary assessment should be performed. This should be done only if the child is stable. If the child remains unstable after the primary assessment, resuscitation should be continued. When physiologic stability is established, it is time to begin the secondary assessment—which is a lower priority component of emergency assessment because immediate critical or life-threatening abnormalities should have already been identified and managed. However, dangerous signs and symptoms that are potentially life-threatening can sometimes escape detection in the primary assessment. The secondary assessment is designed to detect less immediate or occult threats to normal physiologic or anatomical features. The more detailed nature of this portion of the physical assessment allows the clinician to develop a reasonable hypothesis for etiology or clinical diagnosis, helps planning for imaging and ancillary laboratory testing, and assists with providing specific treatment.

There are several specific objectives of the secondary assessment:

- Obtaining a history, including the mechanism of injury or circumstances of the illness
- Performing a physical examination, either focused or detailed, depending on the child's age and type of presenting problem (illness or injury)

KEY POINTS

General Impression and Primary Assessment

- Form a general impression based on the PAT.
- Begin treatment for patients in respiratory distress, respiratory failure, shock, or cardiopulmonary failure based on the PAT.
- Continue your assessment with the ABCDEs.
- Modify or add to management priorities based on findings of ABCDEs.

- Establishing an initial clinical diagnosis or differential diagnosis

The process of history taking is intended to glean information pertinent to the current presentation. The physical examination in the secondary assessment can be focused or detailed. This nomenclature distinguishes potentially different degrees of completeness of the physical examination and was derived from the adult assessment model; it might have less relevance to the infant or young pediatric patient in whom a detailed examination should always be performed. In the adult assessment model, a focused examination is suggested for patients with illness presentations and a more time-consuming detailed examination for patients with injury. This emphasis on a more comprehensive examination in trauma patients derives from the concern about missed injuries and the expectation that a detailed examination will reduce the probability of errors in anatomical assessment. Hence, in emergency pediatric assessment, the requirement for a comprehensive examination during secondary assessment of a nontrauma patient pertains to the age and size of the patient. A more limited or focused examination should be performed in adolescents, who have reached physiologic and anatomical adulthood and should be evaluated in this phase with adult techniques. Infants and young children should always receive a detailed examination during the secondary assessment, regardless of whether the presenting problem is caused by illness or injury.

History Taking

The SAMPLE mnemonic can be used to obtain a history, as suggested in Table 1-14. After the history has been taken, the physical findings from the primary assessment should be reassessed based on the additional information.

Physical Examination

The physical examination is an anatomically oriented sequential evaluation typically conducted in a head-to-toe (or toe-to-head in an infant or young child) manner and designed to detect occult illness or injury that was not identified by the primary assessment. The complexity and thoroughness of the examination are

TABLE 1-14 Pediatric SAMPLE Components	
Component	Explanation
Signs/Symptoms	Onset and nature of symptoms or pain or fever Age-appropriate signs of distress
Allergies	Known drug reactions or other allergies
Medications	Exact names and doses of ongoing drugs Timing and amount of last dose Timing and dose of analgesic/antipyretics
Past medical problems	History of pregnancy, labor, delivery Previous illnesses or injuries Immunizations
Last food or liquid	Timing of the child's last food or drink, including bottle or breastfeeding
Events leading to the injury or illness	Key events leading to the current incident Fever history

Dieckmann R, ed. *Pediatric Education for Prehospital Professionals.* 2nd ed. Sudbury, MA: Jones & Bartlett Publishers, American Academy of Pediatrics; 2006:26.

based on the child's age and whether there is illness or injury. A detailed examination should be performed on all trauma patients of all ages and in infants and young children. Frequent or ongoing reassessment is important. If a child has an apparently minor condition, such as low-grade fever, feeding difficulties, fussiness, or minor trauma, physical signs or clues to possible dangerous underlying conditions should not be overlooked (Table 1-15). Child maltreatment, ingestions, and early systemic infections or sepsis in infants, toddlers, or preschoolers are examples of conditions in which the child might not have any acute physiologic or anatomical alterations or the physical findings are not logically related to the symptom or history.

The thorough physical evaluation of children performed as part of the secondary assessment must include all anatomical areas. Often this portion of the assessment is not possible because of life-saving treatment priorities detected during the primary assessment. Use the toe-to-head sequence for this detailed physical examination of infants, toddlers, and preschoolers. This approach will gain the child's trust and cooperation and will increase the accuracy of the physical findings. Get the assistance of the caregiver in the detailed examination.

Note the following special anatomical characteristics of children when performing a comprehensive examination:

- General observations—observe the clothing for any unusual odors or for stains that might suggest a poison. Remove soiled or dirty clothing and save, and wash the skin with soap and water when there is time. If the infant or child vomits, note whether the vomit contains bile or blood. Bile can suggest obstruction, and blood can suggest occult abdominal trauma or gastrointestinal bleeding.
- Skin—inspect the skin carefully for rashes and bruising patterns that might suggest maltreatment. Look for bite marks, straight line marks from cords or straps, pinch marks, or hand, belt, or buckle pattern bruises. Inspect for nonblanching petechiae or purpuric lesions, and look for any new lesions that occur during your physical examination and reassessment.
- Head—the younger the infant or child, the larger the head in proportion to the rest of the body (Figure 1.16). In the infant, the large head sits atop a small and weak neck. Because of this, the head is very easily injured when deceleration occurs

TABLE 1-15 Potentially Dangerous Signs

Sign or Symptom	Examples of Possible Etiologies
Lethargy	Sepsis, shaken baby, intoxication
Poor feeding, sleeping, or fussiness	Congestive heart failure, sepsis
Bilious vomiting	Midgut volvulus
Unusual odor	Intoxication, metabolic acidosis
Bruising, burns, unusual trauma	Child maltreatment
Petechiae	Sepsis
Nonfrontal hematoma of head	Intracranial hemorrhage
Bulging fontanel	Meningitis, encephalitis
Retinal hemorrhage	Shaken baby
Rhinorrhea after head trauma	Basilar skull fracture
Otorrhea	Basilar skull fracture
Postauricular bruising	Basilar skull fracture
Sweet breath odor	Ketosis, diabetic ketoacidosis
Drooling	Bacterial upper airway infection, foreign body
Stridor with crying	Laryngomalacia
Heart murmur	Ventricular septal defect, atrial septal defect, tetralogy of Fallot
Difficult walking	Septic hip, occult fracture, sepsis, leukemia, slipped capital femoral epiphysis, or Legg-Calvé-Perthes disease

(such as in motor vehicle crashes). Look for bruising, swelling, and hematomas. Significant blood can be lost between the skull and scalp of a small infant. The anterior fontanel in infants younger than 9 to 18 months can provide useful information about pressure within the central nervous system. A bulging and nonpulsatile fontanel can suggest meningitis, encephalitis, or intracranial bleeding. A sunken fontanel suggests dehydration.

- Eyes—a thorough evaluation of pupil size, reaction to light, and symmetry of extraocular muscle movements can be difficult to perform in infants. Gently rocking infants in the upright position will often get them to open their eyes. A colorful distracting object can then be used to look at eye movements. Retinal hemorrhages on ophthalmoscopic examination suggest possible subdural hematoma, often a marker of shaken baby syndrome or child maltreatment.

- Nose—many infants prefer to breathe through their noses, as well as through their mouths, and when the nose is plugged with mucus, they are unable to breathe unless they are crying. The most common cause of respiratory distress in small infants is nasal obstruction from mucus. Gentle bulb or catheter suction of the nostrils can bring relief. In the toddler,

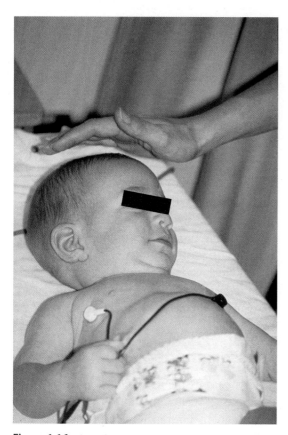

Figure 1.16 The infant's head is disproportionately large compared with older children and adults.

foreign bodies are often the cause of nasal obstruction or unilateral discharge. Peas, beans, paper, plastic toys, and a myriad of small objects find their way into the toddler's nostrils. Leaking fluid (cerebrospinal fluid, rhinorrhea) after head trauma suggests a basilar skull fracture.

- Ears—look for any drainage from the ear canals. Leaking fluid (cerebrospinal fluid, otorrhea) suggests a basilar skull fracture. Check for bruises behind the ear or Battle sign, another sign of basilar skull fracture. The presence of pus can indicate an ear infection or perforation of the eardrum.

- Mouth—avoid looking in the mouth if the child has stridor. A partially obstructed airway in a child with stridor can become completely obstructed if touched. In the trauma patient, look for active bleeding and loose teeth. Note the smell of the breath. Many types of ingestions have specific odors, especially

hydrocarbons. Acidosis can impart a sweet smell to the breath. Drooling suggests a bacterial infection of the upper airway, such as peritonsillar abscess or bacterial tracheitis, or a foreign body.

- Neck—locate the trachea for midline positioning. Listen with a stethoscope over the trachea at the midline. This is a quick and easy way to tell the difference between the sounds of mucus in the mouth, nose, and pharynx versus wheezing and stridor.

- Chest—reexamine the chest for penetrations, bruises, or rashes. If the child is injured, feel the clavicles and every rib for tenderness and/or deformity.

- Heart—listen to the heart for murmurs or abnormal sounds, such as friction rubs, gallops, or muffled heart sound.

- Back—inspect the back for penetrations, bruises, or rashes. Percuss for tenderness.

- Abdomen—inspect the abdomen for distention. Gently palpate the abdomen and watch closely for guarding or tensing of the abdominal muscles, which can suggest infection, obstruction, or intra-abdominal injury. Note any tenderness or masses.

- Pelvis—compress the pelvis, and feel for instability and tenderness.

- Extremities—assess for symmetry. Compare both sides for color, warmth, size of joints, and tenderness. Put each joint through full range of motion while watching the eyes of the child for signs of pain.

- Neurologic examination—do a cranial nerve evaluation. Have children close and open their eyes, smile, and stick out their tongues. If cooperative, hold an object in front of their eyes and track eye movements up, down, left, and right. Doing some simple maneuvers, such as lifting their arms and legs, shrugging their shoulders, pushing against resistance, and squeezing your hand, can test some gross motor functions. Look for a pronator drift with the child's arms extended. If there is no injury and the patient is old enough, have the child walk and observe the gait; is it normal, wide based, or ataxic? Assess for reflexes, especially if the child has back pain or shows signs of motor weakness.

The Tertiary Assessment: Diagnostic Evaluations

After the secondary assessment in a stable child, specific diagnostic tests might be necessary to identify the cause and severity of illness and injury. This component of patient assessment is termed diagnostic assessment or tertiary assessment and uses laboratory and other ancillary procedures (eg, imaging, invasive hemodynamic monitoring) to help establish specific diagnosis. Simple laboratory tests, such as glucose determination, are indicated earlier, during the primary assessment.

Consultations, Admissions, and Transfers

In critically injured or ill children, it might be apparent early in the primary assessment which consultations with other specialists are needed. Predeveloped consultation and admission protocols will facilitate timely access to appropriate in-hospital resources for your critically ill and injured patients. Likewise, transfer and transportation protocols, which specifically address the unique needs of children must be in place (see Online Chapter 15, Emergency Department and Office Preparedness for Pediatric Emergencies).

On completion of the tertiary assessment, an outline of the most likely cause(s) of your patient's condition, the physiologic status, and important issues that need further clarification should be formulated. Check all medication and fluids administered, procedures completed, and documentation by team members. Be alert to detect any medical errors and adverse events. Make a prompt decision about the patient's potential ongoing needs and decide on his or her disposition.

Reassessment

Perform reassessments of all patients to observe responses to treatment and to track the identified physiologic and anatomical problems. Sometimes the reassessment identifies new problems. The reassessment provides necessary guidance about continuing and modifying treatment.

Common Elements in the Reassessment

- PAT
- ABCDEs
- Repeat vital signs
- Reassessment of positive anatomical findings
- Review of the effectiveness and safety of treatment

- Your assessment of an infant or child begins with the primary assessment: the PAT followed by the ABCDEs.

- Form a general impression, then perform the primary assessment or ABCDEs that will drive your management priorities in stabilizing physiologic abnormalities and restoring vital functions.

- Continue assessment with a history and physical examination if your general impression of the child is stable or once initial management steps have begun or the child has been stabilized. Do not miss anatomical abnormalities or signs of occult injury or illness.

- On the basis of the findings in the primary and secondary assessment and your clinical diagnosis, obtain imaging and laboratory testing as part of the tertiary assessment to implement specific treatment.

- Perform reassessments throughout the ED stay.

Check Your Knowledge

1. All of the following are components of the Pediatric Assessment Triangle (PAT) except:

   A. appearance.

   B. circulation.

   C. heart rate.

   D. work of breathing.

2. Abnormalities in which of the following components of the PAT would indicate a decompensated shock state?

   A. Appearance and circulation

   B. Appearance and work of breathing

   C. Circulation

   D. Work of breathing and circulation to skin

3. All of the following are techniques to assess for shock except:

   A. heart rate.

   B. capillary refill time.

   C. pulse quality.

   D. work of breathing.

4. You are about to assess an 8-month-old boy. On the basis of his developmental level, which of the following techniques would be helpful?

   A. Do your assessment from a standing position.

   B. Examine head to toe.

   C. Offer distractions.

   D. Separate infant and mother.

References

1. Dieckmann RA. Epidemiology of pediatric emergency care. In: Dieckmann RA, Fiser DH, Selbst SM. *Illustrated Textbook of Pediatric Emergency and Critical Care Procedures.* St. Louis, MO: Mosby; 1997:3–7.

2. Pitts SR, Niska RW, Xu J, Burt CW, Division of Health Care Statistics. *National Hospital Ambulatory Medical Care Survey: 2006 Emergency Department Summary.* Hyattsville, MD: National Center for Health Statistics; 2008. National health statistics report 7. www.cdc.gov/nchs/data/nhsr/nhsr007.pdf. Accessed March 25, 2011.

3. Schappert SM, Rechtsteiner EA. *Ambulatory medical care utilization estimates for 2006.* Hyattsville, MD: National Center for Health Statistics; 2008. National health statistics report 8. www.cdc.gov/nchs/data/nhsr/nhsr008.pdf. Accessed March 25, 2011.

4. Kellermann A. Crisis in the emergency department. *N Engl J Med.* 2006;355:1.

5. Institute of Medicine. *Hospital-Based Emergency Care: At the Breaking Point.* Washington, DC: Institute of Medicine; June 13, 2006.

6. Institute of Medicine. *Emergency Care for Children: Growing Pains.* Washington, DC: Institute of Medicine; June 13, 2006.

7. Stockwell MS, Findley SE, Irigoyen M, Martinez RA, Sonnett M. Change in parental reasons for use of an urban pediatric emergency department in the past decade. *Pediatr Emerg Care.* 2010;26:181–185.

8. Ben-Isaac E, Schrager SM, Keefer M, Chen AY. National profile of nonemergent pediatric emergency department visits. *Pediatrics.* 2010;125:454–459.

9. Marsh RH, Mollen CJ, Shofer FS, Baren JM. Characteristics that distinguish adolescents who present to a children's hospital emergency department from those presenting to a general emergency department. *Pediatr Emerg Care.* 2009;25:376–379.

10. Bourgeois FT, Shannon MW. Emergency care for children in pediatric and general emergency departments. *Pediatr Emerg Care.* 2007;23:94–102.

11. Shah MN, Cushman JT, Davis CO, Bazarian JJ, Auinger P, Friedman B. The epidemiology of emergency medical services use by children: An analysis of the National Hospital Ambulatory Medical Care Survey. *Prehosp Emerg Care.* 2008;12:269–276.

12. Johnson DW, Adair C, Brant R, Holmwood J, Mitchel I. Differences in admission rates of children with bronchiolitis by pediatric and general emergency departments. *Pediatrics.* 2002;110:e49.

13. American Academy of Pediatrics Section on Orthopaedics, American Academy of Pediatrics Committee on Pediatric Emergency Medicine, American Academy of Pediatrics Section on Critical Care, et al. Management of pediatric trauma. *Pediatrics.* 2008;121:849–854.

14. Miniño AM, Arias E, Kochanek KD, Murphy SL, Smith BL. Deaths: final data for 2000. *Natl Vital Stat Rep.* 2002;50:1–119. www.cdc.gov/nchs/data/nvsr/nvsr50/nvsr50_15.pdf. Accessed March 25, 2011.

15. D'Souza AL, Nelson NG, McKenzie LB. Pediatric burn injuries treated in US emergency departments between 1990 and 2006. *Pediatrics.* 2009;124:1424–1430.

16. Weiss HB, Mathers LJ, Forjuoh SN, Kinnane JM. *Child and Adolescent Emergency Department Visit Data Book.* Pittsburgh, PA: Center for Violence and Injury Control, Allegheny University of the Health Sciences; 1997.

17. Zaritsky A, Dieckmann RA, EMSC Consensus Group, et al. *EMSC Definitions and Pediatric Assessment Approaches.* Washington, DC: Maternal and Child Health Bureau; 2005.

18. Dieckmann RA, Brownstein D, Gausche-Hill M. The Pediatric Assessment Triangle: A novel approach to pediatric assessment. *Pediatr Emerg Care.* 2010;26:312–315.

19. Dieckmann RA, Brownstein D, Gausche M, eds. *Textbook of Pediatric Education for Prehospital Professionals.* 2nd ed. Sudbury, MA: Jones & Bartlett Publishers; 2006.

20. Ralston M, Hazinski MF, Zaritsky AL, Schexnayder SM, Kleinman ME, eds. *PALS Provider Manual.* Dallas, TX: American Heart Association; 2006.

21. Davis D, Barbee L, Ririe D. Pediatric endotracheal tube selection: A comparison of age-based and height-based criteria. *American Association of Nurse Anesthetists Journal.* 1998;66:299–303.

22. Dieckmann RA. The dilemma of pediatric drug dosing and equipment sizing in the era of patient safety [editorial]. *Emerg Med Australasia.* 2007;19:490–493.

23. Sullivan KJ, Kissoon N, Goodwin SR. End-tidal carbon dioxide monitoring in pediatric emergencies. *Pediatr Emerg Care.* 2005;21:327–335.

24. Tobias JD. Transcutaneous carbon dioxide monitoring in infants and children. *Paediatr Anaesth.* 2009;19:434–444.

25. Ward KR, Yealy DM. End tidal CO_2 monitoring in emergency medicine, part 1: Basic principles. *Acad Emerg Med.* 1998;5:628–636.

26. Bhende MS, Thompson AE. Evaluation of an end-tidal CO_2 detector during pediatric cardiopulmonary resuscitation. *Pediatrics.* 1995;95:395–399.

27. Wayne MA, Levine RL, Miller CC. Use of end-tidal carbon dioxide to predict outcome in prehospital cardiac arrest. *Ann Emerg Med.* 1995;25:762–767.

28. Aufderheide TP, Sigurdsson G, Pirrallo RG, et al. Hyperventilation-induced hypotension during cardiopulmonary resuscitation. *Circulation.* 2004;109:1960–1965.

29. Michard F, Teboul JL. Predicting fluid responsiveness in ICU patients: A critical analysis of the evidence. *Chest.* 2002;121:2000–2008.

30. Skippen P, Seear M, Poskitt K, et al. Effect of hyperventilation on regional cerebral blood flow in head-injured children. *Crit Care Med.* 1997;25:1402–1409.

31. Kleinman MC, Chameides L, Schexnayder SM, et al. Part 14: Pediatric advanced life support: 2010 American Heart Association guidelines for cardiopulmonary resuscitation and emergency cardiovascular care. *Circulation.* 2010;122:S876–S908.

32. Fulton JA, Greller HA, Hoffman RS. GCS and AVPU: The alphabet soup doesn't spell "C-O-M-A" in toxicology. *Ann Emerg Med.* 2005;45:224–225.

33. Nayana Prabha PC, Nalini P, Tiroumourougane Serane V. Role of Glasgow Coma Scale in pediatric nontraumatic coma. *Indian Pediatr.* 2003;40:620–625.

34. Hannan EL, Farrell LS, Meaker PS, Cooper A. Predicting inpatient mortality for pediatric trauma patients with blunt injuries: a better alternative. *J Pediatr Surg.* 2000;35:155–159.

35. Gilmore BG, Prashad J. Ultrasonography. In: Baren JM, Rothrock SG, Brennan JA, Brown L, eds. *Pediatric Emergency Medicine.* Philadelphia, PA: Saunders/Elsevier; 2008:1253–1258.

CASE SUMMARY 1

A 6-month-old boy who has had persistent vomiting for 24 hours presents to the emergency department (ED). The infant is lying still and has poor muscle tone. He is irritable if touched, and his cry is weak. There are no abnormal airway sounds, retractions, or flaring. He is pale and mottled. The respiratory rate (RR) is 45/min, heart rate is 170/min, and blood pressure is 50 by palpation. Air movement is normal, and breath sounds are clear to auscultation. The skin feels cool, and capillary refill time is 4 seconds. The brachial pulse is weak. His abdomen is distended.

1. *What are the key signs of serious illness in this infant?*
2. *How helpful are heart rate, RR, and blood pressure in evaluating cardiopulmonary function?*

This infant is severely ill. The PAT indicates poor appearance with diminished tone, poor interactiveness, and weak cry. These are important signals of weakened cardiopulmonary and/or neurologic function in an infant. Work of breathing is normal, although the RR is high, and circulation to skin is poor. The PAT establishes this child as a critical patient who requires aggressive resuscitation. However, the RR, heart rate, and blood pressure are possibly within the normal ranges for age. Therefore, vital signs should be used in the context of findings on PAT and the entire primary assessment. In this case, the PAT tells you that the child has an abnormal appearance and decreased skin circulation, which suggest shock.

The hands-on ABCDE phase of the assessment shows poor skin signs and diminished brachial pulse. These important physical findings confirm the PAT impression of shock. Furthermore, when you review the vital signs in the context of the primary assessment, you might identify that this child has effortless tachypnea, a physiologic attempt to clear acidosis generated by shock.

CASE SUMMARY 2

A 21-month-old girl is brought to the ED after a 911 call. The mother explains that the child, who has a tracheostomy, has had copious secretions and has required more frequent suctioning and breathing treatments for 2 days. The child has severe cerebral palsy. The mother is anxious and demanding immediate hospitalization for the child. The child turns blue and becomes agitated whenever you approach but is easily consoled by the mother. There are no retractions or flaring. Her RR is 50/min, and heart rate is 140/min. You are unable to obtain a blood pressure.

1. *How can the PAT be used to evaluate the severity of illness and urgency for care in a child with special health care needs?*

The PAT is a good way to get a general impression of this child and to judge the degree of illness and urgency for care. Many other conventional assessment methods, such as history taking, auscultation, and blood pressure determinations, would be frustrating to attempt and possibly inaccurate in the first few minutes. The child's appearance is somewhat reassuring, with comfort in her mother's arms and a vigorous cry. There are no retractions or flaring, so work of breathing is normal despite a RR in the highest range for age. Circulation to skin is normal. With these PAT findings, it is highly unlikely that the child has a serious illness. The PAT provides the impression of a relatively well child and allows you to stand back and gain the confidence of the child and mother before rushing to a hands-on evaluation. This child should be placed in the mother's arms to allow the mother to keep the girl on her lap while you proceed with the evaluation. When the child is less agitated, you can approach gently to complete the primary assessment. A toe-to-head sequence should be used.

The PAT is the important first phase of the primary assessment. It does not replace the hands-on assessment of the ABCDEs and vital signs. The PAT for this child should reassure you. Information about the child's baseline neurologic and cardiopulmonary status should be obtained from the mother or primary physician, and physical assessment should be used to compare the presenting condition with the established baseline.

A 7-year-old boy is hit by a car in front of his home. He was thrown 1.5 m (5 ft) and had a brief loss of consciousness. The father decided to take him to the physician's office when he noted the boy becoming sleepy.

In the office, the boy opens his eyes with a loud verbal stimulus but will not speak or interact. There are no abnormal airway sounds, but intercostal retractions and flaring are present. His skin is pale. Respiratory rate is 50/min, heart rate is 145/min, and blood pressure is 90 by palpation. The chest is clear with decreased tidal volume. The skin feels cool, capillary refill time is 4 seconds, and brachial pulse is present. Pupils are equal and reactive. He has a large frontal hematoma.

1. *Does this child's assessment suggest serious injury?*
2. *What actions are required by the physician in the office?*
3. *How should this child be transported to the ED?*

This child's appearance is grossly abnormal, with a serious mechanism of injury. The boy's lethargic appearance, increased work of breathing, and abnormal skin signs on the PAT suggest possible intracranial, chest, and abdominal injuries. The child might have concussion, hemorrhage, or brain edema in conjunction with a chest injury and abdominal hemorrhage. In this child, establishing a baseline neurologic status in the office will help clinicians at the hospital evaluate the trend of neurologic response. The primary assessment suggests an unstable patient who needs rapid treatment in the office with 100% oxygen, crystalloid fluids, and immediate emergency medical services (EMS) transport to the hospital.

chapter 2

The Pediatric Airway in Health and Disease

Phyllis L. Hendry, MD, FAAP, FACEP

Objectives

1 Compare the anatomical and physiologic differences between adult and pediatric airways.

2 Discuss a general approach to pediatric airway emergencies, including the difficult airway.

3 Describe clinical features, diagnosis, and management of upper and lower airway obstruction and diseases of the lung.

Chapter Outline

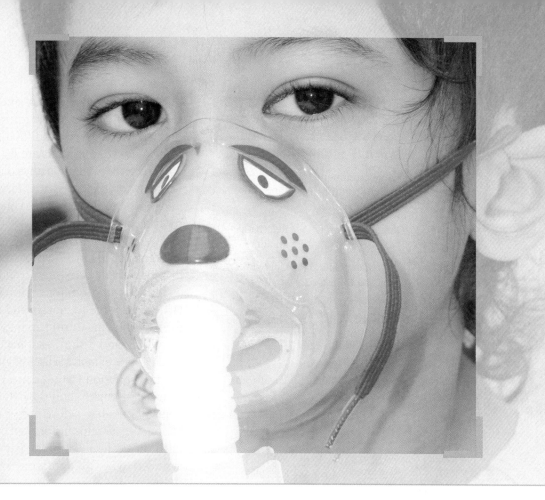

CASE SCENARIO 1

A 6-month-old boy presents to the emergency department (ED) with wheezing, severe retractions, and stridor. The infant has poor tone and is not responsive to his surroundings. He has intercostal retractions, and his color is pale. Vital signs include respiratory rate of 80/min, heart rate of 190/min, temperature (rectal) of 38.6°C (101.5°F), and oxygen saturation of 80% on room air. His mother reveals that he was born at 28 weeks' gestation and was intubated and given mechanical ventilation for 6 weeks before hospital discharge. The patient also has Pierre Robin syndrome.

1. *How would you assess and categorize this patient's airway?*
2. *What special precautions would you take in planning airway management and possible intubation?*

Introduction

The first step toward successful airway management is a thorough understanding of normal pediatric airway anatomy and physiology, differences between adult and pediatric airway anatomy and physiology, and anatomical airway anomalies that occur in children. The infant airway differs significantly from that of the adult; as a child becomes older, the airway becomes more comparable to adult anatomy. By 8 or 9 years of age, the airway is considered similar to the adult airway, with the exception of size. Table 2-1 provides a comparison of infant and adult airways.

These anatomical differences affect all the steps involved in airway management. For example, a small infant lying flat on a gurney might need a towel placed under the back of the shoulders to align the airway and correct for a forward flexion of the head and neck because of the prominent occiput. Also, a straight blade is preferred to a curved blade to accommodate

TABLE 2-1 Comparison of Infant and Adult Airways[1-3]

	Infant	Adult
Head	Large prominent occiput resulting in sniffing position	Flat occiput
Tongue	Relatively larger	Relatively smaller
Larynx	Cephalad position, opposite C2 and C3 vertebrae	Opposite C4 to C6
Epiglottis	Ω shaped, soft	Flat, flexible
Vocal cords	Short, concave	Horizontal
Smallest diameter	Cricoid ring, below cords	Vocal cords
Cartilage	Soft, less calcified	Firm, calcified
Lower airway	Smaller, less developed	Larger, more cartilage

the infant's anterior airway and large tongue. Certain congenital and acquired conditions predispose the airway to difficult management; some of these conditions are listed in Table 2-2.

There are numerous physiologic differences between adult and pediatric airways and respiratory systems. Children have increased rates of oxygen consumption, increased chest wall compliance, lower lung compliance and elastic recoil, and diminished functional residual capacity, predisposing them to respiratory failure.[1-4]

Infants and young children are particularly susceptible to emesis and aspiration due to air swallowing during crying, diaphragmatic breathing, and a short esophagus. Recent oral intake is one of many causes of increased risk for gastric aspiration (Table 2-3). A history of most recent oral intake should be elicited for all patients, if possible, before proceeding with intubation. Because this history can be unobtainable in the critically ill child, all patients should be assumed to be in a nonfasting state.

TABLE 2-2 Selected Conditions Associated With Difficult Intubation

Congenital Anomalies	Anatomical Difference
• Down syndrome	Large tongue, small mouth, frequent laryngospasm
• Goldenhar syndrome	Mandibular hypoplasia
• Robin syndrome	Large tongue, small mouth, mandibular anomaly
• Turner syndrome	Short neck
Tumor/Mass	
• Cystic hygroma	Compression of airway
• Hemangioma	Hemorrhage
Infection	
• Epiglottitis	Inability to visualize cords
• Croup	Airway irritability, edema below cords
Cervical Spine Immobilization	Prevents optimal head and neck positioning
Upper Airway Obstruction	
• Angioneurotic edema	Difficulty visualizing cords
• Peritonsillar abscess	Difficulty visualizing cords
Facial Trauma	Difficulty opening mouth

TABLE 2-3 **Risks for Aspiration of Gastric Contents**
Full Stomach
• Children; less than 6 hours since last meal
• Infants; less than 4 hours since last meal
Unknown History of Last Oral Intake
• Trauma
- Elevated intracranial pressure
- Swallowed blood
• Delayed Gastric Emptying
- Drugs
- Diabetes
- Infection/sepsis
• Intestinal Obstruction
• Esophageal Conditions
- Reflux
- Motility disorders
• Obesity
• Pregnancy
• Pain

Anatomical and Physiologic Responses to Airway Maneuvers

Anatomical and physiologic factors in children affect the performance of airway techniques. These factors include a flexible trachea, a prominent neck, a relatively large tongue for the oral cavity, a profound vagal response to stimulation of the posterior pharynx, and a dependence on diaphragmatic excursion for ventilation.

Bag-Mask Ventilation

Bag-mask ventilation is a technique that requires proper hand placement on the mask and jaw and specific ventilation volumes and rates. Because of flexible tracheal rings, too much pressure on a mask with the thumb and index finger (C component of the E-C clamp) can result in flexion of the head on the neck and possible airway obstruction. Finger placement of the middle, ring, and fifth fingers must be on the angle of the jaw (E component of the E-C clamp) to avoid pushing on the submental soft tissue, which can result in the tongue being forced back into the posterior pharynx, causing airway obstruction (**Figure 2.1**).

The Sellick maneuver (cricoid pressure) has been commonly used to occlude the esophagus and limit gastric distention; however, its use in adults is being questioned in the literature. Excessive cricoid pressure can occlude or distort the airway anatomy and impair laryngoscopic view. Use of the Sellick maneuver is considered optional in adults. There is no current literature to recommend discontinuing the maneuver in pediatric patients, and the maneuver is still recommended by some.[3]

Insertion of a nasogastric tube will decompress the stomach but can induce emesis through stimulation of the oropharynx or by keeping the lower esophageal sphincter open. Maintaining appropriate ventilation rates and providing only the amount of ventilation volume that initiates chest rise (state "squeeze, release, release") are key steps to the proper technique of bag-mask ventilation. If too much volume at too high a pressure is delivered, gastric distention might impede diaphragmatic movement, resulting in hypoventilation.

Laryngoscopy and Intubation

Direct laryngoscopy in a conscious patient is a noxious stimulus that can result in increased intracranial pressure (ICP), pain, emesis, hypoxemia,

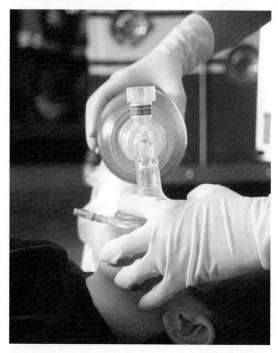

Figure 2.1 E-C clamp positioning for bag-mask ventilation.

hypertension, and cardiac dysrhythmias (**Figure 2.2**). Bradycardia can develop due to a vagal reflex during laryngoscopy, as a direct effect of succinylcholine or other medications, or as a result of hypoxemia. Infants are much more likely to develop bradycardia than are adults.

Intubation trauma can cause significant edema and obstruction of the airway. One millimeter of circumferential edema can result in a several-fold increase in resistance in a 4-mm infant airway.

General Approach to Airway Emergencies

Pediatric patients who need urgent or emergent airway management usually present with little warning; therefore, advance preparation is a key element in the general approach to management. Advance preparation includes selection and stocking of appropriate airway and respiratory equipment, protocols for rapid sequence intubation (RSI) and difficult airway situations, training

of physicians and staff in airway management, and routine practice, or "mock code," scenarios.

Equipment

Airway equipment should be available in all sizes for children ranging from premature newborns to large adolescents. Table 2-4 lists the necessary equipment for basic and advanced airway management. Equipment should be carefully inventoried at regular intervals and checked for proper functioning. Alternative airway equipment should

TABLE 2-4 Equipment for Basic and Advanced Pediatric Airway Management
Uncuffed tracheal tubes in sizes 2.5 to 5.5
Cuffed tracheal tubes in sizes 6.0 to 9
Tracheal tube stylets
Laryngoscope handles in good working order
Laryngoscope blades
• Straight (Miller) in sizes 0 to 3
• Curved (Macintosh) in sizes 2 to 3
Oropharyngeal airways
Nasopharyngeal airways
Pediatric and adult Magill forceps
Nonrebreather oxygen masks (adult and pediatric)
Ventilation masks in all sizes for bag-mask ventilation
Self-inflating ventilation bags (450–1,200 mL) with oxygen reservoir and positive end-expiratory pressure valve
Oxygen source
Suctioning source
Large-bore stiff suction tips (Yankauer)
Flexible suction catheters (French sizes 5 to 16)
Nasogastric tubes (French sizes 6 to 14)
Pulse oximeter
Cardiorespiratory monitor
Tracheostomy tubes
Tracheostomy surgical instrument set
14-gauge needle catheter for needle cricothyrotomy or other commercially available set
Cricothyrotomy tray
End-tidal carbon dioxide monitor or detector
Laryngeal mask airway
Access to video laryngoscopy is ubiquitous and should be strongly considered

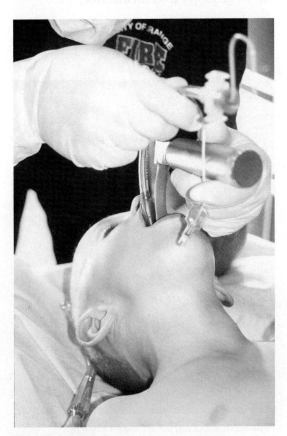

Figure 2.2 Endotracheal intubation of a child.

always be readily available, especially when neuromuscular blocking agents are used or risk factors for a difficult airway exist. Appropriate monitoring during airway management includes cardiorespiratory and blood pressure (BP) monitoring, as well as continuous pulse oximetry and ongoing clinical assessment. Colorimetric end-tidal carbon dioxide ($ETCO_2$) detectors are available for verifying tracheal tube placement in infants and children. Quantitative $ETCO_2$ detectors are used for ongoing monitoring and assessment. (See Online Chapter 26, Critical Procedures.)

Ideally, charts with age- and weight-related equipment sizes and RSI medication dosages should be available. Because there is little time to guess weights and find the correct-sized equipment during a true emergency, intubation equipment should be stocked in an age- or length-related manner with easy access. A pediatric resuscitation tape that relates patient length to weight and precalculates dosages and equipment size can be helpful during an emergency when weight and age cannot be determined accurately (**Figure 2.3**).[5]

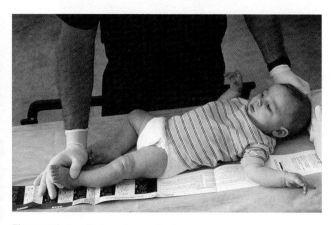

Figure 2.3 Length-based resuscitation tape.

Basic Airway Management

Once it has been determined that an airway or respiratory problem exists, it is important to progress in a calm, stepwise manner, beginning with basic airway skills and frequent reassessment. Before the application of advanced airway techniques, the airway should be assessed and the patient given positive pressure ventilation and oxygen as needed. For the conscious, spontaneously breathing child, it is usually

appropriate to allow the child to assume a position of comfort and to supply oxygen via nasal cannula or mask (**Figure 2.4**). If the child resists, a blow-by technique usually is well tolerated (**Figure 2.5**). In the unconscious child, the airway should be checked for obstruction. If noisy breathing and poor air flow result from obstruction, then the airway should be opened through either the head tilt-chin lift or jaw-thrust maneuver. If cervical spine trauma is suspected, a jaw-thrust maneuver is used, with great care taken to avoid movement of the neck.

If opening the airway does not restore adequate ventilation, begin assisted ventilation with bag-mask ventilation. Place an oral or nasopharyngeal airway as needed to maintain the airway during bag-mask ventilation (**Figures 2.6 and 2.7**). (Refer to Online Chapter 26, Critical Procedures, to review the detailed procedure for bag-mask ventilation and other basic airway procedures.) Suctioning of the airway is often required to remove secretions, blood, or foreign material. Gastric inflation can be reduced by using the correct size of equipment and the proper technique for bag-mask ventilation, as well as by applying cricoid pressure or in some cases insertion of a nasogastric tube. Ventilation with the bag-mask technique using high-flow oxygen should precede endotracheal intubation when the patient is hypoventilating to create an oxygen reserve for the time required to place the tracheal tube and reinitiate ventilation.[1–4,6]

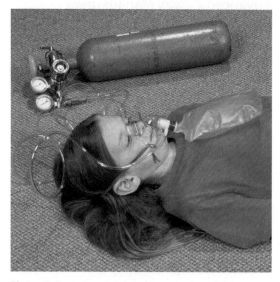

Figure 2.4 Child with partial nonrebreather mask.

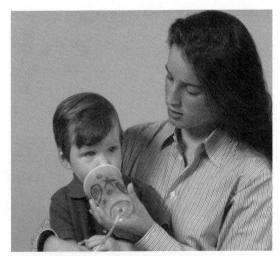

Figure 2.5 If the child resists application of a mask or nasal cannula, administer oxygen through a nonthreatening object, such as a plastic cup.

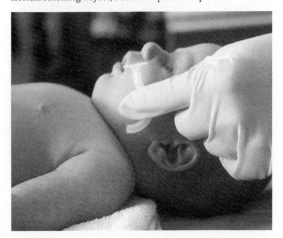

Figure 2.6 Measuring an oropharyngeal airway.

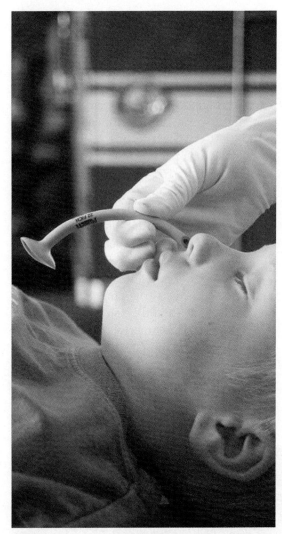

Figure 2.7 Placing a nasopharyngeal airway in a child.

Advanced Airway Management

After basic airway measures have been accomplished, the patient should be reassessed for improvement or the need to progress to advanced airway techniques. The urgency of this progression will be determined by the condition of the patient, the skill of the physician, and the location of the care (out-of-hospital, clinic, or ED). The next step in airway management after bag-mask ventilation is usually endotracheal intubation. This is commonly accomplished using the rapid sequence intubation (RSI) technique. RSI facilitates endotracheal intubation, reduces complications of the procedure, and has become a standard ED procedure for adult and pediatric intubation.[6–10]

If the patient is receiving adequate oxygen and ventilation by the bag-mask ventilation technique, reassess the need for more advanced airway techniques. As in cases of children with a seizure, airway opening techniques and/or bag-mask ventilation might be all that is necessary to manage the airway. If the patient requires prolonged bag-mask ventilation or the physician is not skilled in endotracheal intubation or RSI, then the best course of action is to continue bag-mask ventilation until transfer to definitive care. Gausche et al[11] found no difference in survival or outcome of children when comparing bag-mask ventilation and endotracheal intubation in the out-of-hospital setting.

The physician should be aware of advanced techniques, such as the laryngeal mask airway (LMA), tracheal light, retrograde intubation, video laryngoscopy (GlideScope), and cricothyrotomy (see Online Chapter 26, Critical Procedures). These techniques are rarely needed but might be necessary in cases of a failed difficult airway or unusual airway anatomy. Successful endotracheal intubation for adults and children occurs in tertiary and community ED settings in almost 100% of cases with two attempts. The need for a surgical airway is rare.[3,8–10] Online Chapter 26, Critical Procedures, reviews the procedures for endotracheal intubation, RSI, LMA, cricothyrotomy, and retrograde intubation.

Rapid sequence intubation is an important technique in the treatment of children requiring endotracheal intubation. It is the method of choice for most pediatric emergency intubations performed at academic EDs and is associated with a high success rate and a low rate of serious adverse events.[10]

The following section will briefly review the rationale and general order of RSI. Rapid sequence intubation requires advance preparation.

Rapid Sequence Intubation

The purpose of RSI is to rapidly induce unconsciousness and neuromuscular blockade in preparation for intubation. Rapid sequence intubation facilitates intubation and decreases aspiration, untoward physiologic responses, and psychological trauma associated with awake intubation. The procedure blunts the cardiovascular and ICP responses associated with intubations.[2–4,6,7]

Any patient requiring endotracheal intubation is a potential candidate for RSI. Rapid sequence intubation should be used with caution in the following conditions: significant facial edema, trauma, or fractures; distorted laryngotracheal anatomy; or airway anomalies.

A thorough knowledge of the medications used in RSI, technique of endotracheal intubation, and anatomy of the pediatric airway is essential before attempting intubation with RSI. Ideally, RSI should be attempted before the child develops cardiopulmonary compromise. Early initiation of RSI allows the physician to complete the procedure while the child still has some physiologic reserve.

The sequential steps for RSI are listed below. Health care personnel can perform many of the steps simultaneously. An appointed team leader must direct the sequence and medication selection. The history of the acute illness and the entire medical history influence the choice of medications used in RSI. Frequently, emergency airway scenarios do not allow time for a detailed history. The mnemonic AMPLE has been used to direct the history needed for RSI: A—Allergies; M—Medicines, drugs of abuse; P—Past medical problems, previous anesthesia; L—Last oral intake; E—Events, including out-of-hospital course.

Steps of RSI include the following:
1. Brief history and anatomical assessment
2. Preparation of equipment and medications
3. Preoxygenation
4. Premedication with adjunctive agents (atropine or lidocaine [lignocaine])
5. Sedation and induction of unconsciousness
6. Optional cricoid pressure (Sellick maneuver)
7. Neuromuscular blocking agent for muscle relaxation
8. Intubation
9. Confirmation of tracheal tube placement (clinical, pulse oximetry, and carbon dioxide detection)
10. Postintubation care: tracheal tube secured; chest radiograph; nasogastric tube placement, medical record or procedure note documentation

The Difficult Airway

A crucial step in the evaluation of a child for RSI and emergency airway management is to determine whether there are any features that would make bag-mask ventilation, endotracheal intubation, or cricothyrotomy difficult to achieve. An airway is usually labeled as "difficult" because the patient's normal anatomy is modified due to an acute insult or because the patient has a baseline abnormal airway and requires airway management for an unrelated cause. Clinically, the failed airway can be defined as one of two types: cannot intubate but can oxygenate with bag-mask ventilation or cannot intubate and cannot oxygenate. The difficult, failed airway has been well described in the adult anesthesia and emergency medicine literature. Less is known about predicting and managing the difficult airway in the pediatric population. It has been estimated that 1% to 3% of patients present with difficult airways, leading to difficult intubation under direct visualization. The anesthesia literature indicates that intubation is unsuccessful in 0.1% to 0.4% of patients who were assessed to have no risks for a difficult airway. These statistics do not adequately reflect the emergency medicine airway situation. The National Emergency Airway Registry (NEAR) is a multicenter, prospective, emergency medicine–led registry. The pilot phase included 1,288 patients with an incidence of "rescue" cricothyrotomy of 1%. Additional NEAR studies have confirmed the low rate of cricothyrotomy and the high success rate of endotracheal intubation.[3,9,10]

The most important factor in determining success or failure in airway management is the physician performing the procedure. The physician directing the airway management must attempt to recognize and predict the possibility of a difficult airway, choose the appropriate technique or equipment, have a comprehensive knowledge of the pharmacologic and technical skills for RSI, and be skilled in airway rescue techniques if the initial airway management fails.

In general, the difficult airway is predicted by looking at the patient's unique anatomical features; examining the airway, head, and neck; and assessing for airway obstruction and cervical spine mobility. Mallampati et al[12] classified airways based on the degree of visualization of the pillars, soft palate, and uvula. The classification is an indication of the amount of space in the mouth to accommodate the laryngoscope and tracheal tube. There are four Mallampati grades, with grade I indicating excellent oral access and grade IV indicating difficult access and intubation (**Figure 2.8**). The significance of the Mallampati score in infants and small children is unknown. The developers of the National Emergency Airway Course have developed the LEMON Law for identification of the adult difficult airway as follows[3]:

L—Look externally

E—Evaluate the 3-3-2 rule (three fingers between the patient's teeth, three fingers at the space from the mentum to the hyoid bone, and two fingers between the thyroid notch and the floor of the mouth)
M—Mallampati grade
O—Obstruction
N—Neck mobility

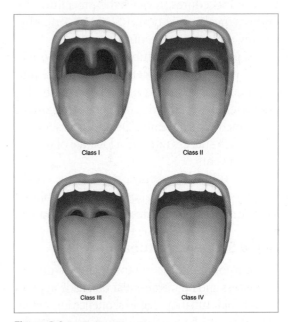

Figure 2.8 Mallampati grades.

Walls RM, Murphy MF, eds. *Manual of Emergency Airway Manage-ment. 3rd ed.* Philadelphia, PA: Lippincott, Williams, & Wilkins; 2008.

Algorithms for management of the difficult airway have been published for adults but not specifically for pediatric patients, although some have been proposed as modifications of adult algorithms (**Figure 2.9**).

Selected conditions associated with the difficult pediatric airway are listed in Table 2-2. Once one of these risk factors has been identified, a stepwise approach should be taken, including calling for anesthesia or surgical assistance and considering other types of airway management, such as awake intubation, video laryngoscopy, LMA, lighted stylet, or cricothyrotomy. Before starting any RSI procedure, it should be established that the patient can effectively receive positive pressure ventilation by the bag-mask ventilation technique and appropriate airway adjuncts or an emergency airway tray should be readily available.

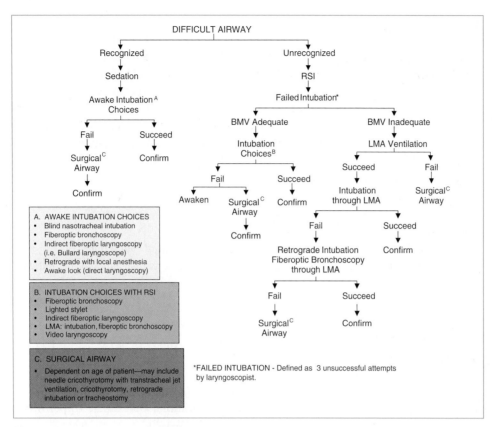

Figure 2.9 Algorithm for management of the difficult airway.

Adapted from Lee BS, Gausche-Hill M. *Pediatric Emergency Airway Management*. Clinical Pediatric Emergency Medicine. WB Saunders, 2001:2:102.

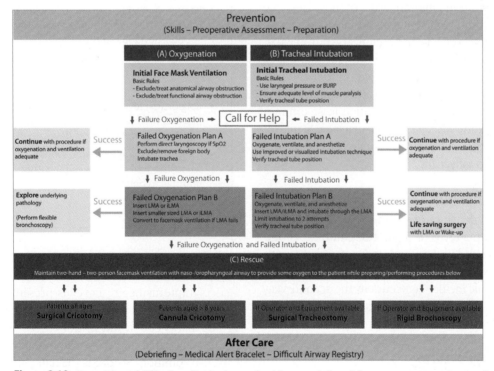

Figure 2.10 Unanticipated difficult pediatric airway algorithm consisting of three parts: oxygenation, tracheal intubation, and rescue.

Weiss M, Englelhardt. Proposal for the management of the unexpected difficult airway. *Pediatric Anesthesia.* 2010;20:454-464.

A 13-month-old boy is brought to the ED by paramedics. The mother found him choking and gagging in the kitchen next to a container of spilled nuts. She immediately called 911. Paramedics note that the child is alert, his work of breathing is increased with audible stridor and subcostal retractions, and his color is normal. Paramedics administer blow-by oxygen and transport the child to the ED. On arrival, the child is awake and alert and in moderate respiratory distress. The patient is placed immediately in a monitored bed. Vital signs are respiratory rate of 60/min, heart rate of 160/min, BP of 88/56 mm Hg, temperature of 37.1°C (98.8°F), and oxygen saturation of 93%.

1. What are your initial management priorities?
2. What diagnostic studies are necessary?
3. What are the possible complications to consider on initial evaluation?
4. What is the definitive management of this condition and disposition of the patient?

Upper Airway Obstruction

Croup

Laryngotracheobronchitis, commonly referred to as croup, is a frequent cause of upper airway obstruction in children. Most of these cases are caused by viral infection of the subglottic airway, producing a characteristic clinical syndrome that consists of a barky cough, stridor, and hoarseness.

Viral origins include parainfluenza virus (accounting for most cases) and influenza A and B. Bacterial infections are much less common and include *Mycoplasma pneumoniae*, *Staphylococcus aureus*, *Streptococcus pyogenes*, and *Haemophilus influenzae*.[13–15]

Epidemiology

The incidence of croup in the United States is approximately 3 to 5 per 100 children. Croup affects children 6 months to 6 years of age, with the incidence sharply decreasing after 6 years of age. Peak incidence occurs in the second year of life. Seasonally, most cases of croup occur during the fall and early winter.[14–16]

Clinical Features

Prodromal symptoms mimic those of an upper respiratory tract infection (URI). Typically,

YOUR FIRST CLUE

Classic Signs and Symptoms of Conditions That Cause Upper Airway Obstruction

- Croup: barking cough, hoarse voice, and stridor develop within several days.

- Foreign-body (FB) aspiration: choking, followed by stridor and decreased breath sounds, develop rapidly in minutes.

- Retropharyngeal abscess (RPA): fever, neck pain/stiffness, drooling, and sore throat develop.

- Epiglottitis: fever, drooling, sore throat, muffled voice, and absence of cough develop within hours to a day.

- Anaphylaxis: angioedema, stridor, wheezing, and shock develop within minutes to hours.

these antecedent symptoms last 1 to 2 days. With the onset of croup, the more characteristic symptoms begin. Fever is present in approximately half of the cases and tends to be low grade. Barky cough and stridor are seen in 90% or more of patients. Hoarseness and retractions are also common. Stridor is the hallmark of upper airway obstruction. In mild cases, stridor is evident only on auscultation with a stethoscope or with agitation. As the disease progresses and airway obstruction becomes more severe, stridor will be more audible and present during the inspiratory and expiratory phases.[14,16] A croup score for determining severity is given in Table 2-5. In general, duration of croup symptoms is 5 to 10 days.

Diagnostic Studies

The diagnosis of croup is made clinically. The utility of laboratory studies and imaging is limited, and routine ancillary studies are not necessary. Plain radiographs of the neck might show a characteristic finding of subglottic narrowing on the lateral view and the "steeple sign" on the anteroposterior view (**Figure 2.11**). Rapid viral testing for parainfluenza is available in some centers but does not change treatment.

Differential Diagnosis

Epiglottitis, bacterial tracheitis, retropharyngeal abscess, peritonsillar abscess, uvulitis, foreign body (FB) aspiration, allergic reaction, and neoplasm are other causes of infectious and non-infectious upper airway obstruction that can present with symptoms similar to croup.

Management

Mist or humidified oxygen has a theoretical benefit of moistening thick secretions and decreasing inflammation of the airway in croup. However, there are few data to support this hypothesis, and trials have not demonstrated significant benefit of this treatment.[14,16–18] If the child becomes more agitated by the mist device and the oxygen saturation level is normal, administration of oxygen should be discontinued.

Nebulized epinephrine (adrenaline) should be promptly administered in all patients with moderate to severe croup. Epinephrine (adrenaline) acts on α- and β-adrenergic receptors, causing vasoconstriction, reduction of mucosal edema,

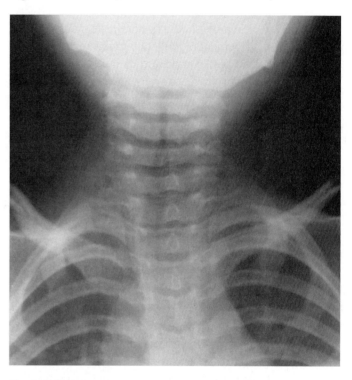

Figure 2.11 Steeple sign in croup.

TABLE 2-5 **Clinical Croup Score***			
	0	1	2
Cyanosis	None	In room air	In 40% oxygen
Inspiratory breath sounds	Normal	Harsh with rhonchi	Delayed
Stridor	None	Inspiratory	Inspiratory and expiratory or stridor at rest
Cough	None	Hoarse cry	Bark
Retractions and flaring	None	Flaring and suprasternal retractions	Flaring and suprasternal retractions plus subcostal and intercostal retractions

*A score of greater than or equal to 4 indicates moderately severe airway obstruction. A score of greater than or equal to 7, particularly when associated with Pa_{CO_2} of greater than 45 mm Hg and Pa_{O_2} of less than 70 mm Hg (in room air), indicates impending respiratory failure.

Adapted from Downes JJ, Raphaely RC. Pediatric intensive care. *Anesthesiology.* 1975;43:238-250.

and bronchial smooth muscle relaxation.[19] Two formulations of epinephrine (adrenaline) can be used for nebulization. The L-epinephrine (L-adrenaline) dose is 0.5 mL/kg of a 1 mg/mL concentration to a maximum of 5 mL. Racemic epinephrine (adrenaline), which contains both stereoisomers of epinephrine (adrenaline), is dosed as 0.05 mL/kg to a maximum of 0.5 mL of a 2.25% solution with a saline diluent. Comparison of these two forms has not demonstrated a significant difference in efficacy.[20]

Steroids should be administered early in the management of moderate to severe croup. Nebulized budesonide and dexamethasone, given intramuscularly or orally, are the two corticosteroids that have been studied for the treatment of croup. Comparison studies have revealed no significant difference in efficacy.[21–23] Dexamethasone is a long-acting corticosteroid with a half-life of 36 to 72 hours. Effective dexamethasone dosages of 0.15 to 0.6 mg/kg per dose either orally or intramuscularly have shown similar benefits. The 0.6-mg/kg dose is more widely used in clinical practice (not to exceed 10 mg).[16,23,24] Benefits of dexamethasone in the hospital setting include faster improvements in symptoms and croup scores, decreased incidence of endotracheal intubation in children admitted for croup, and shorter hospital stays.[19] Safety and efficacy of dexamethasone for mild to moderate croup in the outpatient setting have been demonstrated by fewer return visits and lower hospitalization rates.[21,23,25,26] Budesonide at a dose of 2 mg nebulized in saline solution has shown similar efficacy compared with dexamethasone.[21,22] In a recent study of American freestanding children's hospitals, corticosteroids were prescribed for 82% of children with croup seen in the ED.[27]

Several trials of heliox have demonstrated no advantage over conventional modalities; however, other trials have shown it to be equally effective in moderate-to-severe croup when compared with racemic epinephrine (adrenaline). It has also been shown to improve symptoms in very severe croup that failed to improve with racemic epinephrine (adrenaline). Currently, there is a lack of evidence to establish the effect of heliox inhalation in the treatment of croup in children.[28,29]

General indications for endotracheal intubation in respiratory failure should be used in the treatment of a child with severe croup. Endotracheal intubation or tracheostomy can be necessary in less than 2% of patients. Tracheal tube size should be half to a full size smaller than predicted by size and age to allow for subglottic edema and to reduce the risk of subglottic stenosis.[30]

In the past, treatment with nebulized racemic epinephrine (adrenaline) was a criterion for admission to the hospital. This was due to the "rebound" effect with return of symptoms up to 2 hours after treatment with racemic epinephrine (adrenaline). This dogma was mostly driven by limited data from earlier studies with small sample sizes. Recent literature has refuted this practice and concluded that use of racemic epinephrine (adrenaline) in the ED for outpatient treatment of croup is safe and effective. These studies recommended an observation period of 3 to 4 hours in the ED before discharge, with documentation of periodic croup scores and reevaluation for return of symptoms. During observation, patients who experienced relapse of symptoms were hospitalized but did not have posttreatment croup scores that were worse than on presentation to the ED. No significant complications were seen in patients discharged home. All of the patients included in the studies

KEY POINTS

Management of Croup

- Begin cool mist as long as it does not increase agitation.

- Begin treatment with steroids: dexamethasone, 0.15 to 0.6 mg/kg orally or intramuscularly, or budesonide, 2 mg per 2 mL of saline nebulized.

- Begin epinephrine (adrenaline) for signs of moderate to severe respiratory distress: racemic epinephrine (adrenaline), 0.05 mL/kg, to a maximum of 0.5 mL of 2.25% in 2 mL of saline nebulized, or l-epinephrine (l-adrenaline; 1 mg/mL solution), 0.5 mL/kg nebulized.

- Assist ventilation for signs of respiratory failure.

of outpatient treatment with racemic epinephrine (adrenaline) also received intramuscular dexamethasone.[16, 24]

Guidelines for disposition have been specifically addressed in only one prospective study. Criteria for discharge home of patients were a croup score less than 4, pulse oximetry greater than 90%, and adequate hydration. Hospital admission rates vary widely from 4% to 46%. The average length of hospitalization is 1 to 2 days.[14,16,21,24]

Foreign-Body Aspiration

Foreign-body aspiration is one of the leading causes of unintentional death in infants and young children. In 2000, 160 American children 14 years or younger died secondary to inhaled or ingested FBs. In these fatal cases, 41% were caused by food items and 59% by nonfood objects (Centers for Disease Control and Prevention, unpublished data). In 2001, an estimated 17,537 children 14 years or younger were treated in American EDs for choking episodes, and 10% of those were admitted or transferred to another facility. Sixty percent of nonfatal choking episodes treated in EDs were associated with food items; 31% were associated with nonfood objects, including coins; and in 9% of the episodes, the substance was unknown or unrecorded. Most cases are seen in the 1- to 2-year-old age group, accounting for up to two-thirds of all cases. Foreign-body aspiration can also be seen in older children with developmental delay.[31–35]

Food items are the most commonly aspirated airway FB in children (**Figure 2.12**). Nuts, especially peanuts, are one of the most common foods aspirated into the respiratory tree. Candy was associated with 19% of all choking-related ED visits by children; 65% were related to hard candy; and 12.5% were related to other specified types of candy (chocolate candy, gummy bears, gum, etc). Balloons are a common and often lethal nonfood object associated with choking. This includes blown-up latex gloves in offices and EDs.[32,33,36,37]

Children are more prone to aspirate FBs due to lack of teeth for chewing and developmental issues, such as talking and running while chewing and their exploratory curious nature. Under the Federal Hazardous Substances Act, a toy or object intended for young children must pass a test using a Small Parts Test Fixture (SPTF). The SPTF is a cylinder with a diameter of 3.17 cm and length of 5.71 cm. Any object that can fit inside the SPTF does not pass.[36] An empty toilet paper roll cut in half by length is a convenient household item with roughly the same dimensions.

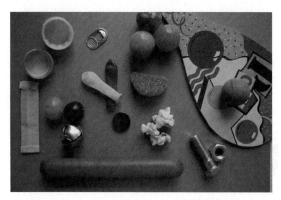

Figure 2.12 Examples of foreign bodies aspirated by children.

Clinical Features

The history and physical examination findings of patients with FB aspiration can be variable. The following are signs and symptoms seen in children with documented FB aspiration listed in order of decreasing frequency: history of choking/aspiration (22%–88%), wheezing (40%–82%), stridor (8%–71%), cough (42%–54%), decreased breath sounds on auscultation (51%), hoarseness (29%), respiratory distress (18%), cyanosis (3%–29%), fever (17%), and respiratory arrest (3%). A history of choking is the most reliable predictor of FB aspiration and should prompt further evaluation and consideration for bronchoscopy.[35,38–42]

Sites of obstruction by FB are as follows: larynx (7%), trachea (14%), right mainstem bronchus (30%), left mainstem bronchus (23%), right bronchus (21%), and left bronchus (5%). Laryngotracheal FBs are the minority but can be immediately life threatening and cause complete airway obstruction.[31,38,39,41]

Delays in diagnosis and treatment can lead to pneumonia, obstructive emphysema, and bronchiectasis. Delays in diagnosis as long as 4 months have been reported. Mortality is uniformly a result of asphyxiation. In rare cases in which an FB lodges in the distal airways and bronchoscopy is unsuccessful, thoracotomy with incisional removal of the FB might be necessary.[34,35,39,41]

Diagnostic Studies

Radiographic studies, including standard chest radiograph, lateral decubitus radiograph, expiratory chest radiograph, lateral neck radiograph, and fluoroscopy, do not have good sensitivity or specificity. Radiopaque FBs are seen in 6% to 15% of films. Other findings suggestive of lower airway FB include air trapping/hyperinflation (38%–63%), atelectasis (8%–25%), pulmonary consolidation (1%–5%), and barotrauma (7%) (**Figure 2.13**).[37-39] Fluoroscopy is diagnostic of FBs when differential ventilation of the lungs causes mediastinal shifting during respiration. Normal plain films are seen in up to one in four cases of FB aspiration and should not lower the clinical suspicion of airway FBs.

Differential Diagnosis

The differential diagnosis for airway FBs includes upper respiratory tract disorders, as listed previously, and lower airway disorders, including reactive airway disease and bronchiolitis.

Management

In the setting of airway FBs, most cases will present with partial airway obstruction. The goal of

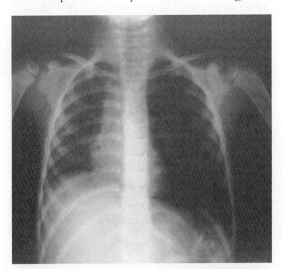

Figure 2.13 Findings associated with foreign-body aspiration. This chest X-ray demonstrates hyperinflation of the left lung.

management in the ED is to support oxygenation and ventilation and to prevent and treat total airway obstruction. Rapid cardiopulmonary assessment is key in patients with suspected airway FBs. A multidisciplinary approach is vital, and airway specialists must be mobilized early.

The therapeutic modality of choice for lower airway FBs is bronchoscopy, preferably performed in the operating room.[34,39] The FB retrieval rate approaches 100%[43] with bronchoscopy, the "gold standard" for diagnosis and treatment. In the absence of respiratory failure or imminent respiratory failure, the child should be left in a position of comfort, with supplemental oxygen as needed. All efforts should be made to limit agitation (ie, intravenous access and unnecessary radiographs should be deferred) until the airway is secured using inhalational anesthesia in the operating room.

In the rare case of complete airway obstruction and respiratory failure, basic life support (BLS) measures should be started immediately. Airway positioning and bag-mask ventilation are the initial intervention. If bag-mask ventilation is adequate for ventilation, then the patient should be rapidly transported to the operating room for definitive therapy. If unable to ventilate with bag-mask ventilation, then five back blows followed by five chest thrusts are done in infants younger than 1 year or repeated abdominal thrusts in children to attempt dislodgement of the impacted FB.[44] Direct laryngoscopy is the next step to attempt visualization of the FB and removal with Magill forceps. If BLS measures fail, options are limited in attempting to provide ventilatory assistance to the patient. Orotracheal intubation can be attempted in an effort to dislodge the FB to a distal bronchus and ventilate one lung or to intubate around the FB. Immediate surgical airway is another option via cricothyrotomy in the older child, tracheotomy, or needle cricothyrotomy with transtracheal jet ventilation in younger children and infants. The mortality rate among patients with FB aspiration and a failed airway attempt is extremely high.

Heliox has been described in a case report as an effective temporizing measure in a child with severe respiratory distress awaiting bronchoscopy. The helium-oxygen mixture is less dense than oxygen or room air and improves ventilation in cases of airway obstruction.[45]

Retropharyngeal Abscess

Retropharyngeal abscess (RPA) is the most common deep space neck infection seen in children. The retropharyngeal space is a potential space that contains lymph nodes, which drain the nasopharynx, adenoids, posterior nasal sinuses, and middle ear. Anatomically, the boundaries of the retropharyngeal space consist of the skull base superiorly, the mediastinum inferiorly, the visceral fascia anteriorly, the carotid sheaths laterally, and the prevertebral fascia posteriorly.[46]

RPA is most commonly caused by suppuration of the lymph nodes after infection of the pharyngeal structures, middle ear, and sinuses. Lymphatic drainage of these areas causes the lymph nodes in the retropharyngeal space to become infected with progression to cellulitis and abscess formation. Uncommon causes of RPA include trauma to the oropharynx caused by penetrating FBs, endoscopic procedures, and endotracheal intubation.[47]

KEY POINTS

Management of FB Aspiration

- Patient alert and able to maintain airway: provide supplemental oxygen and leave patient in a position of comfort.
- Patient with complete airway obstruction:
  - Infant (<1 year old)—perform five back blows followed by five chest thrusts.
  - Child (≥1 year old)—perform abdominal thrusts.
- If BLS maneuvers fail, begin bag-mask ventilation.
- If no chest rise with bag-mask ventilation, perform laryngoscopy and remove FB with pediatric Magill forceps.
- If airway obstruction persists, consider intubation, cricothyrotomy, tracheostomy, or heliox.

Epidemiology

Children younger than 6 years constitute more than 96% of RPA cases, with a peak incidence in 3- to 5-year-old children.[30,48] The incidence of RPA has increased during the past 10 years possibly due to methicillin-resistant *Staphylococcus aureus* (MRSA) or better imaging studies.[49] The incidence of RPA sharply decreases after 6 years of age because the lymph nodes in the retropharyngeal space become obliterated and involute during this age. Older children and adults with RPA have a higher incidence of trauma, intravenous drug abuse, and iatrogenic causes.[50]

Clinical Features

Fever, neck pain, and sore throat are the most common symptoms and are present in most cases of RPA. Hoarse voice, poor oral intake, drooling, cervical adenopathy, and stiff neck are also common symptoms. Frank obstructive symptoms, such as stridor and sleep apnea, are less common.[51] Physical findings can include a visible asymmetric pharyngeal bulge in up to half of the cases of RPA.

Complications in cases of RPA are uncommon in the antibiotic era. Airway obstruction requiring endotracheal intubation or tracheotomy is rare in the pediatric population in contrast to the adult population.[52] In rare cases, RPA can rupture anteriorly into the airway, causing aspiration of pus. Septic jugular vein thrombosis presents with fever, rigors, tenderness, and swelling along the sternocleidomastoid muscle. Septic emboli can travel to distant organs, causing meningitis, lateral sinus thrombosis, pulmonary infarcts, and endocarditis. Diagnosis is confirmed by computed tomography (CT) or magnetic resonance imaging (MRI) of the neck. Carotid artery rupture can result in exsanguination, ipsilateral Horner syndrome, and palsies of cranial nerves 9 through 12. Mediastinitis presents with chest pain, dyspnea, sepsis, and shock and is usually confirmed by CT and MRI. Chest radiography might reveal widening of the mediastinum.[36] Untreated, mediastinitis has a mortality rate that approaches 100%. The overall complication risk and mortality rates associated with RPA are very low.[48] This likely represents early diagnosis, judicious use of antibiotics, and better diagnostic tools, such as CT, in evaluating RPA.

Diagnostic Studies

Cultures of the purulent material from the abscess should be obtained to guide antimicrobial therapy. Group A β-hemolytic *Streptococcus* and *S aureus* are the most commonly cultured bacteria in pediatric neck infections.[47] The incidence of infection with MRSA is increasing.[53] Most deep neck abscesses are also polymicrobial, including anaerobic oral flora, most commonly the *Bacteroides* genus.

Plain radiographs of the neck with special attention to the prevertebral soft tissues are useful in evaluation of RPA (**Figure 2.14**). Normal prevertebral soft tissue dimensions on plain lateral radiographs of the neck are less than 7 mm at C2 and less than 22 mm at the level of C6.[46,54] Sensitivity of a plain radiograph for RPA indicated by thickening of the soft tissue is up to 88% to 100%.[30] The radiograph must be taken during inspiration and with the neck in extension to avoid false-positive results.

Computed tomography with contrast is the test of choice for evaluating deep neck abscesses and is approximately 90% accurate in diagnosing RPA. Computed tomography also identifies the stage of disease from cellulitis to phlegmon to organized abscess, differentiates from retropharyngeal adenitis, and identifies pa-

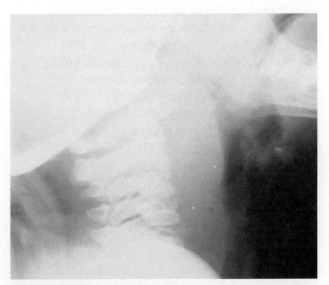

Figure 2.14 Radiograph showing increase in prevertebral soft tissue shadow associated with retropharyngeal infection.

tients with retropharyngeal infections who have a high likelihood of being successfully treated with antibiotics alone, thereby avoiding unnecessary surgical exploration.[48,55] Complications of RPA, such as jugular vein thrombosis, mediastinitis, and carotid artery rupture, can also be diagnosed by CT.[47]

Differential Diagnosis

Other infections of the deep neck spaces to consider in the differential diagnosis of RPA include abscess formation in the lateral pharyngeal space, submandibular and submental space, peritonsillar space, pretracheal space, and epidural space. Ludwig angina and vertebral osteomyelitis should also be included in the differential diagnosis.[36,40] Other less common causes of swelling and upper airway obstruction include superficial neck infections, such as cervical adenitis/abscess, benign and malignant neoplasms, and congenital lesions, such as cystic hygroma, thyroglossal duct cyst, and branchial cleft cysts.[37]

Management

All patients with RPA should receive parenteral broad-spectrum antimicrobial coverage, including MRSA coverage and anaerobic coverage. Antibiotic therapy should be started promptly in the ED when a diagnosis of deep neck infection is suspected. Fifteen percent to 50% of the cases of RPA are successfully treated with intravenous antibiotics alone.[54,56] Many reported cases could actually be retropharyngeal cellulitis and not true RPA.

Definitive management is the adequate drainage of pus from the retropharyngeal space. There is some controversy in the literature about the indications, timing, and type of procedure for drainage of RPA. Needle drainage has been highly successful in some trials in conjunction with antibiotic therapy. The advantage of needle aspiration is the avoidance of an open procedure and general anesthesia. Surgical incision and drainage are recommended as the definitive therapy for all cases of RPA by many head and neck surgeons.[56]

The endotracheal intubation rate in RPA is low preoperatively. If airway obstruction is severe and the child is in danger of imminent respiratory failure, then endotracheal intubation should be performed emergently. As in most cases of upper airway obstruction, this is ideally performed in the operating room. The general indicators for respiratory failure and intubation are the same for RPA as for other causes. The tracheotomy rate is 0% to 8% in children with RPA.[48,56]

Epiglottitis

The incidence of epiglottitis has decreased significantly in the past decade. Before the introduction of the *H influenzae* type b (Hib) vaccine in 1989, the peak incidence of epiglottitis occurred in young children between 1 and 5 years old. Incidence was approximately 10 per 100,000 before 1990. Since 1991, the incidence of Hib-associated epiglottitis in the pediatric population has approached zero. Hence, in the past decade, epiglottitis has become a disease seen predominantly in adults or in unimmunized or immigrant children.[30,57–59]

Clinical Features

Children with epiglottitis typically present with drooling, fever, respiratory distress, muffled voice, and toxic appearance in most cases. Out-of-hospital respiratory arrest is almost always fatal and accounts for most of the mortality in this disease. The rate of mortality from epiglottitis in children is approximately 2% secondary to airway obstruction.[57,58]

Airway obstruction is the most common and severe complication of epiglottitis. Deep neck infections and abscess of the epiglottis itself have been reported.

Diagnostic Studies

Blood cultures should be performed routinely in suspected cases of epiglottitis after the patient's airway has been evaluated. In the postvaccine era, other gram-positive cocci have been found in blood cultures, including group A β-hemolytic *Streptococcus*, *S aureus*, and *S pneumoniae*.[59]

Most patients who can tolerate a radiographic examination will exhibit a swollen epiglottis on lateral radiograph of the neck, classically known

as the "thumbprint" sign (**Figure 2.15**). The results of plain radiographs of the neck are normal in up to 20% of cases.[30] Leukocytosis is present in most cases of epiglottitis, but its presence is not useful in clinical decision making.

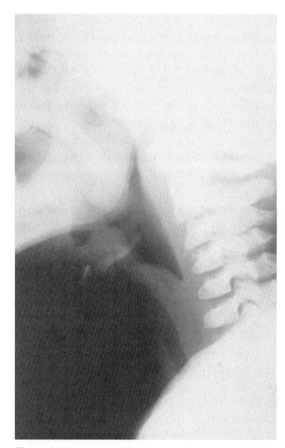

Figure 2.15 Findings with epiglottitis.

Differential Diagnosis

The differential diagnosis for epiglottitis includes pharyngitis, croup, bacterial tracheitis, and other upper airway disorders.

Management

When the diagnosis of epiglottitis is suspected, efforts should primarily be directed at securing the airway. Patients in severe respiratory distress, with complete or near-complete airway obstruction, should undergo endotracheal intubation immediately in the ED. Two-person bag-mask ventilation can be palliative. It might be theoretically advantageous to perform this with the patient in the prone position.

Preparations should be made in advance for surgical airway if orotracheal intubation fails. Patients with signs of airway obstruction but not in severe distress should be prepared for intubation in the operating room. The child should be left in a position of comfort with minimal agitation and transferred to the operating room for laryngoscopy and endotracheal intubation. Patients without respiratory compromise or drooling and minimal inflammation of the epiglottis on laryngoscopy can be medically managed without endotracheal intubation in the pediatric intensive care unit. Laryngoscopy, direct or indirect, does not precipitate complete airway obstruction.[58] Tracheal tubes should be one to two sizes smaller than usually appropriate for the child's age and size.

Intravenous antibiotics should be administered as soon as possible and will be influenced by immunization and immune status. Second- or third-generation cephalosporins are effective against *H influenzae* and also against the less common bacteria seen in epiglottitis. Other effective antibiotics include β-lactamase-resistant penicillins.[59]

Anaphylaxis

Anaphylaxis is a potentially life-threatening condition that can occur through three basic mechanisms. Type 1 hypersensitivity, the most common cause, occurs when an antigen binds circulating IgE from previous antigen exposure. Nonimmunologic direct action on mast cell degranulation is seen typically with contrast media, opiates, and physical stresses, such as cold, vibration, or heat. Complement activation seen in hereditary angioedema (C1 esterase deficiency) can also cause anaphylaxis.

All of these mechanisms have a common final pathway, which is activation and degranulation of mast cells and basophils, causing release of chemical mediators, such as histamine and other vasoactive and chemotactic factors.[50]

Epidemiology

An estimated 29,000 anaphylactic reactions occur in the United States each year, with approximately 150 fatalities.[60] A recent study showed an incidence rate of 49.8 per 100,000 person-years (all ages).[61] Foods cause most anaphylactic reactions in children, with peanuts and other nuts being the most common antigens. Other common food triggers include shellfish, eggs, and milk. Another common cause of anaphylaxis in children is insect stings, especially from the Hymenoptera order (bees, wasps, and fire ants). The most common medications implicated are antibiotics, such as penicillins and cephalosporins. Exercise-induced anaphylaxis is a less common form seen during exercise, frequently after ingestion of certain foods. Risk factors for anaphylaxis are atopic and include asthma, allergic rhinitis, atopic dermatitis, and prior allergy to a substance.[62,63]

Clinical Features

Angioedema is most common in the face and lips. Hypopharyngeal or laryngeal edema is also common and leads to upper airway obstruction with symptoms of throat swelling, dyspnea, stridor, hoarseness, and dysphagia.[64] Lower airway involvement leads to bronchospasm, wheezing, dyspnea, and chest tightness. Cardiovascular effects include hypotension (often severe and refractory), arrhythmias, and cardiogenic and distributive shock. Cutaneous symptoms include generalized flushing from vasodilation, urticaria, and angioedema. Gastrointestinal tract involvement causes nausea, vomiting, diarrhea, and abdominal cramps secondary to intestinal smooth muscle contraction and bowel edema.[62]

> ## KEY POINTS
>
> ### The Management of Epiglottitis
>
> - Patient alert and able to maintain airway: leave in position of comfort and transport to the operating room for airway management.
> - Patient not alert and with signs of respiratory failure: begin bag-mask ventilation (prone position of patient might be advantageous); attempt endotracheal intubation; consider LMA, cricothyrotomy, or tracheostomy.

In July 2005, the National Institute of Allergy and Infectious Disease and Food Allergy and Anaphylaxis Network convened an international consensus meeting to develop universal agreement on the definition of anaphylaxis, the criteria for diagnosis, and treatment.[65]

Diagnostic Studies

The diagnosis of anaphylaxis is made clinically. Routine laboratory studies or radiographic studies are not necessary in the diagnosis or management of anaphylaxis.

Management

Epinephrine (adrenaline) is the treatment of choice in anaphylaxis. The action of epinephrine (adrenaline) is at the α- and β-adrenergic receptors, causing vasoconstriction, increasing cardiac inotropy and chronotropy, and bronchodilation. A dosage of 0.01 mL/kg (0.01 mg/kg) of 1 mg/mL solution to a maximum dose of 0.3 mL (0.5 mg), administered intramuscularly every 5 to 15 minutes as necessary, is the recommended dosage for controlling symptoms and maintaining blood pressure. When the intravenous route is not indicated, the intramuscular route is preferable to the subcutaneous route due to more rapid and reliable absorption. The anterolateral thigh is the preferred site in both children and adults. There is evidence for better absorption at this site compared with a deltoid intramuscular injection or subcutaneous injection.[61,65]

Histamine-1 (H_1)-antagonist antihistamines, such as diphenhydramine, should be given intravenously to all patients with anaphylaxis. These medications are effective in treating the cutaneous symptoms of urticaria and itching. H_2-antagonist antihistamines are also recommended. Bronchospasm is treated with nebulized β_2-agonists, such as albuterol (salbutamol). Parenteral corticosteroids are given routinely to patients with anaphylaxis.[50] Vasopressors should be administered in cases of hypotension refractory to intravenous fluid resuscitation. Dopamine and/or norepinephrine (noradrenaline) is titrated to maintain adequate blood pressure.

Endotracheal intubation is seldom required in the management of anaphylaxis.[64] However, it is important to remember that respiratory arrest

secondary to airway obstruction is the leading cause of death in fatal cases of anaphylaxis.[63,66] In addition to the general indications for endotracheal intubation in respiratory failure, patients in respiratory distress with signs of severe upper airway obstruction, lingual edema, hypopharyngeal edema, or laryngeal edema should be intubated

Management of Anaphylaxis

- Administer epinephrine (adrenaline), 0.01 mL/kg of 1 mg/mL solution, to a maximum of 0.3 mg intramuscularly, repeat every 15 minutes as needed.
- Administer nebulized albuterol (salbutamol).
- Administer H_1- and H_2-antihistamines intravenously.
- Administer methylprednisolone intravenously.
- Consider epinephrine (adrenaline), 0.01 mg/mL or 0.1 mg/mL solution intravenously, only if patient is in cardiopulmonary failure.

early to avoid the dreaded scenario of complete airway obstruction with the inability to intubate or ventilate.

Disposition

No studies have specifically addressed disposition of patients with anaphylaxis from the ED. A reasonable length of time to consider observing the postanaphylactic patient is 4 to 6 hours in most patients, with prolonged observation times or hospital admission for patients with severe or refractory symptoms. More caution should be used in patients with reactive airway disease because most fatalities associated with anaphylaxis occur in these patients.[61] Patients with mild symptoms that resolve after medical therapy can be safely discharged home. Patients who present with moderate to severe anaphylaxis should be admitted to the hospital for observation after treatment in the ED. Biphasic reactions account for up to 50% of fatal cases.[63] In a large pediatric population, biphasic reactions were reported in 6% of patients admitted to the hospital, of which half were serious and required repeat administration of epinephrine (adrenaline) and 1% required intubation. The asymptomatic interval varied widely, from 1 to 28 hours.[67]

Preventive measures are vital in the treatment of anaphylaxis. After an anaphylactic reaction, all patients should undergo skin testing to identify potential allergens. Medical bracelets are recommended for anaphylaxis patients to identify their serious allergies. Epinephrine (adrenaline) self-injection kits should be prescribed to all patients with a history of anaphylaxis. Several studies have demonstrated the deficiencies in proper use of epinephrine (adrenaline) injection kits.[68,69] A review of anaphylaxis deaths reported patients holding an unused kit in hand, use of an expired kit, and one case of a patient who died waiting for the prescription to be filled at a pharmacy.[66]

Radiographic Findings in Conditions Causing Airway Obstruction

Condition	Radiographic Finding
- Croup: posteroanterior and lateral views of the neck	Subglottic edema/ tracheal narrowing, steeple sign
- Foreign-body aspiration: posteroanterior and lateral views of the chest	Lower (air trapping/ hyperinflation, atelectasis, barotrauma) Upper (foreign body visualized, hyperinflation of pharynx)
- Retropharyngeal abscess: lateral view of the neck	Prevertebral thickening of the soft tissues, air fluid level in the prevertebral space; computed tomography scan of the neck is diagnostic
- Epiglottitis: lateral view of the neck	Thumbprint sign (swollen epiglottis and aryepiglottic folds)

A 6-month-old boy presents with acute respiratory distress preceded by a short history of upper respiratory tract symptoms and low-grade fever. He is irritable and feeding poorly. He is alert, but tachypneic, has nasal flaring and intercostal retractions, and is pale. His vital signs include a respiratory rate of 70/min, heart rate of 170/min, temperature (rectal) of 38°C (100.4°F), and oxygen saturation of 90% on room air. Diffuse bilateral wheezing is discovered on physical examination.

1. *What are your initial treatment priorities?*
2. *What diagnostic tests will be helpful?*

Lower Airway Obstruction

Bronchiolitis

Respiratory syncytial virus (RSV) is the most common virus causing lower respiratory tract infection, primarily bronchiolitis, in infants.[70] The terms RSV and bronchiolitis are often used interchangeably. Most children have been infected by RSV before their second birthday.[71] Infants with prematurity and chronic pulmonary and congenital heart disease are at highest risk for severe disease (Table 2-6). Viral shedding generally lasts approximately 1 week; however, in infants with lower respiratory tract disease, it can last up to 4 weeks. Average incubation is 5 days. Apnea can be the presenting manifestation of the infection; however, most infants with RSV present with an upper respiratory infection prodrome, followed by cough and wheezing. Hypoxia is most often due to ventilation/perfusion ($\dot{V}/\dot{Q}$) mismatch, although hypoventilation is seen as fatigue develops. Progression to respiratory failure and shunting can be seen with pneumonia and atelectasis.[70–74]

Immunoprophylaxis is recommended for certain high-risk infants (Table 2-7).

TABLE 2-6 Risk Factors for Severe Respiratory Syncytial Virus Disease[70,71,75]

• Prematurity	• Immunosuppression
• Complex congenital heart disease	• Neuromuscular disease
• Chronic lung disease	• Metabolic disorder

Krilov L. Recent development in the treatment and prevention of RSV infection. Expert Opinion on Therapeutic Patents. 2002; 12:441–449.

Staat MA. Respiratory syncytial virus infections in children. Seminars in Respiratory Infection. 2002; 17:15–20.

TABLE 2-7 Considerations for Immunoprophylaxis of High-Risk Infants and Young Children

- Infants and children younger than 2 years with chronic lung disease (CLD) who have required medical therapy for CLD within 6 months of anticipated respiratory syncytial virus (RSV) season. Some infants with severe disease benefit from prophylaxis for the first 2 years.
- Infants born at ≤28 weeks' gestation and who are younger than 12 months at the start of RSV season.
- Infants born at 29 to 32 weeks' gestation and who are younger than 6 months at the start of RSV season.
- Infants born at 32 to 35 weeks' gestation and who are younger than 3 months at the start of RSV season who attend day care or have a sibling under 5 years of age.
- Infants with congenital abnormalities of the airway or neuromuscular disease born before 35 weeks of gestation
- Infants and children who are 24 months or younger with hemodynamically significant cyanotic or acyanotic congenital heart disease.

Adapted from American Academy of Pediatrics. Respiratory syncytial virus. In: *2009 Red Book: Report of the Committee on Infectious Diseases.* Pickering LK, 28th ed. Elk Grove Village, IL: American Academy of Pediatrics; 2009:560.

Palivizumab, a humanized mouse monoclonal antibody, is licensed for prevention of RSV lower respiratory tract disease in high-risk infants and children, such as those with chronic lung disease (CLD) of prematurity. There is controversy in the literature regarding the cost-effectiveness of prophylaxis therapy and guidelines are complex. No vaccine is currently available.[72,73,75]

Respiratory syncytial virus is a single-stranded RNA virus of the Paramyxoviridae family. Infection is spread by droplets and contact with contaminated surfaces. The eyes and nose are primary sites for inoculation.[71] Respiratory syncytial virus infections tend to occur in fall, winter, and spring in temperate climates. The most severe disease is seen in young infants, especially those younger than 6 weeks. Native Alaskan and American Indian infants have a disproportionately high hospitalization rate for RSV. Approximately 400 deaths related to RSV occur annually. Most deaths that result from bronchiolitis occur in infants during the first 6 months of life; infants with prematurity and underlying cardiopulmonary disease or immunodeficiency are at higher risk.[73]

Clinical Features

The clinical presentation of bronchiolitis varies by age. First infections are more likely to be symptomatic. Premature infants and infants with CLD, immunosuppression, or congenital heart disease are at increased risk for morbidity and mortality. Cough, nasal congestion, otitis media, and fever are commonly seen in these infants. Nonspecific findings can also be seen in this age group and include poor feeding and irritability. Apnea can be seen in infants, especially those born prematurely or who are younger than 6 weeks. Up to 70% of patients will have wheezing or rales with pneumonia. Hypoxia is common to all infants hospitalized with RSV bronchiolitis. Increased work of breathing can manifest as tachypnea, tachycardia, grunting, flaring, supraclavicular and intercostal retractions, and head bobbing in infants. There can be clinical evidence of dehydration if the child has been feeding poorly during the illness.

The most predictive factor for severe disease in a previously healthy infant is oxygen saturation lower than 95%. Other factors associated with severe disease include age younger than 3 months, gestational age younger than 34 weeks, toxic appearance, atelectasis, and tachypnea with respiratory rate greater than 70/min.[71] Diagnosis of bronchiolitis is generally made clinically, taking into account the clinical history, age of the child, time of year, and presence of other cases in the area. Testing for RSV is more frequently performed in those infants who present to the ED during peak RSV season for cohort isolation reasons or for febrile infants.

Complications

Complications of bronchiolitis include apnea, pneumonia, atelectasis, dehydration, respiratory failure, bacterial superinfection, and air leaks. Apnea is a concern in infants with RSV, with the risk being higher in premature and young infants. In a recent study, 2.7% of hospitalized infants had apnea, but all were high-risk cases.[74]

Diagnostic Studies

The primary diagnostic studies for bronchiolitis include oxygen saturation measurements and chest radiograph. The chest radiograph classically shows hyperinflation (**Figure 2.16**).

YOUR FIRST CLUE

Signs and Symptoms of Bronchiolitis

- Cough
- Wheezing
- Nasal congestion
- Otitis media
- Fever
- Tachypnea
- Tachycardia
- Increased work of breathing (grunting, flaring, supraclavicular and intercostal retractions, and head bobbing in infants)
- Hypoxia
- Apnea
- Apparent life-threatening event

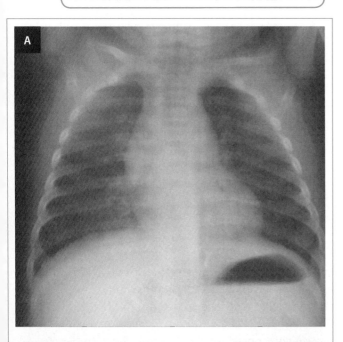

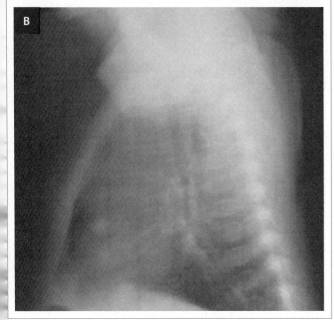

Figure 2.16 Findings of bronchiolitis.

Pneumonia and atelectasis can also be seen. Arterial blood gas (ABG) analysis is needed only in severe cases. Viral antigen detection is available for most of the viral agents that produce a clinical picture of bronchiolitis, but do not usually change treatment or disposition. Rapid antigen detection for RSV is widely available and is best performed on a nasopharyngeal aspirate. Positive detection of RSV is important in the disposition of chronically ill or immunosuppressed infants and febrile neonates.

Differential Diagnosis

The differential diagnosis for bronchiolitis includes pneumonia, reactive airway disease, congestive heart failure, FB aspiration, congenital airway lesion, and viral URI.

Management

General supportive care is the mainstay of management in bronchiolitis and includes antipyretics, suctioning, hydration (intravenously or orally), and ongoing clinical monitoring of vital signs and oxygen saturation. Supplemental oxygen and continuous pulse oximetry are used for infants with signs of respiratory distress and oxygen saturation levels lower than 95%. Mechanical ventilation is rarely necessary. Agitation can worsen hypoxemia and should be prevented.

The most controversial area of management is the use of bronchodilators such as albuterol (salbutamol) or epinephrine (adrenaline). It is often difficult to distinguish bronchiolitis from reactive airway disease with URI. Current literature and guidelines do not support the routine use of bronchodilators but do support a trial dose of an α- or β-adrenergic agonist to be continued only if clinical improvement is noted after treatment. Currently, nebulized epinephrine is not recommended for routine home use.[72,72,76–80]

Ribavirin has in vitro antiviral activity against RSV, and aerosolized ribavirin therapy has been associated with a small but statistically significant increase in oxygen saturation during the acute infection. The aerosol route of administration, concern about potential toxic effects among exposed health care professionals, and conflicting results of efficacy trials have led to decreasing use of this drug. Ribavirin is not recommended for routine use but may be considered for use in select patients with documented, potentially life-threatening RSV infection.[75]

Heliox can also be considered for infants with severe bronchiolitis; however, most studies have been conducted in the intensive care unit setting. There is currently insufficient evidence to consider heliox treatment in the ED setting.[73,81] The use of systemic or inhaled corticosteroids (ICS) has demonstrated no short- or long-term benefits in the acute phase of disease.[72,73,82] The only indications for antibiotics are in cases of a neonate with fever, pending cultures, or when the chest radiograph demonstrates findings consistent with pneumonia or superinfection.

Avoid exposing high-risk infants and children to infants and children with RSV. Nosocomial transmission can be high, and careful attention to standard infection control measures is critical to limit spread.

KEY POINTS

Management of Bronchiolitis

- Supportive care is the mainstay of bronchiolitis treatment.
  - Correction of hypoxia and adequate hydration are basic tools that help to support infants with bronchiolitis.
  - Return to normal respiratory rates in an infant who has been working hard to breathe does not always indicate improvement.
  - It is important to assess the numbers in the context of the child because decreasing respiratory rates might also mean that the child is fatiguing and has impending respiratory failure.
- A trial dose of nebulized albuterol (salbutamol) or epinephrine (adrenaline) can be tried, but studies show limited benefit for routine use.
- Corticosteroids are not recommended.

CASE SCENARIO 4

A 5-year-old boy had an acute asthma episode at school during show-and-tell after a classmate brought in a new kitten. He was given albuterol (salbutamol) by the school nurse but continued to have tachypnea and diffuse wheezing, and his mother was called to take him home. Wheezing continued despite two additional albuterol (salbutamol) nebulizer treatments given consecutively at home. The mother brings him to the ED. On arrival, he is alert, shows increased work of breathing with nasal flaring and retractions, and has normal skin color. Vital signs are respiratory rate of 50/min, a heart rate of 130/min, a blood pressure of 120/80 mm Hg, axillary temperature of 36.6°C (97.9°F), and pulse oximetry of 89% on room air. He is acutely short of breath with poor air entry and no wheezing on auscultation of the chest.

1. *What are your priorities?*
2. *What is the significance of absent wheezing in this scenario?*

Asthma

Asthma is a chronic inflammatory disease of the airways characterized by complete or partial reversible airway obstruction, increased mucous production, and airway edema. It is a common problem in childhood that affects approximately 9% of children in the United States and accounts for more than 750,000 ED visits (3% of all ED visits) and 13 million school absences per year. Asthma is the third major cause of hospitalization in children younger than 15 years. Children younger than 4 years have the highest hospitalization and ED visit frequencies. In 2004, 186 children ages 0 to 17 years died from asthma.[83]

Various aspects of the disease have been proposed to define asthma, including reversible airway obstruction, recurrent cough without clear evidence of airway narrowing, airway hyperresponsiveness, chronic airway inflammation, and altered T-cell function.

Genetics and the environment have influential roles in the development of the phenotypic presentation. Exposure to cigarette smoke, urban and low income environments, and preteen obesity in girls have been associated with increased rates of asthma. Approximately 10% to 25% of asthmatic children seen in the ED are admitted to a hospital. Admission rates are influenced by socioeconomic factors.[83,85] Rapid onset of symptoms (<3 hours) and history of prior intubation are risk factors for deterioration. Table 2-8 reviews important questions to ask about the history.

TABLE 2-8 Abbreviated Asthma History for Emergency Department (ED) Patients

Present Episode

- When did it start?
- Can you identify the trigger?
- What medications have you taken so far (include times)?
- How did you respond to those medications (PEF rate and clinical response)?

Asthma History

- Baseline asthma: What medications do you usually take?
- How often do you wheeze, cough, or have shortness of breath?
- How often do you need to come to the ED? When was your last visit?
- How often were you hospitalized? Did you need to go to the pediatric intensive care unit?
- Have you ever been intubated?
- How often and when were you last taking oral steroids?

Other

- Do you have any other medical problems?
- Do you take any other medications?
- Do you smoke? Are you exposed to tobacco smoke?
- Do you take any herbal remedies?

Clinical Features

The principal presentations of asthma include cough, wheeze, chest congestion, and difficulty breathing. Making the correct diagnosis is sometimes difficult, especially before 12 months of age, when 30% of children with lower respiratory tract illnesses can wheeze. Other respiratory conditions must be considered and excluded.

Decision making is guided by overall clinical impression and is influenced by judgment about the family's ability to care for the child in their environment. Infections are a frequent trigger in children and should be addressed. The most common cause of hypoxia in asthma exacerbations in V/Q mismatch. A complete physical examination should be performed, with special emphasis on determining the mental status and work of breathing of the patient. Documentation should include the position of comfort, respiratory rate, quality of air exchange, presence or absence of grunting, nasal flaring, retractions, wheezes, rhonchi, and crackles. Crackles can also be heard with pneumonia, atelectasis, and heart failure. Pulsus paradoxus correlates with forced expiratory volume and asthma severity in adults; however, in children, it is often difficult to assess and therefore is of limited value.[84] Complications of asthma include recurrent episodes of atelectasis due to mucous plugging, pneumothorax, pneumomediastinum, and respiratory failure.

Diagnostic Studies

Pulmonary function studies are a mainstay of asthma management because asthma is a disease primarily of small and midsized airways. The mean flow rates over the middle 50% of vital capacity is a sensitive indicator of airflow obstruction in children. Peak expiratory flow (PEF) rate is more reflective of larger airways. The forced expiratory volume in 1 second (FEV_1) is also an indicator of airflow obstruction. Peak flow meters are often used as a guide in the ED but are insufficient alone to define the disease and are of limited value in severe exacerbations. Furthermore, they are effort dependent; children younger than 5 years have a difficult time mastering the technique, and some older children require practice to perform accurately. Even under the best circumstances, the peak flow meter might not accurately reflect the degree of obstruction in all children.[85]

Pulse oximetry is an excellent monitoring adjunct to assist in determining baseline status and response to therapy. Keep in mind the various factors that will cause the oxyhemoglobin desaturation curve to shift. Accurate pulse oximetry values depend on adequate blood flow to the monitoring site. Indications for measurement of ABGs include oxygen saturation less than 90% on maximal oxygen therapy, no clinical improvement despite aggressive therapy, and mental status changes. Chest radiographs are not routinely recommended. Considerations for a chest radiograph include first episode of wheezing, fever, and crackles and patients with a poor response to standard therapy.

Differential Diagnosis

The differential diagnosis for asthma includes bronchiolitis, URI, pneumonia, congestive heart failure, congenital airway anomalies, and FB aspiration.

Management

A stepwise treatment approach is recommended. Classification, evaluation, exacerbation management pathways, and medication tables from the most recent 2007 National Institutes of Health guidelines[86] are presented in Tables 2-9 through 2-11 and Figure 2.17. Maintenance and home treatment asthma guidelines are also available and due to medical safety issues are divided into three age groups (0–4 years, 5–11 years, and ≥12 years).[86,87]

Supplemental oxygen and clinical monitoring are appropriate for all patients with respiratory distress. Oxygen saturation levels are useful in assessing exacerbation severity but cannot be used as a sole determinant of the need for hospital admission. Measurement of ABGs should be considered in patients who require maximal oxygen therapy.[88]

Short-acting β$_2$-agonists (SABAs) are considered the main rescue therapy for asthma. Corticosteroids are recommended for moderate to severe exacerbations and for patients who respond poorly or incompletely to β-agonist therapy. Because asthma is an inflammatory disease, early treatment with corticosteroids can help ameliorate an asthma episode. Out-of-hospital emergency medical services agencies should have standing orders to administer oxygen and SABAs to children with signs and symptoms of asthma.

Asthma severity in the ED is categorized as mild, moderate, or severe. Table 2-9 summarizes the signs and symptoms, pulmonary function levels, and clinical course for each category, and Table 2-10 reviews symptom severity for each level. Mild to moderate exacerbations are associated with PEF of 40% or higher. Inhaled SABAs may be given up to three times in the ED and oral steroids administered if no immediate response (after one dose of inhaled β-agonist) or if there is a recent medication history of oral steroids. Severe exacerbations are associated with a PEF of 40% or lower than predicted value. Treatment includes high-dose inhaled SABAs plus ipratropium every 20 minutes or continuously for 1 hour, systemic corticosteroids, and supplemental oxygen to keep oxygen saturations at 90% or greater. Management of ED asthma exacerbations are summarized in Figure 2.17.

YOUR FIRST CLUE

Signs and Symptoms of Asthma Exacerbation

- Cough
- Shortness of breath
- Increased work of breathing (nasal flaring, grunting, intercostal retractions)
- Wheezing
- Chest congestion
- Decreased breath sounds
- Rhonchi
- Crackles
- Decreased expiratory flow rate
- Hypoxia

When these measures are insufficient to control symptoms, adjunct forms of therapy can be considered. Examples for use in severe exacerbations include magnesium sulfate and heliox. Other adjunct therapies to avoid intubation include parenteral β_2-agonists and noninvasive ventilation; however, insufficient data are available to make recommendations regarding these possible adjunct therapies.[86,87]

Evaluation of hydration is important in asthmatic patients. The route of hydration is determined by patient status. Respiratory distress, hypoventilation, and apnea are contraindications for oral hydration. Many children who have had a recent viral illness and respiratory symptoms will not have had adequate oral intake. Adequate hydration helps keep secretions less viscous.[89]

Pharmacotherapy for acute asthma exacerbations is reviewed in Table 2-11.[86]

TABLE 2-9 Classifying Severity of Asthma Exacerbations in the Urgent or Emergency Care Setting			
Note: Patients are instructed to use quick-relief medications if symptoms occur or if PEF decreases below 80% predicted or personal best. If PEF is 50%–79%, the patient should monitor response to quick-relief medication carefully and consider contacting a physician. If PEF is below 50%, immediate medical care is usually required. In the urgent or emergency care setting, the following parameters describe the severity and likely clinical course of an exacerbation.			
	Signs and Symptoms	Initial PEF (or FEV1)	Clinical Course
Mild	Dyspnea only with activity (assess tachypnea in young children)	PEF ≥70% predicted or personal best	• Usually cared for at home • Prompt relief with inhaled SABAs • Possible short course of oral systemic corticosteroids
Moderate	Dyspnea interferes with or limits usual activity	PEF 40%–69% predicted or personal best	• Usually requires office or ED visit • Relief from frequent inhaled SABAs • Oral systemic corticosteroids; some symptoms last for 1–2 days after treatment is begun
Severe	Dyspnea at rest; interferes with conversation	PEF <40% predicted or personal best	• Usually requires ED visit and likely hospitalization • Partial relief from frequent inhaled SABAs • Oral systemic corticosteroids; some symptoms last for >3 days after treatment is begun • Adjunctive therapies are helpful
Severe: Life threatening	Too dyspneic to speak; perspiring	PEF <25% predicted or personal best	• Requires ED/hospitalization; possible ICU admission • Minimal or no relief from frequent inhaled SABAs • Intravenous corticosteroids • Adjunctive therapies are helpful
Abbreviations: ED, emergency department; FEV1, forced expiratory volume in 1 second; ICU, intensive care unit; PEF, peak expiratory flow; SABAs, short-acting β_2-agonists.			
Adapted from: 2007 National Institutes of Health Guidelines, Section 5, Managing Exacerbations of Asthma, Fig. 5-1. p. 375, August 28, 2007.			

TABLE 2-10 Formal Evaluation of Asthma Exacerbation Severity in the Urgent or Emergency Care Setting

	Mild	Moderate	Severe	Severe: Respiratory Arrest Imminent
Symptoms				
Breathlessness	While walking	While walking While at rest (infant— softer, shorter cry, difficulty feeding)	While at rest (infant— stops feeding)	
	Can lie down	Prefers sitting	Sits upright	
Talks in	Sentences	Phrases	Words	
Alertness	May be agitated	Usually agitated	Usually agitated	Drowsy or confused
Signs				
Respiratory rate	Increased	Increased	Often >30/minute	
		Guide to rates of breathing in awake children: Age — Normal rate <2 months — <60/minute 2–12 months — <50/minute 1–5 years — <40/minute 6–8 years — <30/minute		
Use of accessory muscles; suprasternal retractions	Usually not	Commonly	Usually	Paradoxical thoracoabdominal movement
Wheeze	Moderate, often only end expiratory	Loud; throughout exhalation	Usually loud; throughout inhalation and exhalation	Absence of wheeze
Pulse/minute	<100	100–120	>120	Bradycardia
		Guide to normal pulse rates in children: Age — Normal rate 2–12 months — <160/minute 1–2 years — <120/minute 2–8 years — <110/minute		
Pulsus paradoxus	Absent <10 mmHg	May be present 10–25 mmHg	Often present >25 mmHg (adult) 20–40 mmHg (child)	Absence suggests respiratory muscle fatigue

	Mild	Moderate	Severe	Subset: Respiratory Arrest Imminent
Functional Assessment				
PEF percent predicted or percent personal best	≥70 percent	Approx. 40–69 percent or response lasts <2 hours	<40 percent	<25 percent Note: PEF testing may not be needed in very severe attacks
Pao$_2$ (on air) (blood gas)	Normal (test not usually necessary)	≥60 mmHg (test not usually necessary)	<60 mmHg: possible cyanosis	
and/or PCO$_2$ (blood gas)	<42 mmHg (test not usually necessary)	<42 mmHg (test not usually necessary)	≥42 mmHg: possible respiratory failure	
	Hypercapnia (hypoventilation) develops more readily in young children than in adults and adolescents.			
SaO$_2$ percent (on room air) at sea level (pulse oximetry)	>95 percent	90–95 percent	<90 percent	

Key: Pao$_2$, arterial oxygen pressure; PCO$_2$, partial pressure of carbon dioxide; PEF, peak expiratory flow; SaO$_2$, oxygen saturation

Notes:

• The presence of several parameters, but not necessarily all, indicates the general classification of the exacerbation.

• Many of these parameters have not been systematically studied, especially as they correlate with each other. Thus, they serve only as general guides (Cham et al. 2002; Chey et al. 1999; Gorelick et al. 2004b; Karras et al. 2000; Kelly et al. 2002b and 2004; Keogh et al. 2001; McCarren et al. 2000; Rodrigo and Rodrigo 1998b; Rodrigo et al. 2004; Smith et al. 2002).

• The emotional impact of asthma symptoms on the patient and family is variable but must be recognized and addressed and can affect approaches to treatment and followup (Ritz et al. 2000; Strunk and Mrazek 1986; von Leupoldt and Dahme 2005).

From 2007 *National Institutes of Health Guidelines*, Section 5, Managing Exacerbations of Asthma, Fig. 5-3. p. 380, August 28, 2007.

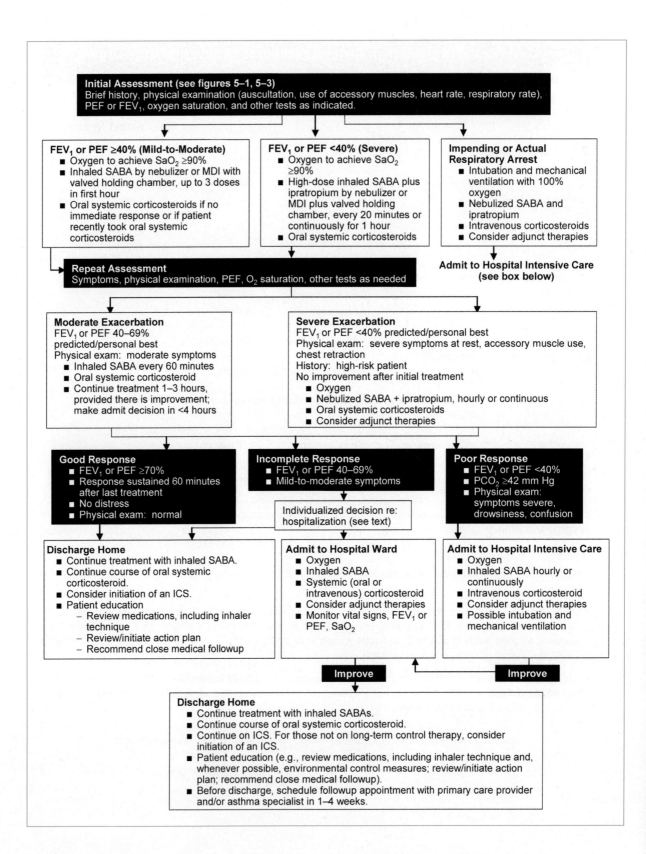

Initial Assessment (see figures 5–1, 5–3)
Brief history, physical examination (auscultation, use of accessory muscles, heart rate, respiratory rate), PEF or FEV$_1$, oxygen saturation, and other tests as indicated.

FEV$_1$ or PEF ≥40% (Mild-to-Moderate)
- Oxygen to achieve SaO$_2$ ≥90%
- Inhaled SABA by nebulizer or MDI with valved holding chamber, up to 3 doses in first hour
- Oral systemic corticosteroids if no immediate response or if patient recently took oral systemic corticosteroids

FEV$_1$ or PEF <40% (Severe)
- Oxygen to achieve SaO$_2$ ≥90%
- High-dose inhaled SABA plus ipratropium by nebulizer or MDI plus valved holding chamber, every 20 minutes or continuously for 1 hour
- Oral systemic corticosteroids

Impending or Actual Respiratory Arrest
- Intubation and mechanical ventilation with 100% oxygen
- Nebulized SABA and ipratropium
- Intravenous corticosteroids
- Consider adjunct therapies

Admit to Hospital Intensive Care (see box below)

Repeat Assessment
Symptoms, physical examination, PEF, O$_2$ saturation, other tests as needed

Moderate Exacerbation
FEV$_1$ or PEF 40–69% predicted/personal best
Physical exam: moderate symptoms
- Inhaled SABA every 60 minutes
- Oral systemic corticosteroid
- Continue treatment 1–3 hours, provided there is improvement; make admit decision in <4 hours

Severe Exacerbation
FEV$_1$ or PEF <40% predicted/personal best
Physical exam: severe symptoms at rest, accessory muscle use, chest retraction
History: high-risk patient
No improvement after initial treatment
- Oxygen
- Nebulized SABA + ipratropium, hourly or continuous
- Oral systemic corticosteroids
- Consider adjunct therapies

Good Response
- FEV$_1$ or PEF ≥70%
- Response sustained 60 minutes after last treatment
- No distress
- Physical exam: normal

Incomplete Response
- FEV$_1$ or PEF 40–69%
- Mild-to-moderate symptoms

Individualized decision re: hospitalization (see text)

Poor Response
- FEV$_1$ or PEF <40%
- PCO$_2$ ≥42 mm Hg
- Physical exam: symptoms severe, drowsiness, confusion

Discharge Home
- Continue treatment with inhaled SABA.
- Continue course of oral systemic corticosteroid.
- Consider initiation of an ICS.
- Patient education
  - Review medications, including inhaler technique
  - Review/initiate action plan
  - Recommend close medical followup

Admit to Hospital Ward
- Oxygen
- Inhaled SABA
- Systemic (oral or intravenous) corticosteroid
- Consider adjunct therapies
- Monitor vital signs, FEV$_1$ or PEF, SaO$_2$

Admit to Hospital Intensive Care
- Oxygen
- Inhaled SABA hourly or continuously
- Intravenous corticosteroid
- Consider adjunct therapies
- Possible intubation and mechanical ventilation

Improve

Improve

Discharge Home
- Continue treatment with inhaled SABAs.
- Continue course of oral systemic corticosteroid.
- Continue on ICS. For those not on long-term control therapy, consider initiation of an ICS.
- Patient education (e.g., review medications, including inhaler technique and, whenever possible, environmental control measures; review/initiate action plan; recommend close medical followup).
- Before discharge, schedule followup appointment with primary care provider and/or asthma specialist in 1–4 weeks.

Figure 2.17 Management of Asthma Exacerbations: Emergency Department and Hospital-Based Care

From 2007 *National Institutes of Health Guidelines*, Section 5, Managing Exacerbations of Asthma, Fig. 5-6. p. 388, August 28, 2007.

TABLE 2-11 Dosages of Drugs for Asthma Exacerbations

Medication	Child Dose	Adult Dose	Comments
Inhaled Short-Acting β₂-Agonists (SABA)			
Albuterol Nebulizer solution (0.63 mg/3 mL, 1.25 mg/3 mL, 2.5 mg/3 mL, 5.0 mg/mL)	0.15 mg/kg (minimum dose 2.5 mg) every 20 minutes for 3 doses then 0.15–0.3 mg/kg up to 10 mg every 1–4 hours as needed, or 0.5 mg/kg/hour by continuous nebulization.	2.5–5 mg every 20 minutes for 3 doses, then 2.5–10 mg every 1–4 hours as needed, or 10–15 mg/hour continuously.	Only selective beta₂-agonists are recommended. For optimal delivery, dilute aerosols to minimum of 3 mL at gas flow of 6–8 L/min. Use large volume nebulizers for continuous administration. May mix with ipratropium nebulizer solution.
MDI (90 mcg/puff)	4–8 puffs every 20 minutes for 3 doses, then every 1–4 hours inhalation maneuver as needed. Use spacing chamber; add mask in children <4 years.	4–8 puffs every 20 minutes up to 4 hours, then every 1–4 hours as needed.	In mild-to-moderate exacerbations, MDI plus spacing chamber is as effective as nebulized therapy with appropriate administration technique and coaching by trained personnel.
Bitolterol Nebulizer solution (2 mg/mL)	See albuterol dose; thought to be half as potent as albuterol on mg basis.	See albuterol dose.	Has not been studied in severe asthma exacerbations. Do not mix with other drugs.
MDI (370 mcg/puff)	See albuterol MDI dose.	See albuterol MDI dose.	Has not been studied in severe asthma exacerbations.
Levalbuterol (R-albuterol)			
Nebulizer solution (0.63 mg/3 mL, 1.25 mg/0.5 mL 1.25 mg/3 mL)	0.075 mg/kg (minimum dose 1.25 mg) every 20 minutes for 3 doses, then 0.075–0.15 mg/kg up to 5 mg every 1–4 hours as needed.	1.25–2.5 mg every 20 minutes for 3 doses, then 1.25–5 mg every 1–4 hours as needed.	See albuterol MDI dose. Levalbuterol administered in one-half the mg dose of albuterol provides comparable efficacy and safety. Has not been evaluated by continuous nebulization.
MDI (45 mcg/puff)	See albuterol MDI dose.	See albuterol MDI dose.	
Pirbuterol MDI (200 mcg/puff)	See albuterol MDI dose; thought to be half as potent as albuterol on a mg basis.	See albuterol MDI dose.	Has not been studied in severe asthma exacerbations.
Systemic (Injected) β₂-Agonists			
Epinephrine 1 mg/mL concentration	0.01 mg/kg up to 0.3–0.5 mg every 20 minutes for 3 doses subcutaneous.	0.3–0.5 mg every 20 minutes for 3 doses subcutaneous.	No proven advantage of systemic therapy over aerosol.
Terbutaline (1 mg/mL)	0.01 mg/kg every 20 minutes for 3 doses then every 2–6 hours as needed subcutaneous.	0.25 mg every 20 minutes for 3 doses subcutaneous.	No proven advantage of systemic therapy over aerosol.

TABLE 2-11 **Dosages of Drugs for Asthma Exacerbations, continued**

Medication	Child Dose	Adult Dose	Comments
Anticholinergics			

Ipratropium bromide
  Nebulizer solution
    (0.25 mg/mL)
	0.25–0.5 mg every 20 minutes for 3 doses, then as needed	0.5 mg every 20 minutes for 3 doses, then as needed	May mix in same nebulizer with albuterol. Should not be used as first-line therapy; should be added to SABA therapy for severe exacerbations. The addition of ipratropium has not been shown to provide further benefit once the patient is hospitalized.

MDI (18 mcg/puff)	4–8 puffs every 20 minutes as needed up to 3 hours	8 puffs every 20 minutes as needed up to 3 hours	Should use with spacing chamber and face mask for children <4 years. Studies have examined ipratropium bromide MDI for up to 3 hours.
Ipratropium with albuterol Nebulizer solution (Each 3 mL vial contains 0.5 mg ipratropium bromide and 2.5 mg albuterol.)	1.5-3 mL every 20 minutes for 3 doses, then as needed	3 mL every 20 minutes for 3 doses, then as needed	May be used for up to 3 hours in the initial management of severe exacerbations. The addition of ipratropium to albuterol has not been shown to provide further benefit once the patient is hospitalized.
MDI (Each puff contains 18 mcg ipratropium bromide and 90 mcg of albuterol.)	4–8 puffs every 20 minutes as needed up to 3 hours	8 puffs every 20 minutes as needed up to 3 hours	Should use with spacing chamber and face mask for children <4 years.
Systemic Corticosteroids		(Dosing applies to all three corticosteroids)	
Prednisone Methylprednisolone Prednisolone	1–2 mg/kg in 2 divided doses (maximum = 60 mg/day) until PEF is 70% of predicted or personal best	40–80 mg/day in 1 or 2 divided doses until PEF reaches 70% of predicted or personal best	For outpatient "burst," use 40–60 mg in single or 2 divided doses for total of 5–10 days in adults (children: 1–2 mg/kg/day maximum 60 mg/day for 3–10 days).

*Children ≤ 12 years of age

Key: ED, emergency department; MDI, metered-dose inhaler; PEF, peak expiratory flow; VHC, valved holding chamber

Notes:

• Albuterol = Salbutamol, Epinephrine = Adrenaline

• There is no known advantage for higher doses of corticosteroids in severe asthma exacerbations, nor is there any advantage for intravenous administration over oral therapy provided gastrointestinal transit time or absorption is not impaired.

• The total course of systemic corticosteroids for an asthma exacerbation requiring an ED visit of hospitalization can last from 3 to 10 days. For corticosteroid courses of less than 1 week, there is no need to taper the dose. For slightly longer courses (eg, up to 10 days), there probably is no need to taper, especially if patients are concurrently taking ICSs.

• ICSs can be started at any point in the treatment of an asthma exacerbation.

From 2007 *National Institutes of Health Guidelines*, Section 5, Managing Exacerbations of Asthma, Fig. 5-5. p. 386-7, August 28, 2007.

Some important things to avoid include feeding the tachypneic child because of the increased risk for aspiration, sedating the anxious child because respiratory difficulty might be a reflection of hypoxia, overhydration, routine use of mucolytics, and administering oral β-agonists during acute episodes because they have a longer and more variable onset of action and more systemic adverse effects.

Routine use of antibiotics for asthma exacerbations has not been shown to be efficacious except when necessary for the treatment of comorbid conditions. Combination of long-acting β-agonists with inhaled steroids is superior to doubling the dose of ICS but there are concerns about the safety of long-acting β-agonists in severe asthma. Inhaled corticosteroids have known benefit in chronic asthma; however, their use in acute episodes is less clear and requires further study. Whether continuous albuterol (salbutamol) is superior to intermittent doses remains controversial, with some studies finding no difference and others reporting decreased ED stays with continuous therapy during the acute ED phase. The combination of ipratropium bromide with SABAs is recommended in the ED but not during hospitalization.[86]

Theophylline is no longer recommended in pediatrics because of its narrow therapeutic range, toxicity profile, and effect on the lower esophageal sphincter, which has been associated with an increased risk for reflux.

Asthma education is important and can be started in the ED with referral to asthma education programs, distribution of patient education materials, and metered-dose inhaler demonstration.

Mechanical ventilation can be administered either invasively with endotracheal intubation or noninvasively with nasal continuous positive airway pressure. Indications for intubation include apnea, coma, and respiratory failure. Permissive hypercapnia is a ventilator strategy recommended by some intensivists.

THE BOTTOM LINE

- Asthma is a chronic condition. It is best managed by a partnership among patient, physician, family, and school or childcare facility.

- Emergency management of the asthma patient should be followed by an asthma action plan individualized for each child and updated regularly by the primary care physician.

- It is incumbent on emergency physicians to expedite affiliation with a medical home for those patients who appear recurrently in the ED for corticosteroid burst therapy.

CASE SCENARIO 5

A 10-month-old infant born at 28 weeks' gestation presents to the ED 4 months after discharge from the hospital neonatal intensive care unit. He is receiving long-term home oxygen therapy and was stable until 2 days ago when he developed URI symptoms followed by increased respiratory rate and increased oxygen requirements. On presentation in the ED, he is alert, shows signs of increase in work of breathing (nasal flaring and retractions), and his color is pale. Vital signs include a respiratory rate of 60/min, heart rate of 160/min, temperature of 37.9°C (100.2°F), and oxygen saturation of 88%. He has diffuse wheezing on examination without rales. Your initial management includes supplemental oxygen and nebulized albuterol (salbutamol) therapy. His oxygen saturation improves to 95% with 4 L of oxygen by nasal cannula. Further assessment shows a right otitis media and clear rhinorrhea on detailed physical examination.

1. *What is your differential diagnosis?*
2. *What are your management priorities?*

Disease of Oxygenation and Ventilation and Disease of the Lungs

Bronchopulmonary Dysplasia

Bronchopulmonary dysplasia (BPD) is a severe form of chronic lung disease. Diagnosis is based on the following three criteria: mechanical ventilation in the neonatal period, continued need for supplemental oxygen at day 28 of life, and pulmonary insufficiency.[90] It is most commonly seen in very low-birth-weight infants. Other factors associated with increased incidence include meconium aspiration syndrome, congenital heart disease (eg, patent ductus arteriosus), perinatal infection (eg, cytomegalovirus), persistent pulmonary hypertension, and high levels of ventilatory support. In all cases, there is a significant inflammatory response in the airways of these infants; most infants with BPD have neutrophils in tracheal aspirates at 11 to 15 days of life. In older infants with BPD, alveolar macrophages are the predominant cell. Up to 50% of infants with BPD require hospital readmission during the first year of life.

Pulmonary infections, especially RSV, and increased frequency of wheezing have been reported in hospitalized infants. Immunoprophylaxis for RSV is indicated for specific groups of infants with BPD.[75]

Since the introduction of surfactant replacement, survival of the most immature infants has improved. However, the stable 25% to 50% survival rates in preterm infants at 23 to 24 weeks' gestation likely reflect the lack of alveolarization and vascular development. Along with other advances in technology and an improved understanding of neonatal physiology, infants with BPD appear to have milder disease today than in years past.[90,91]

Lung function and radiographic findings can improve with age, but some children will have persistent abnormalities. Hyde and English[92] developed prognostic criteria based on the radiographic appearance at day 28. Type 1 infants have patchy or homogeneous opacification without coarse reticulation and generally improve over time. Type 2 infants have coarse reticulation, streaky densities, and areas of emphysema. This type of patient has a less favorable prognosis.

Variations in diagnostic criteria, patient population, and early treatment practices have led to difficulties in defining epidemiology.

Risk factors include prolonged oxygen exposure, mechanical ventilation, and immaturity.[90] Postdischarge pulmonary exacerbations can be complicated by sequelae of prolonged intubation (subglottic stenosis, granulomas, laryngomalacia, and tracheomalacia), which can add to the increase in airway resistance caused by acute airway infections, such as RSV.

Clinical Features

Signs and symptoms of BPD include increased respiratory rate at rest and often increased work of breathing manifested by retractions. The Harrison groove, a depression on the lower edge of the thorax at the insertion of the diaphragm (pear-shaped chest) caused by tug of the diaphragm and sometimes seen in patients with severe dyspnea, can be a result of chronic increased work of breathing. Pulmonary complications of BPD are listed in Table 2-12. Cor pulmonale is seen in infants who are chronically hypoxemic. Other complications of BPD include feeding difficulties, gastroesophageal reflux, failure to thrive, and acute life-threatening events.

Diagnostic Studies

A chest radiograph is important to making the diagnosis, with staging of BPD as reported by Northway et al.[93] Initial radiographic criteria for staging BPD are given in Table 2-13. The chest radiograph in **Figure 2.18** shows classic coarse reticulation with streaky densities and small cystic translucencies.

Comparison with previous radiographs is helpful in diagnosing pneumonia in this group

TABLE 2-12 Pulmonary Complications of Bronchopulmonary Dysplasia

- Cor pulmonale
- Right ventricular hypertrophy and enlargement of the main pulmonary artery reflecting pulmonary hypertension
- Atelectasis
- Segmental or subsegmental collapse
- Hyperinflation

Greenough A. Chronic lung disease in the newborn. In: Rennie JM, Roberton NRC. *Textbook of Neonatology*. 3rd ed. New York, NY: Churchill Livingstone; 1999:608–622. Reprinted with permission.

TABLE 2-13 Radiographic Criteria for Initial Staging of Bronchopulmonary Dysplasia[93]

Stage	Radiographic Criteria
Stage 1: day 1–3	Similar appearance to respiratory distress syndrome
Stage 2: day 4–10	Marked radiopacity
Stage 3: day 10–20	Development of a cystic pattern
Stage 4: >28 days	Hyperexpansion; variable cardiomegaly; streaky densities and areas of emphysema

Adapted from Northway WH, Rosan RC, Porter DY. Pulmonary disease following respiratory therapy of hyaline membrane disease. *New England Journal of Medicine*. 1967, 276:357–368.

of patients. Clinical findings must be correlated with radiographic changes.

Management

If clinical or radiographic deterioration occurs in the patient with BPD, consider pulmonary infection as a cause. Management includes administering supplemental oxygen to keep oxygen saturation at 92% or higher, monitoring hemoglobin level, and obtaining a chest radiograph. If wheezing is present, then a trial of a nebulized bronchodilator is indicated. Apnea is often the only manifestation of infection in patients with BPD. Measurement of ABGs is indicated to evaluate infants in severe respiratory distress. Look for change compared with baseline values.

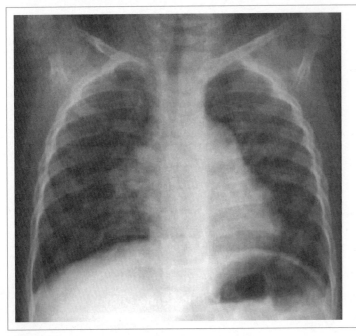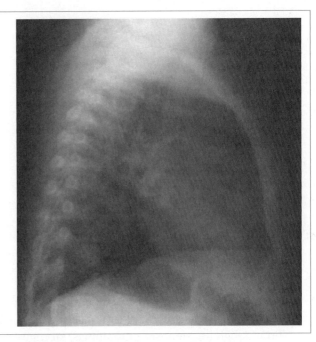

Figure 2.18 Findings of bronchopulmonary dysphasia.

KEY POINTS

Treatment of Infants With BPD

- Increasing supplemental oxygen—titrate to keep oxygen saturation at 92% or higher
- Bronchodilators (see Table 2-11):
  – Albuterol (salbutamol)
  – Ipratropium bromide
- Corticosteroids (inhaled) (see Table 2-14):
  – Budesonide
  – Fluticasone (spacing chamber and metered-dose inhaler)
- Consider trial of diuretics in the following circumstances:
  – Sudden weight gain
  – Sudden deterioration
- Consider antibiotics in the following circumstances:
  – High index of suspicion of bacterial disease
  – Immunodeficiency
  – Recurrent pattern of respiratory infection with frequent exacerbations

These infants often have little reserve and deteriorate rapidly. Send nasopharyngeal or tracheal secretions for viral studies, especially RSV, influenza, and adenovirus, to help determine the cause of the deterioration.[90,91]

Patients requiring long-term oxygen supplementation are a particular challenge in emergency management because it is often difficult to assess the patient's change from baseline pulmonary status. Careful titration of supplemental oxygen is necessary to prevent the infant from retaining carbon dioxide. Nebulized bronchodilator therapy and inhaled or systemic corticosteroids are often used; the efficacy of these therapies is controversial because bronchial smooth muscle might not be fully developed in infants. In cases where the child has shown excessive weight gain, diuretics can be added, and antibiotics are administered in cases of suspected bacterial infection.

Indications for admission are found in Table 2-15 and include persistent tachypnea, hypoxia, inability to feed, new pulmonary infiltrates/pneumonia, or respiratory failure.

Treatment of infants with BPD can be difficult because too aggressive an approach can lead to further complications. Some important things to avoid in the treatment of patients with BPD

TABLE 2-14 Asthma Medications for Long-Term Control: Inhaled Corticosteroids

Estimated Comparative Daily Dosages for Children 12 Years Old or Younger

Drug	Possible Doses	Low Daily Dose	Medium Daily Dose	High Daily Dose
Beclomethasone HFA	40 to 80 mcg/puff	80–160 mcg	160–320 mcg	>320 mcg
Budenoside DPI	200 mcg/inhalation	200–400 mcg	400–800 mcg	>800 mcg
Budenoside for nebulization	0.25 mg 0.5 mg	0.5 mg	1 mg	2 mg
Flunisolide	250 mcg/puff	500–750 mcg	1,000–1,250 mcg	>1,250 mcg
Fluticasone MDI	44, 110, or 220 mcg/puff	88–176 mcg	176–440 mcg	>440 mcg
Fluticasone DPI	50, 100, or 250 mcg/inhalation	100–200 mcg	200–400 mcg	>400 mcg
Triamcinolone acetonide	100 mcg/puff	400–800 mcg	800–1,200 mcg	>1,200 mcg

US Department of Health and Human Services; National Institutes of Health; National Heart, Lung, and Blood Institute; National Asthma Education and Prevention Program. *Expert Panel Report: Guidelines for the Diagnosis and Management of Asthma. Update on Selected Topics 2002.* NIH Publication No. 02-5075, June 2003:115-119, 122-123. (Updates the NAEPP *Expert Panel Report 2*, NIH Publication No. 97-4051.) Available at: www.nhlbi.nih.gov/guidelines/asthma/asthmafullrpt.pdf. Accessed March 2, 2006.

include the following: agitation because it can worsen hypoxia, oral feedings in infants with respiratory difficulty because of increased risk of pulmonary aspiration, overhydration because it can lead to pulmonary edema and worsen the degree of hypoxemia, overuse of digoxin because it can increase pulmonary vascular resistance, and the misconception that parents can be around-the-clock caregivers for a sick child. Consider hospital admission if home support systems are inadequate or stressed.

TABLE 2-15 Indications for Admission in Patients With Bronchopulmonary Dysplasia

- Respiratory rate greater than 70–80/min or a significant change from baseline
- Increasing hypoxia or hypercarbia/increased oxygen requirement
- Poor feeding associated with respiratory symptoms
- Apnea
- New pulmonary infiltrates

CASE SCENARIO 6

A 16-year-old boy who has been followed in the cystic fibrosis (CF) center in the hospital presents to the ED. He has been gradually losing weight and has been admitted for intravenous antibiotic therapy twice in the past 3 months. His lung function studies show a moderate to severe decrease in FEV_1. He presents today with acute onset of sharp chest pain radiating to the right shoulder. He is alert and anxious, sitting in the tripod position; he is tachypneic and has no retractions; and his color is pale with perioral cyanosis. Vital signs include a respiratory rate of 40/min, heart rate of 150/min, and oxygen saturation of 80% on room air. Supplemental oxygen is delivered with a nonrebreather mask. The ABG analysis results are as follows: fraction of inspired oxygen (FIO_2) 0.6, pH 7.4, PCO_2 33 mm Hg, PO_2 83 mm Hg, and bicarbonate 20 mEq/L. He is barrel chested, and breath sounds are significantly decreased on the right side. Hyperresonance is noted to percussion on the right side.

1. What is the most likely cause of his chest pain?
2. What are your management priorities?

Cystic Fibrosis

Cystic fibrosis (CF) is the most common lethal genetic disease in the United States. It is a multisystem disease, associated with abnormalities of the CF transmembrane conductance regulator protein, which results in chronic sinopulmonary disease and pancreatic insufficiency. Pulmonary disease progression is the major determinant of morbidity outside the newborn period. The median age of survival for persons with CF is now more than 37 years, double what it was 25 years ago.[94,95]

Cystic fibrosis is an autosomal recessive disease (mutation of long arm of chromosome 7), affecting approximately 30,000 people in the United States. There are an additional 10 million carriers for the *CF* gene. Frequency estimates in the United States are as follows: whites, 1:3,200; blacks, 1:15,000; and Asians, 1:31,000.[94,96]

The main respiratory manifestation of CF is chronic cough, which becomes productive over time. Sputum is colonized early with *S aureus* and *H influenzae* and later with *Pseudomonas aeruginosa*, mucoid type. It is typically thick and tenacious. During an exacerbation, some patients initially experience fatigue, decreased appetite, and weight loss and later experience increased cough, congestion, and respiratory difficulty. Physical examination findings include fever, increased work of breathing (use of accessory muscles, tachypnea), and new or increased crackles on auscultation. Wheezing can also accompany exacerbations. Sputum is thick and purulent and is often blood streaked. Recurrent infections are the rule rather than the exception in CF. New infiltrates can be seen with acute exacerbations. Bronchiectasis is the result of chronic and recurrent infections. Chronic hypoxemia associated with $\dot{V}/\dot{Q}$ mismatch contributes to the development of pulmonary hypertension.[94–97]

Before newborn screening, children were usually identified by 4 years of age and presented with a history of chronic cough, recurrent episodes of wheezing, recurrent pneumonia, sinus disease, and failure to thrive. Most patients are now identified in infancy. Older children with more advanced disease can have the classic findings of barrel chest and digital clubbing along with failure to thrive. Pulmonary function testing provides a marker for clinical progression; FEV_1 has been used most frequently as a prognostic marker.[94]

Spontaneous pneumothorax is a common complication of patients with CF. Nearly 3.5% of all CF patients will experience a pneumothorax. Pneumothorax is more common in older patients, with approximately 40% having a pneumothorax by the age of 20 years. Recurrent pneumothoraces are common (50%–70%) and result in increasing morbidity and mortality. Clinical factors associated with pneumothorax include severe pulmonary impairment; *P aeruginosa*, *Burkholderia cepacia*, and *Aspergillus*; pancreatic insufficiency; massive hemoptysis; and certain inhaled therapies. Management options include the consideration of whether the patient is a candidate for lung transplantation. A partial pleurectomy has a 95% success rate in treating pneumothorax. Alternatives include intercostal drainage and chemical or limited surgical pleurodesis.[98]

Hemorrhage secondary to hemoptysis is uncommon in young children with CF. Blood-streaked sputum, however, is commonly observed in older children and is generally associated with an acute exacerbation. There is hypertrophy of bronchial vessels as the pulmonary disease progresses with more involved areas of bronchiectasis. Massive hemoptysis is believed to occur because of the increased pressure in the bronchial vasculature. The Cystic Fibrosis Foundation defines severe hemoptysis as the expectoration of more than 100 mL of fresh blood per day for more than 2 days.

Respiratory failure and hypoxia develop in the child with CF as the pulmonary disease progresses with recurrent infections and the development of bronchiectasis and pulmonary fibrosis. Some children compensate by increasing their respiratory rate. With time they will develop dyspnea in addition to hypoxia, and gradual increases in Pco_2 will be seen. The ABG analysis will reveal a compensated respiratory acidosis. Patients with advanced disease and chronic respiratory failure are poor candidates for ventilatory support. Patients with good initial pulmonary function who experience an acute event that results in respiratory failure requiring ventilatory support have a better outcome.[94,98]

Lung transplantation is the most aggressive therapy available for end-stage lung disease due to cystic fibrosis. According to the CF Patient Registry, nearly 1,600 people with CF have received lung transplants since 1991. This constitutes approximately 120 to 150 people per year. The success of lung transplantation

is determined by the recipients' average length of survival after the operation. Successful lung transplantation can increase life expectancy by 4 to 5 years. The emergency physician should be prepared to care for children and young adults with lung transplants. These patients have many challenges related to immunosuppressive drugs and compliance, and improved quality of life can be difficult to determine.[99]

Diagnostic Studies

Hyperinflation is an early finding on chest radiography. With time, peribronchial cuffing, tram lines, recurrent infiltrates, fibrosis, and the formation of blebs and bullae are also seen (**Figure 2.19**). Cor pulmonale develops as the disease progresses. The diagnosis of tension pneumothorax is made clinically. Nontension pneumothorax can be confirmed with an upright posteroanterior chest radiograph. Sputum cultures help guide antibiotic therapy for acute exacerbations. Pulmonary function studies are helpful in making determinations about invasive methods of ventilatory support but are usually unavailable in the ED. Chest CT with high resolution can be used to identify subpleural blebs and evaluate bronchiectasis. Magnetic resonance imaging and arteriography have been used to help identify sources of bleeding. Lipase, glucose, and sweat electrolytes can also be considered.

The classic triad of findings consistent with CF includes chronic pulmonary disease, pancreatic insufficiency, and elevated sweat electrolytes.

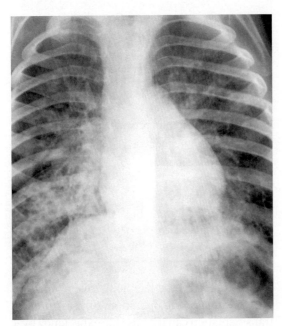

Figure 2.19 Patient with cystic fibrosis.

Management

Management strategies for acute pulmonary exacerbations, hemoptysis, and pneumothorax differ significantly and should be coordinated with the CF care team or pulmonologist.

Acute Pulmonary Exacerbation

Oxygen should be administered to patients who are hypoxic. Some patients who are in the advanced stages of disease will have chronic respiratory failure. Consider respiratory drive when choosing oxygen therapy. If the patient is in moderate to severe respiratory distress or apneic, give 100% oxygen and be prepared to support ventilation if the event is thought to be acute and treatable.

Antibiotic treatment can vary from a short course of one antibiotic agent to a continuous course with multiple antibiotics administered via various routes, including oral, intravenous, or inhalation. Because patients with cystic fibrosis have a larger lean body mass, they often have a higher clearance rate for many antibiotics. Aerosolized antibiotics can reduce symptoms by reducing the organism density in the airways. Initial antibiotic coverage is chosen from two

independent categories to provide synergistic action against the more common CF organisms and to help delay the development of antibiotic resistance. Therapy is continued for 2 to 3 weeks and can be done on an inpatient service combined with home intravenous therapy. Although home therapy is cost-effective, studies suggest added benefits to hospitalization, including more aggressive respiratory therapy than is feasible at home.[96,100]

In infants, endobronchial colonization is generally with *S aureus*, nontypeable *H influenzae*, and gram-negative bacilli. *Pseudomonas aeruginosa* becomes the predominant organism by the age of 10 years.[96] Antibiotic sensitivity profiles from sputum cultures, when available, are more accurate guides to therapeutic choices. Antibiotic doses should be adjusted for the volume of distribution and clearance rate seen in patients with CF. Although not all patients with CF will demonstrate bronchial reactivity, nebulized bronchodilators are often used in conjunction with chest percussion to facilitate pulmonary hygiene and clearance of secretions.

Antibiotic selection can be difficult because of resistant organisms, limited antibiotic sensitivities, and impaired renal or hepatic function. Options should be discussed with the patient's pulmonologist, infectious disease specialist, or primary physician. Although intubation and mechanical ventilation are appropriate for patients with CF with an acute problem and reasonable chance for extubation, outcome in patients with advanced end-stage lung disease is uniformly poor.

Diuresis in patients with CF with cor pulmonale should be done with cautious monitoring of fluid and electrolyte status. Concerns include hypokalemia, hypochloremic metabolic alkalosis, and increased PCO_2.

The management of CF is very complex, and most patients have a rapidly evolving medication list. Recombinant human DNAase (dornase alfa) was developed to degrade the large amount of free DNA that accumulates within CF mucus, thereby improving the viscoelastic properties of airway secretions and promoting airway clearance. Dornase alfa is recommended for patients with CF, 6 years and older, with moderate to severe lung disease to improve lung function.[100]

Pneumothorax

Administer supplemental oxygen to the patient while preparing to place a chest tube. Needle aspiration is not indicated in this circumstance unless there is acute deterioration and shock.

Hemoptysis

Initial management includes administering supplemental oxygen and sending a blood sample for type and crossmatch, complete blood cell count, and prothrombin time. Treatment options will depend on the degree of bleeding. For smaller amounts of bleeding in a stable patient, bed rest, antibiotics, and cough suppression might be sufficient. Fluids and blood are replaced as necessary by clinical evaluation. Vitamin K administration is recommended if the prothrombin time is elevated. For massive hemoptysis, stabilize the patient, intubate, and control bleeding to one lung or one lobe with Fogarty balloon tamponade. Persistent hemoptysis might require bronchial artery embolization or pulmonary resection. Chest percussion should be avoided in patients with hempotysis.[94,95]

THE BOTTOM LINE

Cystic Fibrosis

- Know the natural history of CF.

- Anticipate pulmonary progression and be prepared to identify and treat complications promptly.

- A multidisciplinary team approach is helpful in long-term treatment of patients with CF.

- End-of-life decisions should be discussed in advance with the patient and family to avoid emotional decisions in the ED.

Pneumonia

Pneumonia is a common problem seen in EDs. It has an incidence of 4% per year in children younger than 5 years, 2% in children 5 to 9 years old, and 1% in children older than 9 years.[101] Viral agents are responsible for most pneumonias. Viral pneumonia has its peak incidence between the ages of 3 and 5 years. Boys are more frequently affected. Parainfluenza types 1 and 3, RSV, and adenovirus are common etiologic agents for viral pneumonia. Viruses such as RSV have a seasonal pattern. Although bacterial causes are responsible for only a small percentage of childhood pneumonias, they result in higher mortality (two to three times) and morbidity rates than viral pneumonia.[102]

Approximately 2 million children worldwide die each year from pneumonia. Pneumococcal infection accounts for one-fourth of these deaths. Mortality is rare in the United States; however, pneumococcal pneumonia accounts for more than 500,000 cases of pneumonia each year in children. *Pneumococcus* is the leading cause of community-acquired bacterial pneumonia and carries a risk for significant morbidity, including lobar consolidation, pleural effusion, necrotizing pneumonia, pneumatocele, and lung abscess. The pneumococcal vaccine has decreased radiographically diagnosed pneumonia in children younger than 5 years by 20%.[102,103]

Occult pneumonia has been found in children with fever and no lower respiratory tract signs, tachypnea, or respiratory distress. There is limited utility in obtaining a chest radiograph in febrile children without cough. The likelihood of pneumonia increases with longer duration of cough or fever or in the presence of leukocytosis.[104]

Etiologic considerations are based on the age of the child, immunization status, environment, exposures, and immunologic status. Common pathogens and treatment by age group are listed in Table 2-16.

Clinical Features

The diagnosis of pneumonia is made by integrating the clinical history and the physical examination and radiographic findings. Risk factors are listed in Table 2-17. Viral pneumonia is often preceded by a prodromal phase, including rhinorrhea and cough. These symptoms progress to increasing dyspnea and fever in days. Atypical pneumonias (*Mycoplasma pneumoniae*) generally share common clinical features with the viral pneumonias but can also present with acute symptoms. Bacterial pneumonias often have a more abrupt onset with fever, chest pain, cough, and dyspnea.

The history should include exposures at day care or school and travel history. Classic symptoms include cough, wheeze, dyspnea, fever, chest pain, malaise, vomiting, rhinorrhea, pharyngitis, and diarrhea. Tachypnea out of proportion to the fever should be noted. Physical examination findings can include cough, crackles, or decreased breath sounds. Wheezing might

TABLE 2-16 Pathogens and Empiric Therapy in Pediatric Pneumonia

Age	Bacterial Pathogens	Viral Pathogens	Other Pathogens	Empiric Therapy
<1 month	Group B *Streptococcus*, *Escherichia coli*, *Klebsiella*, *Pseudomonas*, *Listeria*	Varicella, RSV	*Chlamydia**	Ampicillin + aminoglycoside or ampicillin + cefotaxime*
1–3 months	*Haemophilus influenzae*, *Streptococcus pneumoniae*, group A *Streptococcus*, pertussis, group B *Streptococcus*	RSV, parainfluenza, influenza, adenovirus	*Chlamydia**	Ampicillin + cefotaxime*
3 months to 5 years	*S pneumoniae*, *H influenzae*, *Staphylococcus aureus*, group A *Streptococcus*, pertussis	RSV, parainfluenza, influenza, enterovirus, rhinovirus	*Chlamydia**	Cefotaxime or ceftriaxone + antistaphylococcal agent if course indicates*
>5 years	*S pneumoniae*, *H influenzae*, group A *Streptococcus*	Parainfluenza, influenza, adenovirus, rhinovirus	*Mycoplasma*	Cefotaxime or ceftriaxone + antistaphylococcal agent if course indicates or azithromycin if course suggests Mycoplasma

Abbreviation: RSV, respiratory syncytial virus.

*If *Chlamydia* is the suspected pathogen, erythromycin should be added to the treatment regimen.

also be present, especially in those patients with a previous history of asthma. Abdominal pain can be seen with lower lobe pneumonia. Meningismus can be seen in upper lobe pneumonia, with pain radiating to the neck. Pulse oximetry

TABLE 2-17 Risk Factors for Pneumonia

- Young age
- Male
- Pollution
- Nutritional status
- Immunodeficiency
- Anatomical airway abnormalities
- Metabolic disease
- Socioeconomic factors

might reveal decreased values, indicating the need for supplemental oxygen. In patients with chronic lung disease, initial symptoms can be subtle and include fatigue, decreased appetite, weight loss, and increased sputum production.

Complications include secondary bacterial infections after viral pneumonitis, atelectasis, effusion, empyema, abscess, air leaks (pneumothorax, pneumomediastinum), hypoxia, respiratory failure, and dehydration (especially in young children).

Diagnostic Studies

Although pneumonia can be diagnosed solely on clinical findings, most physicians confirm their suspicions with two-view chest radiography. If effusion is suspected, lateral decubitus views are

Signs and Symptoms of Pneumonia
- Cough
- Fever
- Chest pain
- Shortness of breath
- Tachypnea
- Malaise
- Abdominal pain
- Hypoxia

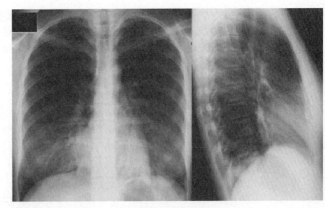

Figure 2.20 Diffuse patchy infiltrates.

helpful. Different patterns of pulmonary infection can be seen on radiographs as follows:
- Diffuse peribronchial thickening, often with hyperinflation from air trapping
- Diffuse, patchy interstitial pattern (**Figure 2.20**)
- Focal lobar consolidation (**Figure 2.21**)

Diffuse patchy infiltrates often with shaggy peribronchial infiltrates in the perihilar regions are commonly seen with viral infections, although bacterial infections can also show a similar pattern. Lobar consolidation can be difficult to distinguish from atelectasis secondary to mucous plugging; however, signs of volume loss with shift of the trachea and unaffected lung to the atelectatic side are usually evident. Focal lobar consolidation sometimes presents as a "round" pneumonia and can be mistaken for a chest mass (**Figure 2.22**). Expiratory radiographs are often misinterpreted as pneumonia, because normal vascular and airway markings will be accentuated if the lungs are underinflated when the film is taken at end expiration.

A complete blood cell count is occasionally helpful in differentiating viral and bacterial infections but is usually not necessary in fully immunized normal hosts older than 6 months. Sputum Gram stain and cultures and skin testing are rarely indicated in the ED. Pleurocentesis might be needed in severe cases with large effusions. Immunofluorescent detection or immunoassay for viral agents such as RSV, rapid

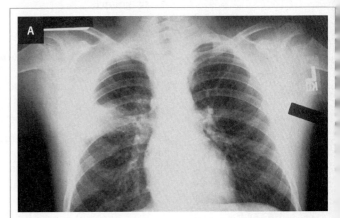

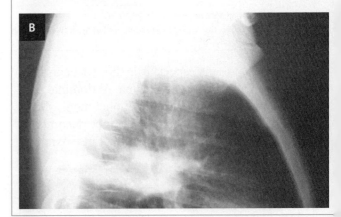

Figure 2.21A and B Focal infiltrates.

antigen tests, and serologic testing with acute and convalescent titers might be indicated in some patients, especially those with chronic illness or immunodeficiency. Single or continuous pulse oximetry is performed in most cases of suspected pneumonia.

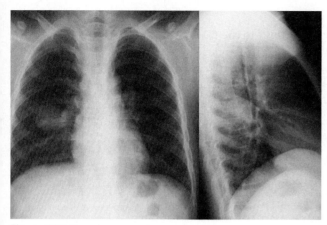

Figure 2.22 Round pneumonia.

Differential Diagnosis

The differential diagnosis for pneumonia includes asthma, bronchiolitis, bronchitis, congestive heart failure, and URI. History, clinical findings, and chest radiography can be helpful in distinguishing these disease processes from pneumonia.

Management

For the previously well child with community-acquired pneumonia and no respiratory compromise, outpatient empiric therapy for the agents most commonly found in the particular age group is an appropriate initial treatment plan. It can be modified after evaluating the child's response to therapy. For the child in respiratory distress, supportive therapy (supplemental oxygen, antipyretics, or bronchodilator therapy as indicated) is given in addition to intravenous antibiotics. Empiric antibiotics are listed in Table 2-16.[101,103,105]

Hospital admission should be considered for infants with lobar infiltrate, respiratory compromise, pleural effusion, dehydration, or failed outpatient treatment. Supportive care includes supplemental oxygen, hydration, nutrition, and rest. Bronchodilators can be a useful adjunct to help facilitate pulmonary hygiene and clearance of secretions. Children with significant effusions or empyema require thoracentesis for diagnosis and therapy.

WHAT ELSE?

Differential Diagnosis for Pneumonia
- Asthma
- Bronchiolitis
- Bronchitis
- Congestive heart failure
- URI

An infant with acute respiratory distress is brought to the ED by his father. The boy was well until yesterday, when he developed a runny nose and low-grade fever. This morning he is irritable, refuses his bottle, and has vomited twice. On examination, he is poorly responsive to his surroundings, he has marked increased work of breathing with stridor and intercostal retractions, and his color is pale to gray with circumoral cyanosis. Vital signs include a respiratory rate of 40/min, heart rate of 60/min, and oxygen saturation of 84% on room air. He has decreased air entry bilaterally and mild end-expiratory wheezes.

1. *What are your initial management priorities?*
2. *What is your differential diagnosis?*

Respiratory Failure

Respiratory failure represents an inability of the body to adequately oxygenate and/or ventilate. It is more common in children than in adults. Certain anatomical factors predispose infants and young children to respiratory failure. These factors include smaller airway size, which increases airway resistance, circular chest wall configuration, more compliant chest wall, horizontal diaphragmatic insertion, and increased number of fatigue-prone type II muscle fibers in the infant diaphragm. Children younger than 3 months and children with neuromuscular disease, chronic lung disease, and complex congenital heart disease might have difficulty compensating by increasing respiratory work consistently over time. Monitoring of clinical status and pulse oximetry will help identify impending respiratory failure.

Respiratory failure is identified by pulmonary insufficiency, hypercarbia, and dyspnea. There are no absolute blood gas values that define this condition. Interpretation of ABG analysis results will be made based on baseline blood gas status, altitude, and ongoing therapy.

Clinical Features

Signs and symptoms of respiratory failure can be categorized as alterations in appearance, muscle tone, mental status, work of breathing, and color of the skin and perfusion. In early or probable respiratory failure (type I—hypoxemia), a child can be anxious, tachypneic, tachycardic, and pale. As respiratory failure progresses to type II (hypoxemia and hypercarbia), the mental status becomes more depressed, muscle tone is decreased, heart rate decreases, and skin color becomes mottled or cyanotic. The progression can lead to cardiopulmonary failure with agonal respirations or apnea and decompensated shock. Finally, cardiopulmonary arrest occurs as all systems fail.

Respiratory distress is often the first clue to the development of respiratory failure. Infants and young children fatigue rapidly with acute respiratory infections and should be monitored appropriately.

YOUR FIRST CLUE

Signs and Symptoms of Respiratory Failure

- Mental status: anxiety, restlessness, confusion, lethargy, coma
- Skin: cyanosis, pallor, diaphoresis
- Breathing: tachypnea → bradypnea → apnea
  - Nasal flaring, grunting
  - Use of accessory muscles
  - Dyspnea, paradoxical abdominal motion
- Respiratory sounds: stridor, wheezing, rales, or decreased breath sounds
- Cardiac: tachycardia, bradycardia, cardiac arrest

Diagnostic Studies

Arterial blood gases, cardiorespiratory monitoring, and pulse oximetry are the main diagnostic tools used in respiratory failure. Complications are usually the result of mechanical ventilation (barotrauma, pneumothorax) or progression to cardiopulmonary failure and arrest. Chest radiographs can help identify cause.

Abnormal blood gas values are as follows:

- $Paco_2$ >50 mm Hg with acidosis (pH <7.25)
- $Paco_2$ >40 mm Hg with severe dyspnea
- Pao_2 <60 mm Hg on Fio_2 0.4

Management

The key to management and prevention of respiratory failure is the recognition of early signs of respiratory distress. See Table 2-18 for normal ranges for respiratory rates. It is often difficult to determine the cause of respiratory failure in the ED. Management follows the guidelines for basic and advanced airway management discussed earlier in this chapter. Infants and children with more severe respiratory distress and impending or actual respiratory failure are usually separated from their parents; however, parents can have a calming effect. Begin ventilatory support when necessary to provide airway protection and administer pressure to improve oxygenation and to assist or control ventilation. Rapid sequence intubation is advantageous in children who are still aware of their surroundings and in those presumed or known to have increased ICP. Initial oxygen setting for children intubated and given mechanical ventilation should be 100%. The most frequent cause of hypoxemia in the clinical setting is $\dot{V}/\dot{Q}$ mismatch. Other causes include hypoventilation, right-to-left shunt, and diffusion abnormality. Oxygen delivery systems are listed in Table 2-19. Adult respiratory distress syndrome can develop in children with acute respiratory failure.[106]

Standard precautions should be followed when handling respiratory secretions. Intravenous fluid therapy should be guided by the underlying cause and clinical assessment.

In children with end-stage lung disease (CF, interstitial lung disease), the benefits of mechanical ventilatory support should be carefully weighed. The child, old enough to participate in decision making, along with the family should have had the opportunity to discuss end-of-life care before the acute event that brought them to the ED. Blood gas values alone are insufficient to make the diagnosis of acute respiratory failure. Such an error might result in intubation of a compensated child with chronic lung disease.

Early identification and treatment are critical to improve outcome in the previously well child with acute respiratory failure. Care should be taken to address patient and family wishes regarding the initiation of ventilatory support when end-stage disease is present.

TABLE 2-18 Normal Resting Respiratory Rate

Age	Respiratory Rate/min
Newborn	30–60
Infant (1–6 months)	30–50
Infant (6–12 months)	24–46
1–4 years	20–30
4–6 years	20–25
6–12 years	16–20
>12 years	12–16

TABLE 2-19 Oxygen Delivery Techniques

Device	Flow, L/min	Oxygen, %
Nasal prongs	2–4	24–28
Simple face mask	6–10	35–60
Face tent	10–15	35–40
Venturi mask	4–10	25–60
Partial rebreathing mask	10–12	50–60
Oxygen hood	10–15	80–90
Nonrebreather mask	10–12	90–95

CHAPTER REVIEW

Check Your Knowledge

1. Which of the following statements about bronchiolitis is correct?
   A. High-risk groups for severe bronchiolitis include infants with congenital heart disease and bronchopulmonary dysplasia (BPD)
   B. Only 20% of children have been infected by respiratory syncytial virus (RSV) by their second birthday
   C. Oral corticosteroids are useful in reducing severity and need for admission
   D. Subsequent RSV infections are more severe than the initial infection

2. Treatment options for croup vary with severity of disease. All of the listed therapies have been shown to improve outcome in patients with croup except?
   A. Dexamethasone intramuscularly or intravenously
   B. Humidified oxygen
   C. L-epinephrine (L-adrenaline)
   D. Racemic epinephrine (adrenaline)

3. Which of the following statements about foreign body (FB) aspiration in children is correct?
   A. Bronchoscopy is the "gold standard" for diagnosis and treatment of FB aspiration
   B. Chest radiographs are highly sensitive for determining the presence of FBs in the airways
   C. Positive physical examination findings are always present after aspiration
   D. Small toys are the most commonly aspirated item
   E. The most common site of obstruction is the larynx

4. Which of the following statements is correct regarding the difference in pediatric and adult airway management?
   A. Adolescents are more likely to develop bradycardia
   B. Adults are more susceptible to air swallowing and emesis leading to aspiration
   C. Infants and children are more likely to experience oxygen desaturation
   D. Rapid sequence intubation (RSI) is not well tolerated by infants

References

1. Berry FA, Yemen TA. Pediatric airway in health and disease. *Pediatr Clin North Am.* 1994;41:153–180.
2. Perkin R, van Stralen D, Mellick LB. Managing pediatric airway emergencies: Anatomic considerations, alternative airway and ventilation techniques, and current treatment options. *Pediatr Emerg Rep.* 1996;1:1–12.
3. Walls RM, Murphy MF, eds. *Manual of Emergency Airway Management.* 3rd ed. Philadelphia, PA: Lippincott Williams & Wilkins; 2008.
4. Sullivan KJ, Kissoon N. Securing the child's airway in the emergency department. *Pediatr Emerg Care.* 2002;18:108–121.
5. Hofer CK, Ganter M, Tucci M, Klaghofer R, Zollinger A. How reliable is length-based determination of body weight and tracheal tube size in the paediatric age group? The Broselow tape reconsidered. *Br J Anaesth.* 2002;88:283–285.
6. Stewart C. Managing the pediatric airway in the ED. *Pediatric Emerg Med Pract.* 2006;3:1–24.
7. Gerardi MJ, Sacchetti AD, Cantor RM, et al. Rapid-sequence intubation of the pediatric patient. Pediatric Emergency Medicine Committee of the American College of Emergency Physicians. *Ann Emerg Med.* 1996;28:55–74.
8. Sakles JC, Laurin EG, Ranatapaa AA, Panacek EA. Airway management in the emergency department: A one-year study of 610 tracheal intubations. *Ann Emerg Med.* 1998;31:325–332.
9. Sagarin MJ, Barton ED, Chng YM, Walls RM, National Emergency Airway Registry Investigators. Airway management by US and Canadian emergency medicine residents: A multicenter analysis of more than 6,000 endotracheal intubation attempts. *Ann Emerg Med.* 2005;46:328–336.
10. Sagarin MJ, Chiang V, Sakles JC, et al. Rapid sequence intubation for pediatric emergency airway management. *Pediatr Emerg Care.* 2002;18:417–423.
11. Gausche M, Lewis RJ, Stratton SJ, et al. Effect of out-of-hospital pediatric endotracheal intubation on survival and neurological outcome: A controlled clinical trial. *JAMA.* 2000;283:783–790.

12. Mallampati SR, Gatt SP, Gugino LD, et al. A clinical sign to predict difficult tracheal intubation: A prospective study. *Can Anaesth Soc J.* 1985;32:429–434.

13. Malhotra A, Drilov LR. Viral croup. *Pediatr Rev.* 2001;22:5–11.

14. Wright RB, Pomerantz WJ, Luria JW. New approaches to respiratory infections in children. *Emerg Med Clin North Am.* 2002;20:93–114.

15. American Academy of Pediatrics. Parainfluenza viral infections. In: Pickering LK, ed. 2009 *Red Book: Report of the Committee on Infectious Disease. 28th ed.* Elk Grove Village, IL: American Academy of Pediatrics; 2009:485–487.

16. Neto GM, Kentab O, Klassen TP, Osmond MH. A randomized controlled trial of mist in the acute treatment of moderate croup. *Acad Emerg Med.* 2002;9:873–879.

17. Bourchier D, Dawson KP, Fergusson DM. Humidification in viral croup: A controlled trial. *Aust Paediatr J.* 1996;20:289–291.

18. Scolnik D, Coates AL, Stephens D, Dasilva Z, Lavine E, Schuh S. Controlled delivery of high vs low humidity vs mist therapy for croup in emergency departments: A randomized controlled trial. *JAMA.* 2006;295:1247–1280.

19. Klasssen TP. Croup: A current perspective. *Pediatr Clin North Am.* 1999;46:1167–1178.

20. Waisman Y, Klein BL, Boenning DA, et al. Prospective randomized double-blind study comparing L-epinephrine and racemic epinephrine aerosols in the treatment of laryngotracheitis (croup). *Pediatrics.* 1992;89:302–306.

21. Johnson DW, Jacobson S, Edney PC, Hadfield P, Mundy ME, Schuh S. A comparison of nebulized budesonide, intramuscular dexamethasone, and placebo for moderately severe croup. *N Engl J Med.* 1998;339:498–503.

22. Klassen TP, Feldman ME, Watters LK, Sutcliffe T, Rowe PC. Nebulized budesonide for children in mild to moderate croup. *N Engl J Med.* 1994;331:285–289.

23. Bjornson CL, Klassen TP, Williamson J, et al. A randomized trial of a single dose of oral dexamethasone for mild croup. *N Engl J Med.* 2004;351:1306–1313.

24. Kunkel NC, Baker MD. Use of racemic epinephrine, dexamethasone and mist in the outpatient management of croup. *Pediatr Emerg Care.* 1996;12:156–159.

25. Cruz MN, Stewart G, Rosenberg N. Use of dexamethasone in the outpatient management of acute laryngotracheitis. *Pediatrics.* 1995;96:220–223.

26. Geelhoed GC, Turner J, Macdonald WB. Efficacy of a small single dose of oral dexamethasone for outpatient croup: A double blind placebo controlled clinical trial. *BMJ.* 1996;313:140–142.

27. Knapp JF, Hall M, Sharma V. Benchmarks for the emergency department care of children with asthma, bronchiolitis, and croup. *Pediatr Emerg Care.* 2010;26:364–369.

28. Vorwerk C, Coats TJ. Use of helium-oxygen mixtures in the treatment of croup: A systematic review. *Emerg Med J.* 2008;25:547–550.

29. Vorwerk C, Coats TJ. Heliox for croup in children. *Cochrane Database Syst Rev.* 2010;2:CD006822

30. Schroeder LL, Knapp JF. Recognition and emergency management of infectious causes of upper airway obstruction in children. *Semin Respir Infect.* 1995;10:21–30.

31. Midulla F, Guidi R, Barbato A, et al. Foreign body aspiration in children. *Pediatr Int.* 2005;47:663–668.

32. CDC injury Center MEdia Relations. Nonfatal chocking-related episodes for children 0 to 14 years of age. http://www.cdc.gov/media/pressrel/fs021024.htm. Updated October 24, 2002. Accessed March 10, 2011.

33. Centers for Disease Control and Prevention. Nonfatal choking-related episodes among children—United States, 2001. *MMWR Morb Mortal Wkly Rep.* 2002;51:945–948.

34. Friedman EM. Tracheobronchial foreign bodies. *Otol Clin North Am.* 2000;33:179–185.

35. Halvorson DJ, Merritt RM, Mann C, Porubsky ES. Management of subglottic foreign bodies. *Ann Otol Rhinol Laryngol.* 1996;105:541–545.

36. Rimell FL, Thome A Jr, Stool S, et al. Characteristics of objects that cause choking in children. *JAMA.* 1995;274:1763–1767.

37. Black RE, Johnson DG, Matlak ME. Bronchoscopic removal of aspirated foreign bodies in children. *J Pediatr Surg.* 1994;29:682–684.

38. Silva AB, Muntz JR, Clary R. Utility of conventional radiography in the diagnosis and management of pediatric airway foreign bodies. *Ann Otol Rhinol Laryngol.* 1998;107:834–838.

39. Even L, Hero N, Talman Y, Samet E, Zonis Z, Kugelman A. Diagnostic evaluation of foreign body aspiration in children: A prospective study. *J Pediatr Surg.* 2005;40:1122–1127.

40. Reilly J, Thompson J, MacArthur C, et al. Pediatric aerodigestive foreign body injuries are complications related to timeliness of diagnosis. *Laryngoscope.* 1997;107:17–20.

41. Monetti S, Monetti C, Meneghini L, Zadra N, Giusti F. Eight years' experience with foreign-body aspiration in children: What is really important for a timely diagnosis? *J Pediatr Surg.* 1999;34:1229–1231.

42. Fontoba JB, Gutierrez C, Lluna J, Vila JJ, Poquet J, Ruiz-Company S. Bronchial foreign body: Should bronchoscopy be performed in all patients with a choking crisis? *Pediatr Surg Int.* 1997;12:118–120.

43. Lee BS, Gausche-Hill M. Pediatric airway management. *Clin Pediatr Emerg Med.* 2001;2:91–106.

44. 2005 International Consensus Conference on Cardiopulmonary Resuscitation and Emergency Cardiovascular Care Recommendations. 2005 international consensus on CPR and ECC science with treatment recommendations: Part 6: Pediatric basic and advanced life support. *Circulation.* 2005;112:III-73–III-90.

45. Brown L, Sherwin T, Perez JE, Perez DU. Heliox as a temporizing measure for pediatric foreign body aspiration. *Acad Emerg Med.* 2002;9:436–437.

46. Weber AL, Sicilian A. CT and MR imaging evaluation of neck infections with clinical correlations. *Radiol Clin North Am.* 2000;38:941–968.

47. Nicklaus PJ, Kelley PE. Management of deep neck infection. *Pediatr Clin North Am.* 1996;43:1277–1296.

48. Kirse DJ, Roberson DW. Surgical management of retropharyngeal space infections in children. *Laryngoscope.* 2001;111:1413–1423.

49. Page NC, Bauer EM, Lieu JE. Clinical features and treatment of retropharyngeal abscess in children. *Otolaryngol Head Neck Surg.* Mar 2008;138:300–306.

50. Kwong KY, Maalouf N, Jones CA. Urticaria and angioedema: Pathophysiology, diagnosis and treatment. *Pediatr Ann.* 1998;27:719–724.

51. Gaglani MJ, Edwards MS. Clinical indicators of childhood retropharyngeal abscess. *Am J Emerg Med.* 1995;13:333–336.

52. Parhiscar A, Har-El G. Deep neck abscess: A retrospective review of 210 cases. *Ann Otol Rhinol Laryngol.* 2001;11:1051–1055.

53. Brooke I. Role of methicillin-resistant Staphylococcus aureus in head and neck infections. *Laryngol Otol.* 2009;123:1301–1307.

54. Lee SS, Schwartz RH, Bahadori RS. Retropharyngeal abscess: Epiglottitis of the new millennium. *J Pediatr.* 2001;138:435–437.

CHAPTER REVIEW

55. Shefelbine SE, Mancuso AA, Gajewski BJ, Oriji H, Stringer S, Sedwick JD. Pediatric retropharyngeal lymphadenitis: Differentiation from retropharyngeal abscess and treatment implications. *Otolaryngol Head Neck Surg*. 2007;136:182–188.

56. Lalakea ML, Messner AH. Retropharyngeal abscess management in children: Current practices. *Otol Head Neck Surg*. 1999;121:398–405.

57. Kickerson SL, Kirby RS, Wheeler JG, Schutze GE. Epiglottitis: A 9-year case review. *South Med J*. 1996;89:487–490.

58. Mayo-Smith MF, Spinale JW, Donskey CJ, Yukawa M, Li RH, Schiffman FJ. Acute epiglottitis: An 18-year experience in Rhode Island. *Chest*. 1995;108:1640–1647.

59. Nakamura H, Tanaka H, Matsuda A, Fukushima E, Hasegawa M. Acute epiglottitis: A review of 80 patients. *J Laryngol Otol*. 2001;115:31–34.

60. Sampson HA. Food anaphylaxis. *Brit Med Bull*. 2000;56:925–935.

61. Decker WW, Campbell RL, Manivannan V, et al. The etiology and incidence of anaphylaxis in Rochester, Minnesota: A report from the Rochester Epidemiology Project. *J Allergy Clin Immunol*. 2008;122:1161–1165.

62. Kagy L, Blaiss MS. Anaphylaxis in children. *Pediatr Ann*. 1998;27:727–734.

63. Sampson HA, Mendelson L, Rosen JP. Fatal and near-fatal anaphylactic reactions to food in children and adolescents. *N Engl J Med*. 1992;327:280–284.

64. Shah UK, Jocobs IN. Pediatric angioedema: Ten years' experience. Arch *Otol Head Neck Surg*. 1999;125:791–795.

65. Sampson HA, Munoz-Furlong A, Campbell RL, et al. Second Symposium on the Definition and Management of Anaphylaxis: Summary Report—Second National Institute of Allergy and Infectious Disease/Food Allergy and Anaphylaxis Network Symposium. *Ann Emerg Med*. 2006;47:373–380.

66. Pumphrey RS. Lessons for management of anaphylaxis from a study of fatal reactions. *Clin Exp Allergy*. 2000;30:1144–1150.

67. Lee JM, Greenes DS. Biphasic anaphylactic reactions in pediatrics. *Pediatrics*. 2000;106:762–766.

68. Gold MS, Sainsbury R. First aid anaphylaxis management in children who were prescribed an epinephrine autoinjector device (EpiPen). *J Allergy Clin Immunol*. 2000;106:171–176.

69. Sicherer SH, Forman JA, Noone SA. Use assessment of self-administered epinephrine among food-allergic children and pediatricians. *Pediatrics*. 2000;105:359–362.

70. Krilov L. Recent development in the treatment and prevention of RSV infection. *Expert Opin Ther Patents*. 2002;12:441–449.

71. Staat MA. Respiratory syncytial virus infections in children. *Semin Respir Infect*. 2002;17:15–20.

72. American Academy of Pediatrics Subcommittee on Diagnosis and Management of Bronchiolitis. Diagnosis and management of bronchiolitis. *Pediatrics*. 2006;118:1774–1793.

73. Zorc JJ, Hall CB. Bronchiolitis: Recent evidence on diagnosis and management. *Pediatrics*. 2010;125:342–349.

74. Willwerth BM, Harper MB, Greenes DS. Identifying hospitalized infants who have bronchiolitis and are at high risk for apnea. *Ann Emerg Med*. Oct 2006;48:441–7.

75. American Academy of Pediatrics. Respiratory syncytial virus. In: Pickering LK, ed. 2009 *Red Book: Report of the Committee on Infectious Disease*. 28th ed. Elk Grove Village, IL: American Academy of Pediatrics; 2009:560–569.

76. Dobson JV, Stephens-Groff SM, McMahon SR, Stemmler MM, Brallier SL, Bay C. The use of albuterol in hospitalized infants with bronchiolitis. *Pediatrics*. 1998;101:361–368.

77. Ngai P, Bye M. Bronchiolitis. *Pediatr Ann*. 2002;31:90–97.

78. Petruzella FD, Gorelick, MH. Current therapies in bronchiolitis. *Pediatr Emer Care*. 2010;26:302–311.

79. Plint AC, Johnson DW, Patel H, et al. Epinephrine and dexamethasone in children with bronchiolitis. *N Engl J Med*. 2009;360:2079–2089.

80. Kellner JD, Ohlsson A, Gadomski AM, Wang EE. Efficacy of bronchodilator therapy in bronchiolitis. A meta-analysis. *Arch Pediatr Adolesc Med*. 1996;150:1166–1172.

81. Martinon-Torres F, Rodriguez-Nunez A, Martinon Sanchez JM. Heliox therapy in infants with acute bronchiolitis. *Pediatrics*. 2002;109:68–73.

82. Corneli, HM, Zorc JJ, Mahajan P, et al. A multicenter, randomized, controlled trial of dexamethasone for bronchiolitis. *N Engl J Med.* 2007;357:331–339.

83. Akinbami LJ. Advance data from vital and health statistics; no 381. *The State of Childhood Asthma, United States,* 1980–2005. Hyattsville, MD: National Center for Health Statistics; 2006.

84. Baren J, Puchalski A. Current concepts in emergency department treatment of pediatric asthma. *Pediatr Emerg Med Rep.* 2002;105–112.

85. Smith S, Strunk RC. Acute asthma in the pediatric emergency department. *Pediatr Clin North Am.* 1999;46:1145–1165.

86. *National Asthma Education and Prevention Program Guidelines for the Diagnosis and Management of Asthma.* Bethesda, MD: US Dept of Health and Human Services, National Institutes of Health; 2007. NIH publication 07-4051.

87. American Academy of Pediatrics. State of childhood asthma and future directions: Strategies for implementing best practices. *Pediatrics.* 2009;123:S129–S214.

88. Keahey L, Bulloch B, Becker AB, Pollack CV Jr, Clark S, Camargo CA Jr; Multicenter Asthma Research Collaboration (MARC) Investigators. Initial oxygen saturation as a predictor of admission in children presenting to the emergency department with acute asthma. *Ann Emerg Med.* 2002;40:300–307.

89. Werner H. Status asthmaticus in children. *Chest.* 2001;119:1913.

90. Greenough A. Chronic lung disease in the newborn. In: Rennie JM, Roberton NRC. *Textbook of Neonatology.* 4th ed. New York, NY: Churchill Livingstone; 2005:608–622.

91. Walsh MC, Szefler S, Davis J, et al. Summary proceedings from the bronchopulmonary dysplasia group. *Pediatrics.* 2006;117: S52–S56.

92. Hyde I, English RE. The changing pattern of chronic lung disease of prematurity. *Arch Dis Child.* 1989;64:448–451.

93. Northway WH, Rosan RC, Porter DY. Pulmonary disease following respiratory therapy of hyaline membrane disease. *N Engl J Med.* 1967;276:357–368.

94. Rowe SM, Miller S, Sorscher EJ. Cystic fibrosis. *N Engl J Med* 2005;352:1992–2001.

95. Ramsey BW. Management of pulmonary disease in patients with cystic fibrosis. *N Engl J Med.* 1996;335:179–188.

96. Rajan S, Saiman L. Pulmonary infections in patients with cystic fibrosis. *Semin Respir Infect.* 2002;17:47–56.

97. Marshall BC, Samuelson W. Basic therapies in cystic fibrosis: Does standard therapy work? *Clin Chest Med.* 1998;19:487–503.

98. Flume PA, Strange C, Xiaobu Y, Ebelind M, Hulsey T, Clark LL. Pneumothorax in cystic fibrosis. *Chest* 2005;128;720–728.

99. Liou TG, Adler FR, Cox DR, Cahill BC. Lung transplantation and survival in children with cystic fibrosis. *N Engl J Med.* 2001;357:2143–2152.

100. Flume PA, O'Sullivan BP, Robinson KA, et al. Cystic fibrosis pulmonary guidelines: Chronic medications for maintenance of lung health. *Am J Respir Crit Care Med.* Nov 15 2007;176:957–969.

101. Vaughan D, Katkin J. Chronic and recurrent pneumonias in children. *Semin Respir Infect.* 2002;17:72–84.

102. Miller MA, Ben Ami T, Daum R. Bacterial pneumonia in neonates and older children. In: Taussig LM, Landau L, eds. *Pediatric Respiratory Medicine.* St Louis, MO: Mosby; 1999:595–664.

103. Tan TQ. Update on pneumococcal infections of the respiratory tract. *Semin Respir Infect.* 2002;17:3–9.

104. Murphy CG, van de Pol AC, Harper MB, Bachur RG. Clinical predictors of occult pneumonia in the febrile child. *Acad Emerg Med.* 2007;14:243–249.

105. Bradley JS. Old and new antibiotics for pediatric pneumonia. *Semin Respir Infect.* 2002;17:57–64.

106. Bateman ST, Arnold JH. Acute respiratory failure in children. *Curr Opin Pediatr.* 2000;12:233–237.

A 6-month-old boy presents to the emergency department (ED) with wheezing, severe retractions, and stridor. The infant has poor tone and is poorly responsive to his surroundings. He has intercostal retractions, and his color is pale. His vital signs include respiratory rate of 80/min, a heart rate of 190/min, temperature (rectal) of 38.6°C (101.5°F), and oxygen saturation of 80% on room air. His mother reveals that he was born at 28 weeks' gestation and was intubated and given mechanical ventilation for 6 weeks before hospital discharge. The patient also has Robin syndrome.

1. *How would you assess and categorize this patient's airway?*
2. *What special precautions would you take in planning airway management and possible intubation?*

This airway is a potentially difficult one. The history of prematurity and previous intubation suggests the possibility of subglottic stenosis or other chronic changes. Robin syndrome includes micrognathia, mandibular hypoplasia, large tongue, and cleft soft palate. This syndrome is associated with difficult airway management due to inadequate visualization. In addition to underlying chronic or past medical problems, this patient is an infant with bronchiolitis. The current disease state and age add the possibility of increased secretions and increased oxygen consumption.

Planning should take the previously stated risks into account. The first step is to ensure the infant can be given adequate bag-mask ventilation. A nasal pharyngeal airway might be helpful in preventing airway obstruction from the large tongue. If airway management is performed in the ED, then anesthesia and surgical backup should be notified. For RSI, only short-acting agents should be used in case intubation is unsuccessful. The laryngeal mask airway has been used successfully in this setting. A needle cricothyrotomy kit should be readily available. In an elective setting, a pediatric anesthesiologist is the best person to intubate this child.

A 13-month-old boy is brought to the ED by paramedics. The mother found him choking and gagging in the kitchen next to a container of spilled nuts. She immediately called 911. Paramedics note that the child is alert, his work of breathing is increased with audible stridor and subcostal retractions, and his color is normal. Paramedics administer blow-by oxygen and transport the child to the ED. On arrival, the child is awake and alert and in moderate respiratory distress. The patient is placed immediately in a monitored bed. Vital signs are respiratory rate of 60/min, heart rate of 160/min, blood pressure of 88/56 mm Hg, temperature 37.1°C (98.8°F), and oxygen saturation of 93%.

1. *What are your initial management priorities?*
2. *What diagnostic studies are necessary?*

3. What are the possible complications to consider on initial evaluation?
4. What is the definitive management of this condition and disposition of the patient?

Rapid cardiopulmonary assessment reveals an awake child with signs of airway obstruction but not in respiratory failure. Airway specialists are mobilized, and an otolaryngologist and anesthesiologist are en route. The patient is given supplemental blow-by oxygen, which he seems to tolerate well without further agitation. The patient is kept in a position of comfort and continuously monitored for deterioration.

No specific diagnostic studies are necessary in this patient. Intravenous access is deferred to prevent agitation. A portable chest radiograph is obtained, and the child remains calm during this procedure. The chest radiograph is normal. The child is in danger of complete airway obstruction, and preparations for orotracheal intubation and needle cricothyrotomy are made. All appropriate equipment sizes and medication dosages are determined and ready at the patient's bedside.

The patient is rapidly transported to the operating room accompanied by the pediatric otolaryngologist. Preparations in the operating room have been made for rigid bronchoscopy and possible emergent tracheostomy. The child undergoes inhalation anesthesia, after which intravenous access is promptly established. Rigid bronchoscopy is performed with successful retrieval of a peanut from the subglottic airway. The patient is then transferred to the pediatric intensive care unit for observation.

A 6-month-old boy presents with acute respiratory distress preceded by a short history of upper respiratory tract symptoms and low-grade fever. He is irritable and feeding poorly. He is alert but tachypneic, has nasal flaring and intercostal retractions, and is pale. His vital signs include a respiratory rate of 70/min, heart rate of 170/min, temperature (rectal) 38°C (100.4°F), and oxygen saturation of 90% on room air. Diffuse bilateral wheezing is discovered on physical examination.

1. What are your initial treatment priorities?
2. What diagnostic tests will be helpful?

Initial treatment priorities are to assess airway patency and position, administer humidified oxygen, and give a trial of albuterol (salbutamol) or another bronchodilator medication. The patient should be reassessed after each intervention.

Helpful diagnostic tests include a chest radiograph to look for classic hyperinflation or other causes or respiratory distress and oxygen saturation readings. Rapid antigen detection for RSV should be considered if the patient is admitted or has chronic disease.

A 5-year-old boy had an acute asthma episode at school during show-and-tell after a classmate brought in a new kitten. He was given albuterol (salbutamol) by the school nurse but continued to have tachypnea and diffuse wheezing, and his mother was called to take him home. Wheezing continued despite two additional albuterol (salbutamol) nebulizer treatments given consecutively at home. The mother brings him to the ED. On arrival, he is alert, shows increased work of breathing with nasal flaring and retractions, and has normal skin color. Vital signs are respiratory rate of 50/min, a heart rate of 130/min, a blood pressure of 120/80 mm Hg, axillary temperature of 36.6°C (97.9°F), and pulse oximetry of 89% on room air. He is acutely short of breath with poor air entry and no wheezing on auscultation of the chest.

1. *What are your priorities?*
2. *What is the significance of absent wheezing in this scenario?*

This child is in acute respiratory distress. Leave the patient in a position of comfort and administer supplemental oxygen. Begin treatment with a short-acting nebulized bronchodilator. Place a catheter and give methylprednisolone (Solu-Medrol), 2 mg/kg intravenously. Consider use of magnesium if the patient does not respond to albuterol (salbutamol) and steroid treatment. Monitor the patient for the need for airway management.

Wheezing is a sound caused by airflow obstruction in the intrathoracic airways. Lack of this sound in a child having an acute asthma episode implies that the airflow is severely decreased. This is a more dangerous sign than audible wheezing.

A 10-month-old infant born at 28 weeks' gestation presents to the ED 4 months after discharge from the hospital neonatal intensive care unit. He is receiving long-term home oxygen therapy and was stable until 2 days ago when he developed upper respiratory tract infection (URI) symptoms followed by increased respiratory rate and increased oxygen requirements. On presentation in the ED, he is alert, he shows signs of increase in work of breathing (nasal flaring and retraction), and his color is pale. Vital signs include a respiratory rate of 60/min, heart rate of 160/min, temperature of 37.9°C (100.2°F), and oxygen saturation of 88%. He has diffuse wheezing on examination without rales. Your initial management includes supplemental oxygen and nebulized albuterol (salbutamol) therapy. His oxygen saturation improves to 95% with 4 L of oxygen by nasal cannula. Further assessment shows a right otitis media and clear rhinorrhea on detailed physical examination.

1. *What is your differential diagnosis?*
2. *What are your management priorities?*

Viral illnesses are common causes of acute pulmonary deterioration in infants with BPD. Respiratory syncytial virus is the most common of these and frequently results in hospitalization. Immunoprophylaxis for RSV is recommended for specific infants with chronic lung disease, and this child fulfills those criteria. Respiratory syncytial virus, influenza, and adenovirus should be considered. Frequently, RSV is associated with otitis media and pneumonia.

Assess airway, work of breathing, and circulation. The oxygen saturation will help you titrate the correct amount of oxygen the child will need. If the child is working hard to breathe, then give nothing orally, establish intravenous access, and consider whether the child will need ventilatory support. Medication options have been described previously.

A 16-year-old boy who has been followed in the cystic fibrosis (CF) center in the hospital presents to the ED. He has been gradually losing weight and has been admitted for intravenous antibiotic therapy twice in the past 3 months. His lung function studies show a moderate to severe decrease in forced expiratory volume in 1 second. He presents today with acute onset of sharp chest pain radiating to the right shoulder. He is alert and anxious, sitting in the tripod position; he is tachypneic and has no retractions; and his color is pale with perioral cyanosis. Vital signs include a respiratory rate of 40/min, heart rate of 150/min, and oxygen saturation of 80% on room air. Supplemental oxygen is delivered with a nonrebreather mask. Arterial blood gas analysis results are as follows: F_{IO_2} 0.6, pH 7.4, PCO_2 33 mm Hg, PO_2 83 mm Hg, and bicarbonate 20.7 mEq/L. He is barrel chested, and breath sounds are significantly decreased on the right side. Hyperresonance is noted to percussion on the right side.

1. *What is the most likely cause of his chest pain?*
2. *What are your management priorities?*

Pneumothorax can be seen in up to 23% of patients with CF with moderate to severe pulmonary disease. Typically, the onset is acute. Pain can radiate to the shoulder, and the patient might be acutely dyspneic. Acute-onset chest pain in a patient with CF should be addressed immediately.

Supplemental oxygen should be given immediately to all patients with respiratory distress. Pneumothorax greater than 10% should be treated with chest tube thoracostomy.

CASE SUMMARY 7

A 2-year-old boy with asthma presents to the ED with a 1-week history of upper respiratory symptoms followed by increased cough and wheezing over the past 2 days. His mother has been giving him albuterol (salbutamol) treatments every 4 hours at home without resolution or significant improvement. On arrival in the ED, he is alert and in no acute distress and has audible wheezes; his color is normal. Vital signs include a respiratory rate of 40/min, heart rate of 150/min, temperature (rectal) of 39°C (102.2°F), and oxygen saturation of 93% on room air. Crackles are heard over the right anterior chest wall.

1. *What are your management priorities?*
2. *What study would be most useful to you in evaluating this child?*

Fever and respiratory difficulty in a child with respiratory disease should raise the possibility of pneumonia. In this child, priorities include administration of supplemental oxygen to keep saturations at 94% and intravenous access for hydration and administration of intravenous corticosteroids. Treatment with a short-acting bronchodilator and appropriate antibiotics is indicated by factors discussed previously.

Pulse oximetry and chest radiography will be most helpful in the evaluation. The oxygen saturation level will help guide oxygen therapy, and the chest radiograph will provide a diagnosis and need for further evaluation and treatment.

CASE SUMMARY 8

An infant with acute respiratory distress is brought to the ED by his father. The boy was well until yesterday, when he developed a runny nose and low-grade fever. This morning he is irritable, refuses his bottle, and has vomited twice. On examination he is poorly responsive to his surroundings, he has marked increased work of breathing with stridor and intercostal retractions, and his color is pale to gray with circumoral cyanosis. Vital signs include a respiratory rate of 40/min, heart rate of 60/min, and oxygen saturation of 84% on room air. He has decreased air entry bilaterally and mild end-expiratory wheezes.

1. *What are your initial management priorities?*
2. *What is your differential diagnosis?*

This case illustrates that a normal respiratory rate does not always signify that a child is breathing well. You would expect that an infant with this history would need to increase his respiratory rate to maintain adequate oxygenation and ventilation. A respiratory rate of 40/min can also indicate that the infant is tiring. This finding, in conjunction with the other clinical findings, suggests respiratory failure. Management priorities include positioning the head, opening the airway, suctioning the airway, beginning bag-mask ventilation with 100% oxygen, and preparing for RSI.

This is likely respiratory failure. Sepsis, occult trauma, and metabolic disease should be considered as possible causes, but this history is most consistent with croup, which develops within a few days, beginning with URI symptoms followed by inspiratory stridor and respiratory decompensation.

chapter 3

Shock

Marianne Gausche-Hill, MD, FAAP, FACEP
Casey Buitenhuys, MD

Objectives

1 Define shock and categorize shock types in children.

2 Distinguish septic shock from other forms of shock, including hypovolemic, distributive, obstructive, and cardiogenic.

3 Outline management of shock based on etiology.

4 Discuss goal-directed therapy for septic shock and identify differences in the treatment of neonates and children.

Chapter Outline

Introduction
Pathophysiology of Circulatory Shock
Hypovolemic Shock
Distributive Shock
Obstructive Shock
Cardiogenic Shock

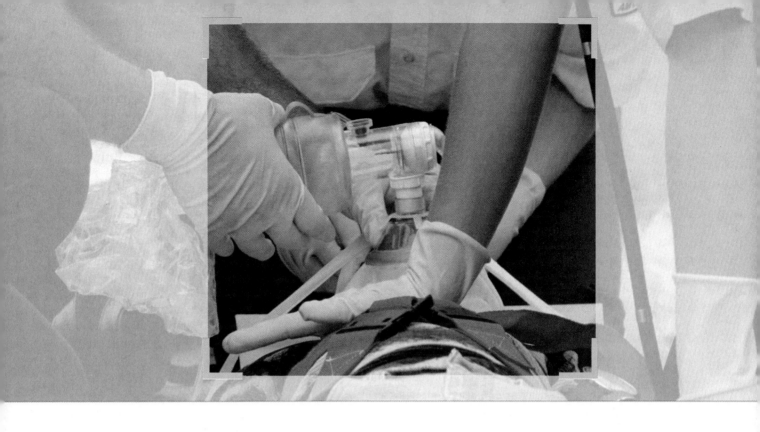

A 9-year-old boy is brought to the emergency department (ED) for joint pain and fever for the last 5 days. He was playing soccer last week and fell. He was initially experiencing left arm and right hip pain but now cannot walk secondary to pain in his ankles and feet. Two days ago he was seen by his pediatrician for a sore throat and then developed nonbloody diarrhea. His past medical history is unremarkable, and he takes no medicine and has no allergies. All childhood immunizations are up to date. He is uncomfortable, but interactive. He is tachypneic, but without retractions or stridor. His skin reveals generalized erythema, almost a "sunburn appearance," yet his hands and feet are cool to the touch and appear cyanotic. His vital signs are heart rate (HR) of 141/min, respiratory rate of 22/min, blood pressure of 94/56 mm Hg, temperature of 39°C (102.2°F), and pulse oximetry of 100% on room air. He has a petechial rash on the soles of his feet, and diffuse swelling and tenderness of the ankles and left wrist, and diffuse muscular tenderness. He is neurologically intact but will not bear weight secondary to pain.

1. What is your initial assessment?
2. What are your initial management priorities?
3. What are the most likely causes based on this assessment?
4. What complications can arise from this condition?

Introduction

At the cellular level, shock results from the inability of the body to use adenosine triphosphate (ATP) to support cellular functions. Without ATP, all organ systems will stop functioning. Plasma glucose is circulated through the body and delivered to all cells. Cells uptake glucose and catabolize it to pyruvate in a process called glycolysis. This process produces a small amount of ATP for the body. Pyruvate is then metabolized through the Krebs cycle to produce an additional small amount of ATP and a large amount of electron donors in the form of flavin adenine dinucleotide and nicotinamide adenine dinucleotide. These electron donors are then transported into the mitochondria of cells, where they release their electrons into the electron transport chain. By reacting with several protein complexes and using oxygen as an electron acceptor, a large amount of ATP is produced, which can then be used for vital cellular functions.

The inability to produce ATP and the resultant multiorgan system failure can be caused by multiple breakdowns in this system. An adequate cardiopulmonary system is necessary for the delivery of oxygen to the plasma and red blood cells and the circulation of bound and unbound oxygen to all cells in the body. An adequate hematologic system is necessary for the adequate binding and delivery of oxygen to the tissues. If there is a failure to deliver oxygen from the lungs and into the bloodstream, as in a severe pneumonia, then despite adequate perfusion, oxygen delivery to cells would cease, and ATP synthesis via the electron transport chain would be minimal. If there is a failure of adequate hemoglobin, as in the case of severe chronic anemia, despite adequate oxygenation and circulation or if the electron transport chain were nonfunctional, as in the case of cyanide poisoning, despite an adequate hemoglobin, oxygenation, and circulatory system, ATP would then be synthesized inefficiently via anaerobic methods and the lactic acid pathway, resulting in hypoxemia, metabolic acidosis, and organ failure.

The most common cause of shock in children, and the focus of this chapter, is failure of circulation (inadequate perfusion) and its resultant multisystem organ failure.

Pathophysiology of Circulatory Shock

Cardiac output (CO) is governed by both the contractility of the heart (stroke volume [SV]) and the rate at which the heart contracts (HR).[1]

$$CO = HR \times SV$$

It is also proportional to the mean arterial pressure (MAP) divided by the systemic vascular resistance (SVR).

$$CO \propto MAP/SVR$$

In the circulatory system, SVR is controlled by adrenergic and cholinergic receptors in the vascular smooth muscle. The MAP is reflective of the SVR but is also an indicator of intravascular volume. Therefore, any state that decreases the contractile rate or strength of the heart, ability of the body to increase SVR, or the intravascular volume will impair CO and cause circulatory shock.

Compensated shock refers to a physiologic insult strong enough to cause shock without end organ dysfunction. The human body has multiple systems in place to compensate for shock. In the cardiovascular system, HR, SV, and SVR all increase. Circulation is diverted away from nonessential structures (eg, skin, skeletal muscle, and splanchnic organs) and toward the brain, heart, kidneys, and adrenal glands.[2]

There are several subtypes of circulatory shock. Hypovolemic shock refers to a state of decreased intravascular volume that results in a decreased CO. The causes are multiple, including hemorrhage, gastrointestinal volume loss, increased insensible water loss, and other causes of severe dehydration. Distributive shock refers to a state of normal intravascular volume and decreased SVR, which results in a decreased CO. Anaphylaxis, sepsis, medication overdose, and spinal cord injury are all causative disease processes. Obstructive shock refers to a state of normal intravascular volume and SVR, whereby a mechanical obstruction causes either decreased venous return to the heart or decreased left ventricular outflow, thereby decreasing CO. Significant causes of obstructive shock include pericardial tamponade, tension pneumothorax, severe pulmonary embolus, severe pulmonary hypertension, and hypertrophic cardiomyopathy. Cardiogenic shock refers to a state of normal to elevated intravascular volume and SVR but decreased CO secondary to poor myocardial contraction. Significant causes include myocarditis, myocardial infarction, severe bradyarrhythmia or tachyarrhythmia, cardiomyopathy, or congenital heart lesions.[1,2]

Clinical Features

In children, differences in total body water percentage, metabolic rate, and mechanisms of compensation make the diagnosis of shock difficult. In children, the main mechanisms for compensation include significant increases in SVR and increases in HR without changes in SV. A child can be in profound shock but have minimal changes to their blood pressure. Despite the higher percentage of total body water, children are metabolically more active than their adult counterparts and can quickly deteriorate with relatively small volume losses. Tables 3-1 and 3-2 differentiate signs and symptoms in various types of shock, and Table 3-2 also describes management strategies.

The methodical approach to the pediatric patient in shock involves a rapid assessment of patients using the Pediatric Assessment Triangle. The Pediatric Assessment Triangle, as described in Chapter 1, Pediatric Assessment, uses a quick impression of patients using three vital components: appearance, work of breathing, and circulation to the skin. Children in compensated shock can present with circulatory abnormalities, such as pale or mottled skin. Further assessment might reveal delayed capillary refill, tachycardia, dry mucous membranes, and poor skin turgor.

They can also appear irritable, agitated, or restless. On respiratory examination, they can have an effortless tachypnea as they attempt to compensate from a metabolic acidosis that is developing. Children in decompensated shock might present with all of these findings, including profound somnolence, lethargy, and listlessness with or without respiratory compromise.

Management

Once a child is identified as possibly being in a state of shock, rapid intravenous access, oxygen supplementation, and directed therapy of the suspected shock subtype should be initiated as soon as possible.

Hypovolemic Shock

The most common type of circulatory failure in children is hypovolemic shock. In developing countries, hypovolemic shock from acute diarrheal illnesses remains a major cause of mortality in children. In the United States, mortality from

TABLE 3-1 Signs and Symptoms of Hypovolemic, Distributive, Septic, and Cardiogenic Shock			
	Hypovolemic Shock	Distributive or Septic Shock	Cardiogenic Shock
Level of consciousness	Early—normal or anxious Late—agitated, confused, lethargic	Early—normal or anxious Late—agitated, confused, lethargic	Early—normal or anxious Late—agitated, confused, lethargic
Respiratory rate and effort	Effortless tachypnea	Effortless tachypnea	Increased rate Increased work of breathing
Breath sounds	Clear	Clear (might have crackles if pneumonia)	Crackles, grunting
Heart rate	Increased	Increased	Increased
Pulses	Weak, thready	Early—bounding Late—weak, thready	Weak, thready
Skin perfusion	Cool, delayed capillary refill time	Early—warm, brisk capillary refill time Late—cool, delayed capillary refill time	Cool, mottled, delayed capillary refill time

American Heart Association. *PALS Provider Manual.* Dallas, TX: American Heart Association; 2002.

TABLE 3-2 Signs, Symptoms, and Management of Hypovolemic, Septic, Distributive, and Cardiogenic Shock

Type of Shock	Pathophysiology	Signs and Symptoms	Treatment
Hypovolemic	↓CO, ↑SVR intravascular with or without interstitial volume loss	↑HR, ↓pulses, delayed CR, hyperpnea, dry skin, sunken eyes, oliguria, BP normal until late	Repeat boluses of 20 mL/kg of crystalloid as indicated. Blood products as indicated for acute blood loss.
Septic*	↑CO, ↓SVR (classic adult, 20% pediatric)	↑HR, ↓BP, ↓pulses, delayed CR, hyperpnea, MS changes, third spacing, edema	Repeat boluses of 20 mL/kg of crystalloid; might need >60 mL/kg in first hour. Consider colloid if poor response to crystalloid. Pharmacologic support of BP with dopamine or norepinephrine (noradrenaline).
	↓CO, ↑SVR (60% pediatric)	↑HR, normal to ↓BP, ↓pulses, delayed CR, hyperpnea, MS changes, third spacing, edema	Repeat boluses of 20 mL/kg of crystalloid; might need >60 mL/kg in first hour. Consider colloid if poor response to crystalloid. Pharmacologic support of CO with dopamine or epinephrine (adrenaline).
	↓CO, ↓SVR (20% pediatric)	↑HR, ↓BP, ↓pulses, delayed CR, hyperpnea, MS changes, third spacing, edema	Repeat boluses of 20 mL/kg of crystalloid; might need >60 mL/kg in first hour. Consider colloid if poor response to crystalloid. Pharmacologic support of CO and BP with dopamine and epinephrine (adrenaline).
Distributive	Anaphylaxis: ↑CO, ↓SVR	Angioedema, rapid third spacing of fluids, ↓BP, respiratory distress	Repeat boluses of 20 mL/kg of crystalloid as indicated. Pharmacologic support of SVR with norepinephrine (noradrenaline) or phenylephrine.
	Spinal cord injury: normal CO, ↓SVR	↓BP with normal HR, paralysis with loss of vascular tone	Pharmacologic support of SVR with norepinephrine (noradrenaline) or phenylephrine. Fluid resuscitation as indicated by clinical status and associated injuries.
Cardiogenic	↓CO, normal to ↑SVR	Normal to ↑HR, ↓pulses, delayed CR, oliguria, JVD, hepatomegaly, BP normal until late in course	Pharmacologic support of CO with dobutamine, milrinone, dopamine. Judicious fluid replacement as indicated clinically.

*In regions with limited access to critical care resources, treat all forms of septic shock with an initial fluid bolus of 20 mL/kg of crystalloid. Additional fluid boluses should be done with extreme caution. The patient should be reassessed after every fluid bolus.

Abbreviations: BP, blood pressure; CO, cardiac output; CR, capillary refill; HR, heart rate; JVD, jugular venous distension; MS, mental status; SVR, systemic vascular resistance.

McKiernan CA, Lieberman SA. Circulatory shock in children: An overview. *Pediatr Rev.* 2005;26:451–460

hypovolemic shock is decreasing steadily but remains an important cause for hospital admission and frequent ED visits.

Hypovolemic shock can be categorized into two major subtypes: hemorrhagic and nonhemorrhagic. The causes of hypovolemic shock are listed in Table 3-3.

Etiology

Hemorrhagic-hypovolemic shock can be caused by trauma or it can be atraumatic. An adult can present after trauma in hemorrhagic-hypovolemic shock with major bleeding into the thorax, abdominopelvic cavity, retroperitoneum, bilateral thigh compartments, and onto "the street." A child can present with significant hemorrhagic-hypovolemic shock by bleeding into all of these locations and with intracranial bleeding. In addition to trauma, hemorrhagic-hypovolemic shock can present after gastrointestinal bleeding or surgery.

Nonhemorrhagic hypovolemic shock most commonly presents after significant vomiting and

TABLE 3-3 Common Causes of Hypovolemic Shock in Children

Hemorrhagic
- Gastrointestinal bleeding
- Surgery
- Trauma
- Hepatic or splenic rupture
- Major vessel injury
- Intracranial bleeding
- Long bone fractures

Nonhemorrhagic
- Vomiting/diarrhea
- Heat stroke/water deprivation
- Pharmacologic (eg, diuretics)
- Burns
- Nephrotic syndrome
- Pancreatitis
- Diabetes mellitus
- Diabetes insipidus

McKiernan CA, Lieberman SA. Circulatory shock in children: An overview. *Pediatr Rev.* 2005;26:451–460

YOUR FIRST CLUE

Signs and Symptoms of Circulatory Shock

- Pale, mottled, or cyanotic skin
- Tachycardia
- Tachypnea
- Delayed capillary refill
- Hypotension
- Altered appearance (irritability, restless, listless, lethargic, somnolent, altered level of consciousness, poor tone)

Clinical Features

Children in hemorrhagic shock will present with signs and symptoms similar to nonhemorrhagic hypovolemic shock, depending on their advanced trauma life support degree of hemorrhage. This hemorrhagic shock classification is listed in Table 3-4. In children with a history of trauma, signs and symptoms might be related to the site of injury and bleeding. Abdominal distention, tenderness, and ecchymosis might indicate an intra-abdominal injury. Decreased breath sounds, chest pain, paradoxical motion, and chest wall trauma can indicate an intrathoracic injury. Altered mental status in a patient with head trauma can

diarrhea. Viral gastroenteritis is the most common cause, but bacterial enteritis, gastrointestinal outflow obstructions, and hepatobiliary causes are also common. In addition to gastrointestinal losses, patients can present in hypovolemic shock with severe diabetic ketoacidosis, diabetes insipidus, burns, water deprivation, and pancreatitis.

TABLE 3-4 Hemorrhagic Shock Classification

Class	Class I	Class II	Class III	Class IV
Estimated blood loss	0%–15%	15%–30%	30%–40%	>40%
Symptoms	• Minimally symptomatic	• Anxiety • Irritable	• Confusion • Agitation	• Lethargic • Comatose
Signs	• Minimal tachycardia • Capillary refill might be prolonged	• Tachycardia • Decreased pulse pressure • Tachypnea • Cool, clammy skin • Normal blood pressure	• Profound tachycardia • Marked tachypnea • Oliguria • Markedly prolonged capillary refill • Decreased blood pressure	• Profound tachycardia • Cold/mottled extremities • Very narrow pulse pressure • Decreased blood pressure • Anuria

Advanced Trauma Life Support. Student Course Manual. 8th ed. American College of Surgeons Committee on Trauma. Chicago: American College of Surgeons, 2008 indicate a significant head injury. Back pain and flank ecchymosis can indicate a retroperitoneal injury, and significant bleeding from any site can be a precipitant of hemorrhagic shock.

Patients who present with nonhemorrhagic hypovolemic shock might have an antecedent diarrheal illness, nausea, or vomiting related to a medical or surgical condition. Patients can present with increased urinary output related to concurrent diabetes mellitus or diabetes insipidus. If patients present acutely, signs and symptoms of hypovolemic shock can be similar to those with hemorrhagic shock.

Diagnostic Studies

Laboratory
Patients with hemorrhagic-hypovolemic shock should undergo serial measurements of their hemoglobin or hematocrit. It is important to be aware that patients presenting with acute life-threatening hemorrhagic shock can have initially normal values. In addition, patient should have renal function tested and serum calcium levels measured to assess a baseline function in preparation for massive transfusion. Blood samples for typing and cross-matching should also be sent to the laboratory but should not delay transfusion in the patient in acute shock. Coagulation profiles should be determined for all patients at risk for coagulopathy.

Radiology
Patients with significant traumatic hemorrhagic shock should undergo imaging dedicated to uncovering the source of hemorrhage. Computed tomography is the study of choice for cranial and retroperitoneal sources. Computed tomography can be selectively used in stable patients with abdominopelvic trauma in mild resolved shock or for patients with signs of severe multisystem trauma. A focused abdominal sonography for trauma (FAST) examination can be performed at bedside to assess for significant abdominopelvic injury. Plain radiographs are usually sufficient for suspected femur fractures or thoracic injuries.

Management
Children presenting with nonhemorrhagic hypovolemic shock require early aggressive fluid re-suscitation. For those children in decompensated shock, multiple 20-mL/kg boluses of isotonic crystalloid can be titrated to normalization of appearance and skin findings or until rales or hepatomegaly develop. Vasopressors are not indicated and generally used only for fluid-refractory shock.

Hemorrhagic hypovolemic shock requires early aggressive resuscitation with blood products and prompt surgical consultation. Two large-bore peripheral intravenous catheters or intraosseous catheters should be placed. Type O negative packed red blood cells should be transfused in aliquots of 10 mL/kg for exsanguinating hemorrhage if fully cross-matched or type-specific blood is unavailable. Children presenting in shock after trauma might require surgical intervention; therefore, an immediate surgical consultation or transfer to trauma center is essential.

Distributive Shock

Distributive shock occurs when SVR and blood pressure decrease despite attempts made to increase CO. There are multiple causes of distributive shock: anaphylactic shock, neurogenic shock, and septic shock.

Anaphylactic Shock

Anaphylactic shock is a severe systemic reaction to an allergic stimulus. An ingested, inhaled, transdermally absorbed, or percutaneously acquired allergen causes preformed IgE to bind the allergen and then activate mast cells throughout the body. Children in anaphylactic shock, as opposed to simple urticaria or allergic reaction, have profound levels of circulating IgE and have widespread mast cell activation. Activated mast cells release histamine and other inflammatory mediators, causing vasodilatation, capillary leak, and angioedema.

Etiology
An estimated 29,000 anaphylactic reactions occur each year in the United States with approximately 150 fatalities. The mortality rate in children is less than 2%.[3] Foods cause most anaphylactic

reactions, with peanuts and other tree nuts being the most common antigens. Insect stings, especially from the Hymenoptera order, are a common cause as well. Medications have been implicated in anaphylactic reactions, with antibiotics being the most common class implicated.

Clinical Features

Children presenting with anaphylactic shock can present with other signs and symptoms of a widespread type I hypersensitivity reaction. Difficulty speaking, throat tingling, stridor, and dysphagia might be present with upper airway angioedema. Nausea, vomiting, and abdominal pain might be present with gastrointestinal angioedema. Diffuse pruritus and urticaria may be present. In addition, anxiety, weakness, tachypnea, wheezing, stridor, and evidence of poor perfusion might be present.

Diagnostic Studies

There are no specific laboratory tests or diagnostic imaging studies necessary when evaluating the patient with anaphylactic shock.

Management

Children presenting in anaphylactic shock should have immediate large-bore intravenous or intraosseous catheter placed. Intravascular crystalloid fluids should be given in 20-mL/kg boluses. In addition to crystalloid, multiple medications can assist in anaphylactic shock. Epinephrine (adrenaline) can be administered intramuscularly or intravenously, depending on severity of symptoms. If administered intramuscularly, 0.01 mg/kg of the 1:1,000 solution can be administered to a maximum of 0.3 mg. If administered intravenously, 0.01 mg/kg of the 1:10,000 solution can be administered to a maximum of 0.5 mg with or without an epinephrine (adrenaline) drip (0.1–1 mcg/kg per minute). Epinephrine (adrenaline) counteracts the vasodilatation caused by the inflammatory cytokines and histamine, raises SVR, improves cardiac inotropy, and decreases capillary permeability and angioedema. Intravenous histamine$_1$ antagonists, such as diphenhydramine (1.25 mg/kg per dose: to maximum of 50 mg), should also be given to decrease further mast cell degranulation. Histamine$_2$ antagonists have also been demonstrated to decrease severity and length of anaphylactoid reactions. Multiple histamine$_2$ antagonists exist in intravenous form. Lastly, intravenous steroids have also been shown to decrease recurrence of symptoms and shorten symptom duration and should be given accordingly.

Neurogenic Shock

Traumatic disruption of the cervicothoracic spinal cord can cause a transient state of hypotension and bradycardia termed neurogenic shock. This constellation of symptoms results from decreased sympathetic outflow to the heart and vasculature, causing a decrease in SVR, HR, and SV. The sympathetic nervous system contains central neurons that start in the reticular system of the brain and then synapse in the lateral gray matter of the thoracolumbar spinal cord. An acute disruption proximal to the thoracolumbar spinal cord decreases all efferent signaling to the sympathetic nervous system. Because the parasympathetic nervous system is controlled above the level of the cervical cord, the end result is unopposed parasympathetic stimulation.

Etiology

Blunt or penetrating trauma to the neck can cause cervical disruption. The degree of sympathectomy depends on the completeness of injury.

YOUR FIRST CLUE

Signs and Symptoms of Anaphylactic Shock

- Pruritus
- Urticaria
- Angioedema
- Tachypnea, wheezing, or stridor
- Delayed capillary refill
- Tachycardia
- Hypotension

Clinical Features

Patients in neurogenic shock present with signs and symptoms of cervicothoracic neurologic disruption. The preganglionic sympathetic neurons are located in the intermediolateral cell column lamina VII, which is in the lateral aspect of the gray matter in the cervicothoracic spinal cord. Spinothalamic and corticospinal tracts are in close proximity to this area, so disruption of these cell bodies might result in paralysis and sensory deficits. In addition, patients present with signs and symptoms of poor perfusion. Hypotension and paradoxical bradycardia are usually present due to the lack of sympathetic tone to the myocardium and vasculature. One should be aware that hypotension and bradycardia in the traumatized patient does not exclude significant hemorrhage as a cause of shock. Patients with significant cord injuries and neurogenic shock can have hemorrhage without significant tachycardia.

Diagnostic Studies

Laboratory

Laboratory tests to exclude and/or manage hypovolemic hemorrhagic shock should be performed. There are no specific tests in the evaluation of neurogenic shock.

Radiology

Cervical computed tomography has largely supplanted plain radiography in the initial evaluation of the neurologically afflicted trauma patient. It provides detailed information regarding cervical spine fractures, ligamentous instability, and subluxations. Magnetic resonance imaging is also indicated in the evaluation of the neurologically afflicted trauma patient for several reasons. First, the incidence of spinal cord injury without radiographic abnormality is 20% to 36% of pediatric patients with traumatic myelopathy. In addition, magnetic resonance imaging can aid in the prognostication of injuries. Cervical cord contusions and ligamentous injuries can have some functional recovery, whereas cervical cord lacerations and transections generally demonstrate poorer outcomes.

Management

Immediate cervical spine immobilization and management of airway and breathing take priority. Circulatory support can be managed with judicious application of intravenous crystalloid fluids in 20-mL/kg boluses initially. However, because the primary problem is a loss of sympathetic tone, use of a vasopressor, such as norepinephrine (noradrenaline) or dopamine, temporarily to increase SVR and improve perfusion to an already injured cord is of greater efficacy. Early use of systemic steroids are controversial, with recent data revealing no significant trend toward benefit.[4]

Septic Shock

Sepsis remains a major cause of morbidity and mortality among children.[5] The sepsis-associated mortality rate decreased from 97% in 1966[6] to 9% among young infants in the early 1990s.[7] Although there have been significant improvements in the treatment of sepsis and septic shock, it still remains a significant cause of childhood mortality, with more than 4,300 deaths annually.[8] This equates to approximately 7% of all childhood mortality and an estimated annual total cost of $1.97 billion.[8] This discussion does not apply to resource-limited settings.

Definitions

Because children differ in their response to an infectious agent, it is useful to qualify age groups so that standardized vital signs and laboratory criteria can be used. In 2005, an expert consensus panel agreed on age group definitions for pediatric patients based on observed differences in vital sign parameters and patterns of organ dysfunction.[9] See Table 3-5 for list of ages and definitions.

TABLE 3-5 Pediatric Age Groups for Severe Sepsis Definitions	
Newborn	0 days to 1 week
Neonate	1 week to 1 month
Infant	1 month to 1 year
Toddler and preschool	2 to 5 years
School-age child	6 to 12 years
Adolescent and young adult	13 to <18 years

Goldstein B, Giroir B, Randolph A, et al. International pediatric sepsis consensus conference: Definitions for sepsis and organ dysfunction in pediatrics. *Pediatr Crit Care Med.* 2005;6:2–8.

To qualify a patient as having septic shock, one needs to understand the requirements for having both sepsis and shock. Shock has already been defined. Systemic inflammatory response syndrome (SIRS) is the nonspecific inflammatory process that occurs after trauma, pancreatitis, infection, and other diseases.[10] Sepsis was then further defined as SIRS criteria with an infectious source.[10] Because the original SIRS criteria were based on adult-specific vital signs and laboratory criteria, an expert consensus panel refined this criteria to their pediatric age-specific groups.[9,11-18] Table 3-6 lists the definitions for SIRS and reflects these expert consensus panel changes. Severe sepsis was even further defined as sepsis plus cardiovascular organ dysfunction or acute respiratory distress or two or more other organ system dysfunctions (renal, hepatic,

neurologic, or hematologic). Septic shock was then defined as sepsis and cardiovascular organ dysfunction.

Age-specific SIRS criteria have been modified by expert panel groups.[9] An abnormal temperature is required for SIRS diagnosis in children. Children with core temperatures higher than 38.5°C (101.3°F) are considered to have fever. Children with core temperatures lower than 36°C (96.8°F) are considered hypothermic. Oral, bladder, rectal, and central catheter probes are considered sufficient locations for temperature acquisition. However, any child with a documented fever at home by a reliable source within 4 hours of presentation can be assumed to be febrile. Tachycardia is age specific and defined as a HR greater than 2 SDs for age in the absence of exogenous stimuli that is sustained for at least

TABLE 3-6 Definitions of Systemic Inflammatory Response Syndrome (SIRS), Infection, Sepsis, Severe Sepsis, and Septic Shock*

SIRS†

The presence of at least two of the following four criteria, one of which must be abnormal temperature or leukocyte count:

- Core temperature of >38.5°C (101.3°F) or <36°C (96.8°F).
- Tachycardia, defined as a mean heart rate 2 SD, above normal for age in the absence of external stimulus, long-term drug use, or painful stimuli; or otherwise unexplained persistent elevation during a 0.5- to 4-hour period **OR for children younger than 1 years: bradycardia, defined as a mean heart rate <10th percentile for age in the absence of external vagal stimulus, β-blocker drugs, or congenital heart disease; or otherwise unexplained persistent depression during a 0.5-hour period.**
- Mean respiratory rate >2 SDs above normal for age or mechanical ventilation for an acute process not related to underlying neuromuscular disease or the receipt of general anesthesia.
  - Leukocyte count elevated or depressed for age (not secondary to chemotherapy-induced leukopenia) or >10% immature neutrophils.

Infection

A suspected or proven (by positive culture, tissue stain, or polymerase chain reaction test result) infection caused by any pathogen OR a clinical syndrome associated with a high probability of infection. Evidence of infection includes positive findings on clinical examination, imaging, or laboratory tests (eg, white blood cells in a normally sterile body fluid, perforated viscus, chest radiograph consistent with pneumonia, petechial or purpuric rash, or purpura fulminans).

Sepsis

- SIRS in the presence of or as a result of suspected or proven infection.

Severe sepsis

- **Sepsis plus one of the following: cardiovascular organ dysfunction OR acute respiratory distress syndrome OR two or more other organ dysfunctions.**

Septic shock

- Sepsis and cardiovascular organ dysfunction.

Abbreviation: SD, standard deviation.

*Modifications from the adult definitions are highlighted in boldface.

†Age-specific ranges for physiologic and laboratory variables; core temperature must be measured by rectal, bladder, oral, or central catheter probe.

Goldstein B, Giroir B, Randolph A, et al. International pediatric sepsis consensus conference: Definitions for sepsis and organ dysfunction in pediatrics. *Pediatr Crit Care Med.* 2005;6:2–8.

30 minutes.[9] In addition, age-specific tachypnea, leukocytosis, and leukopenia are all criteria for inclusion in SIRS. In contrast to the original adult criteria, pediatric SIRS requires both temperature and leukocyte abnormalities. See Table 3-7 for age-appropriate criteria.

The definitions of severe sepsis and septic shock in particular are problematic. Because most children will maintain their blood pressure until they are severely ill,[19] there is no requirement for systemic hypotension to make the diagnosis of septic shock. Shock can occur long before hypotension occurs in children. The current definition includes the following findings despite the administration of 40 mL/kg of isotonic intravenous fluid boluses: tachycardia greater than 2 SDs for age with signs of decreased perfusion, including peripheral pulses compared with central pulses, altered alertness, flash capillary refill or capillary refill greater than 2 seconds, mottled or cool extremities, or decreased urine output.[20] In addition, the use of vasoactive drugs at any time, unexplained metabolic acidosis, elevated arterial lactate level, oliguria, or a core to peripheral temperature gap of greater than 3°C are indicative of shock and cardiovascular dysfunction. Although systemic hypotension is not a requirement for the diagnosis of septic shock, its presence is confirmatory. Current definitions of organ system dysfunction are listed in Table 3-8.

Further definition of septic shock has been suggested by expert panels.[21] Cold shock is defined similarly as described above but is characterized by a high-SVR, low-CO state. Patients in cold shock demonstrate capillary refill of more than 2 seconds, narrow pulse pressures, mottled and cool extremities, and oliguria. Warm shock is defined similarly as described above but is characterized by a low-SVR, high/low-CO state. Patients in warm shock demonstrate flash capillary refill, bounding pulses, and wide pulse pressures. Fluid-refractory septic shock is defined as cardiovascular dysfunction that persists despite 60 mL/kg of fluid resuscitation. Dopamine-resistant septic shock is defined as cardiovascular dysfunction that persists despite adequate fluid resuscitation in addition to administration of dopamine infusion at 10 mcg/kg per minute. Catecholamine-resistant shock is defined as cardiovascular dysfunction that persists despite adequate fluid resuscitation, dopamine infusion,

TABLE 3-7 Age-Specific Vital Signs and Laboratory Variables for SIRS*

Age Group	Heart Rate/min		Respiratory Rate, min	Leukocyte Count, ×10⁹/mcL	Systolic Blood Pressure, mm Hg
	Tachycardia	Bradycardia			
0 days to 1 week	>180	<100	>50	>34	<65
1 week to 1 month	>180	<100	>40	>19.5 or <5.5	<75
1 month to 1 year	>180	<90	>34	>17.5 or <5.5	<100
2 to 5 years	>140	NA	>22	>15.5 or <6	<94
6 to 12 years	>130	NA	>18	>13.5 or <4.5	<105
13 to <18 years	>110	NA	>14	>11 or <4.5	<117

Abbreviation: NA, not applicable.

Goldstein B, Giroir B, Randolph A, et al. International pediatric sepsis consensus conference: Definitions for sepsis and organ dysfunction in pediatrics. *Pediatr Crit Care Med.* 2005;6:2–8.

*Lower values for heart rate, leukocyte count, and systolic blood pressure are for the 5th percentile and upper values for heart rate, respiration rate, or leukocyte count are for the 95th percentile.

TABLE 3-8 Organ Dysfunction Criteria

Cardiovascular dysfunction

Despite administration of isotonic intravenous fluid bolus ≥40 mL/kg in 1 hour

- Decrease in BP (hypotension) less than 5th percentile for age or systolic BP <2 SDs, below normal for age OR
- Need for vasoactive drug to maintain BP in normal range (dopamine >5 mcg/kg per minute or dobutamine, epinephrine [adrenaline], or norepinephrine [noradrenaline] at any dose) OR
- Two of the following:
  - Unexplained metabolic acidosis: base deficit >5.0 mEq/L
  - Increased arterial lactate >2 times upper limit of normal
  - Oliguria: urine output <0.5 mL/kg per hour
  - Prolonged capillary refill: >5 seconds
  - Core to peripheral temperature gap >3°C

Respiratory

- Pao_2/Fio_2 <300 in absence of cyanotic heart disease or preexisting lung disease OR
- $Paco_2$ >65 or 20 mm Hg over baseline $Paco_2$ OR
- Proven need or >50% Fio_2 to maintain saturation ≥92% OR
- Need for nonelective invasive or noninvasive mechanical ventilation

Neurologic

- Glasgow Coma Scale score ≤11 OR
- Acute change in mental status with a decrease in Glasgow Coma Scale score ≥3 points from abnormal baseline

Hematologic

- Platelet count <80,000 mm³ or a decline of 50% in platelet count from highest value recorded during the past 3 days for chronic hematology/oncology patients OR
- International normalized ratio >2

Renal

- Serum creatinine ≥2 times upper limit to normal for age or 2-fold increase in baseline creatinine

Hepatic

- Total bilirubin ≥4 mg/dL (not applicable for newborn) OR
- ALT two times the upper limit of normal age

Abbreviations: ALT, alanine aminotransferase; BP, blood pressure; Fio_2, fraction of inspired oxygen.

Goldstein B, Giroir B, Randolph A, et al. International pediatric sepsis consensus conference: Definitions for sepsis and organ dysfunction in pediatrics. *Pediatr Crit Care Med.* 2005;6:2–8.

and the addition of direct-acting catecholamines (ie, epinephrine [adrenaline] or norepinephrine [noradrenaline]). Refractory shock is defined as cardiovascular dysfunction that persists despite goal-directed use of inotropic agents, vasopressors, vasodilators, and maintenance of metabolic and hormonal homeostasis.[21]

Although the definition of SIRS only incorporates vital sign abnormalities and leukocyte abnormalities, there is current evidence investigating the role of biomarkers in the diagnosis of SIRS and sepsis. Elevated sedimentation rate, C-reactive protein level,[22] base deficit, interleukin 6 level,[23] and procalcitonin level[22–24] have all

been suggested as potential biochemical markers of SIRS. The sensitivity and specificity of each marker, as well as its onset and peak during sepsis, are vastly different. More research is needed to test the efficacy of these markers and their possible use as inclusive or exclusive criteria in a SIRS definition.

Pathophysiology

A site of infection occurs when bacteria, viruses, fungi, or protozoa invade a normally sterile site (eg, blood, urine, or cerebrospinal fluid) or overproliferate in a nonsterile site (eg, colon or skin). Most models of sepsis have used bacteria. Gram-positive and gram-negative bacteria induce a variety of proinflammatory mediators, including cytokines. The bacterial cell wall components are known to cause release of these cytokines. Lipopolysaccharide (gram-negative bacteria), peptidoglycan (gram-positive and gram-negative bacteria), and lipoteichoic acid (gram-positive bacteria) are all known entities to cause cytokine release.

Several cytokines are induced, including tumor necrosis factor, interleukin 6, interleukin 1, interleukin 8, and many others. These cytokines act on the vascular smooth muscle and the immune system. Cytokines with pyrogenic capabilities are released as well.

The complement system is also activated, which causes elevated levels of bradykinin and increases vascular permeability, as well as causing vascular smooth muscle relaxation. Nitric oxide is also activated by cytokines, causing smooth muscle relaxation and decreased SVR.

Metabolic demand increases secondary to direct cytokine activity on cellular activity, thermal regulation, and cardiac contractility. Children, unlike their adult counterparts, lose a disproportionate amount of fluid during periods of increased metabolic demand. Tachypnea as a result of metabolic acidosis and direct stimulation from cytokines contributes to significant intravascular volume depletion. Coupled with decreased oral intake, children generally present to the ED with significant hypovolemia.

Clinical Features

Children with septic shock can present with signs and symptoms of shock, such as delayed or flash capillary refill, oliguria, anxiety, or alterations in mental status and tachypnea. Table 3-7 demonstrates SIRS criteria, which are the minimal criteria for presentation of septic shock.

Neonates with septic shock can present more nonspecifically with signs of irritability, increased crying, poor feeding, lethargy, and changes in bowel and bladder patterns. In addition, children can present with signs and symptoms of an infectious process. An abnormally high or low temperature, changes in the urine characteristics, abdominal distention, vomiting, diarrhea, cough, rhinorrhea, bulging or sunken fontanelle, or rashes might be present.

YOUR FIRST CLUE

Signs and Symptoms of Septic Shock
- Fever or hypothermia
- Tachycardia
- Tachypnea
- Petechiae/purpura
- Altered appearance (irritability, increased crying, lethargy)
- Increased or decreased sleeping
- Decreased feeding

Diagnostic Studies

Laboratory

White blood cell count should be obtained to check for leukocytosis and leukopenia. Serum chemical analyses should be performed to check for a metabolic acidosis. A serum lactate level can be elevated in septic shock. Urinalysis, urine Gram stain, and urine culture should be performed in all patients with septic shock. Blood cultures should be performed in all patients with septic shock. Coagulation function tests, D-dimer test, and fibrinogen measurement should be performed on all patients with septic shock at risk for disseminated intravascular coagulation. Blood typing and cross-matching should be performed on all patients with suspected anemia and shock. Cerebrospinal fluid studies should be performed on all patients with signs or symptoms of meningitis and all patients younger than 2 months regardless of the symptoms if presenting with septic shock.

Radiology

Patients with hypoxia, wheezing, rales, rhonchi, or a productive cough and sepsis should undergo chest radiography. Any child regardless of symptoms with septic shock should undergo chest radiography to look for source of infection. Children with abdominal pain, tenderness, and suspicion for an intra-abdominal surgical emergency should undergo abdominopelvic computed tomography. Otherwise, selected radiologic studies based on signs and symptoms should be performed.

Management

Septic Shock: Initial Management of the Golden Hour

The first goal of management should be maintenance or restoration of the airway, oxygenation, and circulation to predetermined end points within the first 60 minutes of patient care. Rivers et al[25] first described goal-directed therapy in adult septic patients and demonstrated a 15% reduction in mortality. Previous pediatric studies demonstrated improved outcomes and results in those patients who received early immediate resuscitation versus those patients who received delayed resuscitation.[26,27] **Figure 3.1** summarizes the management pathway for pediatric septic shock.

Airway/Breathing High-flow oxygen should be administered regardless of the oxygenation saturation in the patients with suspected sepsis. This can be accomplished with a nonrebreather mask, bag mask ventilation, or blow-by oxygen. The decision to place an endotracheal tube should be based on clinical assessment of increased work of breathing, hypoventilation, or impaired mental status and should be considered in patients with fluid refractory shock. The patient in early sepsis might demonstrate a metabolic acidosis and respiratory acidosis, whereas the patient in advanced sepsis might demonstrate a mixed acidosis. Awaiting confirmatory laboratory tests, such as an arterial blood gas or lactate measurement, is discouraged. Up to 40% of the CO is used for work of breathing; thus, endotracheal intubation can decrease this strain on CO and can reverse shock.

Aggressive fluid resuscitation is recommended before performing intubation because of relative or absolute hypovolemia, cardiac dysfunction, peripheral vasodilatation, and stress hormone suppression that can accompany induction agents.

Ketamine with or without atropine premedication is the induction agents of choice in septic shock.[28] Ketamine is a central acting N-methyl-D-aspartate blocker that preserves CO and suppresses endogenous inflammatory cytokines without adrenal suppression.[29] Etomidate is a popular induction agent because it maintains blood pressure, has a rapid onset, and has a short duration. However, even one dose used during intubation is independently associated with increased mortality in both children and adults with septic shock.[30,31] Therefore, etomidate use is not recommended in the patients with suspected sepsis. Other agents, such as high-dose opioids, barbiturates, and propofol, cannot be recommended for induction because they depress CO, lower SVR, and can worsen an already perilously low perfusion pressure.

A short-acting neuromuscular blocker can be used to facilitate intubation if the physician is confident that he or she can maintain the airway.

Circulation A peripheral intravenous catheter should be placed immediately with the largest diameter possible. If immediate peripheral access cannot be obtained, then an intraosseous catheter or central vein catheter can be placed. In the neonate, an umbilical venous catheter or an intraosseous catheter can be placed if peripheral access is limited.

Early and aggressive fluid therapy has proven to decrease mortality in pediatric shock models[32] and should commence unless hepatomegaly or rales are present. Fluids should be rapidly given in aliquots of 20-mL/kg boluses up to and greater than 60 mL/kg within the first 15 minutes with close monitoring of perfusion status and/or development of fluid overload. Normalization of capillary refill, decreases in HR, improvement in skin turgor, normalization of mental status, and normalization of urine output are all indicators that a patient is no longer in a shock state. Patients who continually display signs of shock despite 60 mL/kg can be considered to have fluid-refractory shock.

The solution used for initial resuscitation should be based on the physician's experience and preference. Although there is some evidence that supports the use of colloid solutions for initial resuscitation,[33–35] the evidence demonstrates mixed results.[36] Whether a physician chooses to use a crystalloid solution (eg, normal saline or lactated Ringer solution) or a colloid solution (eg, hetastarch [hydroxyethyl starch], or albumin), the solution used should be rapidly administered in 5 minutes and repeated until signs of perfusion improve or signs of fluid overload develop. The use of blood as a volume expander

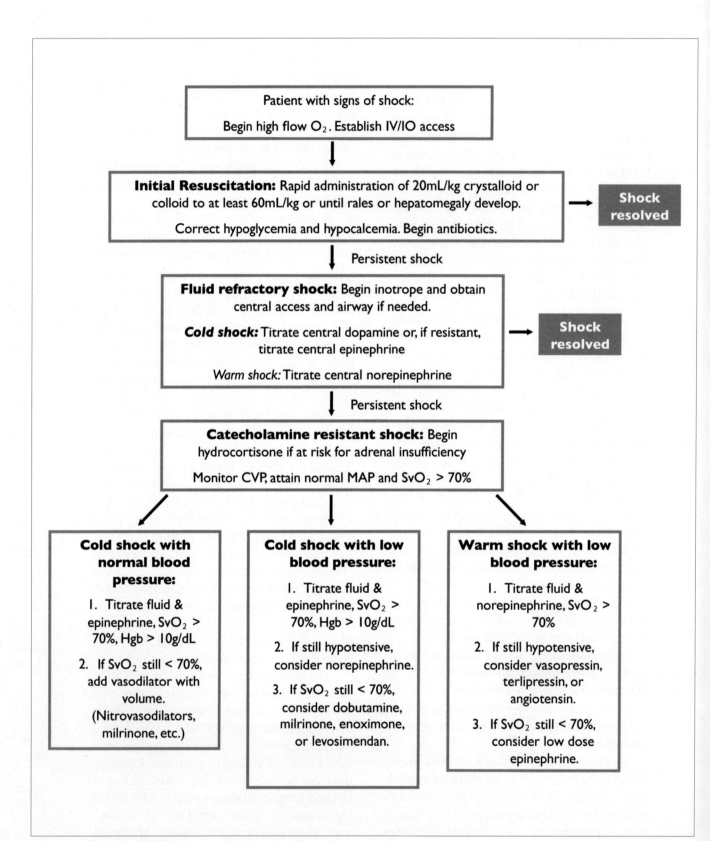

Figure 3.1 Management of pediatric septic shock.

Brierley J, Carcillo JA, Choong K, et al. Clinical practice parameters for hemodynamic support of pediatric and neonatal septic shock: 2007 update from the American College of Critical Care Medicine. *Crit Care Med.* 2009;37:666–688 has been demonstrated to improve oxygen delivery to tissues without improvement in oxygen use.[37] Therefore, no recommendations have been made regarding its routine use. However, transfusions in addition to fluid administration titrated to keep central venous saturation higher than 70% have improved outcomes.[25,38] Transfusion can only currently be recommended in the patient with a hemoglobin level less than 10 g/dL who presents with septic shock and impaired oxygen delivery (SvO_2 <70%).

A patient in fluid-refractory shock should immediately have a second peripheral intravenous catheter placed. If a second peripheral site is unavailable, then an intraosseous or central vein catheter can be used. This second site should immediately be used for initial inotropic therapy. The choice of inotrope should depend on the presentation of the patient.

A patient presenting in fluid-refractory cold shock (high SVR, low CO) will demonstrate delayed capillary refill, cold and mottled extremities, and oliguria. Patients in cold shock should have inotropes directed to improving CO with little effect on SVR. Dopamine infused at a rate of 5 to 9 mcg/kg per minute is a preferred first-line agent with these properties. Dopamine is a catecholamine precursor that binds to dopaminergic receptors at low rates of infusion (2 to 5 mcg/kg per minute), causing renal vasodilatation and improved renal perfusion. At moderate rates of infusion (5 to 10 mcg/kg per minute), it stimulates β-adrenergic receptors, causing increased HR and SV. At high rates of infusion (>10 mcg/kg per minute), it stimulates α-adrenergic receptors, causing arteriolar vasoconstriction and increased SVR.[39] The use of dopamine in adult septic shock has demonstrated worsened mortality rates,[40] but these results have yet to be borne out in pediatric patients. Epinephrine (adrenaline) can be used in fluid-refractory cold shock. Epinephrine (adrenaline) is a naturally occurring catecholamine with β1- and β2-adrenergic receptor affinity with little α-adrenergic affinity. When infused at higher doses (>0.3 mcg/kg per minute), epinephrine (adrenaline) demonstrates significant α-adrenergic activity and increases SVR. Therefore, if epinephrine (adrenaline) is going to be used, then a lower rate of infusion (<0.3 mcg/kg per minute) should be initiated in fluid-refractory cold shock. In very young children (<6 months old), the peripheral stores of epinephrine (adrenaline) and norepinephrine (noradrenaline) are limited, and these patients might be refractory to dopamine infusion. If a patient is presenting with dopamine-refractory cold shock, then epinephrine (adrenaline) should be titrated to effect.

A patient presenting in fluid-refractory warm shock (low SVR, high or normal CO) will demonstrate bounding pulses, flash capillary refill, and warm extremities. Patients in warm shock should have inotropes directed to improving SVR. Norepinephrine (noradrenaline) is a naturally occurring catecholamine with these properties. Norepinephrine (noradrenaline) binds α-adrenergic receptors and β1-adrenergic receptors with little affinity for β2-adrenergic receptors. By binding these receptors, norepinephrine (noradrenaline) causes an increase in HR and SV, as well as arteriolar vasoconstriction and increased SVR. These effects are not rate dependent. (Dose is 0.05-0.1 mcg/kg/min.)

When administering inotropes through a peripheral intravenous catheter, there is a theoretical risk of tissue necrosis should these agents extravasate. It is recommended that these agents be diluted and be administered at the lowest possible rate to achieve physiologic effect. Should an agent extravasate, then its adverse effects can be antagonized by local subcutaneous infiltration with phentolamine, 1 to 5 mg diluted in 5 mL of normal saline. While inotropic support is titrated to physiologic response, patients should have a central catheter placed for further monitoring and administration of vasoactive drugs. Aggressive fluid resuscitation should be continued while inotropic support is titrated. Some septic children require up to 200 mL/kg of fluids before attaining euvolemia.

Cortisol (Adrenal Insufficiency) If a child is at risk for absolute adrenal insufficiency or adrenal pituitary axis failure (eg, purpura fulminans or congenital adrenal hyperplasia) and remains in shock despite norepinephrine (noradrenaline) or epinephrine (adrenaline) infusion, stress-dose steroids should be given.

Hydrocortisone (1 to 2 mg/kg per day for stress dosing to 50 mg/kg per day for shock dosing) can be given in a continual infusion or intermittent boluses. Steroids should not be routinely given to all patients in septic shock. In a large pediatric sepsis trial, no significant improvement was seen in patients administered steroids.[41] In addition, critically ill patients who are given steroids can develop a severe myopathy[42] or hyperglycemia, which has been demonstrated to worsen outcomes in critically ill children.[43,44]

Calcium (Hypocalcemia) Calcium is a cation that acts on smooth, cardiac, and skeletal muscle to increase contractility. When deficient, actin/myosin complexes cannot bind, and muscle is unable to contract sufficiently. It is a not an infrequent cause of cardiac dysfunction in the critically ill child.[45] The resultant dysfunction in the septic patient leads to generalized weakness (skeletal muscle dysfunction), decreased SV and CO (myocardial dysfunction), and decreased arteriolar vasoconstriction with resultant decreased SVR (smooth muscle dysfunction). If a patient presents with decreased ionized calcium, it is recommended to replete those calcium levels with calcium gluconate (peripheral intravenous site) or calcium chloride (central intravenous site).

Dextrose (Hypoglycemia/Hyperglycemia) Young infants have immature glycogen storages, and when metabolic demands increase during septic shock, hypoglycemia can result. Untreated, hypoglycemia can cause neurologic devastation. A rapid bedside glucose should be checked on every septic patient. If hypoglycemia is confirmed (<60 mg/dL in a child or <45 mg/dL in a neonate), then a glucose-containing solution should be administered. If central venous access is available, a dextrose-containing solution of any concentration can be used. If peripheral access or intraosseous access is the only access available, then a 10-25% dextrose-containing solution can be administered. If a child is persistently hypoglycemic, then normal human glucose requirements can usually be met by infusing a 10% dextrose (in water) solution at maintenance fluid rates. Ideally, glucose should be kept between 80 mg/dL and 150 mg/dL.[1]

Septic shock is a stressful event on the human body. As a result of that stress, endogenous stress hormones (eg, cortisol or catecholamines) are released. These stress hormones act secondarily to increase serum glucose concentrations. Hyperglycemia and poor glycemic control lead to poorer outcomes.[43,44] Hyperglycemia should be treated with an insulin drip to maintain normoglycemia. Although tight glycemic control was not associated with improved outcome in adult patients,[46] it is shown to improve mortality rates in pediatric patients.[43,44]

Early Antibiotics Administration of appropriate broad-spectrum antibiotics within the first hour of presentation is recommended. There is a close association between delays in antibiotic administration and increasing mortality.[47] Immediately before or during administration of antimicrobials, cultures should be obtained from the blood, indwelling vascular devices, urine, and/or other appropriate sources. The obtainment of cultures should not delay administration of broad-spectrum antibiotics.[48]

Septic Shock: Beyond the Golden Hour

With demand for emergency services increasing and hospitals becoming increasingly overcrowded, length of stay in the ED has increased.[49] Therefore, critically ill patients can linger in the ED while awaiting admission to the intensive care unit in the hospital. During this time, resuscitative measures still need to be continued. Patients in septic shock can be refractory to all of the initial measures described beforehand, and directed therapies should be pursued.

Catecholamine-Resistant Shock

Patients whose signs of decreased perfusion continue despite aggressive fluid resuscitation and titration of norepinephrine (noradrenaline; for warm shock) or epinephrine (adrenaline) or dopamine/epinephrine (adrenaline; for cold shock) can be considered to have catecholamine-resistant shock.

Those with catecholamine-resistant shock should have a central venous catheter placed if they do not have one already. A central venous pressure should be calibrated from central catheter placement. Central venous pressures calibrated from iliofemoral sites have been shown to be as reliable as those from internal jugular and subclavicular sites.[50] A mixed venous oxygen saturation (SVO_2) should be measured from direct aspiration from a central venous catheter with the tip near the right atrial and superior vena cava/inferior vena cava junction,[51] continual electronic catheter measurement, or noninvasive spectroscopy.

Catecholamine-resistant shock can next be classified as cold shock with normal blood pressure, cold shock with low blood pressure, and warm shock with low blood pressure. See Figure 3.1 for summary and recommendations.

In cold shock with normal blood pressure, the patient has maximum vasoconstriction and an elevated SVR with a significantly depressed CO. Initial recommendations are to maximize oxygen delivery and capacity with existing CO by transfusing to a hemoglobin level greater than 10 g/dL and titrating epinephrine (adrenaline) infusion to an SVO_2 of greater than 70%. If the patient still presents with signs of poor perfusion and a normal blood pressure, decreasing afterload can improve SV by improving the myocardial contractility on the Starling curve. This can be accomplished with a vasodilator, such as sodium nitroprusside, or phosphodiesterase inhibitor, such as milrinone. Both of these types of agents are direct systemic vasodilators, with milrinone having the added benefit of being a direct cardiac inotrope.

In cold shock with low blood pressure, the patient has a poor CO with submaximal vasoconstriction. Initial recommendations are to maximize oxygen delivery and capacity with existing CO by transfusing to a hemoglobin level greater than 10 g/dL and titrating epinephrine (adrenaline) infusion to an SVO_2 70%. If the patient still presents with signs of poor perfusion and a low blood pressure, increasing afterload and inotropy can improve perfusion. This can be accomplished by adding norepinephrine (noradrenaline) and titrating to a normal blood pressure. If after normalization of blood pressure, the CO remains depressed, then an additional inotropic agent, such as a phosphodiesterase inhibitor (eg, milrinone) or β-adrenergic agonist (eg, dobutamine), can be used.

In warm shock with low blood pressure, the patient has a normal CO with severely decreased SVR. Initial recommendations are to titrate norepinephrine (noradrenaline) to a normal oxygen delivery or SVO_2 greater than 70%. If the patient is still hypotensive despite norepinephrine (noradrenaline) titration, then addition of a direct arteriolar vasoconstrictor to increase SVR is warranted. Vasopressin and terlipressin are direct arteriolar vasoconstrictors and act independently of catecholamines and can be administered as initial vasoconstrictors. It is important to continuously monitor CO when infusing vasoconstrictors because these agents can increase afterload significantly, thereby decreasing CO and worsening tissue perfusion.

Refractory Shock

Patients who display signs of poor perfusion despite attaining goals of adequate fluid resuscitation, maximum inotropic use, vasoconstrictors, transfusion, intubation, and maintenance of euglycemia and serum calcium are considered to have refractory shock. These patients should have investigations into other causes of decreased CO, including pericardial effusion, tension pneumothorax, abdominal compartment syndrome, significant bleeding, and massive pulmonary embolus. Patients without any readily reversible condition that remains in refractory shock should be considered a potential candidate for extracorporeal membrane oxygenation. The risks of extracorporeal membrane oxygenation and its associated mortality in the neonatal (80%) and pediatric (50%) populations should be weighed against its potential benefit in conjunction with your pediatric intensivist.[52,53]

Septic Shock in Resource-Limited Settings (no mechanical ventilation, no inotropic support)

Studies have demonstrated improved survival with the use of maintenance fluids alone compared to those who received 20 to 40 mL/kg in the first hour of therapy.[53a] In this setting, an initial fluid bolus of 20 mL/kg of crystalloid is reasonable. Administration of additional fluid boluses should occur with extreme caution. The patient should be reassessed after every fluid bolus.[53b]

Septic Shock: Neonatal Considerations

Neonatal septic shock usually occurs as a result of perinatally acquired bacteremia. A history of chorioamnionitis, maternal fever, prolonged rupture of the membranes, and active genital herpes simplex virus lesions at time of delivery put neonates at higher risk for developing neonatal sepsis.

The most common causative organisms are *Streptococcus agalactiae* (Group B Streptococci),

Escherichia coli, and *Listeria monocytogenes.* However, other organisms have been implicated in neonatal sepsis.

Classically, neonates present with early-onset perinatally acquired sepsis or late-onset perinatally acquired sepsis. The early-onset type is usually within the first week, manifested by fever, irritability, decreased feeding tolerance, increased crying, changes in sleep patterns, and lethargy. Early acquisition of perinatal bacterial flora results in bacteremia, possible meningitis, and sepsis. The late-onset type is usually at 3 weeks of age and manifested by similar symptoms. Neonates are colonized at delivery, usually in the nasopharynx, with translocation of this bacteria into the bloodstream and/or meninges with resultant sepsis.

The presentation of neonatal septic shock can be similar to cardiogenic shock, adrenal crisis, and inborn errors of metabolism. Therefore, care should be taken to entertain all causes in this age group.

There are some significant differences between neonatal and nonneonatal septic shock. First, neonatal sepsis is a vague syndrome that can mimic several other life-threatening processes. Neonates can present with delayed-onset cardiogenic shock after closure of the ductus arteriosus. Presence of rales, hepatomegaly, diaphoresis during feeding, cyanosis/hypoxemia, differential blood pressures, differential extremity pulse oxygenation, and presence of a murmur might indicate this as a possible diagnosis. If the possibility of a ductal-dependent cardiac lesion causing cardiogenic shock is entertained, initiation of a prostaglandin infusion in addition to treatment of shock should be continued. See the section titled Cardiogenic Shock for further details. The presentation of an inborn error of metabolism can mimic or coincide with septic shock. Tests for hyperammonemia and metabolic acidosis should be performed accordingly.

Second, under acidotic and hypoxemic conditions, neonates can exhibit persistent pulmonary hypertension of the newborn. During in utero circulation, fetal CO is maintained by right ventricular outflow through the ductus arteriosus and into the aorta, thereby bypassing the lungs. A hypoxemic and acidotic environment sustains pulmonary vasoconstriction and ductal patency, providing a pressure gradient for circulation between the pulmonary artery and aorta via the ductus arteriosus. Neonates who are septic can develop pulmonary vasoconstriction in response to the acidotic and hypoxemic environment. Resultant pulmonary hypertension can increase patency of a partially closed ductus arteriosus and cause shunting of blood from right-sided to left-sided circulation.

Initial Resuscitation See **Figure 3.2** for a summarized approach to the management of neonatal septic shock. The airway and oxygenation are managed in the same manner as for the pediatric patient. Volume loading should precede any induction for intubation because neonates are generally hypovolemic at the time of presentation. An intravenous access site or intraosseous site is adequate. If central access is needed, an umbilical venous catheter is preferred. Because cardiogenic shock is a possible presentation, crystalloid or colloid fluid boluses should be administered rapidly in smaller increments of 10 mL/kg up to 60 mL/kg until signs of perfusion improve or hepatomegaly or rales develop.

A preductal and postductal pulse oximeter reading and differential blood pressure should be obtained. Any neonate with a significant difference in oximetry and/or blood pressure, presenting in shock, or with cyanosis refractory to oxygen supplementation should be administered a prostaglandin infusion to maintain ductus arteriosus patency until a confirmatory echocardiogram can be obtained. Prostaglandin E_1 (PGE_1), when infused, can cause apnea. Therefore, preparations for advanced airway management should be made before initiation of infusion.

Neonates are considered to be in fluid-refractory shock if they display signs of poor perfusion despite administration of 60 mL/kg of crystalloid or colloid. If a patient is in fluid-

---

WHAT ELSE

Differential Diagnosis of Neonatal Septic Shock

- Inborn error of metabolism
- Cardiogenic shock (congenital heart disease, congestive heart failure)
- Persistent pulmonary hypertension
- Congenital adrenal hyperplasia

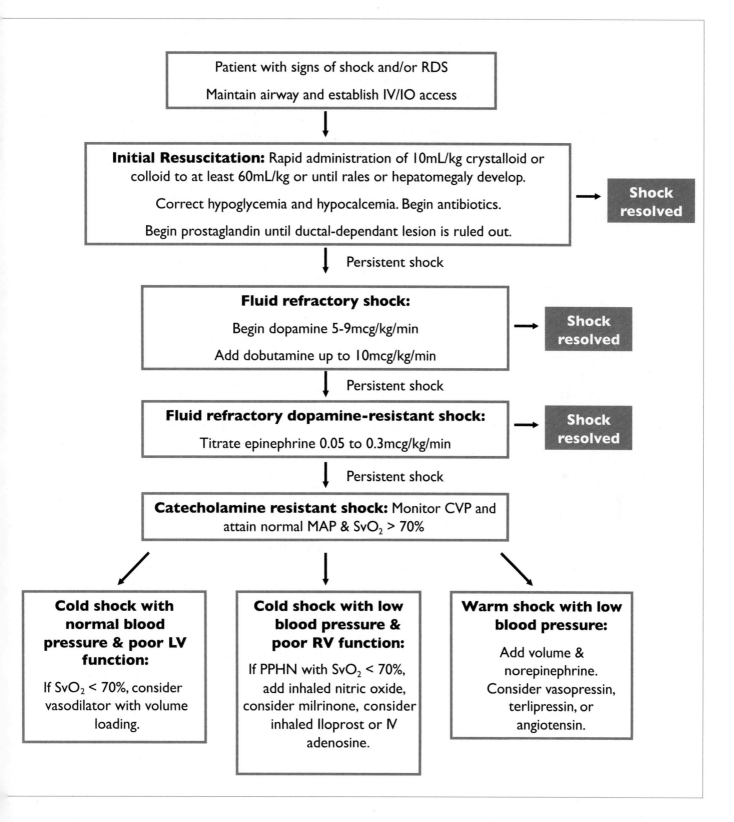

Figure 3.2 Management of neonatal septic shock.

Brierley J, Carcillo JA, Choong K, et al. Clinical practice parameters for hemodynamic support of pediatric and neonatal septic shock: 2007 update from the American College of Critical Care Medicine. *Crit Care Med.* 2009;37:666–688 refractory shock, dopamine infusion should be started at 5 to 9 mcg/kg per minute with 10 mcg/kg per minute of dobutamine added. Administration of dopamine can increase pulmonary vascular resistance, thereby increasing pulmonary hypertension and worsening right to left circulatory shunt. Dobutamine can increase CO without significant changes to pulmonary vascular resistance and mitigate this effect.

Because neonates have immature peripheral stores of epinephrine (adrenaline) and norepinephrine (noradrenaline), it is possible that administration of a procatecholamine, such as dopamine, will not result in sufficient enough levels of epinephrine (adrenaline) and norepinephrine (noradrenaline) to have effect. As a result, in the dopamine-refractory patient, a direct-acting catecholamine is advocated. Epinephrine (adrenaline) infusion should be started at a rate of 0.05 to 0.3 mcg/kg per minute and titrated to signs of perfusion.

Neonates who demonstrate ambiguous genitalia or are at risk for absolute corticosteroid deficiency should be given stress or shock dose hydrocortisone.

In infants with persistent pulmonary hypertension of the newborn, therapies directed at reducing tissue hypoxemia and acidosis should be undertaken. Tissue hypoxemia can be reduced by starting all suspected neonates on 100% oxygen by a nonrebreather mask. The metabolic acidosis can be buffered by starting a sodium bicarbonate drip and alkalinizing the serum to a pH of 7.5. Both of these remedies can be initiated while setting up for nitric oxide administration, a direct pulmonary vasodilator. Nitric oxide should be administered as the first-line treatment when available at each institution.

Shock: Implications for Aggressive Management

Before institution of these guidelines, early and aggressive fluid resuscitation portended improved outcomes.[54] After dissemination of guidelines, the mortality and morbidity rates of patients presenting with shock improved from 15% to 8%.[55] Systematic application of septic shock guidelines has been implemented and demonstrated improved outcomes where applied.[56] However, difficulties in adherence to

THE BOTTOM LINE

- Early aggressive fluid resuscitation improves outcomes.
- Early use of inotropic or vasoactive agents to support perfusion improves outcomes.
- Capillary refill, HR, and blood pressure should be monitored.
- Glucose and calcium should be monitored and administered if deficient.

guidelines resulting in underresuscitated children on arrival to the intensive care unit remain problematic and cause increased mortality.[57]

Obstructive Shock

Obstructive shock is a state of decreased CO with normal cardiac function, intravascular volume, and SVR. Decreased CO is usually caused by mechanical complications, such as acute decreases in preload (eg, massive pulmonary embolus, pericardial tamponade, tension pneumothorax, and air or thrombotic embolus) or acute increases in afterload (eg, hypertrophic cardiomyopathy and atrioventricular myxoma).

Etiology

The etiology of obstructive shock is varied. Any process that decreases preload mechanically or increases afterload mechanically can cause a shocklike state.

Pericardial Tamponade

The incidence of pericardial tamponade is 1 in 10,000, with most of these cases from malignant neoplasms or trauma. In the pediatric population, malignant neoplasms[58] and central venous catheter placement in the neck[59] are associated with pericardial tamponade. Pericardial tamponade is an accumulation of pericardial fluid under high or low pressure. Hemodynamic consequences can be seen as the pericardial fluid pressure increases and becomes greater than myocardial chamber pressures. Right atrial collapse occurs initially when pericardial pressure eclipses the right atrial pressure. Stroke volume decreases as right ventricular filling is limited by lack of end diastole atrial kick. Heart rate increases as a compensatory mechanism. Untreated, pericardial pressure soon eclipses left atrial pressure, which causes a similar effect. Further accumulation of pericardial fluid and pressures greater than right ventricular pressure cause a precipitous decrease in right ventricular filling, decreasing SV to virtually zero, and results in cardiovascular collapse.

Clinical Features

The triad of shock, distended neck veins, and muffled heart sounds should prompt the clinician to investigate this diagnosis. Children can present early with normal blood pressure and tachycardia and tachypnea with positional chest pain as their only symptoms.

Diagnostic Studies

Laboratory

No laboratory data are useful in the acute diagnosis of pericardial tamponade. However, laboratory tests to evaluate for malignant neoplasms, hypothyroidism, renal failure, tuberculosis, and pericarditis can assist in evaluating the cause of the effusion.

Radiology

Emergency physicians can easily diagnose pericardial tamponade with bedside ultrasonography.[60] If not available, transthoracic ultrasonography is the most efficacious diagnostic study. Chest radiography can demonstrate cardiomegaly, and computed tomography is a fairly sensitive test for detecting an effusion but exposes children to a significant amount of radiation.

Tension Pneumothorax

Tension pneumothorax develops when air enters the pleural cavity via a bronchopleural fistula. The fistula is created from traumatic (eg, missile projectile) or nontraumatic (eg, spontaneously from high peak inspiratory pressures in positive pressure ventilation or rupture of a bleb in a child with cystic fibrosis). The fistula acts as a one-way valve so that air accumulates in the pleural space with no path for exodus. Air accumulated under pressure can cause respiratory insufficiency and cardiovascular collapse as intrapleural pressures exceed right ventricular pressures and CO decreases.

Clinical Features

Children with blunt or penetrating thoracic trauma and children with chronic lung disease, cystic fibrosis, asthma, history of prolonged ventilation, tall stature, or history of previous pneumothorax are at risk for pneumothorax. The triad of shock, distended neck veins, and absent or asymmetric ventilation of a hemithorax should cue the physician to a diagnosis of tension pneumothorax.

Diagnostic Studies

Radiology

Although chest radiography is fairly sensitive in the evaluation of tension pneumothorax, it should never delay management.

Embolism

Air embolism and venous thromboembolism are exceedingly rare conditions that can cause rapid-onset obstructive shock in children. Pulmonary venous thromboembolism is a rare condition, with only 300 cases reported during a 20-year period.[61] Virchow described risk factors for venous thromboembolism more than 150 years ago, which are still observed today: venous stasis, vessel endothelial damage, and a hypercoagulable state. When these thrombi form, they are at risk of dislodging and traveling through the venous system on through the right atrium and right ventricle, lodging in the pulmonary arterioles. These thrombi block flow to areas of the lung, causing ventilation/perfusion mismatching and resulting in alveolar dead space. When thrombi become large enough and block proximal pulmonary arteries, right ventricular pressures can become severely elevated. Left ventricular venous return diminishes as right-sided CO decreases. As right ventricular pressures exceed systemic arterial pressure, septal bowing can decrease left ventricular SV with resulting obstructive shock. Air embolism occurs in a similar manner, albeit more rarely than venous thromboembolism. Air introduced into the venous system by traumatic (eg, tracheobronchial injury or penetrating wounds to the vasculature) or nontraumatic (eg, central venous catheter placement or improperly prepared intravenous solutions) can rapidly travel to the right ventricle and pulmonary circulation, where it blocks pulmonary blood flow in a similar mechanism to venous thromboembolism.

Clinical Features and Diagnostic Studies

Rapid-onset hypoxia, poor perfusion, tachycardia, and chest pain in patients at risk for venous thromboembolism (eg, cancer, recent surgery, protein C or protein S deficiency, or factor V Leiden) should prompt one to consider its diagnosis. Computed tomography angiography has supplanted pulmonary angiography for the detection of pulmonary embolus with a negative predictive value of more than 99%.[62] Ventilation perfusion scans have an unclear utility in the pediatric population and tend to perform more poorly in ruling out the diagnosis than computed tomographic angiography.[63] In the patient with obstructive shock and pulmonary embolism, Doppler echocardiography should be expedited to determine whether elevated right-sided cardiac pressures are present.

Rapid onset of the same clinical prodrome in the setting of trauma or recent surgery or vascular instrumentation should prompt one to consider the diagnosis of air embolism. Precordial Doppler ultrasonography is the most sensitive noninvasive method to detecting as little as 0.05 mL/kg of embolized air.[64]

Other Causes

Hypertrophic cardiomyopathy is a disorder of disorganized myocardial growth that can eventually impede left ventricular outflow and cause symptoms of obstructive shock.

Management

Management of obstructive shock should include early vascular access, supplementation with oxygen via a nonrebreather face mask, aggressive fluid resuscitation with 20-mL/kg boluses, and a rapid evaluation and treatment of cause.

In a patient with obstructive shock and pericardial tamponade, decompression of that tamponade should commence immediately. In the nontrauma patient, a pericardiocentesis should be performed (see procedure section on pericardiocentesis for details).

In a patient with obstructive shock and tension pneumothorax, decompression of the akinetic/hypokinetic hemithorax should take place via a needle thoracostomy before any imaging modality (see procedure section on needle thoracostomy for details).

In a patient with obstructive shock and venous thromboembolism, Doppler echocardiography should be performed immediately. Elevated pulmonary artery pressures can indicate right ventricular strain and the needed for thromboembolism decompressive therapy. Immediate surgical or percutaneous thrombectomy or intravenous infusion of tissue plasminogen activator in addition to heparin anticoagulation have been shown to improve mortality in patients with massive pulmonary embolus.[65,66]

In suspected air embolism, the patient should be placed in the left lateral decubitus position with Trendelenburg tilting. This effectively allows the air to collect at the apex of the right ventricle without further air collecting in the pulmonary circulation. Patients should have their airways managed if needed and be placed on 100% oxygen. Because most air emboli are created from communication with room air, 78% of the air bubble's content is nitrogen. Placing the patient on 100% oxygen causes the partial pressures of nitrogen to decrease and facilitates nitrogen absorption, thereby decreasing the size of the air embolus. If persistently unstable, the patient can have attempts at air embolism aspiration only if a central venous catheter is in place.[67] Arrangements should be made for hyperbaric oxygen therapy because its role in decreasing nitrogen bubble size is promising.[68]

Cardiogenic Shock

Cardiogenic shock is a state of decreased CO caused by myocardial dysfunction, manifested as a decreased cardiac index, increased SVR, and impaired tissue perfusion. Cardiogenic shock can be categorized as arrhythmogenic or functional. Arrhythmogenic cardiogenic shock results from a HR that is either too fast or too slow to sustain a sufficient CO despite a normal SV. Functional cardiogenic shock is due to impaired SV secondary to a failing heart.

Etiology

Arrhythmogenic cardiogenic shock can result from an unstable tachyarrhythmia or an unstable bradyarrhythmia. See Table 3-9 for complete listing of possible causes. Functional cardiogenic shock can result from a congenital anomaly, direct infection, ischemia and infarction, toxins and drugs, cardiomyopathy, and sepsis.

Congenital cardiac anomalies can result in congestive heart failure, cyanosis and diminished pulmonary flow, cyanosis and congestive heart failure, and shock (Table 3-10). Because the emphasis of this chapter is shock, we will only discuss the congenital heart defects that cause cardiogenic shock. Congenital lesions that can present in cardiogenic shock are generally

TABLE 3-9 Possible Causes of Bradyarrhythmias and Tachyarrhythmias	
Bradyarrhythmias	Tachyarrhythmias
Sick sinus syndrome	Supraventricular tachycardia
Atrioventricular block (second or third degree)	Ventricular tachycardia
Idioventricular rhythm disturbances	Polymorphic ventricular tachycardia
Toxin-induced (β-blocker, calcium blocker, digitalis, cholinergic toxicity)	Atrial tachycardia (atrial fibrillation, atrial flutter, multifocal atrial tachycardia, atrial tachycardia)
Sinus arrest	Junctional tachycardia
Sinus bradycardia	Preexcitation syndromes (Wolfe-Parkinson-White)
Junctional escape bradycardia	

TABLE 3-10 Congenital Heart Defects That Cause Cardiac Symptoms			
Congestive Heart Failure	Cyanosis and Diminished Pulmonary Flow	Cyanosis and Congestive Heart Failure	Cardiogenic Shock
Ventricular septal defect	Tetralogy of Fallot	Transposition of the great arteries	Hypoplastic left heart syndrome
Atrial septal defect	Tricuspid atresia	Total anomalous pulmonary venous return	Coarctation of the aorta
Atrioventricular canal	Ebstein anomaly	Truncus arteriosus	Interrupted aortic arch
Patent ductus arteriosus	Pulmonary atresia	Double outlet right ventricle	Critical aortic stenosis
Coarctation of the aorta	Severe pulmonary stenosis	Single ventricle	
Critical aortic stenosis	Hypoplastic right ventricle	Hypoplastic left heart syndrome	
	Eisenmenger complex		
	D-transposition of the great arteries with pulmonary stenosis		

obstructive left ventricular outflow lesions. An underdeveloped left ventricle or significant post-ventricular stenosis prohibits CO. These lesions usually present within the first 2 weeks of life after closure of the ductus arteriosus. **Figure 3.3** demonstrates left ventricular outflow obstruction before closure of the ductus arteriosus. In this example of hypoplastic left heart syndrome, most of the CO is maintained by the right ventricle via a patent ductus arteriosus. Whether the left ventricle outflow obstruction is a failed left ventricle, stenotic aortic valve, or critical coarctation of the aorta, they all share the common physiologic trait that they depend on a patent ductus arteriosus for systemic circulation. **Figure 3.4** demonstrates a hypoplastic left heart syndrome with closure of the ductus arteriosus.

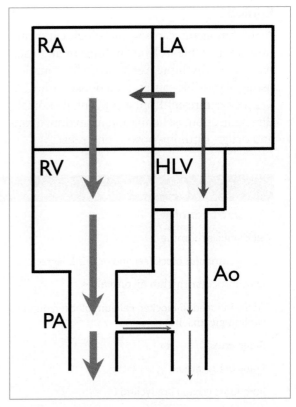

Figure 3.4 Ductus arteriosus closed in hypoplastic left heart syndrome. Cardiac output is severely depressed. Note there is now minimal mixing occurring. Ao, aorta; CDA, closed ductus arteriosus; HLV, hypoplastic left ventricle; LA, left atrium; PA, pulmonary artery; RA, right atrium; RV, right ventricle.

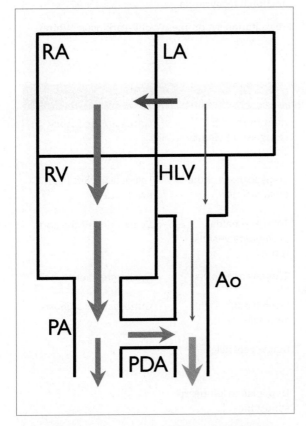

Figure 3.3 Ductus arteriosus open in hypoplastic left heart syndrome. Most of the cardiac output is supplied from the right ventricle via the ductus arteriosus. Note that significant mixing occurs with resulting cyanosis. Ao, aorta; HLV, hypoplastic left ventricle; LA, left atrium; PA, pulmonary artery; PDA, patent ductus arteriosus; RA, right atrium; RV, right ventricle.

Note the diminished CO and likely cardiogenic shock that follows. Many of these patients present in extremis and are initially misdiagnosed as being septic. Physical examination often reveals cyanosis (55%), diminished upper extremity (32%) and lower extremity pulses (70%) with a pulse differential, and a murmur (53%). Chest radiography demonstrates cardiomegaly in 85% of cases, whereas electrocardiography results are abnormal in 80% of cases.[69]

Children who have undergone surgical procedures to repair complex congenital heart diseases can present with cardiogenic shock in the ED as a result of revision failure. Specifically, patients who require surgical correction for single ventricle physiology (eg, hypoplastic left heart syndrome or severe Epstein anomaly) will undergo a Fontan or Norwood procedure. Simply speaking, these procedures bypass a failing ventricle to provide systemic circulation and create direct connection from the venous caval system into the pulmonary artery. Because the cavopulmonary connections are low flow (not propelled by a right ventricular pressure gradient), they are at risk for thrombosis should a patient develop a low flow or hyperthrombotic state (eg, dehydration, illness, trauma, arrhythmia, or sepsis). When these connections thrombose, CO decreases precipitously and patients go into severe shock.[70,71,72]

Myocarditis is an infection of the myocardial tissue. It is usually caused by viruses (coxsackievirus, influenza, or echovirus) but can be parasitic in underdeveloped countries. Inflammation of the myocardial tissue results in hypokinetic or akinetic ventricular function, which might improve after the initial insult or develop into a permanent dilated cardiomyopathy. Patients can present with signs of poor perfusion, congestive heart failure, and chest pain. Abdominal pain and hypotension may be the only presenting signs in a young child or adolescent.[73]

Myocardial ischemia and infarction is an exceedingly rare phenomena in the pediatric patient. However, patients can be predisposed to infarction should they have an anomalous left coronary artery arising from the pulmonary artery (ALCAPA). Constituting approximately 0.5% of all congenital heart disease, ALCAPA is rare. Untreated, ALCAPA portends a 90% mortality rate in the first year of life. Patients are not affected in utero because the anomalous coronary artery is supplied by oxygen-rich blood from the pulmonary artery. However, after birth, the coronary artery is supplied by deoxygenated blood under low pressures. This results in myocardial ischemia during times of feeding, crying, or stress. Neonates can present initially with excessive crying and tachycardia. After 1 month of age, most infants' left-sided pressures have become more dominant. This results in more myocardial demand, worsening myocardial perfusion with the low-flow pulmonary system feeding the coronary artery, and myocardial infarction.[74] Patients with a previous episode of Kawasaki disease might have preexisting coronary artery aneurysms that predispose them to thrombosis and infarction.[75]

Toxins and drugs can cause transient or permanent myocardial dysfunction. Anthracyclines, such as daunorubicin and doxorubicin, can contribute to permanent cardiomyopathy.[76] Medications for human immunodeficiency virus,[77] attention-deficit/hyperactivity disorder,[78] and recreational drug use have all been implicated in the development of cardiomyopathy.

Patients with diagnosed or undiagnosed existing cardiomyopathy can present in cardiogenic shock. Patients with muscular dystrophy, metabolic disorders, endocrinopathies, chronic anemia, collagen vascular disease, and chronic malnutrition can all present with dilated cardiomyopathy. Patients with hypertrophic obstructive cardiomyopathy can all present with severe cardiogenic shock.

Clinical Features

Children presenting with cardiogenic shock can present with signs and symptoms related to their inciting condition. Children with myocardial infarction or myocarditis can present with chest pain, abdominal pain, weakness, and tachycardia. Children with cardiomyopathies can present with dyspnea, tachypnea, decreased exercise tolerance, lethargy, irritability, and hepatomegaly. Neonates with cardiogenic shock can present with diaphoresis during feeding, poor weight gain, tachypnea, cyanosis, and irritability. Physical examination can demonstrate hepatomegaly, tachycardia, pathologic murmurs, a prominent S3, gallop, rales, and displaced heart prominence.

Diagnostic Studies

Laboratory

A complete blood cell count should be obtained to rule out severe chronic anemia and malignant neoplasms as a cause of high-output ventricular failure. Serum electrolytes should be performed and renal function should be checked to rule out renal failure and electrolyte abnormalities. Serum albumin should be measured to assess for diminished oncotic capacity. Serum troponin and creatine kinase MB isoenzyme should be assessed for evidence of myocarditis or myocardial infarction. A B-type natriuretic peptide should be measured if the diagnosis of congestive heart failure is considered. Serum lactate should be measured for all patients with suspected shock. Urinalysis should be assessed to rule out nephrotic syndrome. In neonates, a septic workup should be pursued concomitantly. An electrocardiogram is mandatory and can demonstrate chamber enlargement, arrhythmias, pericarditis, myocarditis, myocardial infarction, channelopathies, and other causes for cardiogenic shock.

Radiology

A chest radiograph can demonstrate cardiomegaly and pulmonary congestion and/or edema, but its absence does not exclude cardiogenic causes of shock. Transthoracic echocardiography is essential in evaluating patients with cardiogenic shock. Detailed assessment of diastolic and systolic function, congenital lesions, segmental hypokinesis, valvular abnormalities, and extracardiac malformations can all be assessed with echocardiography.

Management

Initial treatment of the pediatric patient with suspected cardiogenic shock should proceed in a similar manner to treatment of other types of shock with emphasis on the first hour in the ED.[79]

Airway and Breathing

High-flow oxygen should be initiated via a nonrebreather face mask or noninvasive positive pressure ventilation to maximize oxygen delivery to the underperfused tissues. If intubation is attempted, it should be performed after intravascular resuscitation has occurred because these patients are generally intravascularly depleted. The choice of induction agents depends on the comfort of the physician, but agents that cause less hemodynamic changes are preferred. Neonates in cardiogenic shock are profoundly vasoconstricted with maximally elevated SVR. Any agent that is vasodilatory can have disastrous consequences. Therefore, agents such as propofol, benzodiazepines, barbiturates, and naturally occurring opioids should be avoided. Ketamine, an N-methyl-D-aspartate antagonist as described previously, is a preferred choice secondary to its sparing of hemodynamic changes. Fentanyl, a synthetic opioid, can be used with only mild changes to SVR. Etomidate, acting on γ-aminobutyric acid receptors, is an adequate agent as well because of its short duration, short onset of action, and lack of hemodynamic changes. Caution should be used in the potentially septic patient because etomidate can cause adrenal suppression. Positive pressure ventilation, aside from induction agents, can cause a decrease in blood pressure initially as it decreases preload; therefore, intravascular repletion with crystalloid should be provided.

Circulation

Rapid intravenous access should be obtained and patients should receive crystalloid rehydration. If resuscitated too quickly, these patients can quickly become fluid overloaded and develop pulmonary edema. Instead, quick, serial boluses of 10 mL/kg of isotonic crystalloid is the recommended therapy followed by reassessment at 5- to 10-minute intervals for signs of hepatic congestion or respiratory compromise, indicating volume overload.[79]

Alprostadil (PGE_1) can be potentially lifesaving in patients with congenital heart lesions with a ductal-dependent systemic circulation (eg, hypoplastic left heart syndrome, coarctation of the aorta, critical aortic stenosis, or interrupted aortic arch).[80] Alprostadil is a prostaglandin agonist that acts to maintain the patency of the ductus arteriosus. Although ideal to have echocardiographic confirmation of the specific congenital anomaly and know whether PGE_1 is helpful, acquiring the echocardiogram should not delay infusion of PGE_1 in the neonate with shock.[81] A PGE_1 infusion is started at 0.05 to 0.1 mcg/kg per minute and usually takes effect within 15 minutes. If there is no effect, doses can be increased to a maximum of 0.4 mcg/kg per minute.[82] One of the main adverse effects of PGE_1 infusion is apnea; therefore, active monitoring of the airway or early endotracheal intubation should be considered.[82]

If after 60 mL/kg of intravenous isotonic crystalloid the patient still demonstrates signs of shock or becomes overloaded with fluids (hepatomegaly and rales) before full fluid infusion, inotropic support should be started. Because children are near maximally vasoconstricted when presenting with cardiogenic shock, administration of agents that increase dromotropy, chronotropy, and inotropy should be initiated.

Dopamine, dobutamine, epinephrine (adrenaline), and phosphodiesterase inhibitors are all potential agents. Dobutamine has been shown to be less effective than dopamine in improving blood pressure and signs of shock in the neonate.[83] As noted earlier, neonates can have immature catecholamine stores and be unresponsive to dopamine. However, dopamine is a reasonable first-line agent at 5 to 10 mcg/kg per minute with epinephrine (adrenaline; 0.05 to 0.3 mcg/kg per minute), as a second-line agent if unresponsive to dopamine. Inamrinone and milrinone are phosphodiesterase inhibitors with combined inotropic and vasodilatory properties that might be useful in patients with cardiogenic shock.[84]

Other Considerations

Patients with a history of prior repaired congenital heart disease who present with cardiogenic shock should be assumed to have a conduit thrombosis. In addition to the aforementioned airway and circulatory components, patients with a shunt thrombosis can be treated with heparin anticoagulation, balloon angioplasty, tissue plasminogen activator infusion, or stent replacement.[72] A cardiologist should be consulted before any of these options are used.

Patients with a presentation suggestive of myocarditis should rapidly undergo electrocardiography, chest radiography, and measurement of cardiac enzymes. A normal cardiac enzyme level does not rule out myocarditis.[85] Hemodynamic support should be commenced as illustrated above. Intravenous immunoglobulin (2 g/kg for 24 hours) has shown some promise in decreasing left ventricular dysfunction in acute myocarditis.[86] There is questionable benefit to the role of steroids and immunomodulators in myocarditis,[87] and further evidence is needed.

Patients with myocardial infarction should rapidly undergo electrocardiography and have cardiac biomarkers measured. In children, findings significant for myocardial infarction include Q waves greater than 35 milliseconds, ST-segment elevation greater than 2 mm, and a prolonged QT interval corrected for HR with Q wave abnormalities.[88] Pediatric patients can present with electrocardiographic signs similar to adult myocardial infarction without coronary arterial disease.[89] Cardiac biomarkers can help guide therapy, but little evidence has supported their use in pediatric patients.[90] If the diagnosis is suspected, treatment should be initiated aggressively in conjunction with a cardiologist.

THE BOTTOM LINE

- Pediatric shock is a state of decreased perfusion that should be rapidly identified and treated.
- Children usually do not exhibit frank hypotension unless they are severely ill.
- Early aggressive fluid resuscitation should be initiated within the first hour until signs of tissue perfusion improve or patient becomes overloaded with fluids.
- If the patient is fluid refractory, early inotropic support should be initiated within the first hour.
- During resuscitation, the specific type and cause for shock should be identified and addressed.
- Despite the cause and type of shock, all patients should receive early aggressive fluid resuscitation.
- All patients presenting in shock who do not respond to initial resuscitation should be admitted to a unit capable of invasive pediatric monitoring.

CHAPTER REVIEW

Check Your Knowledge

1. A 2-month-old, previously healthy boy with a history of fever for 2 days at home is brought to the emergency department (ED) by paramedics. On arrival at the ED, the patient is listless and vital signs show his temperature is 39°C (102.2°F), heart rate (HR) is 190/min, respiratory rate is 48/min without retractions, blood pressure is 68/40 mm Hg, and pulse oximetry is 95% on room air. You are concerned the child is in septic shock. What are your initial management priorities?
   A. Place the patient on oxygen, obtain vascular access, and fluid resuscitate up to 60 mL/kg.
   B. Place the patient on a monitor, obtain intravenous access, and administer prostaglandin E$_1$.
   C. Perform rapid sequence intubation, obtain vascular access, and administer antibiotics.
   D. Place the patient on oxygen, place an intraosseous catheter, and administer dopamine.

2. Which of the following types of shock represent a distributive form of shock?
   A. Anaphylaxis
   B. Septic shock
   C. Neurogenic shock
   D. All of the above

3. In a child in septic shock who remains tachycardic with signs of poor perfusion and delayed capillary refill after 60 mL/kg of normal saline, what additional therapy should be initiated next?
   A. Dopamine
   B. Norepinephrine (noradrenaline)
   C. Vasopressin
   D. Milrinone
   E. Nitric oxide

4. In a patient with neurogenic shock, the initial goal of treatment after control of airway and ventilation is to do which of the following?
   A. Increase circulating blood volume.
   B. Increase systemic vascular resistance.
   C. Decrease pulmonary vascular resistance.
   D. Decrease sympathetic tone.

5. Which of the following statements best describes systemic inflammatory response syndrome (SIRS) in children as defined by 2009 published guidelines?
   A. SIRS in children can exist with tachycardia and tachypnea alone.
   B. SIRS requires elevation of procalcitonin or C-reactive protein.
   C. SIRS in children requires abnormal leukocyte count or fever.
   D. SIRS in children requires that hypotension be present.

6. A 4-day-old infant presents in septic shock. The infant remains in shock after repeat boluses of normal saline and dopamine. Echocardiography results are normal. What therapy should be added to this regimen?
   A. 5% Albumin
   B. Epinephrine (adrenaline)
   C. Adenosine
   D. Nitric oxide

7. When should hydrocortisone be given in patients with septic shock?
   A. In patients born prematurely
   B. In patients with hypotension unresponsive to fluid resuscitation
   C. Never
   D. In patients with suspected adrenal insufficiency

8. What is the role of endotracheal intubation and mechanical ventilation in the treatment of children with shock?
   A. Up to 40% of cardiac output might be required to support the work of breathing, and this can be unloaded by ventilation, diverting flow to vital organs.
   B. Decreased intrathoracic pressure also reduces left ventricular afterload that might be beneficial in patients with low cardiac output and high systemic vascular resistance.
   C. Aggressive hyperventilation might be required to compensate for metabolic acidosis by altering the respiratory component of acid-base balance.
   D. Temperature control is prevented and oxygen consumption increased.

References

1. Yager P, Noviski N. Shock. *Pediatr Rev.* 2010;31:311–319.
2. McKiernan CA, Lieberman SA. Circulatory shock in children: An overview. *Pediatr Rev.* 2005;26:445–454.
3. Sampson HA. Food anaphylaxis. *Br Med Bull.* 2000;56:925–935.
4. Hurlbert RJ. Methylprednisolone for acute spine cord injury: An inappropriate standard of care. *J Neurosurg.* 2000;93:1–7.
5. Martinot A, Leclerc F, Cremer R, Leteurtre S, Fourier C, Hue V. Sepsis in neonates and children: Definitions, epidemiology, and outcome. *Pediatr Emerg Care.* 1997;13:277–281.
6. Dupont HL, Spink WW. Infections due to gram negative organisms: An analysis of 860 patients with bacteremia at the University of Minnesota Medical Center, 1959–1966. *Medicine.* 1969;48:301–332.
7. Stoll BJ, Holman RC, Schuchat A. Decline in sepsis-associated neonatal and infant deaths in the United States, 1979 through 1994. *Pediatrics.* 1998;102:e18.
8. Watson RS, Carcillo JA, Linde-Zwirble WT, Clermont G, Lidicker J, Angus DC. The epidemiology of severe sepsis in children in the United States. *Am J Respir Crit Care Med.* 2003;167:695–701.
9. Goldstein B, Giroir B, Randolph A, International Pediatric Sepsis Concensus Conference. International pediatric sepsis consensus conference: Definitions for sepsis and organ dysfunction in pediatrics. *Pediatr Crit Care Med.* 2005;6:2–8.
10. Bone RC, Sprung CL, Sibbald WJ. Definitions for sepsis and organ failure. *Crit Care Med.* 1992;20:724–726.
11. Levin M, Quint PA, Goldstein B, et al. Recombinant bactericidal/permeability-increasing protein (rBPI21) as adjunctive treatment for children with severe meningococcal sepsis: A randomized trial. rBPI21 Meningococcal Sepsis Study Group. *Lancet.* 2000;356:961–967.
12. Krafte-Jacobs B, Brilli R. Increased circulating thrombomodulin in children with septic shock. *Crit Care Med.* 1998;26:933–938.
13. Samson LM, Allen UD, Creery WD, Diaz-Mitoma F, Singh RN. Elevated interleukin-1 receptor antagonist levels in pediatric sepsis syndrome. *J Pediatr.* 1997;131:587–591.
14. Sullivan JS, Kilpatrick L, Costarino AT, Jr, Lee SC, Harns MC. Correlation of plasma cytokine elevations with mortality rate in children with sepsis. *J Pediatr.* 1992;120:510–515.
15. Wong HR, Carcillo JA, Burckart G, Shah N, Janosky JE. Increased serum nitrite and nitrate concentrations in children with the sepsis syndrome. *Crit Care Med.* 1995;23:835–842.
16. Doughty L, Carcillo JA, Kaplan S, Janosky JE. Plasma nitrite and nitrate concentrations and multiple organ failure in pediatric sepsis. *Crit Care Med.* 1998;26:157–162.
17. Spack L, Havens PL, Griffith OW. Measurements of total plasma nitrite and nitrate in pediatric patients with the systemic inflammatory response system. *Crit Care Med.* 1997;25:1071–1078.
18. Krafte-Jacobs B, Carver J, Wilkinson JD. Comparison of gastric intramucosal pH and standard perfusional measurements in pediatric septic shock. *Chest.* 1995;108:220–225.
19. Zaritsky AL, Nadkarni VM, Hickey RW, et al, eds. *Pediatric Advanced Life Support Provider Manual.* Dallas, TX: American Heart Association; 2002.
20. Carcillo JA, Fields AI, Task Force Committee Members. Clinical practice variables for hemodynamic support of pediatric and neonatal patients in septic shock. *Crit Care Med.* 2002;20:1365–1378.
21. Brierley J, Carcillo JA, Choong K, et al. Clinical practice parameters for hemodynamic support of pediatric and neonatal shock: 2007 update from the American College of Critical Care Medicine. *Crit Care Med.* 2009;37:666–688.
22. Enguix A, Rey C, Concha A, Medina A, Coto D, Diéquez MA. Comparison of procalcitonin with C-reactive protein and serum amyloid for the early diagnosis of bacterial sepsis in critically ill neonates and children. *Intensive Care Med.* 2001;27:211–215.
23. Resch B, Gusenleitner W, Muller WD. Procalcitonin and interleukin-6 in the diagnosis of early-onset sepsis of the neonate. *Acta Paediatr.* 2003;92:243–245.
24. Han YY, Doughty LA, Kofos D, Sasser H, Careillo JA. Procalcitonin is persistently increased among children with poor outcome from bacterial sepsis. 2003;4:21–25.
25. Rivers E, Nguyen B, Havstad S, et al. Early goal-directed therapy in the treatment of severe sepsis and septic shock. *N Engl J Med.* 2001;345:1368–1377.
26. Pollack MM, Fields AI, Ruttimann UE. Distributions of cardiopulmonary variables in pediatric survivors and nonsurvivors of septic shock. *Crit Care Med.* 1985;13:454–459.
27. Ceneviva G, Paschall JA, Maffei F, Careillo JA. Hemodynamic support in fluid refractory pediatric septic shock. *Pediatrics.* 1998;102:e19

28. Yamamoto LG. Rapid sequence intubation. In: Ludwig S, Fleisher GR, eds. *Textbook of Pediatric Emergency Care*, 5th ed. Philadelphia, PA: Lippincott, Wilkins & Williams; 2006.

29. Song XM, Li JG, Wang YL, et al. Protective effect of ketamine against septic shock in rats. *Zhongguo Wei Zhuang Bing Ji Jiu Yi Xue*. 2004;16:348–351.

30. Edwin SB, Walker PL. Controversies surrounding the use of etomidate for rapid sequence intubation in patients with suspected sepsis. *Ann Pharmacother*. 2010;44:1307–1312.

31. der Brinker M, Joosten KF, Liem O, et al. Adrenal insufficiency in meningococcal sepsis: Bioavailable cortisol levels and impact of interleukin-6 levels and intubation with etomidate on adrenal function and mortality. *J Clin Endocrinol Metab*. 2005;90:5110–5117.

32. Nhan NT, Phuong CXT, Kneen R, et al. Acute management of dengue shock syndrome: A randomized double-blind comparison of 4 intravenous fluid regimens in the first hour. *Clin Infect Dis*. 2001;32:204–212.

33. Maitland K, Pamba A, English M, et al. Randomized trial of volume expansion with albumin or saline in children with severe malaria: Preliminary evidence of albumin benefit. *Clin Infect Dis*. 2005;40:538–545.

34. Finfer S, Bellomo R, Boyce N, et al. SAFE Study Investigators. A comparison of albumin and saline for fluid resuscitation in the intensive care unit. *N Engl J Med*. 2004;350:2247–2256.

35. Booy R, Habibi P, Nadel S, et al, Meningococcal research group. Reduction in case fatality rate from meningococcal disease associated with improved healthcare delivery. *Arch Dis Child*. 2001;85:386–390.

36. Upadhyay M, Singhi S, Murlidharan J, Kaur N, Majumdar S. Randomized evaluation of fluid resuscitation with crystalloid (saline) and colloid (polymer from degraded gelatin in saline) in pediatric septic shock. *Indian Pediatr*. 2005;42:223–231.

37 Mink RB, Pollack MM. Effect of blood transfusion on oxygen consumption in pediatric septic shock. *Crit Care Med*. 1990;18:1087–1091.

38. de Oliveira CF, de Oliveira DS, Gottschald AF, et al. ACCM/PALS haemodynamic support guidelines for paediatric septic shock: An outcomes comparison with and without monitoring central venous oxygen saturation. *Intensive Care Med*. 2008;34:1065–1075.

39. Gabrielli A, Layon J, Yu M, eds. *Civetta, Taylor and Kirby's Critical Care*. 4th ed. New York, NY: WW Norton & Co; 2008.

40. Beale RJ, Hollenberg SM, Vincent JL, Parrillo JE. Vasopressor and inotropic support in septic shock: An evidence-based review. *Crit Care Med*. 2004;32:S455–S465.

41. Zimmerman JJ, Williams MD. Adjunctive corticosteroid therapy in pediatric severe sepsis: Observations from the RESOLVE study. *Pediatr Crit Care Med*. 2010;11:1–7.

42. Herridge MS. Building consensus on ICU-acquired weakness. *Intensive Care Med*. 2009;35:1–3.

43. Hirshberg E, Larsen G, Van Duker H. Alterations in glucose homeostasis in the pediatric intensive care unit: Hyperglycemia and glucose variability are associated with increased mortality and morbidity. *Pediatr Crit Care Med*. 2008;9:361–366.

44. Yung M, Wilkins B, Norton L, Slater A. Pediatric Support Group, Australian and New Zealand Intensive Care Society. Glucose control, organ failure, and mortality in pediatric intensive care. *Pediatr Crit Care Med*. 2008;9:147–152.

45. Cardenas-Rivero N, Chernow B, Stoiko MA, Nussbaum SR, Todres ID. Hypocalcemia in critically ill children. *J Pediatr*. 1989;114:946–951.

46. Wiener RS, Wiener DC, Larson RJ. Benefits and risks of tight glucose control in critically ill adults. *JAMA*. 2008;300:933–944.

47. Kumar A, Roberts D, Wood KE, et al. Duration of hypotension prior to initiation of effective antimicrobial therapy is the critical determinant of survival in human septic shock. *Crit Care Med*. 2006;34:1589–1596.

48. Dellinger RP, Levy MM, Carlet JM, et al. Surviving Sepsis Campaign: International guidelines for management of severe sepsis and septic shock: 2008. *Crit Care Med*. 2008;36:296–327.

49. Timm NL, Ho ML, Luria JW. Pediatric emergency department overcrowding and impact on patient flow outcomes. *Acad Emerg Med*. 2008;15:832–837.

50. Reda Z, Houri S, Davis AL, Baum VC. Effect of airway pressure on inferior vena cava pressure as a measure of central venous pressure in children. *J Pediatr*. 1995;126:961–965.

51. Fernandez EG, Green TP, Sweenet M. Low inferior vena caval catheters for hemodynamic and pulmonary function monitoring in pediatric critical care patients. *Pediatr Crit Care Med*. 2004;5:14–18.

52. Meyer DM, Jessen ME. Results of extracorporeal membrane oxygenation in children with sepsis. The Extracorporeal Life Support Organization. *Ann Thorac Surg*. 1997;63:756–761.

53. Beca J, Butt W. Extracorporeal membrane oxygenation for refractory septic shock in children. *Pediatrics*. 1994;93:726–729.

53a. Maitland K, Kiguli S, Opoka RO, et al. FEAST Trial Group. Mortality after fluid bolus in African children with severe infection. *N Eng J Med*. 2011;364:2483–2495.

53b. de Caen AR, Berg MD, Chameides L, et al. Part 12: Pediatric advanced life support: 2015 American Heart Association Guidelines Update for Cardiopulmonary Resuscitation and Emergency Cardiovascular Care. *Circulation*. 2015;132(suppl2): 5526–5542.

54. Han Y, Carcillo J, Dragotta M, et al. Early reversal of pediatric-neonatal septic shock by community physicians is associated with improved outcome. *Pediatrics*. 2003;112:793–799.

55. Carcillo JA, Kuch BA, Han YY, et al. Mortality and functional morbidity after use of PALS/APLS by community physicians. *Pediatrics*. 2009;124:500–508.

56. Ferrer R, Artigas A, Levy M, et al. Improvement in process of care and outcome after a multicenter severe sepsis educational program in Spain. *JAMA*. 2008;299:2294–2303.

57. Inwald DP, Tasker RC, Peters MJ, Nadal S. Emergency management of children with severe sepsis in the United Kingdom: The results of the Paediatric Intensive Care Society sepsis audit. *Arch Dis Child*. 2009;94:348–353.

58. Medary I, Steinherz LJ, Aronson DC, La Quaglia MP. Cardiac tamponade in the pediatric oncology population: Treatment by percutaneous catheter drainage. *J Pediatr Surg*. 1996;31:197–200.

59. Nowlen TT, Rosenthal GL, Johnson GL, Tom DJ, Vargo TA. Pericardial effusion and tamponade in infants with central catheters. *Pediatrics*. 2002;110:137–142.

60. Mandavia DP, Hoffner RJ, Mahaney K, Henderson, SO. Bedside echocardiography by emergency physicians. *Ann Emerg Med*. 2001;38:377–382.

61. David M, Andrew M. Venous thromboembolic complications in children. *J Pediatr.* 1993;3:337–346.

62. Quiroz R, Kucher N, Zou KH, et al. Clinical validity of a negative computed tomography scan in patients with suspected pulmonary embolism: A systematic review. *JAMA.* 2005;293:2012–2017.

63. The PIOPED Investigators. Value of the ventilation/perfusion scan in acute pulmonary embolism: Results of the prospective investigation of pulmonary embolism diagnosis (PIOPED). *JAMA.* 1990;263:2753–2759.

64. Mirski MA, Lele AV, Fitzsimmons L, Toung TJ. Diagnosis and treatment of vascular air embolism. *Anesthesiology.* 2007;106:164–177.

65. Konstantinides S, Geibel A, Heusel G, Heinrich F, Kasper W, Management Strategies and Prognosis of Pulmonary Embolism–3 Trial Investigation. Heparin plus alteplase compared with heparin alone in patients with submassive pulmonary embolism. *N Engl J Med.* 2002;347:1143–1150.

66. Meneveau N, Seronde MF, Blonde MC, et al. Management of unsuccessful thrombolysis in acute massive pulmonary embolism. *Chest.* 2006;129:1043–1050.

67. Orebaugh SL. Venous air embolism: Clinical and experimental considerations. *Crit Care Med.* 1992;20:1169–1177.

68. Closon M, Vivier E, Breynaert C, et al. Air embolism during an aircraft flight in a passenger with a pulmonary cyst: A favorable outcome with hyperbaric therapy. *Anesthesiology.* 2004;101:539–542.

69. Pickert CB, Moss MM, Fiser DH. Differentiation of systemic infection and congenital obstructive left heart disease in the very young infant. *Pediatr Emerg Care.* 1998;14:263–267.

70. Jahangiri M, Ross DB, Redington AN, Lincoln C, Shinebourne EA. Thromboembolism after the Fontan procedure and its modifications. *Ann Thorac Surg.* 1994;58:1409–1414.

71. Rosenthal DN, Friedman AH, Kleinman CS, Kopf GS, Rosenfeld LE, Hellenbrand WE. Thromboembolic complications after Fontan operations. *Circulations.* 1995;92:287–293.

72. Ruud E, Holmstrom H, Aagenaes I, et al. Successful thrombolysis by prolonged low-dose alteplase in catheter-directed infusion. *Acta Paediatr.* 2003;92:973–976.

73. Sharieff GQ, Wylie T. Pericarditis, myocarditis, and endocarditis. In: Baren J, Rothrock S, Brennan J, et al, eds. *Pediatric Emergency Medicine.* Philadelphia, PA: Saunders; 2008:500–505.

74. Mancini MC, Weber HS. Anomalous left coronary artery from the pulmonary artery. *Emedicine.com.* 2008. http://emedicine.medscape.com/article/893290-overview. Accessed March 16, 2011.

75. Safi M, Taherkhani M, Badalabadi RM, Eslami V, Movahed MR. Coronary aneurysm and silent myocardial infarction in an adolescent secondary to undiagnosed childhood Kawasaki disease. *Exp Clin Cardiol.* 2010;15:e18–e19.

76. Maradia K, Guglin M. Pharmacologic prevention of anthracycline-induced cardiomyopathy. *Cardiol Rev.* 2009;17:243–252.

77. Oberdorfer P, Sittiwangkul R, Puthanakit T, Pongprot Y, Sirisanthana V. Dilated cardiomyopathy in three HIV-infected children after initiation of antiretroviral therapy. *Pediatr Int.* 2008;50:251–254.

78. Nissen SE. ADHD drugs and cardiovascular risk. *N Engl J Med.* 2006;354:2296.

79. Carcillo JA, Han K, Lin J, Orr R. Goal-directed management of pediatric shock in the emergency department. *Clin Ped Emerg Med.* 2007;8:165–175.

80. Freed MD, Heyman MA, Lewis AB, Roehl SL, Kensey RC. Prostaglandin E1 in infants with ductus arteriosus dependant congenital heart disease. *Circulation.* 1981;64:899–905.

81. Savitsky E, Alejos J, Votey S. Emergency department presentations of pediatric congenital heart disease. *J Emerg Med.* 2003;24:239–245.

82. Sharieff GQ, Wylie TW. Pediatric cardiac disorders. *J Emerg Med.* 2004;26:65–79.

83. Subhedar NV, Shaw NJ. Dopamine versus dobutamine for hypotensive preterm infants. *Cochrane Database Syst Rev.* 2003;3:CD001242.

84. Shipley JB, Tolman D, Hastillo A, Hess ML. Milrinone: Basic and clinical pharmacology and acute and chronic management. *Am J Med Sci.* 1996;311:286–291.

85. Smith SC, Ladenson JH, Mason JW, Jaffe AS. Elevations of cardiac troponin I associated with myocarditis: Experimental and clinical correlates. *Circulation.* 1997;95:163–168.

86. Drucker NA, Colan SD, Lewis AB, et al. Gamma-globulin treatment of acute myocarditis in the pediatric population. *Circulation.* 1994;89:252–257.

87. Schultz JC, Hilliard AA, Cooper LT, Jr, Rihal CS. Diagnosis and treatment of viral myocarditis. *Mayo Clin Proc.* 2009;84:1001–1009.

88. Towbin JA, Bricker JT, Garson A. Electrocardiographic criteria for the diagnosis of acute myocardial infarction in children. *Am J Cardiol.* 1992;69:1545–1548.

89. Gazit AZ, Avari JN, Balzer DT, Rhee EK. Electrocardiographic diagnosis of myocardial ischemia in children: Is a diagnostic electrocardiogram always diagnostic? *Pediatrics.* 2007;120:440–444.

90. Towbin JA. Myocardial infarction in childhood. In: Garson A, Bricker JT, McNamara DG, eds. *The Science and Practice of Pediatric Cardiology.* Vol iii. Philadelphia, PA: Lea and Febiger; 1990:1684–1722.

CHAPTER REVIEW

A 9-year-old boy is brought to the ED for joint pain and fever for the last 5 days. He was playing soccer last week and fell. He was initially experiencing left arm and right hip pain but now cannot walk secondary to pain in his ankles and feet. Two days ago he was seen by his pediatrician for a sore throat and then developed diarrhea (nonbloody). His past medical history is unremarkable, and he takes no medicine and has no allergies. All childhood immunizations are up to date. He is uncomfortable but interactive. He is tachypneic but without retractions or stridor. His skin reveals generalized erythema, an almost "sunburn appearance," yet his hands and feet are cool to the touch and appear cyanotic. His vital signs are HR of 141/min, respiratory rate of 22/min, blood pressure of 94/56 mm Hg, temperature of 39°C (102.2°F), and pulse oximetry of 100% on room air. He has a petechial rash on the soles of feet, diffuse swelling and tenderness of the ankles and left wrist, and diffuse muscular tenderness. He is neurologically intact but will not bear weight to walk secondary to pain.

1. What is your initial assessment?
2. What are your initial management priorities?
3. What are the most likely causes based on this assessment?
4. What complications can arise from this condition?

The initial assessment indicates compensated shock. His tachycardia and cyanotic distal extremities are two forms of compensation. In the initial phase of resuscitation, cardiorespiratory monitoring should be started, supplemental oxygen provided, vascular access established, laboratory studies including cultures ordered, and aggressive fluid resuscitation initiated. Given the temperature and flushed appearance, this is most likely septic shock. The lack of history of heart disease, a murmur, and rales makes a cardiogenic origin unlikely. This child has streptococcal toxic shock syndrome. Many complications can arise, including renal failure, hepatitis, coagulopathy, acute respiratory distress syndrome, necrotizing fasciitis, and myositis.

chapter 4

Cardiovascular System

Laura Fitzmaurice, MD, FAAP, FACEP
Cole Condra, MD, FAAP

Objectives

1 Present the clinical features and emergency management of cardiovascular disorders, including congenital and acquired heart disease

2 Identify pediatric rhythm disturbances.

3 Describe postsurgical complications after cardiac surgery.

Chapter Outline

Introduction
Congenital Heart Disease
Cyanotic Heart Disease
Noncyanotic Heart Disease
Congestive Heart Failure
Acquired Heart Disease
Myocarditis
Acute Rheumatic Fever
Pericarditis
Bacterial Endocarditis
Kawasaki Disease
Rhythm Disturbances
Bradydysrhythmias
Tachydysrhythmias
Cardiomyopathy
Postsurgical Complications

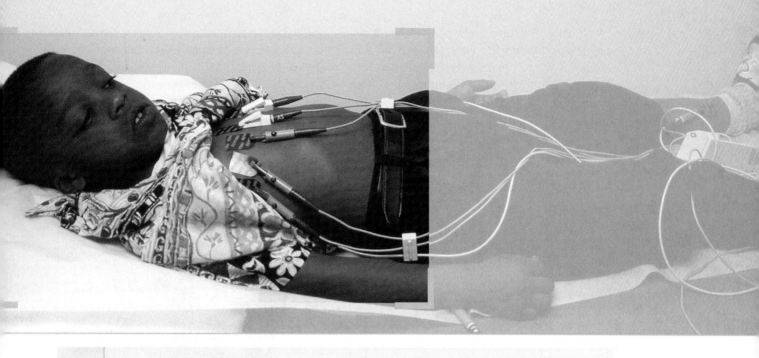

A 10-day-old infant is brought to the emergency department (ED) by his mother. She tells the physician that he seems to be breathing fast and is not eating very well. He is a full-term infant delivered vaginally with a birth weight of 3.2 kg (7 lb). He spent 2 days with his mother in the hospital and then was discharged after an uneventful circumcision. He has been slow to breastfeed since birth, but the mother became more alarmed when she noted that he would gasp and cry after sucking for a short time. He has approximately three or four wet diapers per day. He has no congestion or fever. He does not vomit with feedings and has had two yellow, seedy stools since passing meconium after birth. On initial examination, he is pale, irritable, and breathing fast, has nasal flaring, and is sweaty to touch. Vital signs reveal a respiratory rate of 70/min, heart rate of 170/min, blood pressure of 80/40 mm Hg, temperature (rectal) of 37°C (98.6°F), and weight of 2.9 kg. His lungs sound equal bilaterally with rales in both bases. Cardiac examination reveals a hyperactive precordium with a gallop rhythm. No murmurs are heard. The abdomen is distended with good bowel sounds, and his liver is palpated 4 cm below the right costal margin. Pulses feel weak in the lower extremities. The capillary refill is 3 to 4 seconds in the fingertips, and pulse oximeter reading is 90% on room air.

1. *What is your rapid assessment of this infant?*
2. *On the basis of this assessment, what are your treatment priorities?*
3. *What is the most likely cause of the infant's condition?*
4. *What are the immediate and definitive treatment options?*
5. *What are some complications of this condition?*

CASE SCENARIO 1

Introduction

It is important to recognize children with cardiovascular system (CVS) disorders and distinguish between a congenital anomaly or an acquired disease, as well as to be able to stabilize them and manage their acute problems. An understanding of normal CVS physiology in children and how it changes with growth and development is important in recognizing the early signs and symptoms of CVS dysfunction.

Normal CVS function in pediatric patients is represented by normal vital signs and oxygen saturation, as well as the overall appearance of the child. A normal cardiac output is required to meet the body's needs. It is defined as the amount of blood that the heart pumps each minute and is calculated using a combination of heart rate and ventricular stroke volume. Many physiologic parameters, such as the heart rate, stroke volume, mean arterial blood pressure, and vascular resistance, affect the cardiac output. Stroke volume is the quantity of blood ejected from the heart with each contraction and is a function of the pumping action of the ventricle, which is dependent on preload, afterload, and contractility of the ventricle. Infants and young children rely mainly on the heart rate to increase cardiac output because they have limited capacity to change stroke volume. Children older than 8 to 10 years develop the capacity of adults to change the stroke volume and heart rate to improve cardiac output. Oxygen delivery is the amount of oxygen delivered to the entire body per minute and is an essential component of adequate cardiac function. If the oxygen delivery fails for any reason, supplemental oxygen is required and/or the cardiac output must increase to maintain adequate oxygen delivery to the tissues. Oxygen delivery to the tissues is determined by the amount of blood flow through the lungs, the arterial oxygen content (dependent on oxygenation and hemoglobin concentration), and the cardiac output. Without adequate delivery, the metabolic demand of tissues is not met, and shock (inadequate substrate delivery to meet metabolic demands) begins.

Congenital Heart Disease

Congenital heart disease (CHD) has an incidence of 4 to 50 cases per 1,000 live births.[1] Children of parents who have CHD have an increased incidence from this baseline by a range of 5% to 15%. The most common isolated congenital heart lesion is a bicuspid aortic valve (most cases are asymptomatic and found on adult autopsies at a rate of 1% to 2%). The CHD lesions range from a small ventriculoseptal defect to a complex atrioventricular (AV) canal anomaly.[2–5] Typically, congenital heart lesions are divided into cyanotic and noncyanotic lesions. The child with a congenital anomaly usually does not show cardiovascular problems in utero because the fetal/maternal circulation, as a parallel pumping system via the placenta, provides adequate support to help maintain growth. **Figure 4.1** provides a diagram of normal fetal circulation.

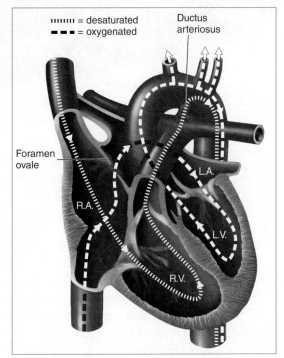

Figure 4.1   Normal fetal circulation

In the normal fetal circulation, oxygenated blood (large broken line in Figure 4.1) returns from the placenta via the ductus venosus, mixing with some systemic venous return blood in the inferior vena cava. This oxygenated blood partially mixes with deoxygenated systemic venous blood (small broken line in Figure 4.1) in the right atrium, but oxygenated blood is preferentially shunted through the foramen ovale to the left atrium and left ventricle, where the most oxygenated blood is pumped to the cerebral and coronary circulations. The right ventricle pumps less oxygenated blood into the pulmonary artery. The pulmonary vascular bed is vasoconstricted, so most of the blood is shunted through the ductus arterious to mix with the systemic arterial circulation in the descending aorta (distal to the coronary and carotid arteries), thus delivering less oxygenated blood to the rest of the systemic arterial circulation.

The placental circulation is interrupted at birth, which increases the systemic arterial blood pressure. The newborn becomes hypoxic with the discontinuation of the placental flow relied on in utero. This causes an increase in blood pressure, heart rate, and the start of spontaneous respirations. The respirations help decrease pulmonary vascular resistance and increase the pulmonary blood flow. The pulmonary artery pressure decreases and there is an increase in pulmonary venous return and left atrial pressure, which closes the foramen ovale. Finally, the increase in systemic arterial pressure and decrease in pulmonary artery pressure cause flow through the ductus arteriosus to reverse. This initial rapid change slows during the first 24 hours of life, and pulmonary artery pressures continue to decrease toward adult levels during the next 6 weeks of life. Some of this change in pressure is aided by the anatomical structure of pulmonary vessels in the fetus and newborn, which have a thicker medial smooth muscle layer with increased vasoreactivity compared with children and adults.[6–8]

Cyanotic Heart Disease

Cyanotic heart disease results from structural and flow anomalies that develop in utero. In children with structural CHD, the changes that occur at birth and the interruption of intrauterine flow place great stress on the infant's CVS. Oxygenation is not possible for the infant who relied on the extraneous shunting (in utero) received from the ductus arteriosus. The normal oxygen saturation is 70% to 75% on the right side and 95% to 98% on the left side. The infant shunts deoxygenated blood into the systemic circulation; this is called right-to-left shunting. Some cyanotic heart disease conditions are highly dependent on shunting through the ductus arteriosus (ie, transposition), in which case complete closure of the ductus is a terminal event. Cyanosis can present shortly after birth, when the ductus arteriosus begins to close. The

lesions most commonly seen that are cyanotic in presentation include the five Ts: truncus arteriosus, tetralogy of Fallot (**Figure 4.2**), transposition of the great vessels (**Figure 4.3**), tricuspid atresia (**Figure 4.4**), and total anomalous pulmonary venous return (**Figure 4.5**), along with severe aortic stenosis, hypoplastic left heart, and severe coarctation of the aorta.

Clinical Features

Cyanosis as a presenting sign can be secondary to respiratory, cardiac, and hemoglobin disorders. Normal newborns will have cyanosis of the hands and feet. This is called acrocyanosis and is caused by cold stress and peripheral vasoconstriction. Generalized, or central cyanosis, is more ominous and is exacerbated by crying. The respiratory rate in children with cyanotic

---

YOUR FIRST CLUE

Signs and Symptoms of Cyanotic Heart Disease

- Pediatric Assessment Triangle:
  - Appearance: ranges in severity from cyanotic but active and vigorous to cyanotic with severe distress or lethargy (shock), with some patients appearing noncyanotic (normal) if the degree of right-to-left shunting is mild
  - Work of breathing: ranges in severity from normal (early, mild) to retractions, tachypnea, or grunting (pulmonary edema or ductus dependent absence of pulmonary flow)
  - Circulation: ranges in severity from cyanotic but well perfused to cyanotic with poor perfusion (shock)
- Other signs and symptoms:
  - Generalized cyanosis
  - Tachypnea
  - Respiratory distress
- Signs of shock
  - Poor distal perfusion
  - Cool extremities
  - Weak cry
  - Tachycardia

heart disease might not be as elevated as one would expect to see as with cyanosis caused by respiratory disorders. The infant can also have signs of shock with poor distal perfusion, cool extremities, weak cry, and a fast heart rate.

Diagnostic Studies

To differentiate between the causes of cyanosis, apply 100% oxygen. In infants with respiratory and hemoglobin disorders, the Pao_2 will increase significantly. The child with cyanotic

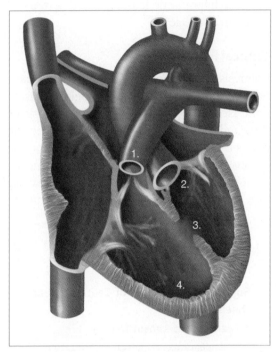

Figure 4.2 Tetralogy of Fallot: 1. pulmonic stenosis; 2. overriding aorta; 3. VSD; 4. RVH.

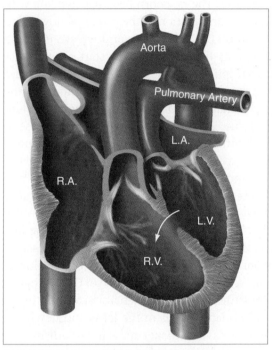

Figure 4.3 Transposition of the great vessels.

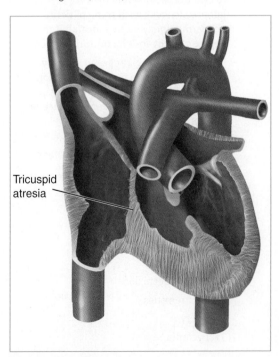

Figure 4.4 Tricuspid atresia.

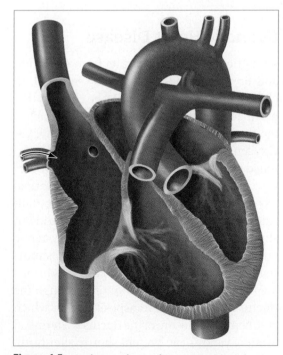

Figure 4.5 Total anomalous pulmonary venous return.

heart disease from a significant right to left shunt will have a low Pao$_2$ to start, which will increase only slightly with 100% oxygen because deoxygenated blood bypasses the lungs and goes directly to the left side of the heart. This dilutes the fully oxygenated blood coming from the lungs with deoxygenated blood. The oxygen saturation of the resultant mixture will never reach 100% (hence, Pao$_2$ will never rise significantly above 100 mm Hg despite 100% inspired oxygen). This is called the hyperoxia test and can help to distinguish cyanotic heart disease from respiratory causes, although severe respiratory illness might also result in low oxygen saturation despite the application of oxygen. In children with cyanotic heart disease, a chest radiograph might show an abnormal cardiac shadow and decreased pulmonary vascularity (**Figure 4.6**). The electrocardiogram (ECG) might show an abnormal axis, QRS, or ST-segment changes. An echocardiogram will give the definitive diagnosis. Poor oxygen delivery can precipitate acidosis and shock, which require rapid intervention with support of the airway, breathing, and circulation (ABCs), as well as monitoring and inotropic drugs.

Differential Diagnosis

The differential diagnosis for cyanotic CHD can be divided into those with increased pulmonary vascularity and those with decreased pulmo-

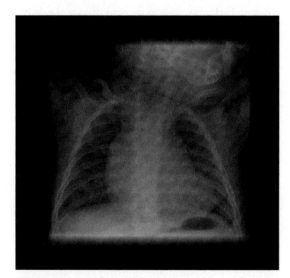

Figure 4.6 Chest radiograph showing a boot-shaped heart in a patient with tetralogy of Fallot.

nary vascularity. A special consideration in cyanotic CHD is ductal-dependent lesions, such as transposition of the great vessels. If the ductus closes, blood flow to the lungs is completely interrupted because of the congenital anomaly.

Management

The primary focus of management in the ED and acute care setting is to optimize oxygenation and support cardiovascular function. The infant should be given high-flow oxygen via a nonrebreather face mask at 10 to 15 L/min and be considered for elective intubation if significant respiratory distress is present. Cardiac, oxygen saturation, and blood pressure monitors are important for following response to therapy and as adjuncts in determining cardiac function. Intravenous (IV) access with maintenance fluid management can be started, and baseline laboratory tests (hemoglobin, hematocrit, and electrolytes) should be performed. Prostaglandin E_1 can be used to keep the ductus open after birth. It is infused at 0.05 to 0.1 mcg/kg per minute with an increase to 0.2 mcg/kg per minute during several minutes, up to a maximum of 0.4 mcg/kg per minute. Adverse effects of the infusion include apnea, pulmonary congestion, fever, hypotension, seizures, and diarrhea.[9–11] The infant should be considered for elective intubation if a prostaglandin infusion is started to secure the airway in case of apnea and to decrease the work of breathing. This can add stress to an already stressed heart. If the infant appears to be in shock, a fluid bolus can be started while monitoring the response to the fluid challenge to assess whether cardiac function worsens. The fluid bolus amount should be 10 mL/kg at a time because of the concern for iatrogenic overloading cardiac function. Diuretics might be needed to treat fluid retention. A dobutamine infusion (2 to 20 mcg/kg per minute) can be used to augment myocardial contractility. Dopamine and epinephrine (adrenaline) also can be used to augment contractility, but they have other effects as well.

Noncyanotic Heart Disease

Noncyanotic CHDs can present with signs of congestive heart failure (CHF) and/or heart murmurs that are heard during physical examination.[12,13] They can be divided into left-to-right shunts and obstructive lesions. The left-to-right shunt lesions, which can show an increase in pulmonary circulation, include atrial septal defects, ventricular septal defects, and patent ductus arteriosus. Obstructive lesions include aortic stenosis, coarctation of the aorta, pulmonary stenosis, and mitral stenosis. Most of these patients present during the first 6 months of life when the shunt or obstruction overwhelms the cardiac compensation and function.

Clinical Features

Clinical features include signs of CHF, such as tachypnea, tachycardia, diaphoresis, decreased feeding, hepatomegaly, various systolic flow murmurs, and gallop rhythms, depending on the specific lesion. The child might present with decreased activity or poor sleeping with respiratory distress.

Diagnostic Studies

Diagnostic studies include chest radiography, ECG, and echocardiography. The chest radiograph will show an abnormal cardiac shadow or increased pulmonary vascular flow. The ECG can show an abnormal axis, QRS changes, ST-segment changes, and chamber enlargement. The definitive test is two-dimensional echocardiography, which will define the abnormality and the degree of CHF. An additional helpful test is to check the blood pressure in all four extremities to assess for a coarctation of the aorta. Blood pressures in the legs are lower than in the arms in children with a coarctation, whereas in healthy children they might be higher.

Differential Diagnosis

The differential diagnosis for noncyanotic CHD includes those entities that have increased pulmonary vascularity and those with normal pulmonary vascularity. The lesions with increased pulmonary vascularity include atrial septal defect, ventricular septal defect, patent ductus arteriosus, and AV septal defect (eg, AV canal or

---

WHAT ELSE?

Differential Diagnosis of Noncyanotic CHD

- Lesions with increased pulmonary vascularity
  - Atrial septal defect
  - Ventricular septal defect
  - Patent ductus arteriosus
  - Arterioventricular septal defect
- Lesions with normal vascularity
  - Aortic stenosis
  - Pulmonary stenosis
  - Coarctation of the aorta

---

endocardial cushion defect). The cardiac lesions with normal vascularity include aortic stenosis, pulmonary stenosis, and coarctation of the aorta. Symptomatic pulmonic stenosis can show pulmonary hypoperfusion.

Management

Management in the acute care setting begins with administration of oxygen for those children with respiratory distress and/or cardiovascular instability. Cardiac, oxygen saturation, and blood pressure monitors should be placed. Intravenous access might be necessary to treat CHF. The drugs of choice for management of this condition include diuretics and digoxin. Laboratory testing should include measurement of blood glucose and electrolytes.

Congestive Heart Failure

Congestive heart failure (CHF) is a clinical syndrome in which the heart is unable to meet the hemodynamic demands and perfusion requirements of the body. The primary cause of CHF in infancy and childhood is from CHD. Congestive heart failure is the most common reason that children who have heart disease receive medical therapy and accounts for at least 50% of referrals for pediatric heart transplantation.[14] One possible uncommon congenital heart lesion is an anomalous left coronary artery that can cause an infant or child to present with a myocardial infarction. The cause is an acute decrease in oxygen flow to the myocardium secondary to deoxygenated blood in the left coronary artery because it originates from the pulmonary artery. The infant typically presents with CHF, vomiting, and cardiomegaly at approximately 2 to 3 months of age. Other causes of CHF to consider include those of acquired heart disease, such as myocarditis, endocrine and metabolic abnormalities, endocarditis, rheumatic fever with rheumatic heart disease, dysrhythmias, and pericardial effusions in older children. The typical problem is pulmonary overflow seen in children with large left-to-right shunts that can be exacerbated by infections such as respiratory syncytial virus. Children with cyanotic CHD can also develop overflow CHF. Other physiologic reasons for CHF are myocardial impairment, outflow obstructive lesions (usually on the left side), and rhythm abnormalities. With myocardial impairment, there is decreased cardiac output and passive venous congestion. The obstructive lesions and arrhythmias can cause CHF because of impaired ventricular function with resultant pulmonary venous congestion.

Clinical Features

Children with CHF present with tachycardia and/or a gallop, tachypnea with rhonchi and wheezing, rales in the lung bases, pallor, and/or cool skin. The extremities will have decreased perfusion, and there might be peripheral edema. Capillary refill will be prolonged, and the lower extremities might be mottled. The abdominal examination might reveal hepatomegaly. If the cardiac problem has been present for awhile, the child will present with growth failure and undernutrition.

YOUR FIRST CLUE

Signs and Symptoms of CHF
- Pediatric Assessment Triangle:
  - Appearance: ranges in severity from normal, to sweaty with feeding (early CHF), to irritability (pulmonary edema), to lethargy (shock)
  - Work of breathing: ranges in severity from degrees of retractions, tachypnea, or grunting (pulmonary edema) to respiratory failure
  - Circulation: ranges in severity from pallor (mild hypoxemia), marginal perfusion (more severe), cyanosis (pulmonary edema), poor perfusion, to mottling (severe shock)
- Other signs and symptoms:
  - Tachycardia
  - Gallop rhythm
  - Respiratory distress
  - Wheezing or rales
  - Hepatomegaly
  - Peripheral edema
  - Shock

Diagnostic Studies

Diagnostic studies include chest radiography, which can show an enlarged cardiac shadow and pulmonary edema (**Figure 4.7**). An ECG can show cardiac chamber dilation and ST-segment changes and/or T-wave abnormalities. Arterial blood gas analysis or pulse oximetry and the hemoglobin and hematocrit will help determine oxygen delivery. Electrolytes (along with the hemoglobin and hematocrit) can estimate the degree of excess fluid, acidosis, and electrolyte imbalance that might need to be corrected. An echocardiogram can be used to determine an underlying congenital cardiac lesion as a cause for CHF and how well the heart is pumping (contractility).

Differential Diagnosis

The differential diagnosis includes all causes of cardiac failure that might be secondary to respiratory failure, such as infection, sepsis, or severe anemia (high-output CHF). Primary cardiac causes of CHF are related to the abnormal anatomical flow and contractility.

Management

Initial management in the ED begins with cardiorespiratory resuscitation and managing the ABCs. The goals of treatment include relief of pulmonary and systemic venous congestion, improvement of myocardial performance, and reversal of the underlying process. Humidified oxygen support is important, as is elevating the head and shoulders approximately 45° to support pulmonary function. Cardiac, oxygen saturation, and blood pressure monitoring provide baseline information. Elective intubation might need to be considered in those children with respiratory distress who do not improve with initial management. Early IV access is important. Baseline electrolytes should be measured because correcting electrolyte abnormalities is important to optimize cardiac function. Diuretics remain a mainstay of therapy for CHF. Diuretic therapy can be used to help increase renal perfusion and sodium delivery to the renal excretion sites, thus helping the body rid itself of excess free water. Furosemide is the most commonly used diuretic for this purpose and is given as an IV dose of 0.5 to 2 mg/kg. Nitroglycerin can cause vasodilatation, which might be useful to reduce the preload and afterload on the right and left ventricles. This decreases cardiac workload and helps the heart pump more efficiently. Digoxin is the most widely used drug for the treatment of heart failure in children. It increases the force and velocity of ventricular contraction. It is given as a loading dose (IV in the case of acute heart failure). The dosage is 25 to 50 mcg/kg IV or orally with a maintenance dose rate of 5 to 15 mcg/kg per day in two divided doses. It has a narrow therapeutic range so serum levels need to be monitored and the potassium level should be kept in a normal range because hypokalemia increases the potential for digoxin toxicity. Other inotropic agents that can be used include dopamine, dobutamine, and epinephrine (adrenaline), which are all infused as a titratable continuous drip. All three of these improve contractility and heart rate. Dobutamine is the most specific for improving

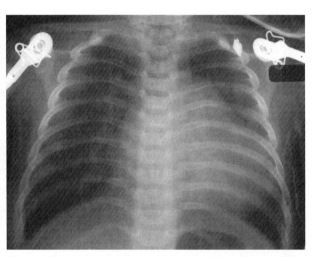

Figure 4.7A Chest radiograph showing cardiomegaly. Note the heart size is greater than 50% of the diameter of the chest. This is a 2-month-old with a ventriculoseptal defect and DiGeorge syndrome with cardiomegaly, without pulmonary edema.

Yamamoto LG. Seizure and VSD in 2 month old infant. In: Yamamoto LG, Inaba AS, DiMauro R, eds. *Radiology Cases in Pediatric Emergency Medicine.* Vol 2. Case 2. Honolulu: Kapiolani Medical Center For Women And Children, Department of Pediatrics, University of Hawaii John A. Burns School of Medicine; 1995.

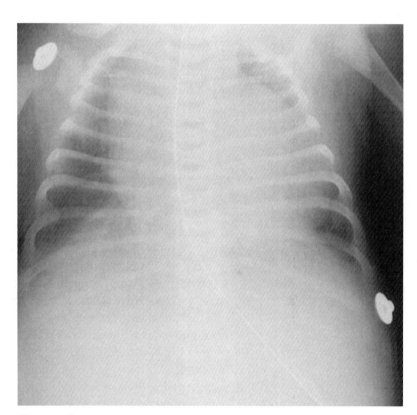

Figure 4.7B This is a 6 week old with high output congestive heart failure and resultant severe cardiomegaly.

Yamamoto LG. Seizure and VSD in 2-month-old infant. In: Yamamoto LG, Inaba AS, DiMauro R, eds. *Radiology Cases in Pediatric Emergency Medicine.* Vol 2, Case 2. Honolulu: Kapiolani Medical Center For Women And Children, Department of Pediatrics, University of Hawaii John A. Burns School of Medicine; 1995.

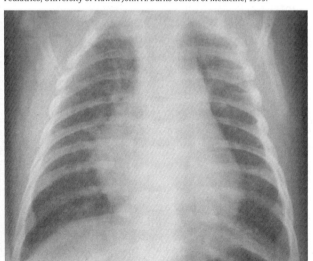

Figure 4.7C This is a 2 month old with mild cardiomegaly and pulmonary edema.

Matsuda JJ. Tachypnea in a 2 month old. In: Yamamoto LG, Inaba AS, DiMauro R, eds. *Radiology Cases in Pediatric Emergency Medicine.* Vol 4. Case 3. Honolulu: Kapiolani Medical Center For Women And Children, Department of Pediatrics, University of Hawaii John A. Burns School of Medicine; 1996.

contractility and increasing the heart rate. Dopamine and epinephrine (adrenaline) also increase systemic vascular resistance, which increases the blood pressure, but excessive vasoconstriction can adversely affect visceral organ perfusion.

CASE SCENARIO 2

A 10-year-old boy presents with chief symptoms of chest pain and shortness of breath. He has had 5 days of cold and cough symptoms. According to his mother, he has been lying around a lot and has missed 1 week of school. He is usually a very active child but states that he is "just too tired" to play. He says that his chest hurts, mostly with cough. He says that he has a hard time catching his breath whenever he gets up to walk around. He has had no medical problems or operations. He is in the fourth grade at school and had been the star basketball player until becoming ill. His only exposure to illness is his aunt, who was recently hospitalized for pneumonia. On initial presentation, he is a thin, pleasant boy who seems tired but talks in complete sentences without difficulty. He is tachypneic with mild retractions and slightly pale with dusky nail beds. His vital signs include a respiratory rate of 30/min, heart rate of 130/min, blood pressure of 90/65 mm Hg, and oral temperature of 37.8°C (100°F). Oxygen saturation is 90% on room air. His weight is 36.4 kg (80 lb). He is lying on the gurney with his head elevated. Capillary refill time is 4 to 5 seconds. His lungs have diminished breath sounds, with an occasional end expiratory wheeze with deep breaths. His heart sounds are present but faint without any murmurs. His abdomen is distended with a palpable liver and spleen.

1. *What is your initial assessment?*
2. *What are the treatment priorities?*
3. *What are the most likely causes based on this assessment?*
4. *What are initial and definitive treatment options?*
5. *What are the complications of this condition?*

Acquired Heart Disease

Myocarditis

Myocarditis is an inflammatory disease of the myocardium that can result from direct infection of the myocardium (eg, viral myocarditis), toxin production (eg, diphtheria), or an immune response as a delayed sequela of an infection (postviral or postinfectious myocarditis). A common type of myocarditis is acute rheumatic fever (ARF).

Clinical Features

Clinical features that might be present with myocarditis include fever, signs of CHF, dysrhythmias, muffled heart tones (ie, distant heart sounds), and systolic murmurs.

Diagnostic Studies

The primary tests to aid in diagnosis include a chest radiograph, ECG, and blood cultures.

YOUR FIRST CLUE

Signs and Symptoms of Myocarditis

- Pediatric Assessment Triangle:
  - Appearance: ranges in severity from normal (early, mild) to sweaty with feeding (early CHF), irritability, or lethargy (shock)
  - Work of breathing: ranges in severity from normal (early, mild) to retractions, tachypnea, or grunting (pulmonary edema)
  - Circulation: ranges in severity from normal (early, mild) to marginal perfusion (more severe), cyanosis (pulmonary edema), or poor perfusion (severe shock)
- Other signs and symptoms:
  - Fever
  - Muffled heart tones
  - Dysrhythmias
  - Heart murmur
  - Gallop rhythm
  - Shock

THE BOTTOM LINE

- Echocardiography is the diagnostic test of choice.
- Consider myocarditis because it can follow a viral infection (someone not getting better or getting worse with respiratory syncytial virus or influenza).

An echocardiogram is indicated to determine the area of enlargement of the heart and to assess contractility and to rule out any underlying congenital heart abnormalities.

Differential Diagnosis

In working up a diagnosis for the child, consider other causes of CHF, which can include sepsis, toxins, CHD, and metabolic abnormalities.

Management

Management in the ED begins with the ABCs, followed by inotropic support for the heart, control of dysrhythmias, and treatment of CHF.

Acute Rheumatic Fever

Acute rheumatic fever is perhaps the most common cause of acquired heart disease in children worldwide. In the United States as a whole, its incidence had decreased, but there has been a resurgence in some areas. Acute rheumatic fever results from an immune response that occurs as a delayed sequela of a group A streptococcal infection.

Clinical Features

The attack rate after this infection ranges from 0.3% to 3% (of those with an untreated streptococcal infection) and is most common in children 6 to 12 years old.[15–17] The rheumatic process affects multiple organs, with carditis being the most serious. The diagnosis is made using the Jones criteria (Table 4-1), which includes major and minor criteria with evidence of previous group A streptococcal infection. The major

TABLE 4-1 Jones Criteria for Guidance in the Diagnosis of Rheumatic Fever	
Major	Minor
Carditis	Fever
Migratory polyarthritis	Arthralgia
Chorea	Previous rheumatic fever/rheumatic heart disease
Erythema marginatum	Elevated erythrocyte sedimentation rate or C-reactive protein
Subcutaneous nodules	Prolonged PR interval

Diagnosis requires two major criteria or one major plus two minor. In addition, there must be evidence of antecedent streptococcal infection for the diagnosis of rheumatic fever. An exception is chorea, which alone (no need for any minor criteria to be present) can make the diagnosis without evidence of streptococcal infection.

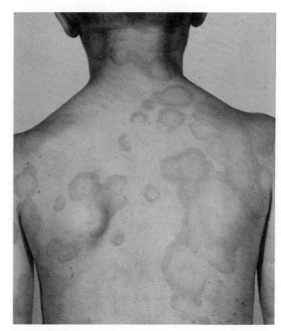

Figure 4.8 Erythema marginatum in a child with acute rheumatic fever.

criteria include carditis, polyarthritis, chorea, erythema marginatum, and subcutaneous nodules (**Figure 4.8**).

Clinically, children present with one of the major Jones criteria. Migratory polyarthritis is the most common. The arthritis is not very impressive on inspection, but it is extremely tender and will render the patient nonambulatory if it involves any of the lower-extremity joints. The arthritis will migrate from one joint to another, often with two or more joints involved simultaneously. Commonly involved joints include the knee, ankle, small foot joints (tarsals), elbow, wrist, shoulder, and small hand joints (carpals); however, any joint can be affected. Arthritis is distinguished from arthralgia in that arthritis has objective findings of inflammation, such as tenderness on palpation, tenderness with range of motion, visible swelling or redness, or limited range of motion. Arthralgia is only a subjective sense of joint pain without these findings. Carditis will often present in an occult manner unless chest pain or CHF is present. Fever might be the chief symptom. The most common manifestation of carditis is valvulitis. However, less

specific manifestations of ARF carditis include myocarditis, second-degree and third-degree AV block, and pericarditis. Valvulitis most often involves mitral insufficiency (holosystolic murmur at the apex radiating to the axilla) and aortic insufficiency (diastolic murmur heart over the base). Acute rheumatic fever valvulitis can result in chronic rheumatic heart disease. As the valves scar, they can develop elements of stenosis as well. Mitral and aortic insufficiency occur in acute rheumatic carditis, whereas mitral stenosis and aortic stenosis are complications of rheumatic carditis commonly seen in rheumatic heart disease (note the difference between ARF carditis and rheumatic heart disease). Sydenham chorea is a subacute presentation of rheumatic fever (ie, it occurs longer after the initial streptococcal infection, so acute phase reactants might no longer be elevated), which manifests as choreiform movements. Subcutaneous nodules and erythema marginatum are rare major criteria that occur with ARF.

Diagnostic Studies

Diagnostic studies include CBC, erythrocyte sedimentation rate (ESR), or C-reactive protein (CRP) to look for Jones minor criteria of acute inflammation. Typically, the ESR and CRP are in the very high range. The CBC is nonspecific. An ECG can show a prolonged PR interval (first-degree AV block), which is a Jones minor criterion and is not indicative of carditis. However, if ECG signs of CHF or advanced-degree AV block are present, these findings are more suggestive of carditis. Chest radiograph can reveal CHF. Doppler echocardiography is the most sensitive indicator of valvulitis. Evidence of preceding group A streptococcal infection is required for the diagnosis. This can include an elevated streptococcal serologic level (antistreptolysin O or a multiple streptococcal antibody assay) or a positive throat culture for group A streptococci. A reliable history indicating a previous episode of scarlet fever might suffice, but streptococcal serologic testing is more objective.

Differential Diagnosis

Differential diagnosis includes other entities that have similar cardiac, central nervous system, and joint involvement, such as Lyme disease, systemic lupus erythematosus, systemic arthritis, bacterial endocarditis, and myocarditis.

Management

Management priorities in the ED are to make a diagnosis when possible and to hospitalize the patient for further management. Although the treatment for polyarthritis is nonsteroidal anti-inflammatory drugs, these patients are usually nonambulatory, making it difficult to discharge them to home. In addition, the diagnosis of ARF has future consequences because penicillin prophylaxis is required until the age of 18 years or for life (depending on risk of recurrence). Thus, establishing an accurate diagnosis as an inpatient is required to commit a patient to such long-term prophylaxis. Carditis might require corticosteroid treatment under the direction of a cardiologist. Congestive heart failure should be treated as noted in the CHF section.

Pericarditis

Pericarditis is an acute or chronic inflammation of the pericardial sac with an increase in the pericardial fluid volume and pressure that causes cardiac stroke volume reduction. The pericardium can be divided into two components: the visceral pericardium (or epicardium) and the parietal pericardium. The parietal pericardium surrounds the heart and limits the diastolic dimensions of the heart. It attaches along the great vessels and has minimal elasticity. The visceral pericardium covers the heart and great vessels with a delicate lining that also includes fat, coronary vessels, and nerves. Between these two layers is a fluid layer to help protect the heart and its contractility. The usual fluid volume in the pericardial sac is 10 to 30 mL. When there is a sudden increase in fluid or constriction of the pericardial sac, this results in restriction of chamber-filling volume, which results in stroke volume reduction and hypotension (a process known as tamponade).[18–20] This increases the end diastolic pressure in the ventricle, which impairs ventricular filling and the ejection volume. The most common cause is infectious, with approximately 30% resulting from a bacterial cause. The most common viral cause is Coxsackie virus. Other causes include autoimmune disease, trauma, and neoplasms. A specific end point condition that can result from the acute or chronic inflammatory process is constrictive pericarditis. It is characterized by thickening of the pericardium adherent to the myocardium, causing restriction of the diastolic expansion of the ventricles. The most common cause of constrictive pericarditis is tuberculosis. Other bacterial causes of pericarditis include pneumococci, staphylococci, and *Haemophilus influenzae* pericarditis.

Clinical Features

Clinically, the child might present with chest pain and respiratory distress. The child who has altered cardiac function from either an increase in pericardial fluid or constriction of the pericardial sac will present with signs of CHF and a precordial "knock" or rub (like the sound of shoes walking on snow). The classic signs include exercise intolerance, fatigue, jugular venous distention, lower-extremity edema, hepatomegaly, poor distal pulses, diminished heart tones, and pulsus paradoxus.

Diagnostic Studies

An ECG is often normal but can show ST-segment elevation in multiple leads (**Figure 4.9**) or signs of tamponade while showing low-voltage QRS complexes or electrical alternans (**Figure 4.10**). A chest radiograph can show a normal or enlarged cardiac silhouette. There is a pleural effusion in 50% of cases. A two-dimensional echocardiogram is the "gold standard" for diagnosis and can differentiate between possible causes of the cardiac enlargement and impairment. Magnetic resonance imaging or computed tomography can be used to determine pericardial thickness but are not needed for acute diagnostic testing unless there is difficulty in obtaining a clear picture with echocardiography.

Differential Diagnosis

The differential diagnosis includes the various causes of pericarditis, including infections (viral and bacterial), autoimmune disorders, rheumatic disorder, systemic lupus erythematosus, and juvenile rheumatoid arthritis. Other causes to consider include traumatic hemopericardium, dysrhythmias, and toxicologic abnormalities.

Management

The management priorities in the acute care setting are pain control, oxygen support, and

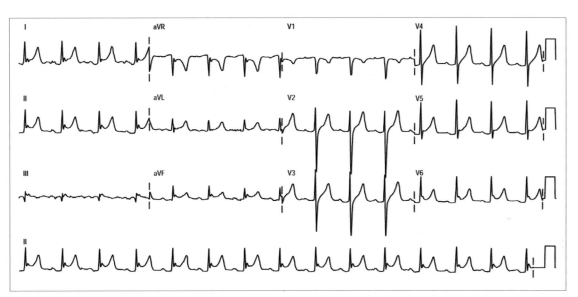

Figure 4.9 Electrocardiogram demonstrating ST-segment elevation in multiple leads consistent with pericarditis.

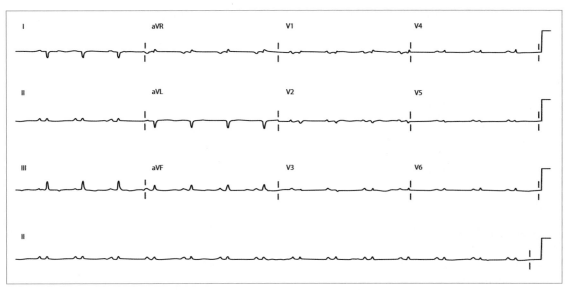

Figure 4.10 Low voltage QRS complexes.

Management of Pericarditis

- Provide supplemental oxygen.
- Perform cardiorespiratory monitoring and pulse oximetry.
- Elevate head of bed.
- Obtain vascular access.
- Administer analgesics and anti-inflammatory medication and consider antibiotic therapy.
- Obtain ECG, chest radiograph, and echocardiogram.
- Obtain cardiology consultation.
- Perform emergent pericardiocentesis for cardiac tamponade.

definitive management of the pericarditis. The child should be supported with head and shoulders elevated. Humidified oxygen should be given while monitoring for dysrhythmias. Oxygen saturation monitoring will help recognize deterioration. Once the diagnosis of pericarditis is made, the pericardial sac should be tapped for fluid (pericardiocentesis) for diagnostic and/or therapeutic reasons. The child should be prescribed anti-inflammatory medication and antibiotics. Emergency pericardiocentesis might be necessary if acute tamponade is present.

THE BOTTOM LINE

- Obtain echocardiography to distinguish pericardial effusion from dilated heart and to determine the degree of constriction and contractility compromise.

Bacterial Endocarditis

Endocarditis, although uncommon, is increasing in incidence, mostly because of the survival of children with CHD with artificial valves and patches and the increased frequency of patients with central catheters for various therapies. Endocarditis is an infection of the endothelial surface of the heart, with a propensity for the valves. Endocarditis can be caused by many different organisms, although 90% of cases are caused by gram-positive cocci. Although α-streptococcus (eg, *Streptococcus viridans*) is the most common organism involved, infections with *Staphylococcus aureus, Streptococcus pneumoniae,* or group A β-hemolytic streptococci can be more virulent.

Clinical Features

Patients typically present with fever, tachycardia, and signs of cardiac failure or dysrhythmia with a history of recent cardiac surgery or indwelling vascular catheter.[21] Other signs include myalgias, heart murmur, petechiae, septic emboli, or splenomegaly. Patients can also present with signs indistinguishable from myocarditis, with poor cardiac contractility and inadequate perfusion

YOUR FIRST CLUE

Signs and Symptoms of Bacterial Endocarditis

- Pediatric Assessment Triangle:
  - Appearance: ranges from tired, with flushed skin and tachycardia, to pale, diaphoresis, and poor perfusion
  - Work of breathing: ranges from slightly tachypneic (early stages), to tachypneic with diaphoresis (in shock)
  - Circulation: cutaneous signs of septic emboli can be visible; pale or mottled skin might be present
- Other signs and symptoms:
  - Fever
  - Heart murmur
  - Splinter hemorrhages
  - Petechiae
  - Septic emboli
  - Splenomegaly
  - Myalgias

with cool extremities, or symptoms similar to pericarditis, with pain in addition to CHF.

Diagnostic Studies

In a child with suspected endocarditis, laboratory tests, including CBC, ESR, CRP, and blood cultures, as well as a chest radiograph and an ECG, should be performed. The echocardiogram is the diagnostic "gold standard" and will help determine cardiac function and differentiate endocarditis from congenital lesions or shunts. Laboratory evaluation will show elevated acute-phase reactants (ESR and CRP), and a blood culture is usually positive. Echocardiography can show the nidus (ie, vegetation) of infection but is only 80% sensitive.[21] A rhythm strip can show premature ventricular contractions.

Differential Diagnosis

Congenital cardiac lesions with bacteremia, myocarditis, and pericarditis should be considered as direct cardiac causes. In addition, septic emboli from IV drug use or indwelling catheter sepsis should be considered.

Management

Treatment involves stabilization of respiratory and cardiac function with oxygen and fluid management. Antibiotic therapy should be started as quickly as possible after two or three sets of blood cultures have been obtained. Penicillin and gentamicin are the drugs of choice in patients who are not allergic to penicillin-based antibiotics. Vancomycin is a penicillin alternative that is empirically preferable because it provides coverage for resistant staphylococci and other resistant organisms. Antibiotic prophylaxis is appropriate for high-risk patients (those with CHD, cardiac surgery, and valvular abnormalities) undergoing dental procedures or other procedures associated with an increased risk of bacteremia. Indwelling catheters, which might be harboring bacteria, should be removed.

Kawasaki Disease

Mucocutaneous lymph node syndrome was first described by Kawasaki in 1967. The etiology is unknown, but it is seen most often in children younger than 5 years, during the winter and spring months. Boys are more susceptible than girls. There is also a predilection for Asian and black children.

Clinical Features

Clinically, the child with Kawasaki disease presents with a history of fever for 5 days or more and is usually irritable or fussy. The diagnostic criteria are the presence of conjunctivitis, cervical lymphadenopathy, erythematous mouth and pharynx, and/or red, cracked lips and strawberry tongue, maculopapular exanthem (called polymorphous, which means that it can have many different patterns), and swelling of the hands with erythema of the palms (**Figure 4.11A** and **Figure 4.11B**).

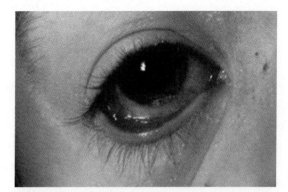

Figure 4.11A Conjunctivitis.

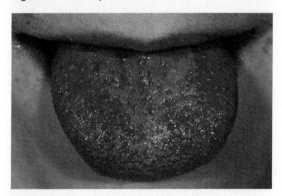

Figure 4.11B Strawberry tongue in a patient with Kawasaki disease.

Habif TP, ed. *Clinical Dermatology: A Color Guide to Diagnosis & Therapy.* 4th ed. St Louis, MO: Mosby; 2004. Copyright 2004, Elsevier. Reprinted with permission.

These patients might present with cardiac abnormalities that present in a manner similar to children with decreased myocardial contractility, myocarditis, or coronary insufficiency. The child might present or go on to develop CHF and shock with chest pain. Without treatment, 15% to 20% of children with Kawasaki disease will develop coronary artery aneurysms within 1 to 3 weeks from the onset of illness, which can eventually lead to a myocardial infarction or ischemia-induced dysrhythmias. A child who presents with a myocardial infarction might have more nonspecific findings than an adult. These patients can present with nausea, vomiting, and abdominal pain. They can be diaphoretic and crying or asymptomatic.

Diagnostic Studies

There are no specific laboratory tests to diagnose Kawasaki disease, but there might be an elevated white blood cell count, elevated platelet count, sterile pyuria, and elevation of liver function test results. There is an elevation of acute-phase reactants (ESR and CRP). An ECG can show nonspecific ST-segment and T-wave changes consistent with strain. A chest radiograph, if abnormal, will show some cardiac enlargement. Group A streptococci infection can mimic many of the signs of Kawasaki disease; therefore, a throat swab for rapid group A streptococci

---

YOUR FIRST CLUE

Signs and Symptoms of Kawasaki Disease

- Pediatric Assessment Triangle:
  - Appearance: fussy but alert
  - Work of breathing: mild tachypnea due to fever and, occasionally, severe respiratory distress due to myocarditis or myocardial infarction
  - Circulation: flushed skin or signs of shock with pallor or mottled skin
- Other signs and symptoms:
  - Red, cracked lips
  - Strawberry tongue
  - Conjunctivitis
  - Cervical lymphadenopathy
  - Rash
  - Swelling of hands and feet
  - Chest pain

THE CLASSICS

Diagnostic Studies in Kawasaki Disease

- Elevated ESR and CRP level
- Elevated white blood cell count
- Thrombocytosis
- Sterile pyuria
- Elevated liver function test results
- Coronary aneurysms revealed by echocardiography

analysis and throat culture should be taken. Once other disease processes are ruled out, the child should undergo echocardiography to examine the coronary arteries.

Differential Diagnosis

The differential diagnosis includes viral or rickettsial exanthems, such as measles, Epstein-Barr virus infection, Rocky Mountain spotted fever, scarlet fever, leptospirosis, and toxic shock syndrome. Other diagnoses to consider are Stevens-Johnson syndrome, drug reaction (eg, serum sickness), and juvenile rheumatoid arthritis. Consider the diagnosis of Kawasaki disease if any of the preceding conditions is also considered as a diagnostic possibility.

Management

The child with Kawasaki disease will need IV fluid support and cardiac monitoring. Once Kawasaki disease is thought to be the diagnosis, the patient should be hospitalized and treated with aspirin and intravenous immune globulin (IVIG). Early IVIG treatment reduces the risk of developing coronary aneurysms. A cardiology consultation should be obtained for echocardiography and follow-up for potential future problems. The initial dose for aspirin is 80 to 100 mg/kg per day orally divided into equal 6-hour doses until the patient is afebrile for 2 to 3 days. Then the dose for aspirin is 3 to 5 mg/kg orally once a day for 6 to 8 weeks. Treatment with IVIG is begun as an infusion at a dose of 2 mg/kg given during 12 hours. Treatment with IVIG can cause hypotension, as well as nausea, vomiting, and seizures. Cardiac monitoring is essential.[22,23]

Rhythm Disturbances

Pediatric patients have three basic types of pathologic rhythm disturbances, which include fast pulse (tachyarrhythmia), slow pulse (bradyarrhythmia), and absent pulse (pulseless) (Table 4-2). These can be further divided into seven classifications based on their anatomical function. Dysrhythmias might be the cause of impaired cardiac function leading to cardiac arrest. Occult dysrhythmias (eg, prolonged QT syndrome or Wolff-Parkinson-White syndrome) might present with intermittent severe symptoms (eg, palpitations or sudden death).

Clinical Features

Clinical features of dysrhythmias are usually nonspecific. The child might present with fatigue or syncope, but many patients are asymptomatic on presentation. Hypoxemia is one of the most frequent causes of bradyarrhythmias, so the child might have cyanosis or respiratory problems as the presenting symptom. Children with tachyarrhythmias usually present with chest or abdominal pain and/or a feeling of the heart racing and the feeling of not being able to catch their breath. Infants with tachyarrhythmias can present with nonspecific symptoms, such as vomiting and irritability.

TABLE 4-2 Classification of Rhythm Disturbances

Fast Rhythms
- Supraventricular tachycardia
- Ventricular tachycardia

Slow Rhythms
- Sinus bradycardia
- Heart blocks

Absent Pulses
- Ventricular fibrillation
- Pulseless ventricular tachycardia
- Asystole
- Pulseless electrical activity

YOUR FIRST CLUE

Signs and Symptoms of Dysrhythmias
- Pediatric Assessment Triangle:
  - Appearance: ranges in severity from normal (sufficient cardiac output), to distress or lethargic (CHF or inadequate cardiac output)
  - Work of breathing: ranges in severity from normal, depending on adequacy of cardiac output, and varying degrees of CHF
  - Circulation: ranges in severity from normal color (sufficient cardiac output), to pale, mottled, and cyanosis; marginal perfusion (insufficient cardiac output, CHF); or poor perfusion (severe shock)
- Other signs and symptoms:
  - Fatigue
  - Irritability
  - Vomiting
  - Chest or abdominal pain
  - Palpitations
  - Respiratory distress
  - Shock

Diagnostic Studies

An ECG is the initial diagnostic test to document the dysrhythmia, followed by ongoing cardiac monitoring and a follow-up ECG to document the effect of any antidysrhythmia agent on establishment of a normal heart rhythm. In addition, monitoring blood pressure will help to determine whether the dysrhythmia is affecting cardiac function. Once the basic type of rhythm disturbance and whether the child is asymptomatic or needs treatment are determined, examination of the ECG will help in differentiating between the various types of fast and slow rhythms. To discriminate between types of fast rhythms, the QRS complex width and the P wave presence should be examined to determine the origin of the dysrhythmia and any aberrant conduction problem. Both the PR interval and beat-to-beat pacing will help differentiate various slow rhythms.

The ECG of patients with Wolff-Parkinson-White syndrome will demonstrate a very short PR interval and a classic delta wave (**Figure 4.12**). These patients are at risk for recurrent paroxysmal supraventricular tachycardia (SVT). Other conditions predisposing patients to paroxysmal SVT might not be as evident on an ECG performed when the patient is nonsymptomatic, requiring long-term (Holter) ECG rhythm monitoring to capture the intermittent abnormal rhythm. Patients with prolonged QT interval will have a prolonged corrected QTc interval. Many QTc intervals are in the borderline prolonged range. Patients with prolonged QTc intervals should be referred to a cardiologist because they are at risk for sudden death.

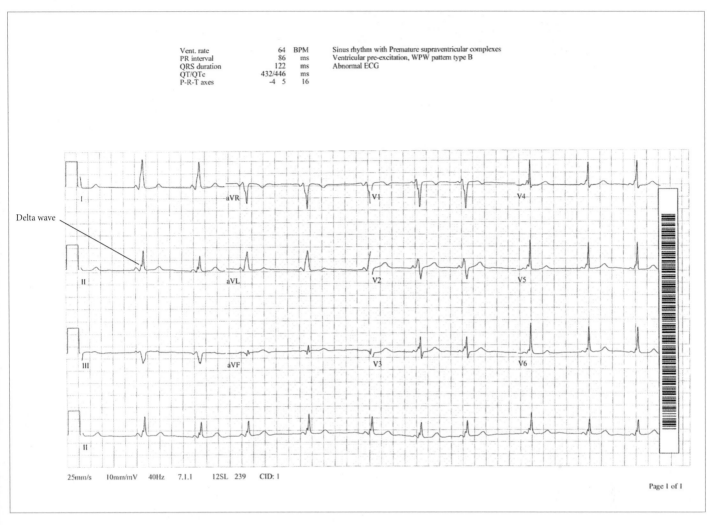

Vent. rate	64	BPM
PR interval	86	ms
QRS duration	122	ms
QT/QTc	432/446	ms
P-R-T axes	-4 5	16

Sinus rhythm with Premature supraventricular complexes
Ventricular pre-excitation, WPW pattern type B
Abnormal ECG

Delta wave

I   aVR   V1   V4

II   aVL   V2   V5

III   aVF   V3   V6

II

25mm/s   10mm/mV   40Hz   7.1.1   12SL   239   CID: 1

Page 1 of 1

Figure 4.12 Twelve-lead electrocardiogram showing Wolff-Parkinson-White syndrome.

Management

The management goal in the ED for any dysrhythmia is to make sure that all reversible causes are addressed, beginning with maintaining oxygenation and ventilation. Thinking of the six Hs and five Ts mnemonic for reversible causes of dysrhythmias will aid in the treatment of any underlying cause and prevent cardiac arrest. The six Hs are hypovolemia, hypoxia, hydrogen ion (acidosis), hypo-/hyperkalemia, hypoglycemia, and hypothermia. The five Ts are toxins, tamponade (cardiac), tension pneumothorax, thrombosis (coronary), and thrombosis (pulmonary) (Table 4-3).[24] To administer antidysrhythmia medications, IV access should be

obtained. If, however, the rhythm is unstable supraventricular or ventricular tachycardia (VT) and requires cardioversion, the nonpharmacologic maneuvers might take precedence over IV access.

Bradydysrhythmias

For bradydysrhythmias, consider hypoxia as a cause first and immediately support the airway, ventilation, and oxygenation. Chest compressions should be started for a heart rate less than 60/min with poor perfusion. The treatment of choice for symptomatic bradydysrhythmias is IV or intraosseous (IO) administration of

TABLE 4-3 Reversible Causes of Pediatric Cardiac Arrest

Six Hs	Five Ts
Hypovolemia	Tension pneumothorax
Hypoxia	Tamponade (cardiac)
Hydrogen ion (acidosis)	Toxins
Hypoglycemia	Thrombosis (pulmonary)
Hypo-/ hyperkalemia	Thrombosis (coronary)
Hypothermia	

Kleinman ME, Chameides L, Schexnayder SM. Part 14: Pediatric advanced life support: 2010 American Heart Association guidelines for cardiopulmonary resuscitation and emergency cardiovascular care. *Circulation.* 2010;122:S876–S908.

epinephrine (adrenaline) at 0.01 mg/kg (0.1 mL/kg of 1:10,000 solution) or tracheal (endotracheal) 0.1 mg/kg (0.1 mL/kg of 1:1,000 solution). Repeat administration of epinephrine (adrenaline) every 3 to 5 minutes. If bradycardia persists or transiently responds, consider an epinephrine (adrenaline) infusion. Atropine can be used to treat bradydysrhythmias if there is a suspicion of increased vagal tone, primary AV block, or cholinergic drug toxicity. The recommended dose is 0.02 mg/kg, with a minimum dose of 0.1 mg and a maximum single dose of 0.5 mg in a child and 1 mg in an adolescent. This can

be repeated in 5 minutes to a maximum total dose of 1 mg in a child and 2 mg in an adolescent. Atropine can be administered tracheally (endotracheally), if IV or IO access cannot be obtained (0.04 to 0.06 mg/kg).[24] Transcutaneous pacing can also be considered in those cases of bradycardia from a congenital or acquired heart disease that has caused a complete heart block or sinus node dysfunction[24] (**Figure 4.13**).

Tachydysrhythmias

Sinus tachycardia is not a dysrhythmia but rather a response by the body to increased cardiac output, so the underlying cause should be identified and treated. Common causes include hypoxemia, hypovolemia, hyperthermia, fever, toxins, poisons, drugs, pain, and anxiety. Supraventricular tachycardia is the most common tachydysrhythmia in children and can produce cardiovascular compromise. The heart rate is usually greater than 220/min but can reach as high as 300/min. Usually the QRS interval is narrow or normal (≤0.09 seconds). The cause is most commonly a reentry mechanism from an accessory pathway. It usually occurs quickly and without a history of volume loss, pain, or fever to suggest sinus tachycardia. In many instances, it might be difficult to distinguish between sinus tachycardia and SVT (Table 4-4). If the child is stable and has good perfusion, the treatment of choice is mechanical vagal interventions. If this is unsuccessful, then IV adenosine

TABLE 4-4 Comparison of Sinus Tachycardia (ST) and Supraventricular Tachycardia (SVT)

ST	SVT
History of underlying problem, such as fever, dehydration, injury, or pain	History incompatible with ST (no history of dehydration, fever) or nonspecific
P waves present	P waves absent
Heart rate varies with activity	Heart rate does not change with activity
Variable R-R interval with respirations	Constant R-R interval with respirations Abrupt rate changes (with conversion)
Infants: heart rate <220/min	Infants: heart rate >220/min
Children: heart rate <180/min	Children: heart rate >180/min

Hazinski MF, Zaritsky AL, Nadkarni VN, et al, eds. *PALS Provider Manual.* Dallas, TX: American Heart Association; 2002:202. Reprinted with permission.

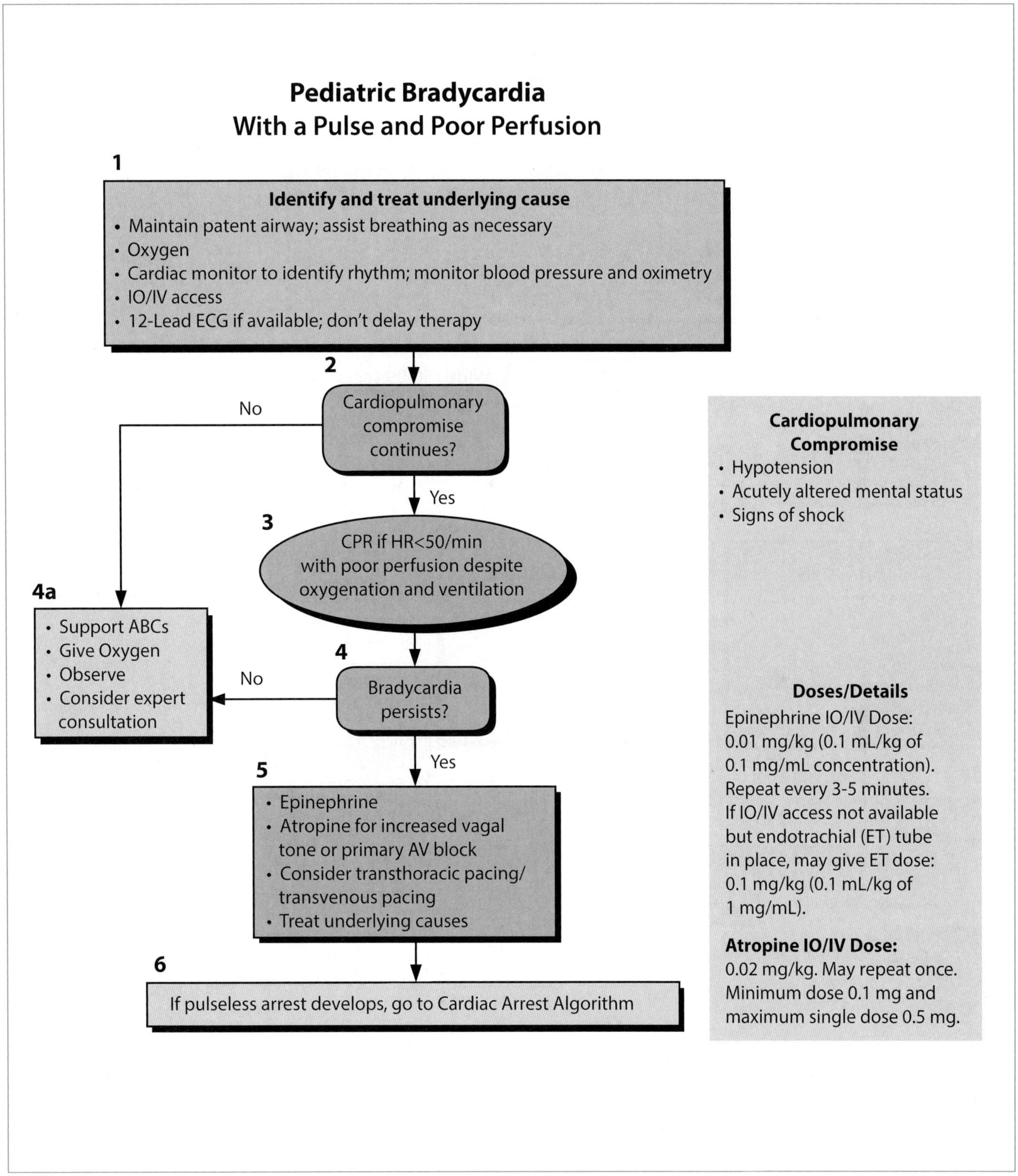

Pediatric Bradycardia
With a Pulse and Poor Perfusion

1

Identify and treat underlying cause

- Maintain patent airway; assist breathing as necessary
- Oxygen
- Cardiac monitor to identify rhythm; monitor blood pressure and oximetry
- IO/IV access
- 12-Lead ECG if available; don't delay therapy

2

Cardiopulmonary compromise continues? — No →

↓ Yes

3

CPR if HR<50/min with poor perfusion despite oxygenation and ventilation

4a

- Support ABCs
- Give Oxygen
- Observe
- Consider expert consultation

← No

4

Bradycardia persists?

↓ Yes

5

- Epinephrine
- Atropine for increased vagal tone or primary AV block
- Consider transthoracic pacing/transvenous pacing
- Treat underlying causes

6

If pulseless arrest develops, go to Cardiac Arrest Algorithm

Cardiopulmonary Compromise

- Hypotension
- Acutely altered mental status
- Signs of shock

Doses/Details

Epinephrine IO/IV Dose: 0.01 mg/kg (0.1 mL/kg of 0.1 mg/mL concentration). Repeat every 3-5 minutes. If IO/IV access not available but endotrachial (ET) tube in place, may give ET dose: 0.1 mg/kg (0.1 mL/kg of 1 mg/mL).

Atropine IO/IV Dose: 0.02 mg/kg. May repeat once. Minimum dose 0.1 mg and maximum single dose 0.5 mg.

Figure 4.13 Pediatric advanced life support bradycardia algorithm.

Reproduced with permission. Kleinman ME, Chameides L, Schexnayder SM. Part 14: Pediatric advanced life support: 2010 American Heart Association guidelines for cardiopulmonary resuscitation and emergency cardiovascular care. *Circulation.* 2010;122:S876–S908.

Pediatric Tachycardia
With a Pulse and Poor Perfusion

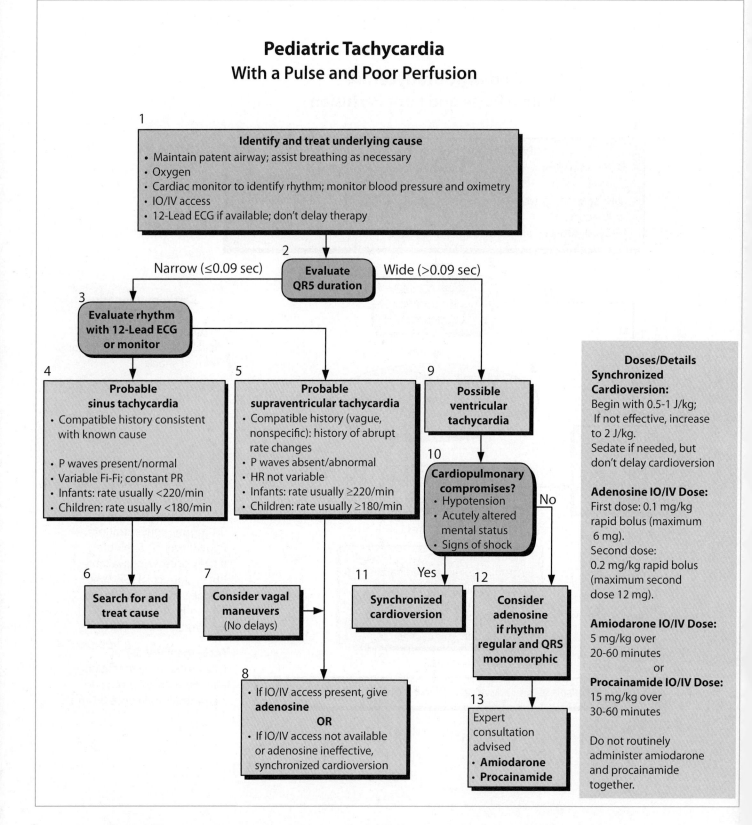

Figure 4.14 Pediatric advanced life support tachycardia algorithm.

Reproduced with permission. Kleinman ME, Chameides L, Schexnayder SM. Part 14: Pediatric advanced life support: 2010 American Heart Association guidelines for cardiopulmonary resuscitation and emergency cardiovascular care. *Circulation.* 2010;122:S876–S908.

is recommended (**Figure 4.14**). Vagal maneuvers include an ice bag to the face (most applicable to infants and young children) or Valsalva maneuvers, such as blowing into a straw or bearing down (most applicable in older cooperative children). Carotid massage and eyeball pressure are poor vagal maneuvers that are potentially harmful and should not be attempted. Adenosine is administered in a dose of 0.1 mg/kg as a rapid IV bolus (maximum initial dose 6 mg). This dose can be doubled on the second attempt to 0.2 mg/kg and increased again to 0.4 mg/kg up to a maximum of 12 mg if initial doses are unsuccessful in converting the rhythm. The rapidity of the adenosine bolus can be an important factor. If a peripheral vein is used, adenosine is most rapidly infused by a fast push followed by an immediate flush of the IV catheter as close to the IV insertion site as possible. If SVT persists and the child remains hemodynamically stable, expert consultation is advised, but amiodarone (5 mg/kg for 20 to 60 minutes) or procainamide (15 mg/kg for 30 to 60 minutes) can be considered. Do not use both.[24] If the child has poor perfusion, then synchronized cardioversion of the rhythm is the treatment of choice[24] (Figure 4.14). Attempts to insert a catheter should occur concomitantly or should be deferred, rather than delaying cardioversion. The cardioversion dose is 0.5 to 1 J/kg, which can be increased to 2 J/kg if the initial attempt is unsuccessful. A baseline ECG and another after electrical or chemical cardioversion should be performed to help determine the cause and assess treatment effectiveness. Ideally, a rhythm strip should be running continuously during rhythm conversion attempts.

Ventricular Tachycardia

Ventricular tachycardia with a pulse is a rare dysrhythmia in pediatrics but is often life threatening.[25] Differentiating VT from SVT is important to initiate the appropriate treatment and prevent deterioration. In VT, typically the heart rate can go as high as 200/min and the QRS complex is wide. Most children with VT have underlying heart disease, either congenital or acquired.

If the child has poor perfusion, signs of shock, or an altered mental status, synchronized cardioversion is the treatment of choice. If the patient does not have cardiopulmonary compromise and it is unclear whether the rhythm is VT but the rhythm is regular and the QRS is monomorphic, adenosine might be helpful in differentiating SVT from VT.[24] Adenosine should not be used in patients with known Wolff-Parkinson-White syndrome. If the VT is confirmed and the patient does not have cardiopulmonary compromise, expert consultation should be obtained and the use of amiodarone (5 mg/kg for 20 to 60 minutes) or procainamide (15 mg/kg for 30 to 60 minutes) considered.[24] These two drugs should not be administered together.

Pediatric Cardiac Arrest

Cardiopulmonary arrest is the end point when the body's compensation mechanisms have been overwhelmed and are unable to overcome dysfunction in respiratory and cardiac systems. In pediatrics, the most common primary cause is respiratory failure, but impaired cardiac output can also lead to arrest. The most common rhythm in an out-of-hospital arrest is asystole, and the likelihood of recovery is less than 1%.[26–31] Other pulseless arrest rhythms include ventricular fibrillation, pulseless ventricular tachycardia, and pulseless electrical activity (PEA) (**Figure 4.15**).

Clinical Features

A child presents with no pulse but might have PEA. Other signs are cool extremities and cyanotic skin. There is no respiratory effort. The underlying cause might not be evident on initial examination, but looking for signs of trauma is important when trying to find a cause.

Diagnostic Studies

Body temperature, ECG, cardiorespiratory monitoring, and blood pH will help determine the cardiac status and provide prognostic indicators for successful resuscitation. A poor prognosis is indicated by PEA or asystole in the absence of underlying causes (six Hs and five Ts)

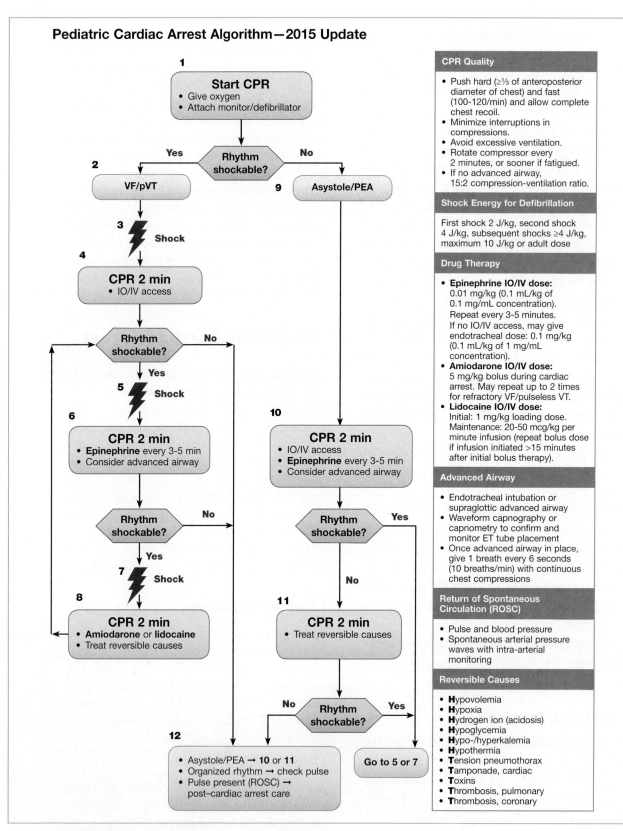

Figure 4.15 Pediatric advanced life support cardiac arrest algorithm.

Reprinted with permission. *Circulation*. 2015;132:S526–S542. © 2015 American Heart Association, Inc.

and/or the presence of severe acidosis (pHL 6.9). A bedside glucose test (rapid test), arterial blood gas analysis, and measurement of electrolytes are important to guide resuscitation.

Once the resuscitation has begun, consider potentially reversible causes. Again, the mnemonic of six Hs and five Ts includes the following: hypoxemia, hypovolemia, hypothermia, hyper/hypokalemia, hydrogen ion (acidosis), hypoglycemia, tamponade, toxins/poisons/drugs, tension pneumothorax, thrombosis (coronary), and thrombosis (pulmonary).[24]

Management

For cardiopulmonary arrest, the first priority is to shout for help, start chest compressions at a rate of at least 100 per minute, and ventilate with 100% oxygen via bag mask. The rate for children less than 8 years is 30 compressions to two ventilations for a single rescuer and 15:2 for two rescuers. For those over 8 years it is 30 compressions to two ventilations. If the patient has an advanced airway in place, the ventilations should be given at 8 to 10 breaths per minute with continuous chest compressions.[24] A monitor/defibrillator or an automated external defibrillator should be attached as soon as possible. The cardiac activity or the effectiveness of chest compressions (measure blood pressure, perfusion, and oxygen saturation) should be monitored and the rhythm assessed. If the rhythm is shockable (ventricular fibrillation/VT), shock or defibrillation should be performed at 2 J/kg and cardiopulmonary resuscitation (CPR) immediately resumed. Either IV or IO access should be obtained during the next five cycles (2 minutes) of CPR, then the rhythm checked. If shockable, CPR should be continued while the automated external defibrillator or monitor/defibrillator is charging, and the patient should be shocked or defibrillated at 4 J/kg. Cardiopulmonary resuscitation should be resumed immediately. During this next cycle of CPR, epinephrine (adrenaline) (0.01 mg/kg IV/IO of 1:10,000 concentration) should be administered and this dose repeated every 3 to 5 minutes. If there is no IV/IO access, but the patient is intubated, 0.01 mg/kg of a 1:1,000 concentration of epinephrine (adrenaline) should be administered by the endotracheal tube. When five cycles (2 minutes) are complete, the rhythm

should be checked and, if shockable, the patient should be shocked or defibrillated with 4 J/kg and CPR resumed. Amiodarone (5 mg/kg IV/IO bolus) or lidocaine (1 mg/kg) therapy should be considered and administered while CPR is provided for five cycles; the rhythm should then be checked. If rhythm is still shockable, the CPR-drug-shock cycle should be repeated with epinephrine (adrenaline) and the patient shocked or administered a 4-J/kg defibrillation energy dose. Amiodarone can be repeated up to two times in this cycle or lidocaine can be maintained at an infusion of 20 to 50 mcg/kg/min (repeat bolus dose if infusion > 15 min after initial bolus therapy).[24a] If torsades de pointes is present, magnesium (25 to 50 mg/kg) administration should be considered during CPR (maximum single dose of 2 g).[24]

If the rhythm shows PEA or asystole (nonshockable rhythm), CPR should be continued for 2 minutes, IV/IO access obtained, and intubation considered. Epinephrine (adrenaline) (0.01 mg/kg IV/IO of 1:10,000 concentration or 0.01 mg/kg endotracheally of 1:1,000 concentration) should be administered and CPR resumed. Epinephrine (adrenaline) can be repeated every 3 to 5 minutes. High-dose epinephrine (adrenaline) can be considered in β-blocker overdose.[24] If at any time there is electrical activity, the pulse should be checked. If a pulse is present, postresuscitation care should begin. If a pulse is absent, CPR should be continued and the asystole/PEA pathway followed.[24]

Termination of resuscitation is a critical issue. Studies show little to no meaningful

---

THE BOTTOM LINE

- Treatment of patients with dysrhythmias is driven by the presence or absence of poor perfusion.
- Sinus tachycardia is not an arrhythmia, but its cause must be determined.
- Provide oxygenation and ventilation for all patients in cardiopulmonary arrest as the primary cause is respiratory failure.
- Once resuscitation has begun, evaluate and treat reversible cause of cardiopulmonary arrest.
- Family presence during resuscitation should be encouraged by the ED staff.

survival if spontaneous circulation has not returned after 30 minutes of resuscitation or after two doses of epinephrine (adrenaline) have been delivered.[28–30] Few children survive out-of-hospital cardiopulmonary arrest, and fewer will have a normal neurologic recovery.[30,31] When asked, parents wish to be present during the resuscitation of their child, and it often can help parents with the grieving process.[32,33]

Cardiomyopathy

The danger of cardiomyopathies is that these conditions can lead to sudden death. Hypertrophic

cardiomyopathy (formerly called idiopathic hypertrophic subaortic stenosis), which can be inherited, and other cardiomyopathies predispose otherwise healthy-appearing children to life-threatening dysrhythmias. These children might have a family history of sudden death, syncope (with or without exercise), and a systolic murmur that increases with certain specific maneuvers. The heart murmur is often a harsh crescendo/decrescendo murmur with an associated S_4 and will increase with standing from the squatting position and Valsalva maneuver. The murmur is heard best at the left sternal border and apex and does not radiate to the carotids, distinguishing it from an aortic stenosis murmur. Chronic cardiomyopathies might cause chronic CHF.

Diagnostic Studies

Diagnostic studies include ECG, chest radiography, and echocardiography. The ECG result can be nonspecifically abnormal in up to 95% of all cases of hypertrophic cardiomyopathy, which might include signs of left ventricular hypertrophy and ST wave changes. The chest radiograph results are often normal. Echocardiography reveals asymmetric septal hypertrophy in 90% of cases.

Differential Diagnosis

The differential diagnosis is that of benign and malignant murmurs, left ventricular hypertrophy due to exercise, and vasovagal syncope.

Management

A child who presents with exercise-induced syncope should be withdrawn from any and all significant physical activity pending a cardiology evaluation. A child who presents with a clinical course suggesting cardiovascular instability (eg, a murmur or palpitations) should be admitted for observation in a monitored bed and undergo an urgent evaluation by a cardiologist (ECG, echocardiography, and exercise stress testing).

Postsurgical Complications

Postsurgical problems in children who have undergone cardiac surgery can include rhythm disturbances, infections (including endocarditis or bacteremia), and pulmonary edema. Most acute problems will occur while the patient is recovering from the surgical procedure.[34–36] However, after discharge, most will still have some pulmonary edema secondary to thoracostomy tube removal and the healing process of the surgical procedure. They might have an acute deterioration during the home recovery stage. If the surgical procedure involved accessing the interior of the heart, the child is also at risk for new dysrhythmias after the surgical procedure while the tissue heals, especially if this is near or over the electrical conduction pathways. Other postsurgical complications include those that occur in multiple-step procedures in which a palliative shunt is placed, which might clot or become dysfunctional. In this case, the child might present with symptoms reflective of the original cardiac lesion.

Clinical Features

Clinically, these patients present with specific features related to their underlying problem, but all might look pale and will have a midsternotomy scar. Febrile children can be tired and tachycardic or tachypneic. They can have either bounding pulses or decreased pulses in the distal extremities. Signs of CHF can be present in those with pulmonary edema and cardiac shunt malfunction.

YOUR FIRST CLUE

Signs and Symptoms of Postsurgical Cardiac Complications

- Pediatric Assessment Triangle:
  - Appearance: ranges in severity from normal (good functional surgical repair), to sweaty with feeding, failure to thrive (CHF), irritability (pulmonary edema), lethargic (shock), or sudden decompensation (clot formation within a shunt or disruption of surgical repair)
  - Work of breathing: ranges in severity from normal (good functional repair), to retractions, tachypnea, or grunting (pulmonary edema)
  - Circulation: ranges in severity from normal (good functional repair) to cyanosis (palliative or inadequate surgical repair) or poor perfusion (shock, sudden decompensation)
- Other signs and symptoms
  - History of CHD and cardiac surgery
  - Presence of sternotomy or thoracotomy scar
  - Fatigue
  - Fever
  - Respiratory distress
  - Dysrhythmia

KEY POINTS

The Management of Postsurgical Cardiac Complications

- Start cardiorespiratory monitoring.
- Provide supplemental oxygen.
- Obtain IV access.
- Manage arrhythmia.
- Manage CHF.
- Obtain ECG and chest radiograph.
- Contact cardiologist or cardiac surgeon.

THE BOTTOM LINE

Postsurgical Cardiac Complications

- Obtain rapid history and assess children in shock or respiratory distress for CHD and postsurgical complications.
- Use the EIF to gather information, contact specialists, and guide therapy.
- Obtain rapid echocardiography and cardiology consultation for definitive diagnosis and cardiac function determination.

Differential Diagnosis

The differential diagnosis is primarily that of problems with the heart itself secondary to the surgical procedure versus the usual childhood illnesses and injuries. The febrile child might have an infection obtained in the hospital or at home. Table 4-5 summarizes the common palliative and definitive surgical procedures typically performed for the listed cyanotic heart disease conditions.

Management

These patients require stabilization of airway, ventilation, and circulation. Oxygen saturation monitoring with humidified oxygen administration is the first step. Cardiac and blood pressure monitoring will help detect dysrhythmias and determine cardiovascular stability. An ECG should be obtained to determine the exact rhythm. A chest radiograph might reveal pulmonary edema or an abnormal cardiac shadow, which should be compared with the postsurgical chest radiograph if possible. An echocardiogram might be indicated if there is concern of pericardial fluid, abnormal cardiac contractility, or an alternation in the surgical repair.

An IV catheter should be placed for fluid management. Depending on the clinical presentation and diagnostic testing, the child might need an intervention for a dysrhythmia or pulmonary edema. The child might require pericardiocentesis. Consultation should be made with the pediatric cardiac surgeon for any postsurgical problems. Information on the type of repair and potential complications with their management can be found on an emergency information form (EIF) (see Chapter 13, Children With Special Health Care Needs). Ask the patient's family whether an EIF is available or note if the patient has a MedicAlert bracelet. If so, contact the MedicAlert Foundation for additional information.

TABLE 4-5 Common Palliative and Definitive Surgical Procedures Typically Performed for the Listed Cyanotic Heart Disease Conditions*

Total Anomalous Pulmonary Venous Return	Truncus Arteriosus
• Obstructive lesion – Balloon atrial septostomy – Complete repair later – Patches and anastomotic procedures to reroute blood flow	• Surgical closure – Closure of the ventriculoseptal defect – Right ventricle–pulmonary artery connection with aortic homograft (Rastelli repair) or conduit with a semilunar valve

Tetralogy of Fallot	Hypoplastic Left Heart
• Palliative repair – Blalock-Taussig—subclavian artery to pulmonary artery – Potts—descending aorta to left pulmonary artery – Waterston—ascending aorta to right pulmonary artery • Surgical repair – Closure of the ventriculoseptal defect – Relief of the pulmonic stenosis	• Surgical palliation—Norwood operation – First stage ▪ Connecting the main pulmonary arterial trunk to the ascending aorta and aortic arch ▪ Dividing the ductus arteriosus ▪ Modified Blalock-Taussig shunt – Second stage ▪ Bidirectional cavopulmonary (superior vena cava and pulmonary arteries) connection (Glenn) ▪ Closing the aortopulmonary window • Modified Fontan procedure—cavopulmonary isolation procedure (anastomosis of the inferior vena cava to the pulmonary arteries) – Completed at 12 to 18 months of age • Transplant protocol

---

TABLE 4-5 **Common Palliative and Definitive Surgical Procedures Typically Performed for the Listed Cyanotic Heart Disease Conditions*, continued**

Transposition of the Great Vessels

- Surgical repair today
  - Arterial switch operation—Jatene operation
- Surgical procedures that are no longer performed
  - Mustard or Senning procedure (intracardiac baffle that diverts blood to the correct side)

Coarctation of the Aorta

- Coaretation repair
- Dividing the ductus

Tricuspid Atresia

- Palliative surgery for relief of hypoxemia
  - Less than 1 month of age
    - Central aortopulmonary shunt
    - Modified Blalock-Taussig shunt
  - 1 to 6 months of age
    - Modified Blalock-Taussig shunt
  - Older than 6 months
    - Modified Blalock-Taussig shunt
    - Bidirectional Glenn anastomosis
  - Surgical repair
    - Staged modified Fontan procedure

*This table does not address surgical repair of mixed cardiac lesions.

Check Your Knowledge

1. Which newborn anatomical structure closes at birth or shortly thereafter to help with the transition from the intrauterine to extrauterine environment?
   A. Coronary sinus
   B. Ductus arteriosus
   C. Pulmonary artery
   D. Ventricular septum

2. Which of the following is a common cyanotic congenital heart lesion?
   A. Patent ductus arteriosus
   B. Tetralogy of Fallot
   C. Pulmonary stenosis
   D. Ventricular septal defect

3. Which of the following drugs can be a lifesaver in a newborn with congestive heart failure (CHF) secondary to closure of the ductus arteriosus?
   A. Digoxin
   B. Dopamine
   C. Furosemide
   D. Prostaglandin E_1

4. Which of the following is a major criterion of the Jones criteria for the diagnosis of acute rheumatic fever?
   A. Arthralgias
   B. Elevated white blood cell count
   C. Erythema marginatum
   D. Positive antistreptolysin O titer

5. Which of the following cyanotic congenital heart lesions show increased pulmonary vascularity on a chest radiograph?
   A. Tetralogy of Fallot
   B. Transposition of the great arteries
   C. Ebstein anomaly
   D. Hypoplastic right heart

6. Without treatment, 15% to 20% of children with Kawasaki disease will develop which of the following?
   A. Fever
   B. Coronary artery aneurysms
   C. Dysrhythmias
   D. Abdominal pain

7. Infants with noncyanotic congenital heart disease can develop hypoxia (and cyanosis) through which of the following mechanisms?
   A. Pulmonary edema
   B. Right to left shunting
   C. Peripheral vasoconstriction
   D. Early onset coronary artery disease

8. Which of the following is not a sign or symptom of congestive heart failure?
   A. Poor feeding
   B. Vomiting
   C. Tachypnea
   D. Soft abdomen
   E. Hepatomegaly

References

1. Pierpont MA, Basson CT, Benson DW, et al. Genetic basis for congenital heart defects: Current knowledge. *Circulation.* 2007;115:3015–3038.
2. Gillum RF. Epidemiology of congenital heart disease in the United States. *Am Heart J.* 1994;127(4 pt 1):919–927.
3. Clark ED. Pathogenetic mechanism of congenital cardiovascular malformations revisited. *Semin Perinatol.* 1996;20:465–472.
4. Hoffman JL. Incidence of congenital heart disease, I. Postnatal incidence. *Pediatr Cardiol.* 1995;16:103–113.
5. Opitz J, Yost HJ, Clark EB. Chapter 55. Heart formation: Evolution and developmental field theory. In: Clark EB, Nakazawa M, Takao A, eds. *Etiology and Morphogenesis of Congenital Cardiovascular Disease: Twenty Years of Progress in Genetics and Developmental Biology.* Armonk, NY: Futura Publishing; 2000:311–321.
6. Teitel DF, Iwamoto HS, Rudolph AM. Changes in the pulmonary circulation during birth-related events. *Pediatr Res.* 1990;27:372–378.
7. Teitel DF, Iwamoto HS, Rudolph AM. Effects of birth-related events on central blood flow patterns. *Pediatr Res.* 1987;22:557–566.

8. Townsend SF, Rudolph CD, Rudolph AM. Changes in ovine hepatic circulation and oxygen consumption at birth. *Pediatr Res.* 1989;25:300–304.

9. Hammerman C, Aramburo MJ, Bui KC. Endogenous dilator prostaglandins in congenital heart disease. *Pediatr Cardiol.* 1987;8:155–159.

10. Calder AL, Kirker JA, Neutze JM, Starling MB. Pathology of the ductus arteriosus treated with prostaglandins: Comparisons with untreated cases. *Pediatr Cardiol.* 1984;5:85–92.

11. Silove ED. Administration of E-type prostaglandins in ductus-dependent congenital heart disease. *Pediatr Cardiol.* 1982; 2:303–305.

12. Rein AJ, Omokhodion SI, Nir A. Significance of a cardiac murmur as the sole clinical sign in the newborn. *Clin Pediatr.* 2000;39:511–520.

13. Klewer SE, Samson RA, Donnerstein RL, Lax D, Zamora R, Goldberg SJ. Comparison of accuracy of diagnosis of congenital heart disease by history and physical examination versus echocardiography. *Am J Cardiol.* 2002;89:1329–1331.

14. Madriago E, Silberbach M. Heart failure in infants and children. *Pediatr Rev.* 2010;31:4–12.

15. Ayoub EM. Resurgence of rheumatic fever in the United States: The changing picture of a preventable disease. *Postgrad Med.* 1992;92:133–142.

16. Dajani AS, Bisno AL, Ching KJ, et al. Prevention of rheumatic fever: A statement for health professionals by the Committee on Rheumatic Fever, Endocarditis, and Kawasaki Disease of the Council on Cardiovascular Disease in the Young, American Heart Association. *Circulation.* 1988;78:1082–1086.

17. Johnson DR, Stevens DL, Kaplan EL. Epidemiologic analysis of group A streptococcal serotypes associated with severe systemic infections, rheumatic fever or uncomplicated pharyngitis. *J Infect Dis.* 1992;166:374–382.

18. Holt JP. The normal pericardium. *Am J Cardiol.* 1970; 26:455–463.

19. Tamburro RF, Ring JC, Womback K. Detection of pulsus paradoxus associated with large pericardial effusions in pediatric patients by analysis of the pulse-oximetry waveform. *Pediatrics.* 2002;109:673–677.

20. Levine MJ. Implications of echocardiographically assisted diagnosis of pericardial tamponade in contemporary medical patients: Detection before hemodynamic embarrassment. *J Am Coll Cardiol.* 1991;17:59–65.

21. Ferrieri P, Gewitz MH, Gerber MA, et al. Unique features of infective endocarditis in childhood. *Pediatrics.* 2002; 109:931–943.

22. Sundel RP. Update on the treatment of Kawasaki disease in childhood. *Curr Rheumatol Rep.* 2002;4:474–482.

23. Lang B, Duffy CM. Controversies in the management of Kawasaki disease. *Best Pract Res Clin Rheumatol.* 2002;16:427–442.

24. Kleinman ME, Chameides L, Schexnayder SM. Part 14: Pediatric advanced life support: 2010 American Heart Association guidelines for cardiopulmonary resuscitation and emergency cardiovascular care. *Circulation.* 2010;122:S876–S908.

24a. de Caen AR, Berg MD, Chameides L, et al. Part 12: Pediatric advanced life support: 2015 American Heart Association Guidelines Update for Cardiopulmonary Resuscitation and Emergency Cardiovascular Care. *Circulation.* 2015;132 (suppl2): 5526–5542.

25. Alexander ME, Berul CI. Ventricular arrhythmias: When to worry. *Pediatr Cardiol.* 2000;21:532–541.

26. Kochanek PM, Clark RS, Ruppel RA, Dixon CE. Cerebral resuscitation after traumatic brain injury and cardiopulmonary arrest in infants and children in the new millennium. *Pediatr Clin North Am.* 2001;48:661–681.

27. Hickey RW, Zuckerbraun NS. Pediatric cardiopulmonary arrest: Current concepts and future directions. *Pediatr Emer Rep.* 2003;8:1–12.

28. Young KD, Seidel JS. Pediatric cardiopulmonary resuscitation: A collective review. *Ann Emerg Med.* 1999;33:195–205.

29. Sirbaugh PE, Pepe PE, Shook JE, et al. A prospective, population-based study of the demographics, epidemiology, management, and outcome of out-of-hospital pediatric cardiopulmonary arrest. *Ann Emerg Med.* 1999;33:174–184.

30. Zaritsky A, Nadkarni V, Getson Kuehl K. CPR in children. *Ann Emerg Med.* 1987;16:1107–1110.

31. Gausche M, Lewis RJ, Stratton SJ, et al. Effect of out-of-hospital pediatric endotracheal intubation on survival and neurological outcome: A controlled clinical trial. *JAMA.* 2000;283:6:783–790.

32. Boie ET, Moore GP, Brummett C, Nelson DR. Do parents want to be present during invasive procedures performed on their children? A survey of 400 parents. *Ann Emerg Med.* 1999; 34:70–74.

33. Meyers TA, Eichhorn DJ, Guzzetta CA. Do families want to be present during CPR? *J Emerg Nurs.* 1998;24:400–405.

34. Turley K, Mavroudis C, Ebert PA. Repair of congenital cardiac lesions during the first week of life. *Circulation.* 1982;66(2 pt 2):1214–1219.

35. Jenkins KJ, Gauvreau K, Newburger J, Spray TL, Moller JH, Iezzoni LI. Consensus-based method for risk adjustment for surgery for congenital heart disease. *J Thoracic Cardiovas Surg.* 2002;123:110–118.

36. Armstrong BE. Congenital cardiovascular disease and cardiac surgery in childhood: Acyanotic congenital heart defects and interventional techniques. *Curr Opin Cardiol.* 1995;10:68–77.

A 10-day-old infant is brought to the emergency department by his mother. She tells the physician that he seems to be breathing fast and is not eating very well. He is a full-term infant delivered vaginally with a birth weight of 3.2 kg (7 lb). He spent 2 days with his mother in the hospital and then was discharged after an uneventful circumcision. He has been slow to breastfeed since birth, but the mother became more alarmed when she noted that he would gasp and cry after sucking for a short time. He has approximately three or four wet diapers per day. He has neither congestion nor a fever. He does not vomit with feedings and has had two yellow, seedy stools since passing his meconium after birth. On initial examination, he is pale, irritable, and breathing fast, has nasal flaring, and is sweaty to touch. Vital signs show a respiratory rate of 70/min, heart rate of 170/min, blood pressure of 80/40 mm Hg, temperature (rectal) of 37°C (98.6°F), and weight of 2.9 kg. His lungs sound equal bilaterally with rales in both bases. Cardiac examination reveals a hyperactive precordium with a gallop rhythm. No murmurs are heard. The abdomen is distended with good bowel sounds, and his liver is palpated 4 cm below the right costal margin. Pulses feel weak in the lower extremities. The capillary refill is 3 to 4 seconds in the fingertips, and pulse oximeter reading is 90% on room air.

1. *What is your rapid assessment of this infant?*
2. *On the basis of this assessment, what are your treatment priorities?*
3. *What is the most likely cause of the infant's condition?*
4. *What are the immediate and definitive treatment options?*
5. *What are some complications of this condition?*

This infant is in respiratory distress and has compensated shock. The infant should be given humidified oxygen and cardiac and oxygen saturation monitoring started. Oxygen administration results in an improvement in the oxygen saturation to 99%. An IV catheter should be started with normal saline or lactated Ringer fluids at a 10-mL/kg bolus for shock, possibly caused by ineffective pumping of the heart. The pulses should be examined in all extremities for color, temperature, and strength. The blood pressure should be measured and the precordium assessed for activity. Murmurs, arrhythmias, and gallop rhythms should be determined. If the respiratory status deteriorates, intubation should be performed. A chest radiograph and ECG should be obtained. Electrolytes and/or arterial blood gas analysis will be helpful in determining the degree of acidosis.

The most likely cause is CHF from congenital heart disease. Oxygen and fluids should be started initially. Then, consider the possibility of starting prostaglandin E_1 (PGE_1) as an IV infusion of 0.05 to 0.1 mcg/kg per minute if deterioration occurs, until the specific congenital heart lesion is determined. Administration of PGE_1 might be held if the infant is stable until echocardiography is performed and a cardiologist is expected to arrive soon. After IV access is established and fluids are being given, furosemide (0.5 to 1 mg/kg) should be administered. Digoxin and PGE_1 can be used to help improve flow dynamics and contractility in ductal-dependent lesions and CHF, respectively. If the blood pressure and perfusion do not improve, the next step is to use inotropic agents, such as a dobutamine infusion at 2 to 20 mcg/kg per minute or an epinephrine (adrenaline) infusion at 0.1 to 1.5 mcg/kg per minute. An echocardiogram will need to be obtained for definitive diagnosis and management.

The infant has CHF, and the underlying cause is important to determine the proper treatment. If the CHF is not addressed, the infant will fall further into shock and become decompensated, leading to cardiorespiratory arrest and death.

The infant was diagnosed as having coarctation of the aorta with the coarctation at the level of the ductus, which made systemic flow ductal dependent. The chest radiograph revealed moderate cardiomegaly with increased pulmonary vascular markings. An echocardiogram gave the definitive diagnosis. After medical management with PGE_1, diuretics, and inotropes, as well as IV fluids for the acidosis, the infant was in a stabilized condition and was scheduled for surgical repair.

A 10-year-old boy presents with the chief symptoms of chest pain and shortness of breath. He has had 5 days of cold and cough symptoms. According to his mother, he has been lying around a lot and has missed 1 week of school. He is usually a very active child but states that he is "just too tired" to play. He says that his chest hurts, mostly with cough. He says that he has a hard time catching his breath whenever he gets up to walk around. He has had no medical problems or operations. He is in the fourth grade at school and had been the star basketball player until becoming ill. His only exposure to illness is his aunt, who was recently hospitalized for pneumonia. On initial presentation, he is a thin, pleasant boy who seems tired but talks in complete sentences without difficulty. He is tachypneic with mild retractions and is slightly pale with dusky nail beds. His vital signs include a respiratory rate of 30/min, heart rate of 130/min, blood pressure of 90/65 mm Hg, and oral temperature of 37.8°C (100°F). Oxygen saturation is 90% on room air. His weight is 36.4 kg (80 lb). He is lying on the gurney with his head elevated. Capillary refill time is 4 to 5 seconds. His lungs have diminished breath sounds, with an occasional end expiratory wheeze with deep breaths. His heart sounds are present but faint without any murmurs. His abdomen is distended with a palpable liver and spleen.

1. What is your initial assessment?
2. What are the treatment priorities?
3. What are the most likely causes based on this assessment?
4. What are initial and definitive treatment options?
5. What are the complications of this condition?

This child is in respiratory distress and cardiogenic shock. He needs immediate oxygen support and cardiac and oxygen saturation monitoring. His oxygen saturation increases to 98% on 15 L/min of oxygen by nonrebreather mask.

He most likely has an acquired cardiac problem. He had a respiratory illness during the winter months, so he might have had influenza or another viral illness that is now causing a secondary myocarditis. He could also have a congenital heart lesion that had been asymptomatic until this illness, possibly an anomalous coronary artery or valvular disease. Pericarditis could also be present but would be somewhat unusual because he does not have chest pain.

He needs gentle diuretic therapy, afterload reduction, and possibly inotropic support. He needs an echocardiogram performed to determine whether he has an intrinsic cardiac lesion, muscle hypertrophy, or fluid in the pericardial sac impeding filling and/or contractility. Without treatment to keep him from progressing into cardiogenic shock, he will deteriorate to a point that cardiac arrest is imminent either from decompensated shock or a fatal dysrhythmia.

Chest radiography revealed an enlarged heart, and an echocardiogram showed poor cardiac contractility. Myocarditis was diagnosed. He was maintained with inotropes and pressor agents and recovered to a point that he could be discharged 2 weeks later. He needs to be followed up by a cardiologist to assess the degree to which he regains his baseline cardiac function.

chapter 5

Central Nervous System

Jennifer L. Trainor, MD, FAAP
Susan Fuchs, MD, FAAP, FACEP
Daniel J. Isaacman, MD, FAAP

Objectives

1 List causes of altered level of consciousness (ALOC) in the pediatric patient.

2 Develop a systematic approach to the emergency department (ED) treatment of the child with ALOC.

3 Recognize the presentations of meningitis and encephalitis.

4 Describe serious signs and symptoms in a child with a headache.

5 Define and describe the evaluation and treatment of children with febrile and afebrile seizures.

6 Describe the initial stabilization and treatment of children in status epilepticus.

Chapter Outline

Altered Level of Consciousness
Bacterial Meningitis
Viral Meningitis and Encephalitis
Headache
Seizures
    Febrile Seizures
    Afebrile Seizures
Status Epilepticus

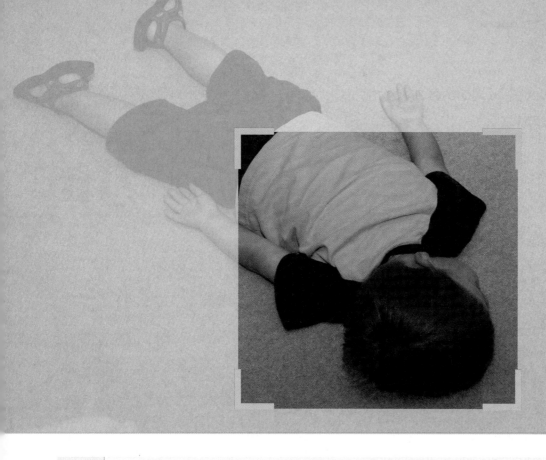

A 2-year-old boy presents to the ED after being found asleep in the garage. His parents were unable to awaken him. He was last seen 30 minutes earlier when his mother let him out to play in the backyard. On examination, the child is somnolent but responds to deep pain. His airway is open and respirations are unlabored. Vital signs include a respiratory rate of 36/min, a heart rate of 116/min, blood pressure of 98/64 mm Hg, and temperature of 38.0°C (100.4°F). Oxygenation saturation measured by pulse oximetry is 98% on room air. Further examination reveals no focal deficits.

1. What is the most important initial intervention in this patient?
2. What are possible causes?
3. What should you include in the management and evaluation?

A 3-month-old boy is brought to the ED by his mother, who says that he is "fussy and not acting right." He was found to be sleepy after returning from a visit to his aunt's home. He is cranky during the examination yet otherwise not lethargic. The patient is afebrile with a respiratory rate of 20/min, a heart rate of 74/min, and a blood pressure of 110/70 mm Hg. His pupils are 4 mm bilaterally and sluggishly reactive. The only abnormality on examination is a small 2-cm hematoma on the occiput, which, according to his mother, was sustained in a fall from a couch.

1. What are your concerns for this patient?
2. What should be done immediately?

Altered Level of Consciousness

The child presenting with ALOC represents one of the most difficult diagnostic and management problems in pediatric emergency medicine. The gravity of the situation, the need to react quickly to avoid irreversible damage, and the wide array of possible diagnoses call for a calm and orderly approach to the problem at hand. The initial management includes immediate attention to the ABCs of resuscitation (airway, breathing, circulation) to sustain life and prevent loss of existing brain function.

Clinical Features

Four pathophysiologic variables help determine the nature of any lesion affecting the brain, the functional level of involvement, and the rate and extent of progression of the disease process. These variables include the pattern of respiration, the size and reactivity of the pupils, spontaneous and induced eye movements, and motor responses.

Respiratory Pattern

Control of ventilation is governed by centers located in the lower pons and medulla and modulated by cortical centers located mainly in the forebrain. Respiratory abnormalities signify either metabolic derangement or neurologic insult in those areas. Several characteristic patterns exist (and are presented in order of rostrocaudal involvement). Postventilation apnea is generally characterized by brief periods of apnea lasting 10 to 30 seconds, followed by voluntary deep breathing. It is generally representative of forebrain injury. Cheyne-Stokes respirations constitute a breathing pattern in which phases of hyperpnea regularly alternate with apnea. The depth of breathing waxes in a smooth crescendo, and then, once a peak is reached, wanes in an equally smooth decrescendo. Cheyne-Stokes respirations usually imply dysfunction of structures deep within both cerebral hemispheres or in the diencephalon. This pattern of ventilation commonly occurs in metabolic encephalopathy. Central neurogenic hyperventilation is manifested by sustained regular and rapid respirations despite a normal PaO_2 and a low $PaCO_2$. This rare and serious finding points to midbrain dysfunction. Apneustic breathing is characterized by brief inspiratory pauses that last 2 to 3 seconds, often alternating with end-expiratory pauses. Clinically, this pattern is characteristic of pontine infarction but occasionally can be seen in anoxic encephalopathy or severe meningitis.

Eye Findings

Pupillary Signs

The pupillary reactions, constriction and dilatation, are controlled by the sympathetic and parasympathetic nervous system. Brainstem areas controlling consciousness are adjacent to those controlling the pupils. In addition, because pupillary pathways are relatively resistant to metabolic insult, the presence or absence of a reaction to light is an important physical finding to distinguish structural from metabolic disease, especially if unilateral. Most metabolic conditions that affect the central nervous system (CNS) lead to constricted pupils that remain reactive to light. (Obviously, pupillary findings are invalid if eye-altering medications have been unintentionally ingested or therapeutically administered). Pupillary responses to structural lesions depend on the primary disturbance site and on the secondary effects of increased intracranial pressure (ICP). Pressure transmitted laterally and downward, generally from mass lesions, can cause a unilaterally fixed and dilated pupil from pressure exerted by the medial aspect of the temporal lobe (uncus) on the third cranial nerve. Transtentorial herniation occurs when pressure forces are transmitted symmetrically downward and exerted on the brainstem. The pupils are initially small, but as herniation continues, the pupils can become asymmetric, then fixed and dilated (**Figure 5.1**).

Induced Eye Movements

Two specific eye maneuvers are helpful in evaluating the comatose child. The oculocephalic or doll's eye reflex is performed by holding the eyelids open and briskly rotating the head from side to side. This test is contraindicated in any child in whom cervical spine injury is a possibility. The normal or positive doll's eye response is conjugate deviation of the eyes opposite of the direction in which the head is turned.

The oculovestibular reflex is evaluated by caloric testing. In the normal awake patient with

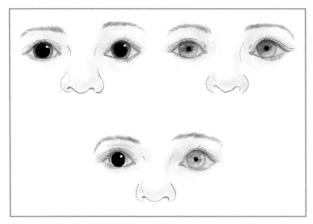

Figure 5.1 Transtentorial herniation sequence.

brainstem intact, the response to ice water testing is nystagmus, with the slow component toward the irrigated ear and the fast nystagmus away from the irrigated ear. In the unconscious patient whose brainstem is intact, the fast nystagmus is abolished, and the eyes move toward the stimulus and remain tonically deviated for a minute or more before slowly returning to the midline.

Deviation of the eyes at rest is also of great diagnostic significance. With cerebral lesions, conjugate deviation is noted *toward* the side of the lesion, whereas with brainstem lesions, conjugate deviation is *away* from the lesion. The setting sun sign, characterized by downward deviation of the eyes, is associated with upper midbrain lesions and hydrocephalus. Third nerve paralysis generally causes the eye to point downward and outward.

Funduscopic Examination

A brief ophthalmoscopic examination should be performed to assess the presence or absence of papilledema or retinal hemorrhages. Papilledema is a late sign of increased ICP. Retinal hemorrhages, thought to be almost pathognomonic of abuse, have also been rarely reported to be caused by other factors.[1–4]

Motor Examination

The motor examination of the comatose patient consists of eliciting various responses to auditory or physical stimuli. Muscle strength, tone, and deep-tendon reflexes should be assessed for normality and symmetry. The ability of the patient to localize, as well as the presence or absence of abnormal posturing, also helps assess the severity of involvement. Decorticate

posturing (flexion of the upper extremities with extension of the lower extremities) suggests involvement of the cerebral cortex and subcortical white matter with preservation of brainstem function. Decerebrate posturing (rigid extension of both the arms and legs) suggests brainstem involvement, usually at the level of the pons. The flaccid patient with no response to painful stimuli has the gravest prognosis and generally has experienced injury deep into the brainstem.

Diagnostic Studies

Laboratory evaluation of the patient with altered mental status can be divided into the routine and the specific. Suggested laboratory tests for the patient with altered mental status of undetermined cause include complete blood cell count (CBC); measurement of electrolytes, blood urea nitrogen, and creatinine; and immediate bedside and serum glucose tests. When a metabolic cause for coma is suspected, liver function testing, serum ammonia, measured and calculated serum osmolality, and toxicology screens should be considered. Arterial blood gas analysis is useful in monitoring the adequacy of ventilation and oxygenation. Focal abnormalities or signs of increased ICP generally mandate a computed tomography (CT) scan once the patient is stabilized. In the patient who remains an enigma, an emergent electroencephalogram (EEG) should be considered because some forms of status

> ### YOUR FIRST CLUE
>
> **Signs of ALOC**
> - Poor responsiveness to environmental cues
> - Abnormal pattern of respiration
> - Size and reactivity of the pupils
> - "Setting sun" pupils pointing downward
> - Papilledema
> - Retinal hemorrhages
> - Abnormal spontaneous and induced eye movements
> - Nonpurposeful motor responses

epilepticus (SE) have little to no motor component and are therefore not clinically obvious. Performance of a lumbar puncture for suspected meningitis should be considered if no signs of increased ICP are present, particularly in the presence of fever. Additional laboratory tests to consider, when clinically indicated, include blood alcohol level, thyroid function tests, blood lead level, blood culture, skeletal survey, and barium or air contrast enema.

Differential Diagnosis

The etiologic possibilities are diverse. The mnemonic AEIOU TIPS has been a useful method for organizing the diagnostic possibilities.

A

Abuse

Child abuse or maltreatment must be considered in any young child presenting in a coma, particularly when the history and physical examination findings are not consistent. The practitioner must look for subtle physical signs of trauma, including bruising, cranial tenderness or swelling, and retinal hemorrhages. Shaken baby syndrome can result in ALOC without external signs of physical abuse.[5]

Alcohol

Alcohol is more commonly encountered in adolescents than younger pediatric patients. However, alcohol is not an infrequent cause of unintentional ingestion in the young child. Young children can exhibit ALOC at serum levels less than 100 mg/dL and can also be obtunded from concurrent hypoglycemia.

E

Electrolytes

Any condition that causes abnormal fluid losses can result in ALOC due to abnormalities in electrolytes, such as sodium, potassium, calcium, and magnesium. Disorders such as adrenal insufficiency and the syndrome of inappropriate antidiuretic hormone can also result in ALOC with abnormal electrolytes.

Encephalopathy

Reye syndrome is a consideration in any child who presents with a history of vomiting leading to altered mental status, particularly when there is a history of an antecedent varicella or flulike illness treated with salicylates. Since 1980, when the association between Reye syndrome and aspirin use was first reported, there has been a sharp decrease in the reported incidence of this disease.[6,7] Furthermore, recent studies have suggested that many cases previously diagnosed as Reye syndrome might represent inborn errors of metabolism not previously recognized.[8,9]

Lead encephalopathy, although unusual, continues to be a concern in the pediatric age group, particularly in children living in older buildings where lead paint might still be present. Children can develop rapid increases in blood lead levels after ingestion of loose paint chips or by mouthing items contaminated with lead paint, dust, and soil. An antecedent history of fatigue, vomiting, or abdominal pain in a child living in an older dwelling should alert the physician to the possibility of this diagnosis. Screening tests include blood lead, free erythrocyte protoporphyrin, and CBC. Occasionally, radiopaque lead chips will be found on abdominal radiography. Treatment involves chelation therapy.[10]

I

Infection

Meningitis and encephalitis are more common in pediatric patients than in adults, and such patients might not always present with fever. Infections outside the CNS, particularly sepsis, can also cause ALOC if associated with cerebral hypoperfusion.

O

Overdose Ingestion

Ingestion is always a strong consideration in the young child with an unexplained alteration in consciousness. A complete history of medications in the household should be obtained early in the evaluation of these patients.

U

Uremia

Hemolytic uremic syndrome is a multisystem disorder characterized by a prodromal phase of gastroenteritis or upper respiratory tract infection followed by acute onset and rapid progression of renal failure, microangiopathic hemolytic anemia, and thrombocytopenia. Other causes of chronic renal impairment in childhood can also lead to uremic encephalopathy.

T

Trauma

Trauma is a major cause of ALOC. It is the leading cause of death in the first four decades of life. Head injuries, chest injuries leading to hypoxia, and blood loss leading to shock all have significant effects on the level of consciousness.

I

Inborn Errors of Metabolism

These are important disorders to keep in mind, particularly when the onset of symptoms is early in life. Presenting signs are somewhat nonspecific and include vomiting, seizures, hypoglycemia, and/or metabolic acidosis. Blood ammonia levels are helpful, and urine screens for organic and/or amino acids are often diagnostic. Inborn errors of metabolism can present past infancy into early childhood.

Insulin and Hypoglycemia

Although patients with known diabetes mellitus are obviously at risk for unintentional insulin overdose, occasionally toddlers will ingest another family member's oral hypoglycemia agent or ingest alcohol or other medications that can cause hypoglycemia. Ketotic hypoglycemia, probably the most common endogenous cause of hypoglycemia in childhood, is actually a diagnosis that compromises a number of disease processes. Children with this problem are often young (18 months to 5 years) and often have histories of low birth weight. Attacks are episodic, most likely occurring in the morning and after prolonged fasting, and are frequently associated with ketonuria. Hypoglycemia episodes, resulting from an inappropriate response to a prolonged fasting state, respond promptly to the administration of glucose.[11]

Intussusception

Intussusception, caused by the prolapse of a portion of small intestine into an adjacent loop, has been known to present with mental status changes before the development of abdominal signs and symptoms. In the child younger than 3 years with unexplained ALOC, intussusception should be entertained. Direct a careful history at any antecedent vomiting, abdominal pain, or blood in the stool and perform repeated examinations of the abdomen with stool testing for blood.[12]

P

Psychogenic

Although factitious ALOC is rare in young children, it is worth considering in older children and adolescents. Careful neurologic examination will often reveal abnormalities inconsistent with an organic cause.

S

Seizures

Postictal states are common causes of ALOC, and an actively seizing infant can appear to be in a coma until close observation reveals continued subtle seizure activity. At times seizure activity is completely occult clinically and can be diagnosed only with an EEG; a high index of suspicion is necessary to make this diagnosis.

Stroke, Shock, and Other Cardiovascular Causes

Cardiovascular abnormalities, such as arteriovenous malformations (AVMs), can present in childhood, resulting in acute CNS symptoms, including ALOC. Poor brain perfusion caused by hypovolemia (eg, from sepsis or severe dehydration) can lead to altered sensorium in the presence of an otherwise normal CNS test result.

Shunt

Patients with ventriculoperitoneal or ventriculoatrial shunts can present with ALOC when the

---

WHAT ELSE?

Differential Diagnosis of ALOC

A	Alcohol, Abuse
E	Electrolytes, Encephalopathy
I	Infection
O	Overdose Ingestion
U	Uremia
T	Trauma
I	Insulin (hypoglycemia), Intussusception, Inborn errors of metabolism
P	Psychogenic
S	Shock, Stroke, Seizure, Shunt

shunt is blocked or infected. Patients are often lethargic and have headache, and they might have difficulty looking upward (sundowning). Rapid evaluation of the shunt is necessary.

Management

Primary Assessment

The initial task is to assess the adequacy of the patient's airway, degree of ventilation, and circulatory status. Patients with a history of trauma should be immobilized with the neck positioned in the midline. A bedside glucose level should be obtained.

Airway and Breathing

Ensure the patency of the airway while protecting the cervical spine if there is a possibility of cervical spine trauma. Open the airway using the chin-lift (if no trauma is suspected) or jaw-thrust maneuver. Avoid hyperextension of the neck so as not to occlude the airway in an infant. Insert a nasal airway as needed (if no basilar skull fracture is suspected); oral airways are best avoided in lightly comatose and conscious patients because of the risk of inducing vomiting and aspiration. Provide supplemental oxygen. If the child is apneic or has respiratory failure, assist ventilatory efforts with bag-mask ventilation or intubation. Intubation will be necessary if the patient has an inadequate gag reflex. If respirations are present but noisy, suction and inspect for foreign material. Mild hyperventilation to a $Paco_2$ of 30 to 35 mm Hg is indicated if there are signs of increased ICP.[13]

Circulation (Cardiovascular Status)

The patient's skin perfusion and capillary refill best estimate circulatory status. Take the patient's pulse and blood pressure, and place the child on a monitor. Achieve venous or intraosseous access, draw diagnostic blood specimens, and perform a rapid estimate of glucose level. The state of hydration as indicated by physical examination should dictate the fluid selection and rate. Shock should be treated as described previously (see Chapter 3, Shock). Check oxygen saturation by pulse oximetry. Only after the ABCs are addressed should attention be directed to the neurologic and general examinations.

Disability (Neurologic Status)

Perform an objective evaluation of the child's level of consciousness using either the AVPU (Alert, Voice, Pain, Unresponsive) system or the Glasgow Coma Scale (see Chapter 6, Trauma). Note pupillary size and reactivity. Look for evolving signs of increased ICP, such as alterations in vital signs (including Cushing triad of bradycardia, hypertension, and irregular respirations), pupillary responses, respiratory pattern, or papilledema. Treat patients with clinical evidence of increased ICP as detailed in Chapter 6, Trauma. Save a tube of blood for later laboratory studies (eg, for inborn errors of metabolism). Infuse glucose, 0.5 to 1 g/kg intravenously (2 to 4 mL/kg of 25% dextrose solution), for documented hypoglycemia. If the child improves, a continuous infusion of 10% dextrose should be initiated at the child's maintenance rate. If intravenous access cannot be obtained, administer glucagon intramuscularly (<20 kg, 0.5 mg; >20 kg, 1 mg). Administer a trial of naloxone (birth to 5 years of age, 0.1 mg/kg intravenously; >5 years of age or 20 kg, 2 mg intravenously) to reverse a potential narcotic-induced mental status alteration.

Exposure

Remove the patient's clothing and other items that hinder full evaluation, and cover with blankets to prevent inadvertent hypothermia.

Secondary Assessment

Once the immediate life-threatening concerns have been addressed, an abbreviated focused history should be obtained. The physician should determine whether the child has had any chronic or recent illness, antecedent fever, rash, vomiting, or trauma. Explore any recent exposure to infection, medications, or intoxicants. Immunization, medical, and family histories should be obtained when time permits. Be alert for any inappropriate responses and delays in seeking care that would arouse the suspicion of child abuse or maltreatment.

The observations in the secondary assessment should attempt to uncover signs of occult infection, trauma, or toxic or metabolic derangements. Important areas to evaluate include the fundi, extraocular movements, anterior fontanel, and the neck for bruits and stiffness. Many afebrile toddlers with altered mental status have unknown ingestions. Signs suggestive of a specific toxidrome should be explored as outlined in Chapter 18, Toxicology Online.

Disposition

The previously described approach might delineate a specific cause of ALOC. When a presumptive diagnosis is confirmed, perform specific management. Definitive therapy can be initiated in the ED. Admit or transfer any patient to a pediatric intensive care unit who does not respond to therapeutic intervention and who will require ongoing monitoring or intensive therapy or in whom the diagnosis is still in question after the initial management.

> **KEY POINTS**
>
> **Management of ALOC**
> - Assess and treat abnormalities in oxygenation and ventilation
> - Place on a monitor
> - Obtain vascular access
> - Obtain blood for laboratory evaluation and test for glucose level
> - Begin specific therapy based on likely differential diagnosis

CASE SCENARIO 3

A 3-month-old girl presents with fever, fussiness, and poor feeding. She is irritable and difficult to console but is breathing comfortably on her own and maintaining a good airway. Vital signs include a respiratory rate of 36/min, heart rate of 120/min, a blood pressure of 90/58 mm Hg, temperature of 39.2°C (102.6°F), and oxygen saturation of 98% on room air. Her fontanel appears full, and her neck appears supple. Capillary refill time is 2 seconds. The remainder of the examination is nonfocal.

1. *Which examination findings in this child are consistent with the diagnosis of meningitis?*
2. *What is the most important therapy to deliver at this time?*
3. *What are possible complications?*

Bacterial Meningitis

Meningitis, an infection of the meninges that surround the brain and spinal cord, remains a significant cause of morbidity and mortality in childhood. Despite major advances in the prevention of serious bacterial infection caused by *Haemophilus influenzae* type B and *Streptococcus pneumoniae* in the past decade, cases of meningitis continue to occur.

Epidemiology

The greatest risk for meningitis occurs in the first year of life. During this time, the bacteriology of the disease shows great change. During the neonatal period, infants are at greatest risk of meningitis from infection with group B *Streptococcus*, *Escherichia coli* (or other gram-negative organisms), and *Listeria monocytogenes*. At approximately 4 weeks of age, *S pneumoniae* and *Neisseria meningitidis* infections become more prevalent, but group B *Streptococcus*, and gram-negative bacilli persist.[14] The peak age-specific incidence of *S pneumoniae* and *N meningitidis* occurs at 6 to 8 months of age, the time at which the immunity afforded by passively acquired maternal IgG antibodies disappears. After 3 years of age, these pathogens become the most prominent organisms.[14] *Streptococcus pneumoniae* meningitis decreased by 55% to 60% after the pneumococcal vaccine gained widespread use, but it still remains the most frequent cause of bacterial meningitis in children.[15]

Clinical Features

The clinical presentation of patients with bacterial meningitis generally involves some combination of fever, irritability, and/or lethargy and, in children older than 18 months, nuchal rigidity. Although some overlap in the signs and symptoms exists between patients with bacterial meningitis and those with viral (aseptic) meningitis, in general, children with aseptic meningitis appear less ill.

Bacterial meningitis can present in two ways. It can develop progressively within days or fulminantly within hours concurrent with sepsis. Most patients generally present with fever and signs of meningeal inflammation, which can include irritability, lethargy, confusion, headache, and neck stiffness.[15] In neonates, temperature instability (fever or hypothermia) and nonfocal neurologic findings, such as irritability, lethargy, poor feeding, tremors, and apnea, can occur with meningitis.[16] In infants younger than 3 months, clinical signs can be particularly subtle, thus arguing for a high index of suspicion for this disease in febrile infants in this age group.

It is important to realize that in children younger than 18 months, neck musculature might not be adequately developed to manifest nuchal rigidity, and thus this sign is unreliable in this age group. In children older than 18 months, physical findings become more reliable. These patients generally have headache, vomiting, and neck pain. Other signs and symptoms occurring with some regularity include anorexia, nausea, focal neurologic signs, and seizures.[15]

On physical examination, alterations in the level of consciousness can be highly variable, extending from extreme lethargy and/or coma to combativeness and irritability. Kernig sign (inability to extend the legs with the hips flexed) and Brudzinski sign (flexion of the neck causes flexion at the hip, knee, or ankle) are indicative of meningeal irritation, but their absence does not exclude the presence of meningitis.[15] A bulging or tense fontanel in an infant suggests increased ICP but can be present in infants with febrile illnesses without meningitis and is therefore neither sensitive nor specific. Petechiae or purpura, hallmarks of meningococcal disease,

can also be seen with other systemic infections such as *S pneumoniae* and *H influenzae*.

Focal neurologic signs might be detected on presentation and are primarily associated with increased ICP or impaired cerebral blood flow. Third and sixth cranial nerve palsies, with accompanying pupillary dilatation and impaired lateral gaze, are indicative of increased ICP and should trigger immediate efforts to lower ICP. Ataxia and hearing loss might be noted because inflammation and infection involving the inner ear affect hearing and balance. Papilledema, generally a late finding, is often suggestive of a complication such as a venous sinus thrombosis, subdural empyema, or brain abscess. Seizures usually occur early in meningitis but are rarely the sole finding.[15]

A search for an underlying condition should always be considered in children presenting with bacterial meningitis. As many as 20% of children with bacterial meningitis have a condition that predisposes them to developing this serious infection. Causes to consider include the presence of a ventriculoperitoneal shunt, cochlear implants, an underlying tumor, head trauma with resultant cerebrospinal fluid (CSF) leak, splenic dysfunction, or other immunodeficiency states.[15]

YOUR FIRST CLUE

Signs and Symptoms Associated With Meningitis
- Apnea
- Bulging fontanel (infant)
- Jitteriness and irritability
- Vomiting
- Hypothermia
- Headache
- Fever
- Meningismus
- Ataxia
- Focal neurologic signs
- Cranial nerve palsy
- Seizures

Diagnostic Studies

The diagnosis of meningitis is made by culturing the spinal fluid. Fluid should be obtained for cell count with differential, glucose and protein, and culture. Classically, bacterial infection yields a high white blood cell (WBC) count with marked polymorphonuclear predominance, elevated protein levels, and low glucose levels. Profiles characteristic of normal CSF and CSF with bacterial and viral meningitis are given in Table 5-1.

Since the decrease in invasive infections caused by *H influenzae* type b, the clinical usefulness of rapid antigen detection in CSF or other body fluids has come into question. Rarely does a positive result alter therapy; however, latex agglutination can be useful in cases of partially treated meningitis or in cases in which the Gram stain is consistent with meningococci. Clarifying the serotype quickly can have implications for providing meningococcal vaccine (types A and C) to classmates. Latex agglutination of urine should be avoided because of the very high occurrence of false-positive results.

Polymerase chain reaction (PCR) of CSF has been used to detect microbial DNA in patients with bacterial meningitis. Primers are available for simultaneous detection of the most common organisms, including *S pneumoniae, N meningitidis,* and *H influenzae.*[17] Another, perhaps more useful, application of PCR is documentation of the presence of specific viral gene products present in CSF (eg, enterovirus). In these cases, PCR results are often more rapid and more sensitive than culture, offering the possibility of earlier diagnosis of equivocal cases, which might lead to shortened hospital stays.

Other laboratory tests that should be obtained in the patient with suspected meningitis include blood culture, serum glucose measurement, and electrolytes measurement. Obtaining a peripheral blood culture is critical because the CSF culture can occasionally be negative. Hypoglycemia resulting from poor intake and increased metabolic demand and hyponatremia from syndrome of inappropriate antidiuretic hormone secretion (SIADH) are important complications to consider.

Because of the decrease in incidence of bacterial meningitis, a CSF result showing pleocytosis (WBC count >10/mcL) is still more likely to be indicative of viral meningitis than bacterial. A clinical decision rule called the Bacterial Meningitis Score was developed and validated in the United States and overseas to help classify children at very low risk (0.1%) of bacterial meningitis who have not been pretreated with antibiotics. The risk of bacterial meningitis is very low if a child older than 2 months meets all of the following criteria: negative CSF Gram stain result, CSF absolute neutrophil count less than 1,000/L, CSF protein level less than 80 mg/dL, peripheral blood absolute neutrophil count less than 10,000/L, and no history of seizure before or at the time of presentation. The Bacterial Meningitis Score was 100% sensitive and 63% specific in identifying those children with bacterial meningitis older than 2 months.[18]

TABLE 5-1 Common Cerebrospinal Fluid Findings	Normal[a]	Bacterial	Viral
Appearance	Clear	Clear to cloudy	Clear
WBC count, mcL	<10	>100–20,000	>10–500
Differential, % PMNs	0	>90	0–30[b]
Glucose, mg/dL	50–90	<40	50–90
Protein, mg/dL	15–45	>250–500	50–150
Gram stain (bacterial)	Negative	Positive	Negative

Abbreviations: PMNs, polymorphonuclear cells; WBC, white blood cell.

[a]In the neonatal period, these normal values can vary as follows: WBC count, less than 22/mcL with less than 60% PMNs; glucose, 30 to 119 mg/dL; and protein, 20 to 100 mg/dL.

[b]Can be predominantly PMNs early in the illness.

Physicians often question the effect of antibiotic pretreatment on CSF results in children with bacterial meningitis. Although antibiotics can induce a negative CSF culture result, in a large, multicenter, retrospective study, the CSF WBC count or absolute neutrophil count was not affected if antibiotics were given 24 hours before the lumbar puncture. However, the CSF glucose level was higher, and the CSF protein level was lower, with pretreatment, especially greater than 12 hours later.[19]

Differential Diagnosis

Although the constellation of irritability and high temperatures should always prompt consideration for meningitis, other entities can present with similar profiles. Infants and young children with cervical or retropharyngeal adenitis can present with fever and a reluctance to move the head, generally with accompanying head tilt or difficulty in turning the head from side to side rather than difficulty with flexion and extension. Children with retropharyngeal cellulitis or abscess can also present with irritability and frank nuchal rigidity, often with accompanying poor oral intake or severe dysphagia. Other disease entities to consider include sinusitis, mastoiditis, CNS tumor or abscess, and encephalitis. Muscular torticollis, although often leading to painful head rotation, is generally distinguished from meningitis by the lack of irritability and the absence of fever. Acute dystonia, often linked with the administration of phenothiazines or other cholinergic agents, is often associated with characteristic muscular rigidity and, again, with intact mental status and the absence of fever. Children with subarachnoid hemorrhages will generally have a history of trauma and/or severe headache and are also less likely to present with fever than those with meningitis. Other conditions capable of producing meningismus include severe pharyngitis, arthritis, osteomyelitis of the cervical spine, and upper lobe pneumonia.

Management

Successful management of bacterial meningitis involves rapid diagnosis; attention to airway, breathing, and circulation; administration of antibiotic therapy; and careful monitoring for potential complications.[20] Once the diagnosis of bacterial meningitis has been entertained and CSF collected, antibiotic therapy should be rapidly started. In cases in which the diagnosis is suspected and the child is deemed too unstable to undergo lumbar puncture or there is a delay due to a necessary CT scan, antibiotic therapy should be administered. Initial antibiotic coverage is often empiric with subsequent therapy guided by Gram stain and culture results. Infants in the first 4 to 6 weeks of life with suspected meningitis should be treated with ampicillin (300 mg/kg per day) and cefotaxime (150 to 200 mg/kg per day) or ampicillin and gentamicin (7.5 mg/kg per day) to cover for gram-negative enteric organisms, group B streptococci, and *L monocytogenes*.[21] In children older than 4 to 6 weeks, local resistance patterns to *S pneumoniae* should dictate the use of single coverage (300 mg/kg per day of cefotaxime or 100 mg/kg per day of ceftriaxone) or double coverage (vancomycin, 60 mg/kg per day, plus cefotaxime or ceftriaxone) for gram-positive organisms until culture results and sensitivities are known.[20] Gram-negative infection in this age group should be covered adequately with cefotaxime or ceftriaxone.

The role of corticosteroids in the treatment of bacterial meningitis continues to be a source of considerable debate. The theoretical goal of steroid use in meningitis is to decrease meningeal inflammation and thus lower the incidence and severity of cerebral edema and resultant brain injury. Although existing data

WHAT ELSE?

Differential Diagnosis of Neck Stiffness
- Cervical adenitis
- Retropharyngeal abscess/cellulitis
- CNS tumors
- Encephalitis
- Pharyngitis
- Torticollis
- Cervical spine trauma

suggest a reduction in sensorineural hearing loss in patients with *H influenzae* meningitis, disease from infection with this organism is now rare. No clear-cut benefit has been demonstrated for dexamethasone in protecting against neurologic deficits from infection with all other organisms. Some experts have expressed concern that the use of corticosteroids might decrease the CSF penetration of some antimicrobials, such as vancomycin, thus offering a potential disadvantage to steroid use in cases of penicillin-resistant pneumococcal meningitis. If dexamethasone (0.15 mg/kg per dose every 6 hours for 2 to 4 days) is used for suspected *H influenzae* type B infections or if the decision is made to give it for other types of meningitis, it should be given before or at the same time as the first dose of antibiotics. It is probably not beneficial if given more than 1 hour later.[20, 21]

Complications

The patient with meningitis is at risk for a number of serious and life-threatening complications. Bacterial meningitis with accompanying bacteremia can lead to a systemic inflammatory response with septic shock, respiratory distress syndrome, and disseminated intravascular coagulation. Intracranial complications can have devastating results. Familiarity with these allows the physician to anticipate the development of complications and thereby institute immediate interventions as needed.

Increased Intracranial Pressure

Acute bacterial meningitis can be associated with increased ICP, which can result in cerebral herniation or other life-threatening complications. Cerebral edema, whether vasogenic, cytotoxic, or interstitial in origin, is the major element contributing to raised ICP. Increases in ICP result in decreased cerebral perfusion pressure, with accompanying impairment in autoregulation of cerebral blood flow. Raised ICP should be anticipated, identified, and treated promptly. Some late manifestations of increased ICP are ALOC, a dilated or poorly reactive pupil, abnormalities of ocular motility, and the Cushing triad of hypertension, bradycardia, and irregular respirations.

Several methods are available to reduce ICP. Simple measures, such as elevating the bed to

> ## KEY POINTS
>
> **Management of Suspected Bacterial Meningitis**
>
> - Assess and treat abnormalities in oxygenation or ventilation
> - Monitor hemodynamics (heart rate, respiratory rate, blood pressure, pulse oximetry)
> - Establish intravenous access
> - Obtain blood samples for laboratory evaluation and bedside glucose testing
> - Treat hypoglycemia
> - Obtain urine cultures in young infants (but do not wait for urine to give antibiotics)
> - Obtain CT scan as indicated
> - Perform lumbar puncture
> - Begin antibiotic therapy based on age (4 to 6 weeks, cefotaxime or gentamicin plus ampicillin; 4 to 6 weeks, cefotaxime or ceftriaxone with or without vancomycin)
> - Treat complications
> - Admit patient

30° and positioning the head midline, should be routinely adopted. Endotracheal intubation and intratracheal suctioning can precipitate a significant increase in ICP, which can be minimized by prior administration of lidocaine (lignocaine). Antipyretic agents should be administered to reduce additional metabolic demand produced by core temperatures above 38°C (100.4°F). Mild hyperventilation can be used immediately to decrease the $Paco_2$ to 30 to 35 mm Hg, which results in cerebral vasoconstriction and reduced cerebral blood volume. The effectiveness of this approach beyond 24 hours is limited. Hyperosmolar agents, such as mannitol, decrease ICP by transiently raising the osmolarity of the intravascular space and pulling water from intracellular brain tissues into the extracellular intravascular compartment. When other modalities have failed to control ICP, high-dose barbiturate therapy can be useful.

Seizures

Approximately 20% to 30% of children with bacterial meningitis have a seizure before admission or at some time during their hospital course. Seizures can occur early or late in the illness or manifest as a late complication after apparent recovery. Hypoglycemia and electrolyte abnormalities (especially sodium) must be excluded as causes of seizures. Early, brief seizure activity might not warrant initiation of anticonvulsant therapy. Prolonged or recurrent seizures require aggressive treatment, as outlined later in this chapter.

Syndrome of Inappropriate Antidiuretic Hormone Secretion

Infections of the CNS can result in increased secretion of antidiuretic hormone from the posterior pituitary gland. The result of this is retention of body water, hyponatremia, and expansion of the extracellular fluid space. The reported incidence of SIADH in bacterial meningitis varies greatly. In addition, central diabetes insipidus (hypernatremia) has also been reported in children with CNS infections.

Subdural Effusion and Empyema

The pathogenesis of subdural effusion in meningitis remains poorly understood. Clinical features include persistent or recurrent fever, seizures, and a variety of neurologic abnormalities. Whether these features are secondary to the effusion or due to meningeal inflammation is unclear. The overall incidence of subdural effusion ranges from 15% to 40%. It seems that young age, low peripheral WBC count, and high CSF levels of protein are associated with a higher likelihood of developing effusion. Because most subdural effusions resolve spontaneously, a noninvasive approach in an otherwise improving patient is appropriate. In those patients in whom the effusion has been related to a clinical deterioration or in whom a subdural empyema is suspected, subdural evacuation should be performed.

Viral Meningitis and Encephalitis

Because the causative organisms of viral meningitis and encephalitis in children are similar, it is beneficial to discuss them together. The major difference between viral meningitis and encephalitis is that viral meningitis only involves the meninges and does not produce the neurologic dysfunction present in encephalitis. Viral meningitis is often termed aseptic meningitis because both cause meningeal irritation, but no bacterial origin is identified.[22]

Encephalitis is an inflammation of the brain associated with neurologic dysfunction that results in a variety of possible manifestations: altered mental status; change in behavior or personality; or motor, sensory, speech, or movement deficits or disorders.[23] Meningoencephalitis is an inflammation of both the brain and meninges.

Encephalitis is usually viral, but it can also be caused by bacteria, fungi, and parasites. Numerous serotypes of enteroviruses, including polioviruses, nonpolioviruses, coxsackieviruses, and echoviruses, account for most cases of viral meningitis and encephalitis, especially in the summer months in the United States.[22,23] Arboviruses are arthropod (mosquito or tick)–borne viruses that are the most common causes of encephalitis worldwide. In the United States, these viruses include Eastern equine encephalitis virus, Western equine encephalitis virus, St. Louis encephalitis, West Nile virus, California encephalitis virus, and La Crosse virus.[22,23] Because common natural reservoirs include birds (Eastern and Western equine, St. Louis, West Nile) and rodents (California, La Crosse), disease first noted in the animal population can be an early clue to an epidemic.[24,25]

Multiple human herpesviruses have been identified as causative agents in CNS infections. Herpes simplex virus 2 (HSV-2) is a leading cause of severe encephalitis in neonates and is acquired through vertical transmission through the vaginal canal. Herpes simplex 1 infection occurs in all ages, including neonates. Other viruses in the herpes family include varicella-zoster, cytomegalovirus (CMV), human herpesvirus 6, and Epstein-Barr virus. Influenza A and B viruses have also been associated with aseptic meningitis and encephalitis. Numerous other viruses, such as measles, mumps, and lymphochoriomeningitis virus, have all been identified as causing CNS infection.[22]

Bacterial causes of encephalitis include *Borrelia burgdorferi* (Lyme disease), *Bartonella henselae* (cat scratch disease), *Rickettsia rickettsii* (Rocky Mountain spotted fever), *Mycoplasma pneumoniae*, and *Treponema pallidum* (syphilis).[25–27] Fungal origins include *Cryptococcus*, *Coccidioides*, and *Histoplasma*. Parasitic causes include *Taenia solium* (cysticercosis), *Plasmodium falciparum* (malaria), and *Toxoplasma gondii*.[25–27]

Clinical Features

The clinical features of an infant or child with viral meningitis are similar to those of bacterial meningitis. Neurologic findings in infants include irritability and lethargy, whereas headache, photophobia, and nuchal rigidity are more common in older children. Nonspecific findings, such as rash, respiratory symptoms, and diarrhea, can occur. The progression to advanced signs of neurologic dysfunction, such as altered mental status, seizures, and focal neurologic findings, occur with and help define encephalitis.[26]

Neonatal HSV-2 meningoencephalitis typically develops 2 to 30 days after delivery, with lethargy, poor feeding, irritability, tremors, or seizures; however, early in the illness, fever can be the sole manifestation. Vesicular lesions noted on the presenting part (scalp or buttocks) are helpful but not universally visible. Other physical findings include temperature instability, a bulging fontanel, pyramidal tract signs, seizures, and systemic signs of infection (eg, jaundice, respiratory distress, bleeding, or shock). The long-term prognosis for these infants is poor.[26] Older children with HSV encephalitis present with fever, altered mental status, and seizures. Mucosal lesions often precede CNS infection by a week.[26]

Specific viruses can have specific features that can assist in diagnosis. Children with enteroviruses have a fever associated with anorexia, rash, myalgias, conjunctivitis, pharyngitis, upper and lower respiratory tract symptoms, nausea, vomiting, headache (frontal or retro-orbital), and photophobia. Children older than 1 to 2 years commonly have nuchal rigidity.[26] The characteristic rash of hand-foot and mouth lesions or herpangina can be seen in coxsackievirus infections. Progression to encephalitis can also be associated with pulmonary edema, cranial nerve palsies, and flaccid paralysis.[26]

Diagnostic Studies

A child with encephalitis or viral meningitis requires basic laboratory investigation, including a CBC, electrolytes measurement, glucose measurement, blood cultures, and a lumbar puncture.[26] If the child has signs of increased ICP or focal neurologic findings, CT should be performed before the lumbar puncture. Additional studies that might prove useful include viral studies from the throat, stool, or nares (adenovirus, influenza). Specific tests for serum IgM help diagnose St. Louis encephalitis, West Nile virus, Western equine encephalitis, and mycoplasma. Enzyme-linked immunosorbent assay and Western blot are useful for detecting Lyme disease, and a serum rapid plasma reagin is helpful in diagnosing syphilis.[28]

Cerebrospinal fluid analysis in viral encephalitis usually shows a lymphocytosis or monocytosis, elevated protein content, and normal or slightly low glucose level.[26,29] An elevated CSF red blood cell count also can be found in herpesvirus encephalitis. Six percent to 15% of patients with

---

YOUR FIRST CLUE

Signs and Symptoms of Encephalitis

- Altered mental status
- Fever
- Headache
- Psychiatric symptoms
- Seizures
- Vomiting
- Focal weakness
- Photophobia
- Dysphasia
- Ataxia
- Hemiparesis
- Cranial nerve deficits
- Visual field loss
- Papilledema

HSV-1 encephalitis have completely normal CSF study results.[25] Children with encephalitis due to other types of viruses (eg, enterovirus, CMV, Epstein-Barr virus, human herpesvirus 6) usually have normal CSF or only mild elevation in protein level or WBC counts.[29]

Polymerase chain reaction of CSF is the "gold standard" for diagnosing HSV encephalitis, with sensitivity of 95%.[28] Polymerase chain reaction of CSF also can be diagnostic in cases of enterovirus, varicella, CMV, and human herpesvirus 6.[28] In neonates, cultures of CSF, conjunctivae, skin, or mucosal vesicular lesions will yield the HSV in only half of cases, whereas cultures of urine or saliva are nearly 100% sensitive for congenital CMV. Varicella can be cultured from skin vesicles in most cases.

Although magnetic resonance imaging (MRI) of the brain is the preferred diagnostic imaging study if encephalitis is highly suspected and the patient is clinically stable, it might not be readily available. Typical findings of herpes encephalitis in children include hypointensity on T1-weighted sequences and hyperintensity on T2-weighted sequences within the medial temporal and inferior frontal lobes.[28,30] With contrast, enhancement of the meninges, cortex, and white matter can occur.[30] The MRI or CT findings in congenital CMV encephalitis can include intracranial calcifications, usually periventricular, cerebral dysgenesis, or other degenerative findings.[29,31] An MRI of congenital toxoplasmosis can show calcifications, whereas a patient with human immunodeficiency virus and toxoplasmosis will show multiple ring-enhancing lesions.[28] In cysticercosis, the CT or MRI reveals cystic lesions, some with calcifications. If ring enhancement is present, this suggests cyst degeneration.[28]

Differential Diagnosis

A number of life-threatening disorders must be considered in patients who present with a clinical picture of encephalitis (before diagnosis by lumbar puncture). Hypoglycemia and hypoxia can be excluded with immediate bedside tests. Other metabolic disorders (eg, inborn errors of metabolism, hepatic encephalopathy, and uremia) require measurement of ammonia or

---

THE CLASSICS

Diagnostic Features of Encephalitis

- CSF profile: lymphocytosis or monocytosis, elevated protein content, and normal or slightly low glucose level; can be completely normal

- MRI: hypointensity on T1-weighted sequences and hyperintensity on T2-weighted sequences within the medial temporal and inferior frontal lobes (herpes); enhancement of the meninges, cortex, and white matter; basal ganglia calcifications

- CT: normal; temporal or frontal lobe attenuation changes, petechial hemorrhages, or edema

---

specific metabolic byproducts. Sepsis, systemic bacterial infections, bacterial meningitis, viral (aseptic) meningitis, and intracranial abscesses, masses, and bleeding can all cause nonfocal alterations in mental status. Lumbar puncture, CT, MRI, radiography, or blood cultures might be required to distinguish among these possibilities. Unsuspected toxins that cause fever and an altered mental status can easily be confused with encephalitis (eg, amphetamines, anticholinergics, arsenic, cocaine, lysergic acid diethylamide, phencyclidine, phenothiazines, salicylates, theophylline, and thyroxine). Clues to a toxin-induced encephalopathy include the presence of other classic toxidrome features (eg, anticholinergic symptoms, sympathomimetic symptoms with cocaine or amphetamines, and respiratory alkalosis with salicylate toxicity). Other considerations in patients with clinical features of encephalitis include postinfectious disease (eg, acute cerebellar ataxia), nonconvulsive status, vasculitis, stroke, and acute confusional migraine.

Management

Most patients with encephalitis present with altered mental status, ill appearance, seizures, or focal neurologic deficits. Apply a cardiac monitor and pulse oximeter and obtain venous access. Perform a bedside glucose test, and immediately treat any life-threatening complications (eg, seizure, airway compromise, hypoxia, hyperthermia, or shock).

Neuroimaging should precede lumbar puncture in all patients with impaired consciousness, signs of increased ICP, focal neurologic signs, impending shock, or suspected bleeding diathesis (eg, petechiae). Although MRI is more accurate in diagnosing encephalitis, CT without contrast will identify tumors, masses, or bleeding that precludes performing a lumbar puncture. If neuroimaging and diagnostic lumbar puncture are delayed, administer broad-spectrum intravenous antibiotics after appropriate bacterial cultures are obtained (urine and blood). For patients with encephalitis, prompt administration of intravenous acyclovir, 20 mg/kg per dose (three times a day for neonates through children younger than 12 years) and 10 mg/kg per dose (three times a day for those 12 years or older), is indicated until herpes or varicella-zoster is excluded.[21,27]

Send CSF samples for Gram stain, culture, glucose, protein, cell count, and differential count. If Gram stain result is negative and features suggestive of bacterial meningitis are not present, order PCR and culture for enterovirus and herpes. Obtain concurrent viral cultures from any vesicles, mucous membranes, and urine for herpes and enterovirus. Consider CSF IgM for arboviruses. Other specialized testing might be required, depending on the clinical presentation. If Rocky Mountain spotted fever, cat scratch disease, or mycoplasma pneumonia are possible causes of encephalitis, give doxycycline for those of any age for Rocky Mountain spotted fever but only for those older than 8 years for cat scratch or mycoplasma. For the latter two diseases, azithromycin is a better choice.[27,28] For those suspected of Lyme disease encephalitis, administer ceftriaxone (75 to 100 mg/kg intravenously once a day). Oseltamivir is indicated for influenza.[27,28] Admit patients to units capable of continuous cardiorespiratory monitoring (ie, intensive care or stepdown unit), and closely monitor neurologic status.

WHAT ELSE?

Differential Diagnosis of Encephalitis
- Metabolic disorders
- Sepsis
- Meningitis
- Intracranial lesion (abscess, mass, and bleeding)
- Toxins

KEY POINTS

Management of Encephalitis
- Apply a cardiac monitor and pulse oximeter
- Obtain venous access
- Send blood and urine samples to the laboratory for diagnostic testing and bacterial culture
- Perform a bedside glucose test
- Perform CT of the head or MRI (if immediately available)
- Obtain lumbar puncture and send for analysis, bacterial culture, PCR testing, and IgM measurement
- Administer antibacterials and acyclovir
- Admit patient

A 13-year-old boy presents with a sudden onset of excruciating headache. He has not been ill recently, does not have a history of headaches, and has no recent history of fever or trauma. Family history is negative for migraines. Vital signs include a respiratory rate of 20/min, heart rate of 98/min, blood pressure of 106/68 mm Hg, and a temperature of 37.0°C (98.6°F). Examination reveals an uncomfortable, white, male teenager with severe headache. The results of neurologic examination are nonfocal and remarkable only for pain with terminal neck flexion. No papilledema is noted.

1. What is the appropriate management strategy for this patient?

Headache

Clinical Features and Differential Diagnosis

Headache is a common condition in children, occurring in more than 82% of children by the age of 15 years.[32] Headaches are also a frequent concern of children who present to the ED. One study of acute headaches in children presenting to an ED revealed that 55% were diagnosed as having febrile upper respiratory tract infection, 18% as having a primary headache syndrome (migraine or tension), 7% as having viral meningitis, and 2.5% as having a brain tumor, 2% were postictal after a seizure, 2% were postconcussive, 2% had a ventricular shunt malfunction, and 7% had an undetermined cause.[33] All of the children with serious causes had neurologic signs.[33]

Headaches are often classified as either primary or secondary. A primary headache, such as a migraine, tension, or cluster headache, is diagnosed based on symptoms and pattern of the headache and is usually self-limited.[34] On the other hand, secondary headaches have identifiable causes, some benign (virus, sinusitis, dental infections, and temporomandibular joint dysfunction) and others more serious (tumor, bacterial meningitis, encephalitis, orbital abscess, intracranial bleed, hypertensive encephalopathy, and carbon monoxide poisoning).[34]

Parents are frequently concerned that a headache is a harbinger of a tumor or mass. However, a malignant mass is a rare cause of headache (3 per 100,000) in children.[35] Several clues should raise the suspicion of a brain tumor. One study found that the following were predictors for space-occupying lesions: sleep-related headache (worse with lying down or on arising in the morning), absence of family history of migraine, vomiting, confusion, abnormal neurologic examination results, absence of vision symptoms, and headache duration of less than 6 months.[36]

Most children with brain tumors have additional symptoms indicating intracranial disease, and nearly all children with brain tumors and headache have signs of intracranial disease.[37] The Childhood Brain Tumor Consortium evaluated 3,291 children with brain tumors and found that 62% had headaches. More than 99% of these children had another symptom before their first hospitalization, including vomiting (72% to 86%); personality, speech, or school problems (81% to 87%); weight loss (66% to 79%); difficulty walking (if 2 years or older) (77% to 92%); upper extremity weakness (63% to 79%); seizures (6% to 23%); and diplopia (if older than 4 years) (60% to 63%), depending on whether the tumor was infratentorial or supratentorial.[37] Abnormal physical examination results were present in 98% with supratentorial and 99% with infratentorial tumors. Lethargy or confusion was present in 72% to 77%, papilledema in 65% to 81%, and head tilt in 50% to 76%.[37] Even though many pediatric brain tumors have a midline origin, lateralizing neurologic signs might be absent, but other signs and symptoms mentioned will still occur.[38,39] Nontraumatic brain hemorrhage and intracranial vascular malformations are rare but important causes of headache in children. The most common causes of spontaneous intracranial bleeding in children are AVMs, arteriovenous fistulas, systemic hematologic disorders (eg, thrombocytopenia, hemophilia, or sickle cell disease), and aneurysms.[34] Acute onset headache and vomiting are the most prominent symptoms in these patients.[35] Other signs include seizures, hemiparesis, and ALOC (Glasgow Coma Scale score < 15).[36,40]

Systemic disease with neurologic manifestations can be an important cause of headache in children. Hypertensive encephalopathy occurs in the setting of severe hypertension (diastolic above 95th percentile for age) with loss of cerebral autoregulation or vasospasm. Almost all children with hypertensive encephalopathy will have headache, seizures, or vision changes.[41] Hypertensive encephalopathy in children is usually secondary to renal disease, although occasional causes include coarctation of the aorta, pheochromocytoma, or neuroblastoma.[41] History and diagnostic evaluation can identify the cause of hypertension (eg, drugs, Wilms tumor, renal disease, coarctation, phakomatosis, or hyperthyroidism) and the presence of complications (eg, CNS bleeding, renal failure, or congestive heart failure).[41] Treatment of hypertensive emergencies is addressed in Chapter 12, Medical Emergencies.

Intracranial abscesses are rare and occur most commonly in patients with cyanotic heart disease, those who are immunocompromised, and those with partially or untreated sinus and otologic infections.[34] Other causes to consider include toxin exposure (eg, carbon monoxide, lead) and environmental (eg, high altitude) exposures.

Diagnostic Studies

All children with headache require a thorough history, physical, and neurologic examination to identify features associated with serious disease. A good headache history should include age of onset, frequency, duration, time of onset (eg, day, night, or schooldays), presence or absence of aura, location (eg, frontal, temporal, occipital, or retro-orbital), quality of pain (eg, stabbing, thunderclap, or pressure), radiation of pain, associated signs or symptoms (eg, nausea, vomiting, or photophobia), family history of migraines,

precipitating or relieving factors, association with food, recent history of trauma, change in family or home environment (eg, divorce or new child), change in weight or vision, recent change in exercise or diet, and therapies tried at home.[34,38,39]

The physical examination should include blood pressure, temperature, height and weight, and head circumference for infants. Examination of the eyes should include evaluation of extraocular movements, pupil reactivity, a funduscopic examination, and visual acuity. Examination of the ears, teeth, pharynx, and temporomandibular joint, palpation over the sinuses, and evaluation of the neck for tenderness or rigidity should be included.[34,38,39]

The skin should be thoroughly examined for signs of neurocutaneous syndromes (eg, neurofibromatosis or tuberous sclerosis).[34,39] The neurologic examination should include a complete cranial nerve examination, strength testing, observation of gait, tandem gait testing, deep tendon reflexes, Romberg test, and cerebellar and coordination tests.[34,38,39]

Laboratory studies should be based on specific causes. Those with hypertension deserve an evaluation of renal function as noted above, including electrolytes, blood urea nitrogen, creatinine, and urinalysis. Children with abnormal neurologic examination results, signs of increased ICP, any of the seven signs of a tumor mentioned previously, a ventricular shunt, known coagulopathy, or signs of a neurocutaneous disease should undergo neuroimaging with CT or MRI.[32,34,38,39] A CT scan is often easier to perform and can provide information about most space-occupying lesions, bleeds, hydrocephalus, and abscesses. An MRI is preferred for better delineation of aneurysms, AVMs, and some posterior fossa lesions but might require sedation and might not be immediately available.[39] A child with recurrent headaches and a normal neurologic examination result does not require neuroimaging.[32]

If a child is suspected of having meningitis or encephalitis, a lumbar puncture is required to obtain CSF for analysis. If there is a concern about a subarachnoid hemorrhage, a lumbar puncture can be diagnostic (red cells in the CSF with a nontraumatic tap). In addition, measuring the opening pressure of the lumbar puncture can be helpful when idiopathic intracranial hypertension (pseudotumor cerebri) is suspected (ie, normal CT or MRI result or papilledema).[34] If there are concerns about increased ICP or if there are focal findings, CT should be performed before the lumbar puncture.[34]

Management

In many cases, reassurance and patient education are all that are necessary. In those patients who are suspected of having a primary headache, the patient should keep a headache diary and try to avoid any precipitating factors.[39] Provide appropriate therapy for those with a secondary headache in which the cause has been determined.

For those with a serious cause of the headache, including ALOC, focal findings, or signs of increased ICP, apply a cardiorespiratory monitor. Patients with profoundly altered mental status are at risk for aspiration and rapid deterioration; therefore, control the airway with endotracheal intubation as appropriate. Immediate neurosurgical consultation is required for patients with increased ICP amenable to surgery (eg, AVM, mass, bleeding, or shunt obstruction). Intracranial infections (eg, abscess, cavernous sinus thrombosis, or meningitis) require intravenous antibiotics. These patients, as well as most with a brain tumor, require hospital admission and inpatient monitoring to evaluate for signs of neurologic deterioration.

CASE SCENARIO 5

A 2-year-old, previously healthy child with a generalized clonic seizure is brought to the ED by emergency medical services. The parents estimate that he had been seizing for 5 minutes before arrival of the paramedics. Paramedics noted that the child was having a generalized seizure and was blue around the lips. The patient was given 100% oxygen by face mask, and the result of a rapid assay for glucose was 80 mg/dL. Rectal diazepam was administered, and the child continues to seize on arrival in the ED.

1. What is the most important initial intervention for this patient?
2. What medications can be used to stop the seizure?
3. What are some of the possible causes of this child's seizure?

CASE SCENARIO 6

A 26-month-old boy is brought to the ED by his parents after a generalized clonic seizure at home. The child had been previously healthy and, other than feeling a little warm before the seizure, had not been ill. The seizure lasted 5 minutes. The parents are not aware of any trauma or ingestion. The child slept on the ride to the hospital, awoke at triage, and is crying vigorously as you approach. Vital signs include a respiratory rate of 32/min, heart rate of 170/min, blood pressure of 95/65 mm Hg, and temperature of 39.8°C (103.6°F). The history reveals that the child has had no previous seizures and has a normal developmental history. Upper respiratory tract symptoms started the day of presentation. His physical examination reveals clear rhinorrhea, an erythematous pharynx without exudates, and clear lungs. He is alert and playing with toys on the bed.

1. What is the most appropriate initial intervention?
2. What is the most appropriate diagnostic evaluation at this time?
3. What is appropriate counseling for the parents?

Seizures

A seizure is the clinical manifestation of an abnormal and excessive electrical discharge from neurons in the brain. Although this definition is narrow, the clinical spectrum of illness associated with seizures is wide, occurring from infancy through adolescence. Their diagnosis, management, and treatment will vary widely, depending on age, presence of preexisting neurologic abnormalities, presence or absence of acute coexisting illness, and pattern of seizure activity. A careful history and physical examination are critical to making the diagnosis, distinguishing among the various causes, and directing evaluation and management.

Febrile Seizures

Epidemiology

Febrile seizures are the most common convulsive disorder of childhood. According to data extrapolated from population-based studies, approximately 3% to 5% of children will experience a febrile seizure before their fifth birthday, with the peak onset in the second year of life.[42,43] Approximately two-thirds of the patients are male, with a median age of onset of 19 to 23 months. The risk of febrile seizure increases when there is a history of febrile seizures in first-degree relatives, as does the risk of recurrence.[44]

Clinical Features

By definition, febrile seizures occur in children 6 months to 5 years of age who do not have evidence of intracranial infection or known seizure disorder. Eighty percent of these seizures are simple febrile seizures (generalized, lasting less than 15 minutes, occurring only once in a 24-hour period), which carry few risks of complications and have an excellent short- and long-term prognosis. Children whose seizures have focal features, last more than 15 minutes, or occur more than once in a 24-hour period are classified as having complex febrile seizures. Children with complex febrile seizures have higher rates of recurrent febrile seizures and epilepsy than do children with simple febrile seizures.[44]

The seizure will be the first sign of febrile illness in approximately 25% to 50% of cases. Most febrile seizures occur during the first 24 hours of illness. According to a multicenter, retrospective review of 455 patients with first-time simple febrile seizures, the most common associated infectious illnesses were otitis media (34%), upper respiratory tract infection (12%) or viral syndrome (6%), and pneumonia (6%). Urinary tract infection (3%), gastroenteritis (2%), varicella (2%), and bronchiolitis (1%) were identified in a smaller subset of patients. Thirty-four percent of patients had no infectious diagnosis identified at the time of ED discharge, presumably because they were so early in their illness.[45] In this population, bacteremia occurred in 1.3% of children in whom blood cultures were drawn. These studies precede widespread use of the pneumococcal vaccine, and rates are likely to be significantly lower.

Diagnostic Studies

The cornerstone of diagnosis remains a carefully performed history and physical examination. The body of evidence to date indicates that routine diagnostic evaluation of children with simple febrile seizure is not indicated.[46] Children should be evaluated as if they were simply presenting with uncomplicated fever. Children who have meningeal signs and symptoms, have been pretreated with antibiotics, who have focal seizures, or whose seizure occurs after several days of illness should be carefully evaluated to rule out meningitis and other significant bacterial infections.[46]

YOUR FIRST CLUE

Signs and Symptoms of Simple versus Complex Febrile Seizures

Simple
- 15-minute duration
- Generalized; nonfocal neurologic examination
- No recurrence for <24 hours

Complex
- >15-minute duration
- Focal seizure or focal neurologic examination
- Repeated seizures within 24 hours

In patients whose level of consciousness has not returned to baseline or who are lethargic or irritable, lumbar puncture should be performed to exclude meningitis. Febrile seizures are infrequently the sole sign of viral meningitis; in a comprehensive retrospective review of patients with bacterial meningitis, seizure was never the sole presenting sign.[47] The threshold for performing lumbar puncture varies based on individual patient characteristics, the accessibility of follow-up care, and the physician's comfort level with infants and young children. The practice of routinely performing a lumbar puncture on a child between 6 and 18 months with a simple febrile seizure is not supported by evidence.[46,48] Even in children with complex febrile seizures (eg, more than one seizure in 24 hours), the utility of routine lumbar puncture has come into question.[49] However, children younger than 6 months are outside the usual age group susceptible to febrile seizures. These infants warrant a more careful evaluation with attention to metabolic derangements and possible underlying neurologic disorders, such as meningitis or encephalitis.

An EEG is not indicated for evaluation of simple febrile seizures, either in the ED or as an outpatient.[46] Both CT and MRI should be reserved for the child with a focal seizure, focal neurologic findings, history of head trauma, or failure to return to baseline neurologic status.

Differential Diagnosis

Children with chills associated with high temperatures can be mistakenly identified as having had a febrile seizure. A careful history can help distinguish between these two entities. Children with febrile seizures are a distinct patient group from children with epilepsy who have intercurrent febrile illnesses. Fever is known to lower the seizure threshold in such children. These children might require additional anticonvulsant medication during febrile illnesses, unlike children with febrile seizures.

Management

Antibiotics are not indicated unless there is a focus of infection documented on physical examination or by laboratory evaluation. Anticonvulsants have no role in the treatment of simple febrile seizures because the potential risks of their use outweigh the potential benefits.[50] The practice of using around-the-clock or alternating acetaminophen (paracetamol) and/or ibuprofen does not prevent febrile seizures and can contribute to parental fever phobia.[50] There is no evidence that children with recurrent febrile seizures have any adverse neurologic or intellectual outcome.[50]

Afebrile Seizures

Epidemiology

Between 25,000 and 40,000 children per year in the United States will experience a first afebrile seizure.[51] Epilepsy is characterized by recurrent unprovoked seizures and is not diagnosed until the patient has two or more afebrile seizures. The overall incidence of epilepsy in childhood is between 4 and 9 per 1,000 from population-based studies. The reported percentage of children who have epilepsy after a single afebrile seizure varies between 29% and 82% based on the cohort cited and whether the patient population was studied prospectively or retrospectively. In population-based studies, more children with developmental delay or learning disability develop epilepsy compared with children with normal development.[52]

Clinical Features and Differential Diagnosis

Seizures can be divided into categories based on motor and sensory involvement, as well as the presence or absence of alteration of consciousness (see Table 5-2). A careful history of the event will often give clues to the seizure type and help distinguish seizures from other paroxysmal events, such as breath-holding spells, gastroesophageal reflux with apnea, vasovagal syncope, arrhythmias, and pseudoseizures (see Table 5-3). Although there can be substantial overlap between behavioral descriptors of seizure and nonseizure events, in one prospective study, 13 descriptors were found to differentiate between seizure and nonseizure events. They include jerking/twitching, stiffening, changes in breathing, staring off, biting or chewing the tongue, glassy eyes, unresponsiveness, mumbling or slurring words, eyes/head turned to one side, and lack of memory of the event. All of these were significantly more common in patients with seizures.[53] When in doubt as to the nature of the event, a broader workup might be necessary.

TABLE 5-2 Categorization of Seizures

Generalized Seizures	Description
Tonic-clonic	Rhythmic stiffening and jerking of trunk and extremities
Tonic	Stiffening without jerking of trunk and extremities
Atonic	"Drop attacks"
Absence	Staring or brief loss of consciousness without postictal depression
Myoclonic	Sudden, brief muscle jerks, either unilateral or bilateral
Infantile spasms	Cluster of sudden, tonic contractions of head, trunk, and extremities ("Salaam")
Partial Seizures	
Simple partial seizure	Motor, somatosensory, or autonomic symptoms without alteration of consciousness during or after seizure
Complex partial seizure	Motor or autonomic symptoms with altered level of consciousness; often preceded by aura and followed by postictal depression; might generalize

Adapted from: Reuter D, Brownstein D. Common emergent pediatric neurologic problems. *Emerg Med Clin North Am.* 2002;20(1):155–176.

TABLE 5-3 Outline for Seizure Assessment

Associated Factors	Ictal Symptoms	Postictal Symptoms
Age	Aura—subjective sensations	Amnesia for events
Family history	Behavior—mood or behavior change before the seizure	Confusion
Developmental status		Lethargy
Behavior	Vocal—cry or grasp, slurring of words, garbled speech	Sleepiness
Health at seizure onset—fever, symptoms of acute illness, sleep deprivation	Motor—head/eye turning or deviation, posturing, jerking, stiffening, automatisms, focality	Headaches and muscle aches
Exposure to trauma or toxins	Respiration—change in breathing pattern, apnea, cyanosis	Transient focal weakness (Todd paralysis)
	Autonomic—pupillary dilatation, drooling, change in respiratory or heart rate, incontinence, pallor, vomiting	Nausea or vomiting
	Loss of consciousness, inability to understand or speak	

Hirtz D, Ashwal S, Berg A, et al. Practice parameter: Evaluating a first nonfebrile seizure in children. *Neurology.* 2000;55(5):616–623. Reprinted with permission.

Diagnostic Studies

Routine laboratory investigation in children older than 6 months has not been shown to be helpful in elucidating the cause of seizures or influencing their management. In the absence of a history of illness, vomiting and/or diarrhea, or suspected ingestion, they are not generally indicated.[51] In infants younger than 6 months, hyponatremia and hypocalcemia are known precipitants of seizures. Hypoglycemia is strongly associated with seizure activity at any age in association with alcohol ingestion, oral hypoglycemic agents, and insulin administration. A rapid assay for glucose is important in a child who is actively seizing or who is in the immediate postictal period.

Otherwise, laboratory testing should be based on individual clinical circumstances or the failure to return to baseline mental status. There is no evidence to indicate that lumbar puncture should be routinely performed on the child with an afebrile seizure. Toxicology screening should be considered if there is any question of intentional or unintentional toxin exposure; most toxicology screens only screen for a limited panel of drugs of abuse. In children with persistent alteration of mental status of unknown origin or with meningeal signs, lumbar puncture should be considered for the evaluation of meningitis or encephalitis. Head imaging should be performed before lumbar puncture.

For children with known epilepsy who are currently taking antiseizure drugs, consider measuring drug levels to determine compliance and therapeutic concentrations. Nontrough levels have limited diagnostic value to the treating neurologist unless they clearly show toxic levels or absence of drug.

In a child with new-onset seizure, an EEG can be helpful in neurologic follow-up to help differentiate seizure from nonseizure events, determine seizure type or epilepsy syndrome, and better define the risk for recurrent seizures. It is not necessary to perform the EEG as part of the initial ED evaluation in an otherwise well child. In fact, if it is performed shortly after the seizure (<48 hours), the EEG might show diffuse postictal slowing without prognostic significance. The absence of abnormal EEG findings does not exclude the diagnosis of seizure or epilepsy, and the presence of an abnormal EEG in isolation does not confirm that a seizure occurred.[51]

Although abnormalities in neuroimaging can be found in up to one-third of children with first-time afebrile seizures, in well-designed studies, few (approximately 2%) revealed clinically significant findings that contribute to clinical management. In their practice parameter, Evaluating the First Nonfebrile Seizure in Children, the American Academy of Neurology, the Child Neurology Society, and the American Epilepsy Society do not recommend routine neuroimaging in these children.[51] They recommend emergency neuroimaging only for children with focal postictal deficits not rapidly resolving (ie, Todd paralysis) or those who do not return to their baseline mental status within several hours of the incident. Nonurgent MRI should be considered in several patient groups: children younger than 1 year, those with focal seizures, and children with unexplained neurologic abnormalities or undiagnosed cognitive or motor impairments. Children in whom head trauma is suspected or known represent a separate patient group and should undergo emergent imaging as outlined in Chapter 6, Trauma.[51]

Management

If the child is not actively seizing in the ED, no treatment is indicated at the time of the evaluation. Appropriate consultation with a pediatric neurologist and outpatient follow-up care should be arranged for all children suspected of having a first-time afebrile seizure. In a child with a recurrent seizure who has previously been evaluated with EEG and who is not taking anticonvulsants, neurologic consultation and initiation of therapy should be considered. If an epileptic child undergoing antiseizure therapy has breakthrough seizures, therapy adherence and acute illness history should be carefully reviewed. Decisions regarding alteration of current therapy should be made in consultation with the patient's pediatric neurologist. During febrile illnesses, many children with known epilepsy will have an increase in seizure frequency because the seizure threshold is lowered with intercurrent illnesses. One successful approach to this problem has been to prophylactically prescribe rectal diazepam to break the seizure cluster.[51] It can be used either in the ED or at home by the parents in a commercially available rectal gel preparation (Diastat).

Children who have an obvious precipitant to the seizure should be treated in accordance with the underlying injury or illness process. Table 5-4 indicates common causes of toxin-mediated seizures and any specific recommendations unique to the toxicologic agent. Benzodiazepines remain the drugs of first choice in terminating seizure activity in children. They are effective, potent, rapidly acting, and easily administered in the field and the ED (see Table 5-5). Recurrent seizures should be managed according to the SE pathway outlined in **Figure 5.2**.

Status Epilepticus

Epidemiology

Every year in the United States, approximately 120,000 individuals will experience SE. More than half of these will be children. One-third of the episodes will be the initial event in a patient with new-onset epilepsy,[54,55] one-third will occur in children with established epilepsy, and one-third will occur as an isolated event at the time of an acute insult.[54,55] Up to 70% of children with epilepsy presenting before 1 year of age will experience an episode of SE in their lifetimes.[55]

Historically, high rates of mortality have been associated with SE, especially in the adult population. Seizure duration of greater than 1 hour, especially in association with hypoxia, has been associated with permanent neurologic injury and increasing rates of mortality.[56] However, more recent reports indicate that the mortality rate in children is related to the prolonged seizure itself and is probably only 1% to 3%.[55,57,58]

Clinical Features

Although SE has been classically defined as continuous or repetitive seizure activity of at least 30 minutes,[59] almost all self-limited seizures stop within 5 minutes. Therefore, the Working Group on Status Epilepticus of the Epilepsy Foundation of America recommends that any patient with

TABLE 5-4 **Mnemonic for Toxin-Induced Seizures (OTIS CAMPBELL)**	
Toxic Substance	Antidotes, Special Instructions (benzodiazepines are the initial drug of choice for all conditions)
Organophosphates	Atropine, pralidoxime
Tricyclic antidepressants	Avoid phenytoin
Isoniazid	Pyridoxine (grams per grams of isoniazid ingested); might not respond to anticonvulsant drugs
Insulin	Glucose
Sympathomimetics	
Camphor, Cocaine	
Amphetamines	
Methylxanthines (theophylline, caffeine)	Use pentobarbital if no response
PCP, Propoxyphene, Phenol, Propranolol	
Benzodiazepine withdrawal, Botanicals	
Ethanol withdrawal	Magnesium sulfate
Lithium	
Lidocaine (lignocaine)	Avoid phenytoin second-degree arrhythmia risk
Lindane	
Lead	Bronchoalveolar lavage, calcium disodium edetate

Erickson TB, Aks SE, Gussow L, Williams RH. Toxicology update: A rational approach to managing a poisoned patient. *Emergency Medicine Practice,* August 2001, Vol 6, Number 8.

TABLE 5-5 Drugs Used to Terminate Status Epilepticus[a]

Drug	Dose	Maximum Dose	Onset of Action	Duration of Action	Rate
Lorazepam	0.05–0.1 mg/kg IV	4 mg	2–3 min	12–24 h	≤2 mg/min
Diazepam	0.1–0.3 mg/kg IV 0.5 mg/kg PR	10 mg	1–3 min	5–15 min	≤2 mg/min
Midazolam	0.05–0.15 mg/kg IV/IM	6 mg	2–3 min (IV) 10–20 min (IM)	30–60 min (IV) 1–2 h (IM)	≤2 mg/min
Phenytoin	20 mg/kg IV	1,000 mg	10–30 min[a]	12–24 h	≤1 mg/kg/min ≤50 mg/min
Fosphenytoin	20–30 mg/kg PE˅ IV/IM	1,000 mg	10–30 min[a]	12–24 h	≤3 mg/kg/min ≤150 mg/min
Phenobarbital	20 mg/kg IV	1,000 mg	10–20 min	1–3 days	≤1–2 mg/kg/min ≤60 mg/min

Adapted from: Pellock JM. Status epilepticus in children: Update and review. *J Child Neurol.* 1994;9(suppl):2S27–2S35; Hanhan UA, Fiallos MR, Orlowski JP. Status epilepticus. *Pediatr Clin North Am.* 2001;48(3):1–12; and Haafiz A, Kissoon N. Status epilepticus: Current concepts. *Pediatr Emerg Care.* 1999;15(2):119–129. Abend N, Dlugos D. Treatment of refractory status epilepticus: Literature review and a proposed protocol. *Pediatr Neurol.* 2008;38(6):277–390.

Abbreviations: IM, intramuscular; IV, intravenous; PE, phenytoin equivalents; PR, per rectum.

[a]After infusion

seizure duration of longer than 10 minutes have anticonvulsant therapy initiated.[60] By extension, any child presenting to the ED actively seizing should be considered to be in SE and treated accordingly. The earlier the attempt to control the seizure, the easier it will be to stop.

Diagnostic Studies

Diagnostic studies should be tailored to rapidly determine metabolic, toxicologic, or neurologic derangements that might have precipitated SE. The American Academy of Neurology published a practice parameter in 2006 outlining the evidence to support the diagnostic assessment of a child with SE. They reviewed all the published studies on pediatric SE in an attempt to formulate recommendations for these children.[59] They found that electrolyte levels were measured as part of routine practice and were abnormal in approximately 6% of cases. Of those investigated for meningitis or encephalitis, CNS infection was found in 12.8% of cases. When anticonvulsant drug levels were measured in children with known epilepsy, the levels were low 32%

of the time. Evidence of toxicologic ingestion was present in 3% to 6% of children. Inborn errors of metabolism were identified in 4% of cases in which a metabolic etiology was sought. Abnormalities on EEG were identified in 43% of studied children, and findings frequently helped determine the nature and localization of the seizure. At least 8% of children in whom neuroimaging was obtained had abnormalities that might have explained the cause of the SE.[59]

Rapid bedside assay for glucose is indicated in all patients. Depending on the clinical scenario, serum levels of sodium, calcium, and phosphorus are indicated for children with ongoing seizure activity. Tests of renal and hepatic function can be useful in selected cases. Anticonvulsant drug levels should be checked in children with known epilepsy. Specific serum toxicologic levels should be directed by the history, including the presence of drugs in the home or surroundings that are known to cause seizures (eg, isoniazid). A urine toxicology screen, usually only available for drugs of abuse, has a rapid turnaround time in most

Management Protocols for Status Epilepticus

Stabilize the Patient (0–10 minutes)
Evaluate the airway (position, suction)
Provide 100% oxygen by face mask
Assess ventilation and support as needed (consider oral or nasal airway)
Measure and monitor vital signs
Establish vascular access
Obtain blood for rapid glucose assay and other specimens as indicated by history and physical
Control hyperthermia (rectal acetaminophen 15 mg/kg)

Begin Therapy (10–45 minutes)
1) Glucose 0.5 mg/kg if hypoglycemic (2 mL/kg D25, 5 mL/kg D10)
2) Lorazepam 0.10 mg/kg IV, max 4 mg/dose, may repeat × 1 in 5–10 minutes
   OR
Diazepam 0.1–0.3 mg/kg IV, max 10 mg/dose, may repeat × 1 in 5 minutes
   OR if no IV access Diazepam 0.5 mg/kg per rectum, max 20 mg
FOLLOWED BY
IF CHILD:
3) Fosphenytoin 20 mg/kg IV or IM, 3 mg/kg/min, max 1,000 mg
   OR
Phenytoin 20 mg/kg IV, 1 mg/kg/min, max 1,000 mg
IF NEONATE:
4) Phenobarbital 20 mg/kg IV, 1 mg/kg/min. BE PREPARED TO VENTILATE.
5) If seizure activity continues 10 minutes after infusion of phenobarbital in a neonate, consider repeated doses of phenobarbital at 10 mg kg dose, up to a maximum of 40 mg/kg.
6) If seizure activity continues after 2 doses of benzodiazepine and an appropriate antiepileptic drug load, move to therapy for refractory SE.

Initiate Therapy for Refractory Status Epilepticus (>45–60 minutes)
1) Rapid sequence intubation and mechanical ventilation.
2) Consider continuous EEG monitoring.
3) Optimal placement in critical care ICU setting with consideration for central venous pressure monitoring, especially if using pentobarbital.
4) Midazolam drip 0.2 mg/kg IV load, followed by 1 mcg/kg/min drip, increase 1 mcg/kg/min every 15 minutes until burst suppression
   OR
Pentobarbital drip 5–15 mg/kg IV load, followed by 0.5–5 mg/kg/hr infusion
   OR
Propofol drip 1–2 mg/kg IV load, followed by 2–10 mg/kg/hr drip
   OR
Valproic Acid 15–20 mg/kg IV load over 1–5 min, may repeat q 10–15 minutes to max of 40 mg/kg or 5 mg/kg/hr infusion

Figure 5.2 Management protocol for status epilepticus.

Adapted from: Pellock JM. Status epilepticus in children: Update and review. *J Child Neurol*. 1994;9(suppl):2S27–2S35; Hanhan UA, Fiallos MR, Orlowski JP. Status epilepticus. *Pediatr Clin North Am*. 2001;48(3):1–12; and Haafiz A, Kissoon N. Status epilepticus: Current concepts. *Pediatr Emerg Care*. 1999;15(2):119–129.

institutions and might influence management. If head trauma is suspected based on the history or physical examination results, emergent CT scan of the head is indicated.

In their 2006 practice parameter, the American Academy of Neurology and the Practice Committee of the Child Neurology Society suggest that neuroimaging be considered after stabilization if there are specific clinical indicators or if the precipitant is unknown, but evidence to support a recommendation of routine neuroimaging was insufficient. They also found that evidence was lacking to support routine blood culture or lumbar puncture in the absence of a clinical suspicion of systemic or CNS infection. They recommend EEG in cases of suspected pseudo-SE (nonepileptic SE), or nonconvulsive SE, as well as to help guide treatment in cases where it is unclear whether the cause was focal or generalized.[59]

Differential Diagnosis

The differential diagnosis of SE includes complex febrile seizures, toxic ingestion or drug withdrawal, intercurrent febrile illness, or subtherapeutic anticonvulsant levels in a child with known epilepsy, meningitis or encephalitis, intracranial injury, or progressive neurodegenerative disorder. Status epilepticus can be classified into five broad categories (listed in Table 5-6): acute symptomatic, remote symptomatic (with or without acute precipitant), progressive encephalopathic, febrile, and cryptogenic (idiopathic). Table 5-6 lists the relative frequency of different causes in pediatric patients with SE.

Management

Management of this life-threatening condition mandates the usual resuscitative measures before specific therapy for seizures. Airway, breathing, and circulation should be assessed first; much of the morbidity and mortality associated with SE can be attributed to hypoxia and its ensuing complications. Hypoxia associated with SE is multifactorial: impairment of mechanical ventilation secondary to tonic-clonic activity, increased salivation, increased tracheobronchial secretions, and increased oxygen consumption by tissues. The combination of seizure activity and hypoxia in turn causes a decrease in brain adenosine triphosphate activity, a decrease in serum glucose, and an increase in lactic acidosis. Acidosis and hypoxia superimposed on ongoing seizure activity lead to impaired cardiovascular function, decreased cardiac output, and hypotension. The acidosis of SE is mixed respiratory and metabolic. The metabolic component is primarily due to the buildup of lactic acid secondary to impaired tissue oxygenation and perfusion in the face of increased metabolic needs and energy expenditure.[60]

TABLE 5-6 Classification of Status Epilepticus

Type	Definition	Examples
Acute symptomatic (26%)	SE occurring during an acute illness (an acute CNS insult) (an acute encephalopathy)	Meningitis, encephalitis, electrolyte disturbance, sepsis, hypoxia, trauma, intoxication
Remote symptomatic (33%)	SE occurring without an acute provocation in a patient with a prior history of a CNS insult (a chronic encephalopathy)	CNS malformation, previous traumatic brain injury or insult, chromosomal disorder
Remote symptomatic with an acute precipitant (1%)	SE occurring with chronic encephalopathy but with an acute provocation	CNS malformation or previous CNS insult with concurrent infection, hypoglycemia, hypocalcemia, or intoxication
Progressive encephalopathy (3%)	SE occurring with an underlying, progressive CNS disorder	Mitochondrial disorders, CNS lipid storage diseases, amino or organic acidopathies
Febrile (22%)	SE occurring when the only provocation is a febrile illness, after excluding a direct CNS infection, such as meningitis or encephalitis	Upper respiratory tract infection, sinusitis, sepsis
Cryptogenic[a] (15%)	SE occurring in the absence of an acute precipitating CNS insult, systemic metabolic disturbance, or both	No definable cause

Adapted from: Riviello J, Ashwal S, Hirtz D, et al. Practice parameter: Diagnostic assessment of the child with status epilepticus (an evidence-based review): Report of the Quality Standards Subcommittee of the American Academy of Neurology and the Practice Committee of the Child Neurology Society. *Neurology.* 2006;67(9):1542–1550. Reprinted with permission.

Abbreviations: CNS, central nervous system; SE, status epilepticus.

[a]The category cryptogenic is now used instead of idiopathic, which had been used in the original classification.

In the first 30 minutes of seizure activity, there is massive catecholamine release and sympathetic discharge. This results in an increase in heart rate, blood pressure, central venous pressure, cerebral blood flow, and serum glucose level. After 30 minutes of generalized tonic-clonic activity, blood pressure begins to decrease, and cerebral blood flow, although still increased above baseline, decreases to the point where it might be unable to supply adequate substrate and oxygen to meet increased cerebral metabolic demands. This results in impaired cortical oxygenation.[60]

Systemic effects of prolonged seizure activity include an increase in body temperature, a decrease in serum glucose level, an increase in serum potassium level, and elevations in creatine kinase levels. As a result of muscle breakdown, myoglobinuria and acute renal failure can ensue.[60]

The mainstays of management involve continuous attention to the ABCs of resuscitation to prevent systemic and cerebral hypoxia. The goals are to maintain adequate vital functions to prevent systemic complications, terminate seizure activity as quickly as possible while minimizing morbidity from treatment, and evaluate and treat the underlying cause of SE.[60]

The risk of respiratory failure is high throughout the entire resuscitation and can be due to the medications used to terminate seizures, the seizure activity itself, and postictal hypoventilation. Proper positioning of the patient, supine on the bed with the head in midline or left lateral decubitus position, to prevent aspiration of emesis is essential. The use of a neck and shoulder roll for airway positioning, a jaw-thrust maneuver, or the placement of a nasal airway are often all that is needed to open an obstructed upper airway. One hundred percent oxygen via a nonrebreather mask should be administered to all patients. Suction equipment and an appropriately sized bag-mask device should be immediately available at the bedside.

Next, an IV catheter should be placed and blood drawn as previously outlined. If hypoglycemia is documented, 0.5 to 1 g/kg of glucose should be given as a bolus (2 to 4 mL/kg of 25% dextrose or 5 to 10 mL/kg of 10% dextrose). Glucagon can be given via the intramuscular route if no intravenous access has been established.[60] Tubes of blood can be drawn and set aside in case further evaluation is required.

After the initial resuscitative measures have been accomplished, specific therapy aimed at terminating seizure activity and preventing its recurrence should begin (see Table 5-7). Benzodiazepines are the first-line drugs for the treatment of SE.[54,61,62] As a class, they act rapidly and are highly effective. Most children will stop seizing with one or two doses. All benzodiazepines cause some degree of respiratory depression, which can be reduced by slowing infusion rates and waiting appropriate intervals before giving additional doses. Lorazepam and diazepam have rapid onsets of action. The median times to cessation of seizure activity are 2 and 3 minutes, respectively. Lorazepam has a much longer duration of action secondary to its smaller volume of distribution and produces less respiratory depression. Effective brain levels can persist for 12 to 24 hours. For these reasons, it is favored as the initial treatment of SE in most centers.[54]

In the absence of intravenous access, rectal diazepam (Diastat) can be initiated at a dose of 0.5 mg/kg. Respiratory depression is not commonly seen via this route, probably because of slightly slower absorption, which makes this a good medication to use at home and in the field to safely terminate seizure clusters or SE. Diazepam is rapidly redistributed, and seizures can recur in 15 to 20 minutes.[54] Therefore, when diazepam is used for SE, it should be immediately followed by a long-acting anticonvulsant, such as fosphenytoin.[63]

Fosphenytoin is a phosphate-ester prodrug of phenytoin that has several advantages over the parent compound. In contrast to phenytoin, it is compatible with any intravenous solution and can be administered with dextrose.[54] The side effect profile has been substantially improved by removing the ethylene glycol base used as a diluent for phenytoin. This decreases the possibility of arrhythmias associated with phenytoin. In addition, it is not tissue toxic and can even be given via the intramuscular route if necessary. In addition, it can be given at triple the maximal rate of phenytoin.[60]

In neonates, phenobarbital should be substituted for fosphenytoin because it has a higher likelihood of terminating seizure activity in this age group. It should be dosed at 20 mg/kg and given at maximal rate of 0.5 to 1 mg/kg per minute. The combination of a benzodiazepine plus phenobarbital in a neonate carries a significant risk of respiratory depression, apnea, and hypotension. Respiratory and hemodynamic support should be immediately available. Another consideration in a neonate with SE is pyridoxine-dependent seizures, a rare autosomal-recessive condition. The diagnosis is made when seizure activity ceases after administration of intravenous pyridoxine (100 mg, up to five doses). Some experts recommend a trial of pyridoxine in all infants without a clear symptomatic cause of SE.[64]

If seizure activity continues for 5 to 10 minutes beyond the initial dose, a second dose of benzodiazepines should be given.[54,60] The managing physician should remain alert to the possible ongoing need for airway intervention because cumulative doses of benzodiazepines carry higher rates of respiratory depression. If the child has had one or two appropriate doses of benzodiazepine and has been loaded with either fosphenytoin or phenobarbital and

seizure activity has persisted, the child should be considered to be in refractory SE. Many of these patients will need to be paralyzed, intubated, and mechanically ventilated. They require careful monitoring (including continuous EEG monitoring) in a critical care setting.

Refractory SE can be difficult to terminate, and there is no consensus as to the optimal management of these patients. Table 5-7 outlines the various pharmacologic interventions currently in favor. Larger prospective studies need to be performed using these drugs to better define the optimal management strategy for the pediatric patient. Historically, pentobarbital, a short-acting barbiturate, was the preferred drug to terminate SE. However, significant complications are associated with the ongoing use of this drug, including hypotension, myocardial depression, low cardiac output, and delayed neurologic recovery.[56,60,62,64] For these reasons, many centers have switched to treating refractory SE with the water-soluble benzodiazepine midazolam as a continuous infusion. It is lipophilic at physiologic pH, has a rapid onset of action, and quickly passes the blood-brain barrier. The

TABLE 5-7 Drugs Used for Refractory Status Epilepticus

Drug	Loading Dose	IV Drip	Adverse Effects	Neurologic Recovery
Midazolam	0.1–0.5 mg/kg IV bolus Maximum of 10 mg	0.1 mg/kg/h, may increase to 0.2 mg/kg/h after additional bolus	Somnolence, respiratory depression	Quick
Pentobarbital	5–15 mg/kg IV over 1 h or 20 mg/kg over 2 h	0.5–5 mg/kg/h	Hypotension, myocardial depression, cardiac output	Slow
Propofol	1–2 mg/kg load	2 mg/kg/h may be titrated up to 10 mg/kg/h if hemodynamics tolerate	Bradycardia, apnea, hypotension with fast infusion, "propofol infusion syndrome"	Quick
Valproic acid	15–20 mg/kg at 5–6 mg/kg/min, maximum of 40 mg/kg	5 mg/kg/h	Isolated case reports of hypotension, hepatotoxicity	Quick
Levetiracetam[a]	20–30 mg/kg IV at 5 mg/kg/min Maximum of 3 g or 80 mg/kg/d		Sedation, irritability	

Adapted from: Part I: Definitions. In: Gastauf H, ed. *Dictionary of Epilepsy.* Geneva, Switzerland: World Health Organization; 1973; Maytal J, Bienkowski RS, Patel M, Eviatar L. The value of brain imaging in children with headaches. *Pediatrics.* 1995;98(3 pt 1):413–416; Dreifuss FE, Rosman NP, Cloyd JC, et al. A comparison of rectal diazepam gel and placebo for acute repetitive seizures. *N Engl J Med.* 1998;338(26):1869–1875; Abend N, Dlugos D. Treatment of refractory status epilepticus: literature review and a proposed protocol. *Pediatr Neurol.* 2008;38(6):277–390; and Singh RK, Gaillard WD. Status epilepticus in children. *Curr Neurol Neurosci Rep.* 2009;9(2):137–144.

Abbreviation: IV, intravenous.

[a]Not currently approved for IV use in children.

major advantage of midazolam is the absence of significant cardiovascular depression, especially in comparison with pentobarbital.[60,62,64–66] It is unclear why patients who have not previously responded to other benzodiazepines respond to midazolam.

Propofol is another highly effective, lipid-soluble drug. It is a nonbarbiturate anesthetic with hypnotic and anticonvulsant properties, a rapid onset of action, and quick recovery times. Case reports and small studies have reported cessation of seizure activity or inducement of burst suppression after a propofol bolus followed by continuous infusion. Known adverse effects include bradycardia, apnea, and hypotension with rapid infusion. It produces less cardiorespiratory depression than pentobarbital. Initial case reports described unexplained acidosis,[60] and others have described "propofol infusion syndrome," which consists of cardiac failure, rhabdomyolysis, metabolic acidosis, renal failure, and rarely death. Although components of this syndrome can occur with SE itself and not be directly attributable to the propofol, concerns regarding this complication have limited its use in children for refractory SE.[64]

The newest drugs in the armamentarium for refractory SE are valproic acid and levetiracetam (Keppra). Valproic acid is known to be effective in partial and generalized epilepsy syndromes in childhood. It can be administered intravenously as a bolus of 15 to 20 mg/kg and continued as a continuous infusion at a rate of 5 mg/kg per hour. In one study involving 41 children, SE was successfully terminated in 78% of cases. Two-thirds of the patients responded within 6 minutes of the initial bolus. The biggest advantage of valproic acid is that it is significantly less sedating, has less respiratory depression than the other drugs mentioned, and has an excellent cardiovascular profile.[60,62,64] Currently, the intravenous formulation of levetiracetam is not approved for use in children; however, small case series have reported efficacy in terminating refractory status.[62,64] Further study of this drug is warranted.

Children with SE should be transferred to a facility capable of providing pediatric critical care. These patients belong in a unit where they can be monitored for the development of cerebral and systemic complications of SE. Consultation with a pediatric neurologist is essential in the ongoing treatment and follow-up care of these patients.

KEY POINTS

Management of Seizures

- ABCs (airway, breathing, circulation)
- Cardiorespiratory and pulse oximetry monitoring
- Obtain vascular access
- Perform rapid glucose test and treat hypoglycemia
- Terminate seizure
- Evaluate and treat identified underlying causes

CHAPTER REVIEW

Check Your Knowledge

1. A child presents to the emergency department (ED) with lethargy after consuming 84 g of his mother's perfume. Which of the following studies is the most helpful bedside test for the evaluation of this patient's altered mental status?
   A. Hemoglobin
   B. Serum electrolytes
   C. Serum glucose
   D. Toxicology screen

2. Of the following options, which is the best method for acutely lowering increased intracranial pressure (ICP)?
   A. Hyperoxygenation
   B. Intravenous steroids
   C. Midline positioning of the neck
   D. Mild hyperventilation

3. All of the following are common complications of bacterial meningitis except:
   A. acute renal failure.
   B. seizures.
   C. syndrome of inappropriate antidiuretic hormone secretion (SIADH).
   D. subdural effusion.

4. All of the following are criteria of simple febrile seizures except:
   A. age 6 months to 5 years.
   B. associated with no neurologic deficit.
   C. temperature greater than 40°C (104°F).
   D. lasting less than 15 minutes.

References

1. Christian CW, Taylor AA, Hertle RW, Duhaime A. Retinal hemorrhages caused by accidental household trauma. *J Pediatr.* 1999;135:125–127.
2. Mei-Zahav M, Uziel Y, Raz J, Ginot N, Wolach B, Fainmesser P. Convulsions and retinal haemorrhage: Should we look further? *Arch Dis Child.* 2002;86:334–335.
3. Gilliland MG, Luckenbach MW. Are retinal hemorrhages found after resuscitation attempts? A study of the eyes of 169 children. *Am J Forensic Med Pathol.* 1993;14:187–192.
4. Odom A, Christ E, Kerr N et al. Prevalence of retinal hemorrhages in pediatric patients after in-hospital cardiopulmonary resuscitation: A prospective study. *Pediatrics.* 1997;99:E3.
5. Duhaime AC, Christina CW, Rorke LB, Zimmerman RA. Nonaccidental head injury in infants—"The shaken baby syndrome." *N Engl J Med.* 1998;338:1822–1829.
6. Belay ED, Bresee JS, Holman RC, Khan AS, Shahriari A, Schonberger LB. Reye's syndrome in the United States from 1981 through 1997. *N Engl J Med.* 1999;340:1377–1382.
7. Monto AS. The disappearance of Reye's syndrome—A public health triumph. *N Engl J Med.* 1999;340:1423–1424.
8. Orlowski JP. Whatever happened to Reye's syndrome? Did it ever really exist? *Crit Care Med.* 1999;27:1582–1587.
9. Gauthier M, Guay J, Lacroix J, Lortie A. Reye's syndrome: A reappraisal of diagnosis in 49 presumptive cases. *Am J Dis Child.* 1989;143:1181–1185.
10. Kim D, Buchanan S, Noonan G, McGeehin M. Treatment of children with elevated blood lead levels. *Am J Prev Med.* 2002;22:71.
11. Bodamer OA, Hussein K, Morris AA, et al. Glucose and leucine kinetics in idiopathic ketotic hypoglycemia. *Arch Dis Child* 2006;91:483–486.
12. Birkhahn R, Fiorini M, Gaeta TJ. Painless intussusception and altered mental status. *Am J Emerg Med.* 1999;17:345–347.
13. Mazzola CA, Adelson PD. Critical care management of head trauma in children. *Crit Care Med.* 2002;30:S393–S401.
14. Nigrovic LE, Kuppermann N, Malley R. Children with bacterial meningitis presenting to the emergency department during the pneumococcal conjugate vaccines. *Acad Emerg Med.* 2008;15:522–528.
15. Kaplan SL. Epidemiology, clinical features and diagnosis of acute bacterial meningitis in children. In: Rose BD, ed. *UpToDate.* Waltham, MA: UpToDate; 2010.
16. Edwards MS, Baker CJ. Clinical features and diagnosis of bacterial meningitis in the neonate. In: Rose BD, ed. *UpToDate.* Waltham, MA: UpToDate; 2010.
17. Corless CE, Guiver M, Borrow R, Edwards-Jones V, Fox AJ, Kaczmarski EB. Simultaneous detection of *Neisseria meningitidis, Haemophilus influenzae,* and *Streptococcus pneumoniae* in suspected cases of meningitis and septicemia using real-time PCR. *J Clin Microbiol.* 2001;39:1553–1558.
18. Nigrovic LE, Kuppermann N, Macias CG, et al. Clinical prediction rule for identifying children with cerebrospinal fluid pleocytosis at very low risk of meningitis. *JAMA.* 2007;297:52–60.
19. Nigrovic LE, Malley R, Macias CG, et al. Effect of antibiotic pretreatment on cerebrospinal fluid profiles of children with bacterial meningitis. *Pediatrics.* 2008;122:726–730.
20. Kaplan SL. Treatment and prognosis of acute bacterial meningitis in children. In: Rose BD, ed. *UpToDate.* Waltham, MA: *UpToDate;* 2010.
21. American Academy of Pediatrics. In: Pickering LK, ed. *Red Book: 2009: Report of the Committee on Infectious Diseases.* 28th ed. Elk Grove Village, IL: American Academy of Pediatrics; 2009.
22. DiPentima C. Viral meningitis: Epidemiology, pathogenesis, and etiology in children. In: Rose BD, ed. *UpToDate.* Waltham, MA: UpToDate; 2010.
23. Hardarson HS. Acute viral encephalitis in children and adolescents: Pathogenesis and etiology. In: Rose BD, ed. *UpToDate.* Waltham, MA: UpToDate; 2010.
24. Horga MA, Fine A. West Nile virus. *Pediatr Infect Dis J.* 2001;20:801–802.
25. Whitley RJ, Gnann JW. Viral encephalitis: Familiar infections and emerging pathogens. *Lancet.* 2002;359:507–513.

26. DiPentima C. Viral meningitis: Clinical features and diagnosis in children. In: Rose BD, ed. *UpToDate*. Waltham, MA: UpToDate; 2010.

27. Hardarson HS. Acute viral encephalitis in children and adolescents: Treatment and prevention. In: Rose BD, ed. *UpToDate*. Waltham, MA: *UpToDate*; 2010.

28. Tunkel AR, Glaser CA, Bloch KC, et al. The management of encephalitis: Clinical practice guidelines by the Infectious Diseases Society of America. Clin Infect Dis. 2008;47:303–327.

29. Bales JF. Human herpesviruses and neurological disorders of childhood. *Semin Pediatr Neurol*. 1999;6:278–287.

30. Leonard JR, Moran CJ, Cross DT III, Wippold FJ II, Schlesinger Y, Storch GA. MR imaging of herpes simplex type 1 encephalitis in infants and young children: A separate pattern of findings. *AJR Am J Roentgenol*. 2000;174:1651–1655.

31. Bales JF. Viral infections of the central nervous system. In: Berg BO, ed. *Principles of Child Neurology*. New York, NY: McGraw Hill; 1996:839–858.

32. Lewis DW, Ashwal S, Dahl G, et al. Practice parameter: Evaluation of children and adolescents with recurrent headaches: Report of the quality standards subcommittee of the American Academy of Neurology and the Practice Committee of the Child Neurology Society. *Neurology*. 2002;59:490–498.

33. Lewis DW, Qureshi F. Acute headache in children and adolescents presenting to the emergency department. *Headache*. 2000;40:200–203.

34. King C. Emergency evaluation of headache in children. In: Rose BD, ed. *UpToDate*. Waltham, MA: UpToDate; 2010.

35. Al-Jarallah A, Al-Rifai MT, Riela AR, Roach ES. Nontraumatic brain hemorrhage in children: Etiology and presentation. *J Child Neurol*. 2000;15:284–289.

36. Medina LS, Pinter JD, Zurakowski D, Davis RG, Kuban K, Barnes PD. Children with headaches: Clinical predictors of surgical space-occupying lesions and the role of neuroimaging. *Radiology*. 1997;202:819–824.

37. Childhood Brain Tumor Consortium. The epidemiology of headache among children with brain tumor. *J Neuro-Oncol*. 1991;10:31–46.

38. Bonthius DJ, Lee AG. Approach to the child with headache. In: Rose BD, ed. *UpToDate*. Waltham, MA: UpToDate; 2010.

39. Fuchs S. Headache. In: Strange GR, Ahrens WR, Schafermeyer RW, Wiebe R, eds. *Pediatric Emergency Medicine*. 3rd ed. New York, NY: McGraw Hill Medical; 2009:489–494.

40. Jakobsson KE, Saveland H, Hillman J, et al. Warning leak and management outcome in aneurysmal subarachnoid hemorrhage. *J Neurosurg*. 1996;85:995–999.

41. Wright RR, Mathews KD. Hypertensive encephalopathy in childhood. *J Child Neurol*. 1996;11:193–196.

42. Verity CM, Golding J. Risk of epilepsy after febrile convulsions: A national cohort study. *BMJ*. 1991;303:1373–1376.

43. Nelson K, Ellenberg J. Prognosis in children with febrile seizures. *Pediatrics*. 1978;61:720–727.

44. Trainor JL. Evaluating and treating the child with a febrile seizure. *Clin Pediatri Emerg Med*. 1999;1:13–20.

45. Trainor JL, Hampers LC, Krug SE, Listernick R. Children with first-time simple febrile seizures are at low risk of serious bacterial illness. *Acad Emerg Med*. 2001;8:781–787.

46. American Academy of Pediatrics Subcommittee on Febrile Seizure. Clinical Practice Guideline: neurodiagnostic evaluation of the child with a first simple febrile seizure. *Pediatrics*. 2011;127:389–394.

47. Green SM, Rothrock SG, Glem KJ, Zurcher RF, Mellick L. Can seizures be the sole manifestation of meningitis in febrile children? *Pediatrics*. 1993;92:527–534.

48. Kimia AA, Capraro AJ, Hummel D, Johnston P, Harper MB. Utility of lumbar puncture for first simple febrile seizure among children 6 to 18 months of age. *Pediatrics*. 2009;123:6–12.

49. Kimia A, Ben-Joseph E, Rudloe T, et al. Yield of lumbar puncture among children who present with their first complex febrile seizure. *Pediatrics*. 2010;126:62–69.

50. American Academy of Pediatrics Steering Committee on Quality Improvement and Management, Subcommittee on Febrile Seizures. Febrile seizures: Clinical practice guideline for the long-term management of the child with simple febrile seizures. *Pediatrics*. 2008;121:1281–1286.

51. Hirtz D, Ashwal S, Berg A, et al. Practice parameter: Evaluating a first nonfebrile seizure in children. *Neurology*. 2000;55:616–623.

52. Verity CM, Ross EM, Golding J. Epilepsy in the first 10 years of life: Findings of the child health and education study. *BMJ*. 1992;305:857–861.

53. Williams J, Grant M, Jackson M, et al. Behavioral descriptors that differentiate between seizure and nonseizure events in a pediatric population. *Clin Pediatr (Phila)*. 1996;35:243–249.

54. Pellock JM. Status epilepticus in children: Update and review. *J Child Neurol*. 1994;9(suppl):2S27–2S35.

55. Hauser WA. Status epilepticus: Epidemiologic considerations. *Neurology*. 1990;40(suppl 2):9–13.

56. DeLorenzo RJ, Towne AR, Pellock JM, Ko D. Status epilepticus in children, adults and the elderly. *Epilepsia*. 1992;33(suppl 4):S15–S25.

57. DeLorenzo RJ, Pellock JM, Towne AR, Boggs JG. Epidemiology of status epilepticus. *J Clin Neurophysiol*. 1995;12:316–325.

58. Chin RF, Neville BG, Peckham C, Bedford H, Wade A, Scott RC. Incidence, cause, and short-term outcome of convulsive status epilepticus in childhood: Prospective population-based study. *Lancet*. 2008;368:222–229.

59. Riviello JJ, Ashwal S, Hirtz D, et al. Practice parameter: Diagnostic assessment of the child with status epilepticus (an evidence-based review): Report of the quality standards subcommittee of the American Academy of Neurology and the Practice Committee of the Child Neurology Society. *Neurology*. 2006;67:1542–1550.

60. Hanhan UA, Fiallos MR, Orlowski JP. Status epilepticus. *Pediatr Clin North Am*. 2001;48:1–12.

61. Lewena S, Pennington V, Acworth J, et al. Emergency management of pediatric convulsive status epilepticus: A multicenter study of 542 patients. *Pediatr Emerg Care*. 2009;25:83–87.

62. Singh RK, Gaillard WD. Status epilepticus in children. *Curr Neurol Neurosci Rep*. 2009;9:137–144.

63. Part I: Definitions. In: Gastauf H, ed. *Dictionary of Epilepsy*. Geneva, Switzerland: World Health Organization; 1973.

64. Abend NS, Dlugos DJ. Treatment of refractory status epilepticus: Literature review and proposed protocol. *Pediatr Neurol*. 2008;38:377–390.

65. Pellock JM. Use of midazolam for refractory status epilepticus in pediatric patients. *J Child Neurol*. 1998;13:581–587.

66. Igartua J, Silver P, Maytal J, Sagy M. Midazolam coma for refractory status epilepticus in children. *Crit Care Med*. 1999;27:1–10.

CASE SUMMARY 1

A 2-year-old boy presents to the ED with a history of being found asleep in the garage. His parents were unable to awaken him. He was last seen 30 minutes earlier when his mother let him out to play in the backyard. On examination, the child is somnolent but responds to deep pain. His airway is open and respirations are unlabored. Vital signs include a respiratory rate of 36/min, a heart rate of 116/min, blood pressure of 98/64 mm Hg, and temperature of 38.0°C (100.4°F). Oxygenation saturation measured by pulse oximetry is 98% on room air. Further examination reveals no focal deficits.

1. What is the most important initial intervention in this patient?
2. What are possible causes?
3. What should you include in the management and evaluation?

The initial treatment of this patient should include attention to his airway. Because he is breathing well on his own, oxygen should be provided for support to maximize oxygen delivery to the tissues. The child described in this case is of toddler age—the age of exploration. Leading causes of altered mental status at this age include infection, poisonings, and trauma. Because he was well appearing with no prodrome and no history of fever, infection becomes less likely. Because the child was found in the garage, a search for the possible toxins in that area should be undertaken. To that end, tests assessing any potential metabolic derangement and hypoglycemia are important. The vital signs in this patient are normal, the neurologic examination results are nonfocal, and the laboratory values show an elevated anion gap acidosis, thus suggesting the possibility of methanol, ethanol, or ethylene glycol. Because oxalate crystals are seen in the urine and are associated with ethylene glycol, a major ingredient found in antifreeze, poisoning by this substance is the most likely diagnosis.

CASE SUMMARY 2

A 3-month-old boy is brought to the ED by his mother, who says that he is "fussy and not acting right." He was found to be sleepy after returning from a visit to his aunt's home. He is cranky during the examination yet otherwise lethargic. The patient is afebrile with a respiratory rate of 20/min, a heart rate of 74/min, and a blood pressure of 110/70 mm Hg. His pupils are 4 mm bilaterally and sluggishly reactive. The only abnormality on examination is a small 2-cm hematoma on the occiput, which, according to his mother, was sustained in a fall from a couch.

1. *What are your concerns for this patient?*
2. *What should be done immediately?*

This patient has an unexplained hematoma on the occiput and an acute alteration in mental status. Head injury, either unintentional and unwitnessed or intentional, should be at the top of your list. The vital signs, although normal for an adult, are abnormal for an infant: the blood pressure is too high and the pulse is too low. The combination of a high blood pressure, a low pulse, and irregular respirations (Cushing triad) is a finding compatible with increased ICP. Coupled with an altered mental status, this presentation requires immediate intervention. This patient should be electively intubated, making sure not to use pharmacologic agents that raise ICP, 2 to 3 minutes after administration of intravenous lidocaine (lignocaine). Routine hyperventilation for long-term control is contraindicated, but mild hyperventilation is still recommended for acute increases in ICP. Once stabilized, a thorough secondary assessment should be performed, including a good ophthalmoscopic examination to look for retinal hemorrhages. A complete blood cell count, urinalysis, and liver function tests should be performed because occult intra-abdominal injury with resultant blood loss can accompany these injuries. A computed tomographic (CT) scan of the head without contrast will be helpful in identifying any acute or chronic intracranial bleeding.

A 3-month-old girl presents with fever, fussiness, and poor feeding. She is irritable and difficult to console but is breathing comfortably on her own and maintaining a good airway. Vital signs include a respiratory rate of 36/min, heart rate of 120/min, a blood pressure of 90/58 mm Hg, temperature of 39.2°C (102.6°F), and oxygen saturation of 98% on room air. Her fontanel appears full and her neck appears supple. Capillary refill time is 2 seconds. The results of the remainder of the examination are nonfocal.

1. *Which examination findings in this child are consistent with the diagnosis of meningitis?*
2. *What is the most important therapy to deliver at this time?*
3. *What are possible complications?*

The infant is manifesting many of the classic aspects of an acute presentation of bacterial meningitis. The patient is irritable, is highly febrile, and has a bulging fontanel. The fact that the patient has a supple neck should not dissuade the examiner from the overall impression of meningitis. Children younger than 18 months frequently lack sufficient neck musculature to manifest nuchal rigidity. Because the patient is well oxygenated and at present has stable vital signs, the most pressing intervention is the rapid delivery of intravenous antibiotics. With a gram-positive organism and morphologic findings consistent with *Streptococcus pneumoniae*, administration of cefotaxime (or ceftriaxone) and vancomycin should be started. Potential complications of meningitis include seizures, SIADH, and increased ICP.

A 13-year-old boy presents with a sudden onset of excruciating headache. He has not been ill recently, does not have a history of headaches, and has no recent history of fever or trauma. Family history is negative for migraines. Vital signs include a respiratory rate of 20/min, heart rate of 98/min, blood pressure of 106/68 mm Hg, and a temperature of 37.0°C (98.6°F). Examination reveals an uncomfortable, white, male teenager with severe headache. Neurologic examination results are nonfocal and remarkable only for terminal neck flexion tenderness. No papilledema is noted.

1. *What is the appropriate management strategy for this patient?*

Because of the excruciating headache, the boy underwent an immediate noncontrast CT. Because his examination showed terminal neck flexion tenderness, he was empirically given cefotaxime, 100 mg/kg intravenously, before the CT scan. The CT scan revealed a large subarachnoid hemorrhage. A cerebral aneurysm from the posterior aspect of the circle of Willis was detected by cerebral angiography. Neurosurgical consultation was arranged, and definitive clipping of the aneurysm was conducted.

A 2-year-old previously healthy child with a generalized clonic seizure is brought to the ED by emergency medical services. The parents estimate that he had been having a seizure for 5 minutes before arrival of the paramedics. Paramedics noted that the child was having a generalized seizure and was blue around the lips. The patient was given 100% oxygen by face mask, and a rapid assay for glucose was 80 mg/dL. Rectal diazepam was administered, and the child continues to seize on arrival in the ED.

1. What is the most important initial intervention for this patient?
2. What medications can be used to stop the seizure?
3. What are some of the possible causes of this child's seizure?

The most important intervention in a seizing child is assessment of the ABCs. This includes opening the airway, suctioning, applying 100% oxygen, and placing the child on cardiac monitors. Then, there are several drugs that can be used initially to stop the seizure, including rectal diazepam, intravenous lorazepam, or intravenous diazepam. The workup should be based on further history and physical examination. Possible causes include infection, toxins, metabolic causes (eg, hypoglycemia), trauma, or tumor.

A 26-month-old boy is brought to the ED by his parents after a generalized clonic seizure at home. The child had been previously healthy and, other than feeling a little warm before the seizure, had not been ill. The seizure lasted 5 minutes. The parents are not aware of any trauma or ingestion. The child slept on the ride to the hospital, awoke at triage, and is crying vigorously as you approach. Vital signs include a respiratory rate of 32/min, heart rate of 170/min, blood pressure of 95/65 mm Hg, and temperature of 39.8°C (103.6°F). The history reveals that the child has had no previous seizures and has a normal developmental history. Upper respiratory tract symptoms started the day of presentation. His physical examination reveals clear rhinorrhea, an erythematous pharynx without exudates, and clear lungs. He is alert and playing with toys on the bed.

1. What is the most appropriate initial intervention?
2. What is the most appropriate diagnostic evaluation at this time?
3. What is appropriate counseling for the parents?

In a child who has had a seizure but is now awake, the most important aspect is a detailed and complete history and physical examination. Because the results of these examinations are unremarkable, the most likely diagnosis for this patient is a simple febrile seizure. Diagnostic studies should be those that can provide a clue to the cause of the fever. Appropriate counseling for the parents includes instructions on what to do in the event of a recurrent seizure, explanation of the risks of recurrent seizures and epilepsy, and reassurance of the benign nature of simple febrile seizures.

chapter 6

Trauma

Stephen R. Karl, MD, NREMTP, FAAP, FACS

Objectives

1 Describe unique anatomical and physiologic characteristics of the pediatric age group that affect response to injury and management.

2 Define concepts of the primary and secondary surveys and systematically discuss patient evaluation using these tools.

3 Establish and discuss management priorities based on life-threatening injuries identified in the primary survey.

4 Discuss the identification and initial treatment of life-threatening injuries to major organ systems.

5 Review relevant issues of injury prevention.

Chapter Outline

Introduction
Pathophysiologic and Anatomical Considerations
Assessment and Management
Primary and Secondary Surveys
Central Nervous System Injuries
Cranial and Intracranial Injuries
Seizures
Extracranial Head Injuries
Spinal Injuries
Chest Injuries
Abdominal Injuries
Burns
Electrical Trauma
Other Burns
Summary

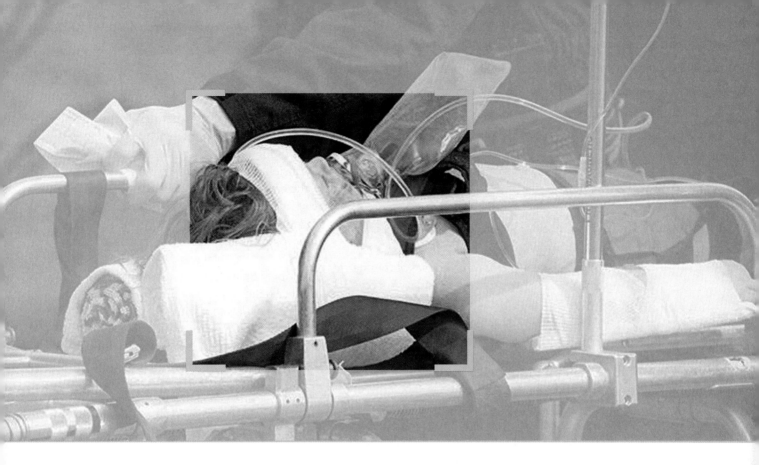

A 5-year-old boy is struck by a car while crossing the street. Paramedics find the boy unconscious and lying in the middle of the street about 5 m from the vehicle. They begin an initial assessment using the Pediatric Assessment Triangle: Appearance: unconscious, not responsive to surroundings; work of Breathing: tachypneic, with no retractions; and Circulation: pale color and delayed capillary refill time. The paramedics stabilize the cervical spine, administer 100% oxygen by face mask, obtain intravenous (IV) access in the right antecubital fossa en route to the hospital, and infuse 500 mL of normal saline (NS).

On arrival in the emergency department (ED) the patient's airway is open; there are increased secretions, and the trachea is midline. There is symmetric chest wall motion and poor tidal volume with no retractions, and breath sounds are equal. The child's color is pale and the skin is diaphoretic. There is no jugular venous distention and capillary refill time is 4 seconds. The heart rate is 160/min with a thready peripheral pulse quality. Blood pressure is 75 by palpation. The abdomen is distended and tense on palpation, and the pelvis is stable. The anal sphincter is intact and the stool is negative for occult blood. The patient remains unconscious. There is no spontaneous eye opening. He responds to painful stimuli with flexor posturing. Pupils are midposition, 4 mm bilaterally, and sluggishly reactive to light. He has a contusion on the forehead, an abrasion on the left arm with swelling at the level of the elbow, an abrasion on the left flank, and deformity on the left femur.

1. *What is the physiologic status of this child?*
2. *What are your initial management priorities?*
3. *Does this patient meet an indication for surgery?*

Introduction

Trauma remains a major threat to the children of our world and is responsible for more than half of all childhood deaths in the United States. As infectious diseases and malnutrition become more effectively prevented and treated, injury is emerging as the major cause of pediatric morbidity and mortality throughout the world.[1,2] To effectively treat an injured child, one must understand and use the basic principles of trauma care. Use of the primary and secondary surveys provides for rapid evaluation and resuscitation. The purpose of this chapter is to describe the process of initial assessment and resuscitation of the injured child. What is accomplished in the minutes and hours after injury can determine survival and quality of life. The core of the process is knowledge of injury patterns, injury recognition, intervention, evaluation of response, and continuous reassessment. Each of these critical areas will be addressed in detail.

Pathophysiologic and Anatomical Considerations

Size, age, and health status set the stage for a patient's physical and emotional response to an injury. The younger the child, the more emotional support will be needed and the less he or she will be able to help with his or her assessment. It is challenging to elicit reliable signs and symptoms from a scared and crying 3-year-old child. Children sustain multiorgan system injury more often than adults. Patience and experience on the part of the practitioner is required to avoid missing injuries.

As children grow and mature, they become more adultlike not only in size but also in anatomical and physiologic development. A child's head occupies a larger relative body surface area and mass than does the head of an adult. Not surprising, head injuries in children are extremely common and account for a great percentage of serious morbidity and mortality. More than 80% of fatalities recorded in the National Pediatric Trauma Registry (NPTR) are the result of traumatic brain injury (TBI).[3]

There are age-specific differences in epidemiology, pathology, and outcome of TBI.[4] The central nervous system of children younger than 3 years is in a state of dynamic development. The increase in head circumference during the first years of life reflects tremendous brain volume expansion. By the age of 6 months, the weight of the brain has doubled; by 2 years of age, it has reached 80% of adult weight. During this period, ongoing myelination, synapse formation, dendritic arborization, increasing neuronal plasticity, and biochemical changes take place. Injury to the developing brain can arrest these processes and produce deficits that become apparent only at a later stage of development.

The head is a major source of heat loss and contributes to the child's increased sensitivity to thermoregulatory stress. Occipital prominence decreases from birth until approximately 10 years of age and is responsible for relative neck flexion and a more anterior position of the airway in small children. The cranial sutures are open at birth and gradually fuse by 18 to 24 months of age. Palpation of the anterior and posterior fontanelles can be an important source of information. The ability of the cranial sutures to spread can also dissipate some of the adverse effects of increased intracranial pressure (ICP).

The type of injury varies with the age of the child. Child abuse is a major cause of severe head injury in infants. In some studies, 95% of all injuries that result in intracranial hemorrhage in children younger than 1 year are due to child abuse.[4] Children who are ambulatory and younger than 5 years are likely to sustain head injuries as a result of falls at home. Those older than 5 years are more likely to be involved as pedestrians or cyclists in crashes with motor vehicles. At any age, head trauma can be sustained by passengers in motor vehicle crashes.

A child's neck is shorter and supports a relatively greater mass than does the neck of an adult. Distracting forces more frequently disrupt the upper cervical vertebrae or their ligamentous attachments. Active growth centers and incomplete calcification make radiologic assessment especially challenging. Many children with cervical spinal cord injury can have no abnormality on conventional radiographs of the neck (spinal cord injury without radiographic abnormality [SCIWORA]),[5] emphasizing the importance of an accurate and thorough initial physical examination and subsequent advanced imaging when indicated. The young child has a short neck, which can make evaluation of neck veins and tracheal position difficult.

The younger the child, the more the position of the larynx is cephalad and anterior. The epiglottis is tilted nearly 45° in a child and is more floppy than that of an adolescent or adult. In an adult patient, the glottis (or the level of the true vocal cords) is the narrowest portion of the upper airway and therefore the limiting factor in tracheal tube size. In the child younger than 8 years, the cricoid cartilage is the narrowest portion of the airway and also the site of abundant loose columnar epithelium. This epithelium is more susceptible to pressure necrosis, which can stimulate exuberant scar tissue, which can lead to stenosis. The size of the tracheal tube thus becomes a critical consideration.

In children, the thorax is more pliable than in adults. The ribs are more cartilaginous and therefore more flexible. There is much less overlying muscle and fat to protect the ribs and underlying structures, so blunt force applied to the chest is more efficiently transmitted to underlying tissues, resulting in pulmonary contusion or pneumothorax. Multiple rib fractures in a child is a sign of massive force. The diaphragm inserts at a nearly horizontal angle in a newborn and maintains this angle until approximately 12 years of age. This is in contrast to the oblique insertion of the diaphragm in an adolescent or adult. Children are diaphragmatic, or belly-breathers, which means they are dependent on effective diaphragmatic excursion for adequate ventilation. In addition, the diaphragmatic muscle is much more distensible in the child. A child's mediastinum is mobile and therefore subject to sudden, wide excursions. As a result, a simple pneumothorax can become a life-threatening tension pneumothorax literally within seconds.

A child's abdomen is less well protected by overlying ribs and muscle. Viscera are more prone to injury (**Figure 6.1**). Seemingly insignificant forces can cause serious internal injury. Although the connective tissue and suspensory ligaments of the child are more elastic and can absorb more energy, the paucity of insulating fat

allows more potential motion of these organs at impact. Significant internal injury can be present despite minimal external evidence of trauma.

Bone growth in children occurs at the growth plates of the long bones. These areas and the epiphyseal-metaphyseal junction (physis, growth plate) are sites of relative weakness.

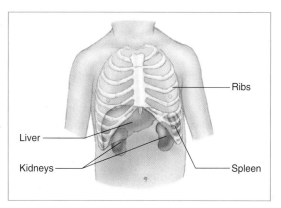

Figure 6.1 Viscera in a child's abdomen are more prone to injury because they are less well protected by overlying ribs and musculature.

In most cases, the ligamentous structures near the epiphyseal region actually are stronger than the growth plate itself; this explains the frequency of physeal and epiphyseal fractures seen in children. A separate classification system (Salter-Harris) is used to describe these injuries because of the implications of disturbances of the growth plate. In addition to the potential impact of growth plate fractures on long-term bony growth, changes in blood flow to the extremity can result in significant limb length discrepancy. Anatomical and physiologic differences between children and adults that affect trauma management are outlined in Table 6-1.

Assessment and Management

Time is critical in the assessment and treatment of the trauma patient. Use of the Pediatric Assessment Triangle gives a first look at the severity of the patient's condition. The primary survey follows with evaluation of airway, breathing, circulation, and neurologic status with treatment/resuscitation initiated as indicated. The secondary survey is the more comprehensive assessment with diagnostic testing as necessary. Reassessment continues throughout the stabilization period.

TABLE 6-1 Anatomical and Physiological Differences Between Children and Adults

Central Nervous System
- Pediatric brain is in state of dynamic development.
  - Myelin is in the process of forming.
  - Pediatric brain has more gray matter.
- Head is a source of heat loss.
- Pediatric skull has expandable sutures until 18 to 24 months of age.
- Prominent occiput causes the head to flex forward on the neck.
- Short neck makes jugular venous distention (JVD) and tracheal deviation assessment challenging.

Cervical Spine
- Neck supports greater weight, making cervical spine fractures and injury more likely in upper cervical spine.
- Cervical spine fractures are uncommon. Ligamentous injury is more common.
- Flatter joint facets and more elastic cervical ligaments lead to spinal cord injury without radiographic abnormality.

Airway
- Larynx is more anterior and cephalad.
- Cricoid is narrowest portion of the airway versus the vocal cords.
- Epiglottis is floppy and Ω-shaped.

Respiratory
- Pliable chest wall implies great force needed to break ribs and more force transmitted to lungs and other intrathoracic structures.
- Horizontal ribs and weak intercostal muscles lead to greater dependence on the diaphragm for breathing.
- Mobile mediastinum can result in rapid transition from pneumothorax to tension pneumothorax.

Abdominal
- Anterior placement of intra-abdominal organs and less subcutaneous fat make them more susceptible to injury.

Skeletal
- Long bones with growth plates that fracture can result in extremity length discrepancies.

Aggressive management of the airway and breathing is the foundation of pediatric trauma resuscitation. Brain injury is the main driver of mortality and morbidity in childhood as reflected by NPTR data. Effective initial management of TBI mandates airway control to support precise ventilation and adequate oxygenation. Only 6% of 92,000 patients registered in the NPTR initially presented with a systolic blood pressure less than 90 mm Hg. Mortality in this group was 18% and represented 42% of all children who died of their injuries. Severe shock must be aggressively treated with rapid intubation and ventilatory control, rapid resuscitation with isotonic crystalloid, and restoration of red cell mass to deliver adequate tissue oxygenation. Children in comas without shock need identical airway control and confirmation that volume resuscitation and red cell mass are adequate to support neuronal oxygenation.

Evaluation of the pediatric trauma patient begins with the same initial assessment of the child presented in Chapter 2, Pediatric Assessment. It includes all of the elements of the Pediatric Assessment Triangle (**Figure 6.2A** and **Figure 6.2B**):

- Appearance (mental status and muscle tone) suggests the level of consciousness.
- Work of breathing (increased, labored, or decreased) indicates the adequacy of ventilation and oxygenation.
- Circulation (skin and mucous membrane color) reflects the adequacy of oxygenation and perfusion.

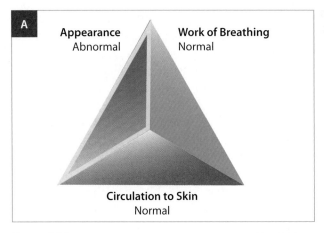

Figure 6.2A Pediatric Assessment Triangle in isolated head injury.

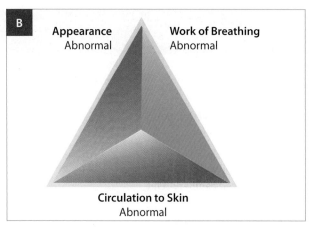

Figure 6.2B Pediatric Assessment Triangle in multisystem injury.

Beware that immediate evidence of circulatory abnormalities is not always present in hemodynamic instability and/or multisystem injury.[6]

Primary and Secondary Surveys

The primary survey and initial resuscitation usually require the first 5 to 10 minutes and focus on treating immediate threats to life. The secondary survey continues and broadens the scope of treatment based on a more thorough physical examination and appropriate diagnostic testing. Ideally, this phase should be completed within the first hour so definitive care and/or safe transport can begin. Life-threatening conditions must be recognized promptly and addressed before treatment of less threatening problems. The sequence for evaluation is always the same. If sufficient expert personnel are available for assistance, many of these tasks can be done simultaneously.

The primary survey consists of an initial assessment of the status of the patient's airway, oxygenation, ventilation, circulation, and overall neurologic status. Primarily, it is a physiologic survey of the patient's vital systems. It is not uncommon to encounter serious physiologic alterations during the primary survey, necessitating interruption of the survey to perform resuscitative care.

In contrast, the secondary survey (focused history and detailed physical examination) is a timely, directed evaluation of each body area, usually performed in a head-to-toe manner. The secondary survey is an anatomical survey in which the physician attempts to define the presence, type, and severity of injury to each anatomical area. The secondary survey essentially begins the child's definitive care. It is important to understand that children with multiple injuries require continual reassessment. The secondary survey must be performed while continuing to reevaluate all of the elements of the primary survey and the effects of initial interventions. Vital signs must be reevaluated continually on all seriously injured pediatric patients, at least every 5 minutes during the primary survey and every 15 minutes during the remainder of the evaluation.

Primary Survey

The steps in the primary survey include assessment of the following:

- Airway, with cervical spine stabilization
- Breathing and emergency treatment of immediately life-threatening chest injuries
- Circulation, with external control of hemorrhage and fluid resuscitation
- Disability (neurologic screening examination)
- Exposure and thorough examination

The most important goals during the primary survey and resuscitative phase should be accomplished within 5 to 10 minutes (Table 6-2).

TABLE 6-2 Goals of the Primary Survey and Resuscitative Phase

Assessment

Airway
- Obstruction

Breathing and ventilation
- Decreased rate
- Decreased breath sounds
- Decreased excursion
- Decreased capillary refill

Circulation
- Neck vein distention
- Distant heart sounds
- Tachycardia
- Hemorrhage

Therapy

Airway
- Relief of obstruction with jaw thrust
- Use of oral or nasopharyngeal airway
- Endotracheal intubation
- Needle cricothyrotomy

Ventilation
- Administration of 100% oxygen
- Treatment of apnea with ventilation/intubation
- Stabilization of flail thorax with positive pressure ventilation
- Aspiration of tension pneumothorax
- Nasogastric tube placement to relieve gastric dilatation
- Chest tube insertion for hemothorax/pneumothorax

Circulation
- Pressure to control hemorrhage
- Two large-bore (14- to 18-gauge) intravenous catheters
- Intraosseous infusion if needed
- Normal saline or lactated Ringer's solution at 20 mL/kg for volume replacement
- Relief of pericardial tamponade
- Thoracotomy when indicated (rare)

Airway and Cervical Spine

The first step in the primary survey is to ensure that the patient's airway is patent and ventilation is adequate. A variety of maneuvers from suctioning to endotracheal intubation or needle cricothyrotomy (also known as cricothyroidotomy) might be needed. Until cervical spine injury is excluded, the cervical spine must be protected, especially during airway manipulation. Adequate stabilization can be accomplished with gentle but firm manual support until a cervical immobilization device or semirigid collar can be provided. Lateral cervical spine radiographs are obtained as rapidly as feasible but must not be permitted to delay or interfere with emergency airway management or rapid assessment and management of shock. Even in cases in which the initial cervical radiography results are normal, stabilization must be maintained if neurologic injury is suspected on the basis of the history or physical examination. Some children with cervical spinal cord injury have symptoms of transient paresthesia, numbness, or paralysis, with no radiographic abnormality. This can occur in any child with a significant injury above the level of the clavicles. Cervical spine precautions may be discontinued only if three views of the cervical spine are normal; the child is awake, reliable, and asymptomatic; and if there is no evidence or history of a neurologic abnormality.

Airway

To open the airway of a child who does not have a suspected neck or spine injury, the head is placed in the sniffing position, with the neck slightly flexed on the chest and the head slightly extended on the neck (**Figure 6.3**). This position is easily accomplished by placing a folded towel or the rescuer's hand under the child's neck. To open the airway of a child with a possible neck or spine injury, the head is placed in the neutral position, with cervical spine elements fully aligned, using bimanual cervical spine stabilization. In infants and young children, the prominence of the occipital region can force the neck into slight flexion when the patient is placed supine, and it might be necessary to place a 1- to 3-cm layer of padding beneath the torso. Maintain cervical spine stabilization during any airway maneuvers if cervical injury or neurologic abnormality has not been ruled out, and immobilize the neck with an extrication collar once the airway is controlled. The mandible is relaxed in the unconscious patient. Posterior displacement of the tongue will produce airway obstruction. This is treated with the jaw-thrust maneuver, which is accomplished by placing hands at the angles of the mandible and applying gentle forward pressure. Remove any foreign matter present in the airway quickly with gentle suction. Neonates are preferential nasal breathers, so relieve nasal obstruction quickly through gentle suction to allow spontaneous ventilation.

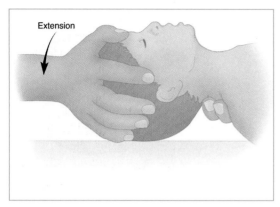

Figure 6.3 Head positioning in the pediatric patient with trauma. The "sniffing position" is optimal, but spine stabilization must be maintained with all airway maneuvers.

Endotracheal Intubation

Indications for endotracheal intubation in the trauma patient are as follows:

- Inability to ventilate the child using bag-mask ventilation
- Need for prolonged control of the airway, including prevention of aspiration in a comatose child
- Need for controlled ventilation in a patient with a serious head injury
- Flail chest
- Shock unresponsive to volume infusion

When intubation is necessary, proper preparation is a requirement. The critical first step is preoxygenation with 100% oxygen. Gentle suction will usually clear the oropharynx of secretions and foreign matter. Unless contraindicated, emergency intubation of the child should always be accomplished using the oral approach. The acute angle of the posterior nasopharynx, the anterior and cephalad position of the larynx, necessity for additional tube manipulation, and probability of causing or increasing pharyngeal bleeding due to prominent adenoids/tonsils make nasotracheal intubation unacceptably hazardous in trauma situations. Oral endotracheal intubation in the pediatric trauma patient begins by maintaining inline stabilization of the cervical spine with the head and neck in a neutral position. A complete review of the procedure can be found in Online Chapter 26, Critical Procedures.

If airway obstruction prevents adequate ventilation, there might be a direct injury to the larynx or trachea. In this unusual circumstance or in any situation in which effective ventilation is impossible, the preferred method for airway control is needle cricothyrotomy. A 14-gauge over-the-needle catheter placed through the cricothyroid membrane and high flow or jet oxygen flow of 15 L/min can provide 30 to 40 minutes of temporary oxygenation (**Figure 6.4**).

Breathing and Emergency Treatment of Immediate Life-Threatening Chest Injuries

The signs and symptoms of potentially serious airway and chest injury can be subtle, and children can deteriorate rapidly after injury. Administer supplemental oxygen to all major trauma pediatric patients in the initial stages of care, even if they have no apparent airway or breathing difficulty. Supplemental oxygen given via face mask at a flow rate of 12 to 15 L/min is well tolerated by most children.

In assessing the adequacy of the pediatric airway, remember the adage, "Look, listen, and feel." Once the airway has been opened, look at both sides of the thorax to determine whether there is symmetric chest wall rise. Children have small tidal volumes, and chest wall movement can be subtle. Carefully note suprasternal, intercostal, or subcostal retractions that can indicate increased work of breathing and respiratory distress. After tracheal tube insertion, listen for breath sounds on both sides of the chest (**Figure 6.5**). Breath sounds can be transmitted easily through the chest wall and adjacent structures in small children, and it is dangerous to rely solely on breath sounds to determine adequacy of ventilation. Use an end-tidal carbon dioxide monitor and confirm tracheal tube position with a chest radiograph.

In addition to assessing the adequacy of bilateral chest wall movement, it is important to confirm that the patient's respiratory rate is sufficient to provide oxygenation and ventilation. Any child who is hypoxic on room air (arterial oxygen saturation <90%) or tachypneic needs additional respiratory support and careful evaluation for injury. A child in respiratory distress with unilateral absent breath sounds and tracheal deviation should be suspected of

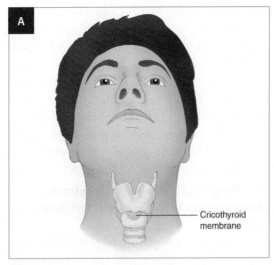
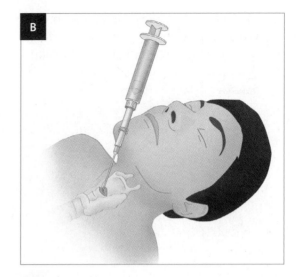
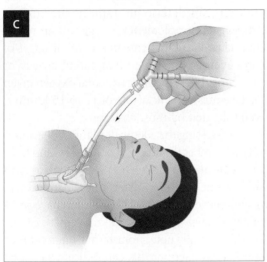
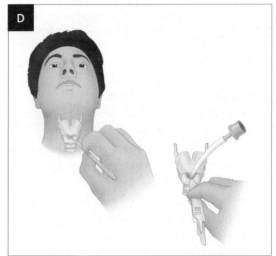

Figure 6.4 A. Locate the cricothyroid membrane. B. Puncture the cricothyroid membrane with an over-the-needle catheter or commercially available cricothyrotomy device. C. Pass the catheter into the membrane and remove the needle. Attach a Y-connector for instillation of oxygenation. D. Surgical cricothyrotomy can be performed and an endotracheal tube placed to keep the airway open.

having a tension pneumothorax. Signs of poor perfusion are often present as the mediastinal structures are shifted to the opposite side due to the expanding pneumothorax.

Needle thoracostomy using a 14-gauge angiocatheter, followed immediately by tube thoracostomy (20 to 30 Fr, depending on patient size), can be lifesaving and is indicated without a preliminary chest radiograph (**Figure 6.6**). The unstable child with an open pneumothorax should have an impermeable dressing with three sides occluded placed directly over the wound (**Figure 6.7**). Cardiac tamponade is associated with penetrating trauma to the parasternal area. Signs of cardiac tamponade include hypotension, distended neck veins, and muffled heart sounds.

Children suspected of having cardiac tamponade should undergo immediate pericardiocentesis. A child with a penetrating injury to the chest who develops cardiac arrest on arrival or during resuscitation might benefit from an emergency thoracotomy if an appropriately trained and credentialed physician is present. See Online Chapter 26, Critical Procedures, for an outline of how to perform needle and tube thoracostomy, ED thoracotomy, and pericardiocentesis.

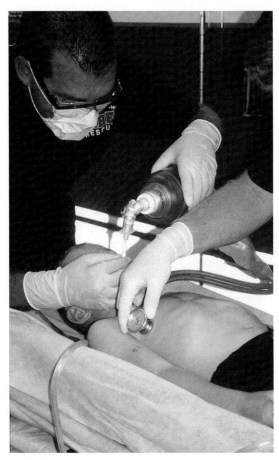

Figure 6.5 After tracheal tube insertion, listen for breath sounds on both sides of the chest.

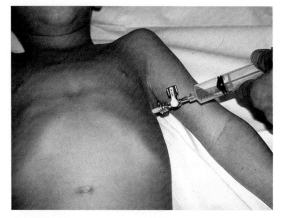

Figure 6.6 Needle thoracostomy can be performed before a chest radiograph to treat suspected tension pneumothorax.

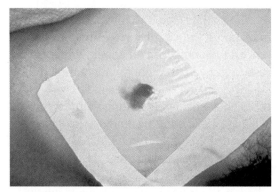

Figure 6.7 Cover chest wounds with an occlusive dressing taped on three sides.

Circulation

During the primary survey, the major goals of circulatory assessment and treatment are as follows:

- Assessment of the overall circulatory status of the injured patient
- Diagnosis and control of both external and internal hemorrhage
- Immediate intervention to provide appropriate vascular access and circulatory support

Circulatory assessment should include evaluation of the 3 Ps. Circulatory efficiency is directly dependent on the performance of the myocardium (pump), the integrity of the vascular system (pipes), and the sufficiency of circulating volume (prime). The most common threats to the pump are ischemia from hypovolemia, hypoxia, or direct contusion. Disruption of the pipes can be catastrophic, which usually leads to exsanguination or subtle, subclinical ooze from

a broken bone or damaged abdominal organ(s). It is the latter that is most common. This ongoing gradual loss of blood, if replaced with only crystalloid solutions, will result in hemodilution, decreased oxygen carrying capacity, and

YOUR FIRST CLUE

Signs and Symptoms of a Tension Pneumothorax

- Respiratory distress
- Unilateral decreased or absent breath sounds
- Tracheal deviation
- Signs of poor perfusion (late)

inadequate tissue oxygenation. Both the quality and quantity of the prime must be ensured.

Crystalloid bolus is an essential first step in restoring lost circulatory volume. In the absence of decompensated shock, which is the case in most injured children, continued fluid management must represent a judicious balance between adequate circulating volume and red cell mass while avoiding fluid overload by inappropriate volumes of crystalloid. It is during the initial resuscitation phase that this issue should be first considered. The recurring question is whether the intravascular volume is adequate and, if not, should the patient be given isotonic crystalloid, hypertonic saline, or blood?[7] Management of brain injury is much more effective if the first 48 hours are not complicated by inadequate fluid resuscitation or by the need to diurese excessive fluid from the cerebral and pulmonary interstitium.

Palpation of the pulse for quality (ie, weak or strong), rate, and regularity remains a reliable initial clinical assessment tool. Capillary refill in and of itself is not a reliable indicator of perfusion, but when combined with heart rate and pulse quality can be a valuable adjunct in the detection of hypoperfusion.[7] Capillary refill time should be less than 2 seconds and is generally assessed by gentle compression of the nailbeds or skin over the sternum in younger children.

Tachycardia is one of the first signs of hypovolemia and is a compensatory mechanism by the body to respond to a decrease of circulating blood volume. Pain and anxiety can also cause tachycardia; however, it will be more prolonged in children without adequate resuscitation. With continued hemorrhage, hypotension will eventually occur when compensatory mechanisms fail, followed by bradycardia and finally cardiopulmonary arrest. The younger the child, the more fixed is the stroke volume and the more dependent is cardiac output on heart rate. Be familiar with the usual heart rates for children by age (Table 6-3). A weak and thready pulse is an indication of cardiovascular instability and impending cardiovascular collapse.

The assessment of perfusion is the basis for the early diagnosis and recognition of shock. Inadequate tissue perfusion (shock) can be recognized by an altered level of consciousness or decreased urine output. Central nervous system injuries are common in children and can cloud the assessment of perfusion. Urine output is an accurate measure of renal perfusion, but it is of little benefit in the very early phases of patient assessment.

TABLE 6-3 Usual Ranges for Awake Heart Rate and Blood Pressure for Children

Age	Heart Rate/min	Blood Pressure, mm HG
Neonate	100–160	60–80 by palpation
1 y	100–130	80/40–105/70
5 y	80–110	80/50–110/80
10 y	70–100	90/55–130/85
15 y	60–80	95/60–140/90
Adult	60–80	100/60–140/90

Vascular Access

While circulatory status is being assessed, reliable vascular access must be established. The choices for vascular access include the following:

- Percutaneous peripheral venous cannulation with large-bore lines placed at one or two sites
- Intraosseous infusion
- Percutaneous ultrasonography-guided cannulation of peripheral or central veins

Peripheral venous cutdowns are slow and destroy whole venous beds. They have all but disappeared, replaced by intraosseous access. Never waste time attempting IV access in a clinically critically ill patient; go directly to intraosseous access (see Online Chapter 26, Critical Procedures for intraosseous and cut-down techniques). Newer intraosseous systems have improved successful placement while decreasing pain and time of insertion. The anterior tibial marrow can be accessed quickly and used as an infusion site for fluids and medications (**Figure 6.8**). Complications are rare and usually involve subcutaneous infiltration of fluid or leakage from the puncture site after the needle has been removed. More serious complications, such as compartment syndrome, tibial fracture, osteomyelitis, and subcutaneous infections, have been reported. However, these occur mainly when the intraosseous infusion is maintained for extended periods (>24 hours), hypertonic fluids are infused, or evidence of limb edema is ignored. Intraosseous infusion must never be used in a fractured extremity. Whenever this means of access is used, it is to be regarded as a temporizing measure while attempts at direct vascular access are continued.

Ultrasound imaging devices have become much more common in the acute care setting. Some are specifically designed to identify arterial and venous structures. They greatly improve the safety, success, and speed of cannulation of peripheral and central veins. Many patients with multiple injuries will eventually need central venous catheterization using the Seldinger technique. If this is to be done during the initial resuscitation phase, the femoral approach is preferred unless major intra-abdominal injuries are suspected.

Hemorrhage Control

Blood loss (hemorrhage) can be external and/or internal. The whole body must be inspected for signs of both. Meaningful information about blood loss at the scene and what maneuvers were used to control the bleeding should be obtained from family and emergency medical services personnel. Any laceration can result in significant bleeding, but scalp and facial wounds are particularly prone to profuse hemorrhage. Begin measures to decrease external bleeding by applying direct pressure over bleeding sites with sterile dressings (**Figure 6.9**). Once pressure has been applied, maintain it with either manual pressure or pressure dressings. Ensure that pressure dressings do not occlude distal pulses. Elevate the bleeding areas to decrease the amount of blood

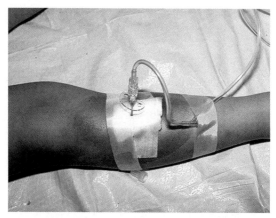

Figure 6.8 Intraosseous needle in the anterior tibia for rapid vascular access.

loss if feasible. In most cases, the combination of direct pressure and elevation will arrest external hemorrhage. If direct pressure does not control extremity bleeding, then use of a tourniquet should be considered.[7] A blood pressure cuff or a military-style tourniquet should be used to decrease bleeding from the underlying tissue. The limb distal to the tourniquet will be ischemic and lactic acid and other metabolic byproducts will build up. Once applied, the tourniquet should not be let down until the patient is stable and a team is available to control the bleeding directly.

In virtually every area of the body except the scalp, major nerves are in proximity to major blood vessels. Blind clamping of vessels can therefore result in peripheral nerve damage. Hemostats should only be used to clamp spurting vessels on the hair-bearing areas of the scalp.

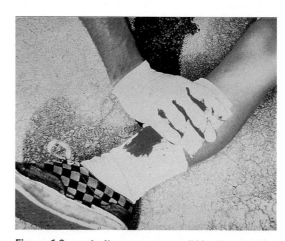

Figure 6.9 Apply direct pressure on all bleeding wounds.

Recognition of internal bleeding requires astute observation, a thorough physical examination, and attention to the subtle changes that sometimes occur with major internal hemorrhage. Life-threatening internal hemorrhage can occur in five body areas: chest, abdomen, retroperitoneum, pelvis, and thigh. Be alert to pain or swelling in any of these areas because this might be the first objective indication of internal hemorrhage. Intracranial bleeding in newborns and very young infants can also result in shock.

Shock and Circulatory Failure

During the initial phase of care of the trauma patient, shock is nearly always hypovolemic in nature. Other causes of shock include cardiac tamponade, tension pneumothorax, and spinal cord injury. Rapid hemorrhage, in contrast to catastrophic exsanguination, proceeds along a predictable course that begins with tachycardia, progresses to clinical signs of sluggish peripheral circulation with decreasing pulse pressure, and evolves into deepening obtundation. The high incidence of TBI in children confuses the last of these findings because this can be a primary cause of decreased level of consciousness. Regardless of the presence of potential brain injury, any child who is tachycardic and has a decreasing systolic pressure and poor peripheral perfusion has lost at least 25% of normal blood volume. This child needs immediate restoration of circulating volume with isotonic crystalloid and

possibly transfusion of packed red blood cells (PRBCs). When blood loss exceeds 25% to 30% of total blood volume, compensatory vasoconstriction can abruptly and catastrophically fail. Hypotension, confusion, decreased urine output, and acidosis can emerge rapidly. At this point, irreversible vascular collapse can be imminent.

Patients with hypotension might have lost 25% or more of their total blood volume and probably have injuries that will cause these losses to continue. They usually require multiple boluses of fluid. Although these boluses can transiently restore circulating volume, they dilute red blood cell concentration and soon undermine rather than improve oxygen delivery. When more than two crystalloid boluses are required, immediate blood transfusion therapy is usually necessary.

Volume Replacement

Normal saline (NS) or lactated Ringer's (LR) solution is the fluid of choice for initial resuscitation of the pediatric trauma patient. In the face of evolving cerebral edema, excess free water is to be avoided. Fluid replacement is divided into two phases: initial therapy and total replacement. When necessary, fluids are administered rapidly via IV push with a 60-mL syringe or a pressure infusion bag so larger volumes of fluid can be administered in as short a period as possible. Vital signs are evaluated carefully before and after bolus therapy. If vital signs do not improve immediately, more volume is given.

The following guidelines are only for initiation of therapy. If a child does not respond appropriately, suspect internal hemorrhage and look for other causes of refractory shock. Typically, approximately 3 mL of crystalloid replacement will be required to replace each milliliter of shed blood. Bolus infusion of 20 mL/kg (NS or LR solution) should be initiated for all patients who have sustained significant trauma or have signs of compensated or decompensated shock. If the initial bolus produces no improvement, it should be immediately repeated with another 20 mL/kg. If there is still no improvement, PRBCs should be immediately transfused and urgent surgical intervention considered.

If crystalloid bolus produces a sustained improvement in pressure and perfusion, NS or LR solution should be infused at 5 mL/kg per hour for several hours. If the child remains stable, the IV infusion rate should be adjusted to maintenance levels listed below, and NS or LR solution can be replaced by standard fluid maintenance solutions. Below are listed maintenance fluid volume requirements by weight.

- weight = 10 kg: 100 mL/kg per 24 hours
- weight = 10 kg: to 20 kg: 1,000 mL plus 50 mL/kg above 10 kg per 24 hours
- weight = >20 kg: 1,500 mL plus 20 mL/kg above 20 kg per 24 hours

There is growing interest in the use of hypertonic saline for resuscitation, especially in the patient with a TBI. The administration of hypertonic saline raises the serum osmolality and draws water from the interstitial and intracellular spaces, supporting intravascular volume and perfusion while reducing brain swelling. Infusion rates from 0.1 to 1.0 mL/kg per hour of 3% sodium chloride solution are delivered centrally to avoid venous injury. The target is a serum sodium level of 145 to 155 mEq/L. This approach appears to be safe, but there are no definitive trials in children that show it to be superior.[7]

Monitoring Fluid Resuscitation

It is critical to assess and record accurately the initial indicators of circulatory status (pulse, respirations, blood pressure, pulse pressure, and mental status). Follow these findings closely to track response to intervention.

Pneumatic Antishock Garment

The pneumatic antishock garment is no longer recommended for the treatment of shock. It might have some benefit in patients with unstable pelvic and lower extremity fractures; however, it might be no more effective than a properly applied external pelvic compression wrap.

Disability

Glasgow Coma Scale

The Glasgow Coma Scale (GCS) score is useful for the neurologic assessment of a trauma patient and also has predictive value for outcome. It involves an assessment of three components of neurologic function: eye opening, motor response, and verbal response. It can be used to assess both verbal and nonverbal children. Age-related modifications are listed in Table 6-4.

AVPU

A rapid neurologic evaluation is part of the primary survey. This neurologic evaluation should include assessment of only pupillary response, patient's level of consciousness, and any localizing finding, such as paralysis or paresis of an extremity. A simple method for evaluating level of consciousness involves the mnemonic AVPU:

A: Alert
V: Responds to verbal stimuli
P: Responds to painful stimuli
U: Unresponsive

A more in-depth neurologic assessment should be performed during the secondary survey.

Exposure and Examination

The child's clothing must be removed completely to allow full assessment of injury and a complete examination. A small child can develop hypothermia quickly after exposure. A radiant warmer, warming blanket, or air convection unit might be required to maintain the child's temperature at 36° to 37°C (96.8° to 98.6°F). This part of the primary survey should include the log roll to examine the back and spine, assessment of the perineum for signs of injury, and a rectal examination to assess rectal tone and the presence of blood in the rectal vault. If there is suspected urethral injury, as is often associated with a pelvic fracture, or blood at the meatus, complete integrity of the urethra must be confirmed by urethrogram before a bladder catheter is placed. If there are no signs of urethral injury, an indwelling urinary catheter should be placed on any moderately to severely injured trauma patient to assess for hematuria and to monitor urine output. Urine present in the bladder at the time of the insertion usually was produced before injury and does not reflect current output.

A nasogastric tube (or orogastric tube if there is evidence of a midfacial or basilar skull fracture) should be placed in every child with multiple injuries whose level of consciousness precludes accurate evaluation. For practical purposes this includes children with a GCS score less than or equal to 9. Children with signs and symptoms of TBI who are obtunded but not comatose will often become severely agitated when any invasive maneuver is attempted.

TABLE 6-4 Pediatric Glasgow Coma Scale

Modified Glasgow Coma Scale

Child	Infant
EYES:	
4 Opens eyes spontaneously	Opens eyes spontaneously
3 Opens eyes to speech	Opens eyes to speech
2 Opens eyes to pain	Opens eyes to pain
1 NO RESPONSE	NO RESPONSE
_____ = Score (Eyes)	
MOTOR:	
6 Obeys commands	Spontaneous movements
5 Localizes	Withdraws to touch
4 Withdraws	Withdraws to pain
3 Flexion	Flexion (decorticate)
2 Extension	Extension (decerebrate)
1 NO RESPONSE	NO RESPONSE
_____ = Score (Motor)	
VERBAL:	
5 Oriented	Coos and babbles
4 Confused	Irritable cry
3 Inappropriate words	Cries to pain
2 Incomprehensible words	Moans to pain
1 NO RESPONSE	NO RESPONSE
_____ = Score (Verbal)	
_____ = Total Score (Eyes, Motor, Verbal) will range from 3 to 15	

James HE, Anas NG, Perkin RM. *Brain Insults in Infants and Children.* Orlando, FL: Grune & Stratton; 1985. Reprinted with permission.

In these patients, the benefit of relevant information or therapeutic effect must be balanced against the risk of additional injury from avoidable agitation. Similar clinical judgment should guide timing of insertion of a urinary catheter.

Secondary Survey

The secondary survey is a more comprehensive evaluation of each body area proceeding from head to toe. It should answer the following questions:

- Is an injury present in the anatomical area under evaluation?
- If so, what type of injury is present, and which organ is injured?
- What is the anatomical and physiologic derangement of each organ?
- What is the appropriate definitive care for the injury?
- What is the priority of therapy for this injury compared with other injuries identified in the secondary survey?

The components of the secondary survey are:

- History (SAMPLE)
- Complete examination

Critical Steps in the Treatment of the Pediatric Trauma Patient

Primary Survey

- Airway: open with jaw thrust; suction; intubate if respiratory failure or decompensated shock.

- Breathing: add supplemental oxygen; assist ventilation if respiratory failure; perform needle or tube thoracostomy for pneumothorax.

- Circulation: compress and elevate external bleeding sites; obtain vascular access (peripheral, central, intraosseous); resuscitate with 20 mL/kg of NS or LR solution; begin PRBC transfusion if more than 40 mL/kg of crystalloid is needed to maintain perfusion.

- Disability: assess level of consciousness, pupillary response, and motor response; calculate GCS score.

- Exposure: remove clothing; keep infant or child warm.

- Laboratory studies
- Radiographic studies
- Problem identification

During this phase, complete the history and perform a thorough physical examination. Pay attention to the adequacy of cervical stabilization obtained during the primary survey and continue aggressive resuscitation.

History Taking

The history is actually best obtained from the emergency medical technician who transported the patient unless key witnesses are available. In most states, the emergency medical technician is required to leave a run sheet, which becomes a permanent part of the hospital record. This document should contain event history and details of how the patient was found and his/her initial physiologic status. The history should include the mechanism of injury, time, status at the scene, changes in status, and patient concerns. Obtain a focused history using the mnemonic SAMPLE:

S: Signs and symptoms (What hurts?)
A: Allergies
M: Medications
P: Past illnesses
L: Last meal
E: Events preceding the injury (What happened?)

The child's parents can be useful not only for the history but also in assessment of the child's interactions with them. Check whether immunizations are up to date.

Physical Examination

Head

Begin the secondary survey with an evaluation of the eyes, including conjunctiva, pupillary size and reaction, retinal appearance, and vision, if possible. Examine the face for evidence of maxillofacial trauma by palpating bony prominences. Check the teeth for injury, loss, and alignment. Examine the scalp carefully for lacerations or underlying soft tissue injury. Suspect basilar skull fracture if Battle sign or raccoon eyes are seen or if hemotympanum, cerebrospinal fluid (CSF) rhinorrhea, or otorrhea is present. Check for symmetric voluntary movement and neurologic function of the facial muscles.

Neck

Examine the neck for subcutaneous emphysema, abnormal tracheal position, hematoma, or localized pain. Palpate the cervical spine for step-offs, swelling, or tenderness. Neck vein distention also should be assessed.

Chest

Reevaluate the chest visually for adequacy of respiratory excursion, asymmetry of chest wall motion, or the presence of a flail segment. After observation, carefully palpate the chest for tenderness or crepitus and auscultate the lung fields and heart sounds.

Abdomen

Examine the abdomen next. It is important to remember that specific diagnoses usually are not immediately obvious. Examination of the abdomen includes inspection for ease of movement with respiration, bruises, seatbelt marks, tire marks, and lacerations; auscultation of bowel sounds; and gentle palpation for localized findings. Observe and palpate the flanks. The abdomen might need to be examined several times to make an accurate assessment.

Pelvis

Compress the pelvis bilaterally to evaluate for tenderness or instability. If stable, palpate bony prominences of the pelvis to assess for tenderness. Carefully examine the perineum for laceration, hematoma, or active bleeding. Check the urethral meatus for blood.

Rectum

A rectal examination is necessary if not already completed; evaluate the integrity of the wall, displacement or distortion of the prostate, sphincter muscle tone, and occult gastrointestinal hemorrhage.

Extremities

Examine the extremities for signs of fracture, dislocation, abrasion, contusion, or hematoma formation. Note preferred limb positions and bony instability. Assess pulses, perfusion, sensation, and motor function.

Back

Examination of the back should not be neglected. With the neck immobilized, if spinal injury or paralysis has not been excluded, gently roll the patient to examine the entire back and spine.

Skin

Examine thoroughly for evidence of contusions, burns, and petechiae, as in traumatic asphyxia.

Neurologic

Perform an in-depth neurologic examination, including motor, sensory, and cranial nerves, as well as level of consciousness. Examine the fundi. Check the nose again for CSF rhinorrhea.

Diagnostic Studies

For the child with severe injury and an uncertain circulatory status, the first laboratory study should be a type and cross-match of blood for possible transfusion. If immediate transfusion is necessary, O negative blood should be infused. Do not exacerbate injury severity and physiologic stress in the bleeding child by delaying transfusion until cross-matched blood is available. Laboratory assessment of any injured child is highly individualized and driven by clinical judgment, suspected injuries, and anticipated critical care therapy. At a minimum, assessment of hematocrit or hemoglobin, white blood cell count, glucose, and urinalysis are needed. Serial determinations can be helpful in the seriously injured child. Coagulation studies should be sent when possible. Trauma-induced coagulopathy might be the result of consumption and dilution of clotting factors.

For any critically ill trauma patient, obtaining a rapid chest and anterior-posterior pelvic films is a priority to assess for injuries that result in blood loss. A cervical spine radiographic series is required if a neck injury is suspected or if the child cannot be fully evaluated clinically. This can be delayed in the critical patient. Other radiographs are obtained as directed by physical findings and history. More sophisticated studies for severely injured children usually include computed tomography (CT) of the head, abdomen with IV contrast, and often the cervical spine.

Continuously monitor and frequently reevaluate the patient. A high index of suspicion and constant vigilance for signs of deterioration or the development of new problems will allow early diagnosis and management of ongoing pathophysiologic complications. Remember the mnemonic (I Vote For Idiots) for Initial or primary survey, Vital signs, Focused examination of injuries, and evaluation of Interventions performed.

It is important that those involved with emergency treatment of seriously injured children understand the principles of care and priorities of treatment in multiple trauma. The person who performs the initial evaluation and stabilization should retain full responsibility for therapy until direction of the child's total care is accepted by another qualified practitioner. One physician with appropriate credentials and experience must serve as the trauma team leader. This is especially critical for coordination of consultative support, implementation of therapy, and assurance that the transition from initial assessment to definitive therapy is a seamless continuum of communication and care. One of the most common problems identified by performance improvement screening is inadequate, inaccurate, or missing documentation of critical information. Initial assessment and all resuscitation procedures must be immediately and completely recorded. Such records are essential in monitoring improvement or deterioration. Avoid this problem by planning the assignment of recordkeeping to experienced personnel.

Critical Signs and Symptoms in the Pediatric Trauma Patient

- Tension pneumothorax: tachypnea, hypoxemia, hypotension, with or without JVD, with or without absent breath sounds
- Pericardial tamponade: tachypnea, hypoxemia, hypotension, with or without JVD, muffled heart sounds
- Shock:
  - Compensated: decreased peripheral pulses, tachycardia, cool extremities, normal or increased blood pressure
  - Decompensated: absent peripheral pulses, tachycardia or bradycardia, delayed capillary refill, hypotension
- Basilar skull fracture: Battle sign, raccoon eyes, hemotympanum, CSF otorrhea, or rhinorrhea
- Increased ICP: headache, vomiting, altered level of consciousness, bulging fontanel (infant), pupillary dilation, cranial nerve deficit, seizure, abnormal posturing, respiratory irregularity, bradycardia
- Spinal injury: altered level of consciousness, abnormal neuromotor or neurosensory examination, report of neurologic abnormality at any time after injury, neck or back tenderness, crepitus or pain on palpation or movement, limitation of neck or back motion, or unexplained hypotension
- Neurogenic shock: hypotension with warm, flushed skin, and spinal shock (decreased deep tendon reflexes, decreased sensory level, flaccid sphincters, and hypotonia)
- Traumatic asphyxia: petechiae of the head and neck, subconjunctival hemorrhages, and, occasionally, depressed level of consciousness

Central Nervous System Injuries

The goal of emergency care of TBI is the prevention of secondary cerebral insults. Bruce et al[8] demonstrated that children have an exaggerated cerebrovascular response to injury compared with adults. Hence, children are more prone to develop diffuse brain swelling, putting them at risk for intracranial hypertension. Brain insults can occur at the time of impact due to damage sustained as a result of direct trauma to the skull and intracranial structures. These injuries include scalp lacerations and skull fractures, as well as traumatic neuronal and vascular injuries. Primary injuries sustained at the time of impact are rarely influenced by therapeutic interventions; however, secondary brain injury can occur as a result of the ongoing pathophysiologic derangements, principally hypoxia and ischemia. Failure to recognize and treat respiratory failure and shock can further exacerbate brain injury.[9] Overzealous hydration can also contribute to cerebral swelling (**Figure 6.10**). Increased ICP and decreased cerebral perfusion pressure (CPP) result in secondary brain injury. Maintenance of adequate CPP relies on maintenance of an adequate blood pressure with appropriate volume expansion and inotropic support when necessary, as well as maneuvers to maintain ICP within acceptable limits.

Determinants of CPP

Cerebral perfusion pressure is calculated as the mean arterial pressure minus ICP. Increased ICP is the most common cause of decreased CPP in the head-injured child older than 1 year. This occurs because of the fixed volume of the cranial vault and relative low compliance of the intracranial contents. The intracranial cavity has three components: CSF, brain, and cerebral blood.

Intracranial volume is represented by the following formula:

Intracranial Volume = CSF Volume + Blood Volume + Brain Volume

Under normal circumstances, the intracranial volume is maintained relatively constant because of compensatory adjustments in these three components. ICP is kept relatively constant (<15 mm Hg) and fluctuates minimally with the Valsalva maneuver, respiration, pulse, and position. Once the compliance of the intracranial vault is exceeded, however, small changes in volume can cause massive increases in ICP (**Figure 6.11**).

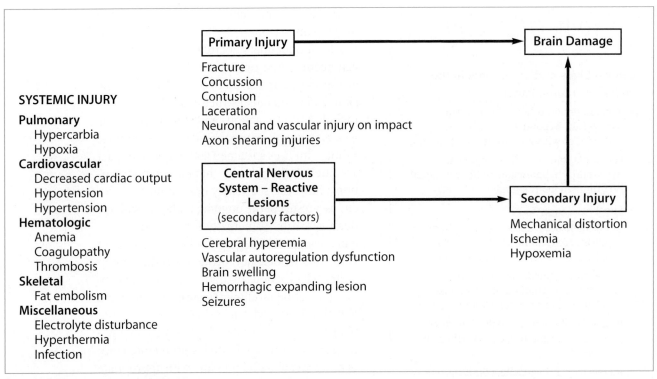

SYSTEMIC INJURY

Pulmonary
Hypercarbia
Hypoxia
Cardiovascular
Decreased cardiac output
Hypotension
Hypertension
Hematologic
Anemia
Coagulopathy
Thrombosis
Skeletal
Fat embolism
Miscellaneous
Electrolyte disturbance
Hyperthermia
Infection

Primary Injury

Fracture
Concussion
Contusion
Laceration
Neuronal and vascular injury on impact
Axon shearing injuries

Central Nervous System – Reactive Lesions (secondary factors)

Cerebral hyperemia
Vascular autoregulation dysfunction
Brain swelling
Hemorrhagic expanding lesion
Seizures

Brain Damage

Secondary Injury

Mechanical distortion
Ischemia
Hypoxemia

Figure 6.10 Dynamics of traumatic brain damage.

Buffering Mechanisms

Cerebrospinal Fluid

The CSF is an important early buffer for the maintenance of ICP. The CSF is approximately 10% of the intracranial volume, and most is displaced easily into the spinal subarachnoid space when brain or intracranial blood volume increases. With further brain swelling, the ventricular system is compressed. This causes further displacement of CSF, which again diminishes the intracranial CSF volume. When CSF volume is almost totally displaced, intracranial compliance is minimal. At this point, small changes in brain or blood volume can produce marked and sustained rises in ICP. In most cases, patients presenting with increased ICP have exhausted the CSF compensatory mechanism, so therapy to decrease ICP relies on other mechanisms, including manipulation of cerebral blood volume.

Cerebral Blood Volume

Intravascular blood is approximately 8% of the intracranial volume. Most of the cerebral blood is in thin-walled venous capacitance vessels. Extrinsic pressure from a mass lesion can displace blood from these vessels. However, cerebral blood flow (CBF) can be increased in response to head trauma in childhood. This global increase in CBF (cerebral hyperemia) can occur shortly after injury. Although the underlying reasons for this increase in CBF and intracranial blood volume are unknown, it is well established that autoregulation of CBF is responsive to changes in $Paco_2$ and Pao_2 (**Figure 6.12** and **Figure 6.13**).

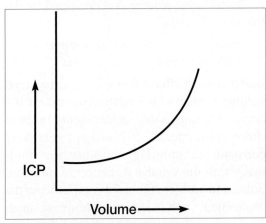

Figure 6.11 Relationship of expanding intracranial volume to intracranial pressure.

Children with severe head injury can hypoventilate and become hypercapnic, with resultant cerebral hyperemia. Conversely, hypocapnia of 25 to 30 mm Hg reduces cerebral blood volume by approximately 50% from baseline levels at Pa_{CO_2} of 40 mm Hg. The carbon dioxide response is the rationale for hyperventilating the child with severe head injury and increased ICP. However, recent evidence suggests that prolonged hyperventilation to Pa_{CO_2} levels of less than 35 mm Hg offers little benefit and that levels of less than 25 mm Hg are potentially hazardous as a result of reduction in global CBF achieved mainly by decreasing flow to undamaged brain tissue.[10] Neurons that are already injured can be particularly sensitive to this hypoxia and hypoperfusion. Seizure activity or hyperthermia increases cerebral metabolic rate and oxygen demand and can potentiate neuronal injury if metabolic demands are not met.

Brain

The brain parenchyma occupies approximately 80% of the intracranial volume. It is minimally compressible and contributes little to the intracranial volume/pressure-buffering system. In children with no significant underlying brain lesions, rapid recovery will occur if CPP is maintained within normal limits. However, in children with diffuse impact injuries, initial control of hyperemia will maintain a normal ICP, but delayed elevation of ICP can occur as the result of progression of cellular edema. Control of this edema can be achieved in part through avoidance of overhydration. Use of hypertonic saline for resuscitation is theoretically appealing to prevent this progressive swelling. Water restriction is no longer recommended because its effects on ICP can be countered by untoward effects on mean arterial pressure, thereby decreasing CPP.

Comprehensive Neurologic Examination

A neurologic flow sheet facilitates an objective and serial recording of the patient's status. This is best accomplished initially using the GCS or the AVPU system. The three variables that correlate best with the degree of coma are adjusted to reflect their relative importance: motor (6—maximum Glasgow Coma Scale score for this category), verbal (5—maximum Glasgow Coma

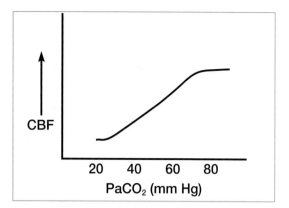

Figure 6.12 Relationship of Pa_{CO_2} to cerebral blood flow.

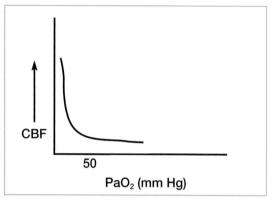

Figure 6.13 Relationship of hypoxemia to increase in cerebral blood flow.

Scale score for this category), and eye opening (4—maximum Glasgow Coma Scale score for this category). When recording motor response as an indication of the functional state of the brain as a whole, the best or highest response from any limb is recorded. However, any difference between the responsiveness of one limb and that of another can indicate focal brain damage, and for this purpose, the worst (most abnormal) response also should be noted. For motor response, it is best to pinch the medial aspect of each arm or leg or apply pressure to a nailbed with a pencil. This can result in either flexion or extension. If flexion is observed, stimulation (eg, sternal rub) is applied to the head and neck or trunk above the nipple line to test for localization. Raising the hand above the chin in response to supraorbital pressure is a localizing response. The eye-opening response to speech does not necessarily require a command to open the eyes.

The neurologic examination includes an assessment of the cranial nerves, eyes, brainstem, motor system, sensory system, and cerebellum. The olfactory nerve (cranial nerve I) is one of the most commonly involved in traumatic injuries, but this is usually of little clinical significance. The abducens (cranial nerve VI), facial (cranial nerve VII), and vestibulocochlear (cranial nerve VIII) nerves are most commonly involved in craniofacial trauma because of their relatively long intraosseous course through the skull. Injuries to these nerves are frequently seen in association with skull fractures, particularly temporal bone fractures. Assessment of acute facial nerve injuries, especially peripheral injuries, should include specialty evaluation (otorhinolaryngology, plastic surgery, or neurosurgery). Hearing loss is common in children who have sustained skull fractures. This should be excluded with audiometric evaluations on a nonurgent basis in all children with moderate or severe traumatic brain injuries and/or basilar skull fractures.[11]

Eyes

Eye examination is a crucial component of the neurologic examination. This examination includes the eye opening response as part of the GCS score, as well as pupillary size and reactivity, light reflex, movement of the extraocular muscles, and examination of the fundus. Pupillary size and reactivity are controlled by cranial nerves II (optic, afferent limb) and III (oculomotor efferent limb), sympathetic fibers (via carotid artery), and parasympathetic fibers (via cranial nerve III). The most significant ocular finding in the trauma setting is an evolving unilateral cranial nerve III palsy, presenting as pupillary dilation and lateral deviation of the eye (blown pupil). This is a sign of uncal herniation, in which the cranial nerve is compressed by brain swelling against the brainstem at the level of the tentorial notch. Further swelling can result in brainstem herniation and death.

A normal light reflex is a brisk pupillary constriction to light shone in the eye. An absent light reflex can be indicative of brainstem dysfunction, second or third cranial nerve injury, or retinal detachment. Light shone into one eye produces constriction of both eyes. This is the consensual reflex, and its absence might be due to interruption of the afferent limb of cranial nerve II, brainstem relay, or efferent limb of cranial nerve III.

Ophthalmoscopic examination is especially important when child abuse is suspected. Retinal hemorrhages are frequently seen in cases of shaken baby syndrome. Papilledema is a late finding of elevated ICP. The absence of papilledema does not exclude the presence of raised ICP.

Brainstem

Brainstem reflex disturbances are indicative of severe TBI. They include pupillary response (cranial nerves II and III), doll's eyes (cranial nerves III, VI, and VIII), corneal reflexes (cranial nerves V and VII), and gag reflex (cranial nerves IX and X). Testing of these reflexes is part of the brain death evaluation. All reflexes must be absent before the patient can be declared brain dead. Other components of the brain death evaluation include a failed apnea test and a GCS score of 3 after the presence of hypothermia and toxic substances has been excluded.

Motor/Sensory

The motor system examination consists of testing the power, reflexes, and tone of the major muscle groups. Classically, upper motor neuron (brain, spinal cord) injuries result in hyperactive reflexes, increased muscle tone (spasticity), and a positive Babinski sign (upgoing plantar reflex), whereas lower motor neuron (peripheral nerves) injuries result in hypoactive reflexes and reduced muscle tone (flaccidity). However, in the acute phase of injury (as would be encountered in the ED), upper motor neuron injuries initially result in hyporeflexia (or areflexia) and flaccidity. Over time, these evolve to the classic findings of hyperreflexia and spasticity.

The sensory system examination is perhaps less important than the motor system in the setting of acute TBI. An isolated sensory loss is usually found in spinal cord or peripheral nerve injuries. Cerebellar examination primarily consists of testing coordination of movement and balance.

Cranial and Intracranial Injuries

Skull Fractures

Skull fractures can involve the cranial vault or base. They are described as open if associated with an overlying scalp laceration and as closed if not. Open skull fractures are usually treated with surgical debridement, especially if there is a depressed skull fracture and the underlying dura or brain is lacerated.[12]

Linear Skull Fractures

Most skull fractures that occur in children are linear and extend across the cranial vault. These children frequently are asymptomatic, except for swelling and tenderness over the fracture site. In younger children, even if the external signs are minimal but a skull fracture is suspected, radiographic evaluation should be undertaken for documentation. This is usually best accomplished by CT scan to identify the extent of the fracture and assess the status of underlying intracranial contents.

Depressed Skull Fractures

Depressed skull fractures usually are more obvious on physical examination. They are commonly the result of significant traumatic force acting on a small cross-sectional area (eg, a blow from a hammer). Depressed skull fractures can be associated with underlying brain injury and, occasionally, dural tears. Depressed fractures can in some instances be compound or comminuted. Neurosurgical evaluation is mandatory in all cases.

Basilar Skull Fractures

Basilar skull fractures involve the basal portion of the skull and can occur in the anterior, middle, or posterior cranial fossa. These fractures usually are characterized by periorbital subcutaneous hemorrhages (raccoon eyes), CSF rhinorrhea or otorrhea, cranial nerve palsies, hemotympanum, or postauricular ecchymosis (Battle sign). These signs might appear at the initial assessment but also develop during stabilization; hence, serial examinations are important. In the young child, the dura closely adheres to the basilar skull and can lead to meningeal tears in basilar fractures. Children with CSF rhinorrhea or otorrhea should be evaluated by a neurosurgeon. Initial definitive treatment entails inpatient bed rest with the head of the bed elevated. Children whose cervical spines have not been cleared will require reverse Trendelenburg positioning. More than 95% of these injuries will heal spontaneously with this therapy. Antibiotic treatment is not needed. Any child who is suspected of having an anterior fossa basilar skull fracture is at risk for intracranial penetration with nasogastric tubes, so orogastric intubation is preferred for gastric decompression.

Concussions

Most patients with a GCS score higher than 13 and a mild TBI will be assigned concussion as the diagnosis. It was once thought to be a transient state of neuronal dysfunction resulting from trauma with no long-term consequences. The last decade has seen a great deal of research and attention focused on concussions, particularly those that are sports related.[13] A concussion results from rotational and acceleration/deceleration forces applied to the brain not necessarily by a direct blow to the head. What follows is a diffuse impairment of the neuronal membrane with depolarization and suppression of neuronal activity. Recovery can be prolonged. Signs and symptoms of concussion go far beyond loss of consciousness and confusion. They can be categorized as physical, cognitive, emotional, and sleep related (Table 6-5). A formalized approach, such as the Sport Concussion Assessment Tool 2, will facilitate the diagnostic process. Neuropsychological testing is an even more sensitive tool for following up a concussed patient, especially if a pre-event test has been taken. This is currently done in both the National Hockey League and the National Football League. Repetitive concussions can have a profound long-term effect on brain structure and function.

In the infant and young child, there is a characteristic concussion syndrome seen minutes to hours after a fall. Consciousness rarely is lost; however, the child becomes pale and sleepy and might begin to vomit. Examination usually reveals a pale infant or child with tachycardia, clammy skin, normal blood pressure, no evidence of focal neurologic deficit, and a soft fontanelle. The level of consciousness varies from spontaneous movements of all extremities to deep stupor with responses to pain only. These symptoms and signs usually subside rapidly. Occasionally, however, hospitalization and judicious administration of IV fluids will be necessary for 24 hours. This is mandatory if the GCS score falls below 15. An older child

TABLE 6-5 Signs and Symptoms of Concussion
Physical
Headache, nausea, vomiting, balance problems, visual problems, fatigue, sensitive to light, sensitive to noise, dazed, stunned
Cognitive
Feeling mentally "foggy," feeling slowed down, difficulty concentrating, difficulty remembering, forgetful of recent information, confused about recent events, answers questions slowly, repeats questions
Emotional
Irritability, sadness, more emotional, nervousness
Sleep
Drowsiness, sleeping more than usual, sleeping less than usual, difficulty falling asleep

TABLE 6-6 Criteria for Discharge From Emergency Department in Neurologically Intact Children
• Brief or no loss of consciousness*
• History compatible with only minor injury
• GCS score of 15
• Normal radiographic findings (if imaging ordered)
• Reliable caregivers, informed about warning signs of neurologic deterioration
• Easy access to hospital should there be any deterioration

*The period "brief" is controversial and not well defined in the literature. Judgment should be used in individual cases.

Adapted from: American Academy of Pediatrics. The management of minor closed head injury in children. *Pediatrics.* 1999;104:1407–1415 and Mitchell KA, Fallat ME, Raque GH, Hardwick VG, Groff DB, Nagaraj HS. Evaluation of minor head injury in children. *J Pediatr Surg.* 1994;29:851–854.

might present with headache, irritability, and vomiting. Amnesia of the events leading to the trauma (retrograde amnesia) or posttraumatic (antegrade) amnesia is fairly common in older children. The clinician must decide who should be studied, what the treatment should be, and when the child can return to full activity.

Using the Pediatric Emergency Care Applied Research Network (PECARN), Kuppermann et al[14] developed an algorithm to identify those patients with mild TBI who are likely to benefit from a CT scan (**Figure 6.14**). They had 42,412 patients and divided them into two groups: those younger than 2 years and those 2 years and older. They further divided them into derivation and validation groups. They looked for clinically important brain injuries (TBI) identified by CT scan.

Observation and rest are the mainstays of concussion treatment. In-hospital observation should be determined on an individual basis. If it is to be done at home (Table 6-6), the parents should be given instructions concerning head injury observation and precautions before discharge (Table 6-7). Rest should be both physical and cognitive. Television, videogames, and schoolwork can exacerbate symptoms. If vomiting persists, hydration might be necessary. Aspirin and nonsteroidal anti-inflammatory drugs should not be used for treatment of persistent

headache early on because of their effect on platelet function and risk of bleeding.

No concussed player should return to play the day of injury. Until recovery is complete, abnormal balance, reaction time, and thought processing put the player at increased risk of injury. Once symptoms have fully resolved with-

TABLE 6-7 Instructions to Parents or Caregivers for Home Observation of Children Who Have Sustained Head Trauma
Immediately bring the child to the ED if any of the following signs or symptoms appears within the first 72 hours after discharge:
• Any unusual behavior
• Disorientation as to name and place
• Unusual drowsiness and sleepiness
• Inability to wake child from sleep
• Increasing headache
• Seizures, twitching, or convulsions
• Unsteadiness on feet
• Clear or bloody drainage from ear or nose
• Vomiting more than two or three discrete episodes
• Blurred or double vision
• Weakness or numbness of face, arms, or legs
• Fever

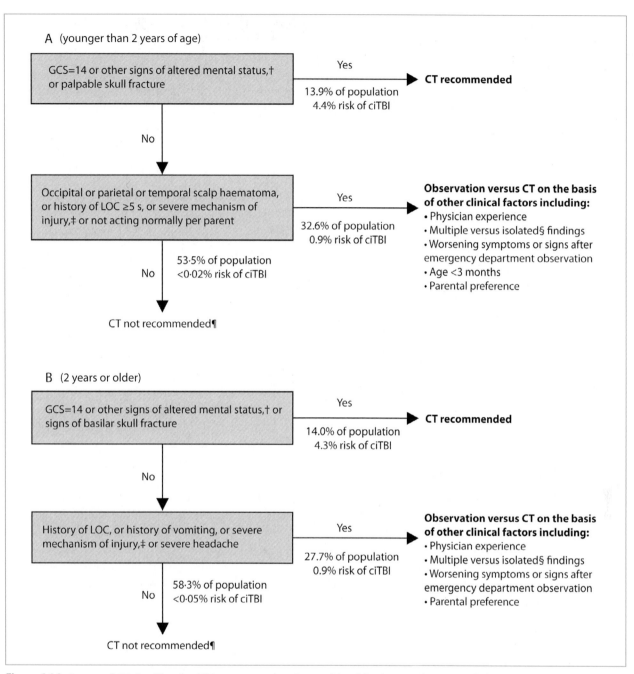

Figure 6.14 Suggested CT algorithm for children younger than 2 years (A) and for those aged 2 years and older (B) with GCS scores of 14–15 after head trauma.*

GCS=Glasgow Coma Scale. ciTBI=clinically-important traumatic brain injury. LOC=loss of consciousness.

*Data are from the combined derivation and validation populations.

†Other signs of altered mental status: agitation, somnolence, repetitive questioning, or slow response to verbal communication.

‡Severe mechanism of injury: motor vehicle crash with patient ejection, death of another passenger, or rollover; pedestrian or bicyclist without helmet struck by a motorized vehicle; falls of more than 0.9 m (3 feet) (or more than 1.5 m [5 feet] for panel B); or head struck by a high-impact object.

§Patients with certain isolated findings (ie, with no other findings suggestive of traumatic brain injury), such as isolated LOC,[39,40] isolated headache,[41] isolated vomiting,[41] and certain types of isolated scalp haematomas in infants older than 3 months,[31,42] have a risk of ciTBI substantially lower than 1%.

¶Risk of ciTBI exceedingly low, generally lower than risk of CT-induced malignancies. Therefore, CT scans are not indicated for most patients in this group.

Kuppermann N, Holmes JF, Dayan PS, et al. Identification of children at very low risk of clinically-important brain injuries after head trauma: A prospective cohort study. *The Lancet*. 2009;374:1160–1170. Reprinted with permission.

out medications, gradual return to activity can be begun. If symptoms return, activity should be reduced. Ideally, a concussed player should have returned to baseline on neuropsychological tests and be asymptomatic even with exertion.

Second-impact syndrome describes the rare event where a child sustains a second head injury before fully recovered. The second impact might be mild; however, rapid and fatal cerebral swelling can ensue.

Diffuse Axonal Injury

Diffuse axonal injury in children younger than 1 year is usually the result of child maltreatment (abusive head trauma, also known as shaken baby syndrome). Pathologically, there is tearing of the anterior bridging veins, petechial hemorrhage in the white matter and deep gray structures with shearing of myelin and axons, contusions of the corpus callosum, subarachnoid hemorrhage, and acute intracranial hypertension. These children often are brought to medical attention after hours of coma and usually have sustained several previous but less severe injuries. On examination, there often is no evidence of external trauma but perhaps some bruising or pinch marks on the upper arms. Infants present in several ways, including deep coma with decorticate posture or flaccidity, fixed dilated pupils, and apnea or bradycardia. They can sometimes be aroused by painful stimulation, move all extremities, and breathe well spontaneously. In severe cases, the fontanel is full and tense. In almost all cases, retinal hemorrhages can be detected on ophthalmoscopic examination.[15]

Diffuse axonal injury in the older child can result from primary impact injury. The pathological patterns range from areas of disruption of the blood brain barrier and small intracranial hemorrhages to significant contusions and lacerations as a result of shearing forces. The most common picture is that of bilateral diffuse swelling produced by vasodilatation and hyperemia after trauma. This swelling is produced mainly by an increase in intracerebral blood volume; however, redistribution of blood from the subarachnoid and pial vessels into the intraparenchymal regions is a contributory factor. Significant brain edema can be superimposed on this hyperemia. A child with a deteriorating neurologic status after a period of lucency is more likely to have generalized cerebral swelling than intracranial hemorrhage. Children who present in deep coma, suggesting a significant degree of neuronal injury at impact, frequently have white matter edema caused by disruption of the blood brain barrier. Treatment of diffuse axonal injury is primarily directed toward control of cerebral swelling and elevated ICP.

Epidural Hematoma

Epidural hematomas are relatively rare (<3%), even in severe trauma in children. Epidural hematomas in adults commonly originate from a hemorrhaging middle meningeal artery that quickly separates the meningeal dura layer from the inner table of the skull. In children, however, most epidural hematomas are due to meningeal and diploic vein hemorrhage. These hematomas occasionally occur in the posterior cranial fossa due to a bleeding deep venous sinus. In contrast to the adult, the dura mater in the young child is tightly adherent to the skull. This factor is probably responsible for the varying and occasional subacute presentation of epidural hemorrhages in children. Epidural hematomas are true surgical emergencies, although small venous epidural hematomas can be managed conservatively.

In the infant and young child, an epidural hematoma usually results from a high fall onto a hard surface or a motor vehicle crash. Acute epidural hematoma in infancy can be associated with anemia and shock because a large amount of blood can accumulate in the head. This is due to the greater compressibility of the brain and the expandable nature of the cranial vault when cranial sutures have not yet fused. If an associated skull fracture is present, the hematoma can decompress into the subperiosteal galea with an even greater blood loss. This is an exception to the general rule that hypovolemic shock does not result from head injury alone.

Children younger than 5 years with epidural hematomas rarely present with the classic pattern of a lucid period followed by rapid neurologic deterioration occurring within hours of injury. The period of lucidity usually is not a totally asymptomatic interval but rather a stable or improving level of consciousness. Many children at this age never become deeply unconscious but present within 48 hours of injury with papilledema, bradycardia, continued moderate lethargy, and sometimes recurrent vomiting over several days. These are signs of increased ICP and impending transtentorial herniation. Cranial vault fractures are present in only approximately 50% of children with epidural hemorrhages. In a child, epidural hemorrhage can also occur in the posterior cranial fossa after occipital trauma, resulting in nuchal rigidity, cerebellar signs, vomiting, and continued impaired consciousness. The outcome from epidural hematomas relies on prompt recognition and treatment. **Figure 6.15** demonstrates the CT findings of a child with an epidural hematoma.

Subdural Hematoma

Posttraumatic subdural hemorrhages are a significant source of neurologic disease in children. Subdural hematomas occur 5 to 10 times more frequently than bleeding in the epidural space and tend to occur in infants more often than in older children. These hemorrhages are almost exclusively venous in origin, mostly due to cerebral bridging vein disruption between the dura and brain. In a young infant, the onset of symptoms can be relatively slow due to the relative plasticity of the skull. Infants can present with nonspecific symptoms, such as vomiting, irritability, and low-grade fever. Some infants, however, will not present with symptoms until the subacute or chronic phase of subdural collection. In the subacute phase, the subdural blood organizes into a hemorrhagic cyst over several weeks and expands in size due to the osmotic pressure of red blood cell breakdown products. The usual presentation is that of a child with an enlarged head and no history of trauma. Occasionally, infants present with focal or generalized seizures. Physical examination reveals an irritable, lethargic infant with a bulging fontanel, "sunsetting" eyes, retinal and preretinal hemorrhages, and hypertonic muscle tone. Older children with subdural bleeding tend to present more acutely with symptoms and signs of increased ICP and impending transtentorial herniation. **Figure 6.16** demonstrates CT findings of a child with a subdural hematoma.

Cerebral Contusions

Brain contusions are commonly seen in deceleration injuries, where brain substance momentum exceeds the suddenly stationary cranium as occurs in high-speed automobile crashes. The brain is subjected to shear stresses that result in varying

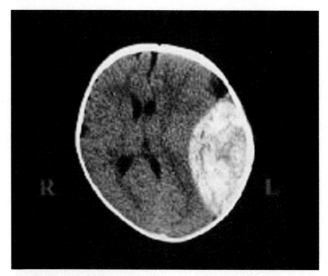

Figure 6.15 Computed tomographic findings of a child with epidural hematoma.

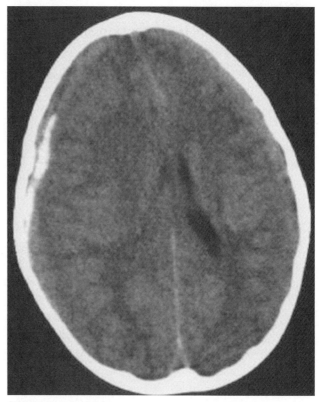

Figure 6.16 Computed tomographic findings of a child with subdural hematoma.

degrees of brain tearing, contusion, and frank intracerebral hematoma formation. Cerebral edema is almost universally associated with intracerebral contusions. These injuries tend to occur near the tips (rostral extent) of the frontal and temporal lobes. A temporal lobe contusion is potentially lethal because of its close proximity to the brainstem, where swelling can quickly result in lateral herniation and death. Larger intraparenchymal hematomas frequently require surgical evacuation. **Figure 6.17** demonstrates CT findings of a child with intracerebral hemorrhage.

Brainstem Injuries

The brainstem is subject to shearing injuries and compression by a swollen, adjacent traumatized brain. Differences in pressure between the supratentorial and infratentorial compartments will place stresses on brainstem tissue as the pressure dissipates between these compartments. If the brainstem moves through the tentorial notch (central herniation), tearing of vessels within the brainstem causes intraparenchymal hematomas known as Duret lesions or hemorrhages. This is a lethal condition.

Intracranial Hypertension and Herniation

Intracranial hypertension is common in children with severe head injury, even in the absence of a mass lesion. The ICP can be elevated early or become elevated after several days because of persistent or uncontrollable cerebral hyperemia or vasogenic or cytotoxic cerebral edema. Symptoms of increased ICP occur only after the compensatory mechanisms for maintaining normal ICP have been exhausted. Early symptoms and signs of increased ICP include headache, vomiting, altered mental status, respiratory irregularity, and abnormal posturing. Prompt therapy should be instituted to avoid further increases in ICP, decreased CPP, or brain herniation (**Figure 6.18**). The diagnosis of elevated ICP should be established well before the onset of the late manifestations of hypertension, bradycardia, and pupillary dilatation. Herniation of the brain can take place at any of three anatomical sites: tentorial incisura, inferior edge of the falx cerebri, and foramen magnum The most common herniation is a central

transtentorial herniation of diffusely swollen cerebral hemispheres. When this occurs, the diencephalon and upper brainstem are compressed initially, causing deterioration in level of consciousness, respiratory irregularity, pupillary dilatation, upward gaze limitation,

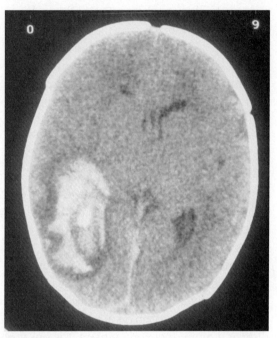

Figure 6.17 Computed tomographic findings of a child with cerebral contusion.

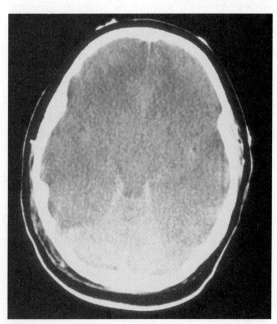

Figure 6.18 Head injury with subarachnoid hemorrhage, diffuse cerebral edema, and impending herniation.

and progressive hypertonia. With continued caudal progression, decorticate posturing, pupillary dilatation, and hyperventilation develop. Basilar artery compression and brainstem ischemia also will develop and lead to further deterioration.

Management

Moderate TBI

The child with a moderate TBI (GCS score of 8 to 12) presents in a less acute manner than one with a severe TBI, but the consequences of these injuries remain substantial in terms of the patient's short- and long-term disabilities. All patients with moderate TBI are admitted to the hospital, and at least one head CT scan is obtained. A neurosurgery consultation is obtained. The patient is closely observed with serial neurologic examinations for at least 24 hours. The family is given information on head injuries, and at least one follow-up appointment with a neurosurgeon is advisable, usually within 2 weeks of injury. Parents of all children who sustain a TBI should be educated about postconcussive syndrome (Table 6-7) and the possible neurobehavioral consequences of a head injury.

Critical Pathway for the Treatment of Established Intracranial Hypertension

Table 6-8 outlines emergency measures for treatment of intracranial hypertension. Patients with severe TBI (GCS score <8) should be admitted to a tertiary care facility and evaluated by a trauma surgeon, neurosurgeon, and/or critical care specialist with pediatric expertise. However, cardiorespiratory stabilization and treatment of ICP should be instituted immediately and are more important than immediate referral. If the child presents to a nontertiary care center, consultation with a trauma surgeon, neurosurgeon, and/or critical care physician at the referral center is advisable before transfer. These patients are best transported expeditiously by an advanced life support service or by a critical care transport team.

Severe TBI

Guidelines for the management of severe head injury were published in 1995 and revised in 2000 and again in 2007 by the Brain Trauma Foundation as a joint initiative of the major national neurosurgical organizations.[16]

TABLE 6-8 Emergency Therapy for Children Who Have Increased Intracranial Pressure Caused by Head Trauma

- Establish controlled ventilation (PaCO$_2$ of 35 to 40 mm Hg).
- Maintain oxygenation.
- Stabilize the cervical spine.
- Keep head and neck in midline position.
- Minimize stimuli (ie, suctioning and movements).
- Institute fluid resuscitation for shock and hypovolemia.
- If not in shock, provide fluids at a maintenance rate.
- Monitor heart rate, respirations, blood pressure, cardiac rhythm, and, if indicated, pulse oximetry.
- Consider mannitol or hypertonic saline if patient deteriorates despite above measures.

This large-scale literature meta-analysis examined 14 specific management topics and classified standards, guidelines, or options as level I, II, or III recommendations based on class I, II or III evidence, respectively. The topics and recommendations pertinent to this course are summarized in Table 6-9.

Seizures

Seizures have been reported in some series in as many as 10% of children seen in EDs after experiencing head trauma. Posttraumatic seizures can be temporally divided into those of immediate, early, and late onset. An immediate seizure occurs within seconds of impact and can represent a traumatic depolarization of the cortex. This seizure can occur with mild trauma, is brief, and has no prognostic significance.

Early seizures account for approximately 50% of posttraumatic seizures. They take place within the first week of the traumatic event and are usually due to focal brain injury. Young children are more susceptible to the development of early posttraumatic seizures within the first 24 hours after trauma. Generalized and focal seizures occur with equal frequency, and 10% to 20% develop status epilepticus. Approximately 25% of children with early seizures continue to have seizures after the first week.

Late posttraumatic epilepsy probably reflects cortical scarring. The severity of head

TABLE 6-9 **Summary of Recommendations From** *Guidelines for the Management of Severe Traumatic Brain Injury* (These are not pediatric-specific guidelines, so they should be adjusted accordingly.)

Issue	Level I	Level II	Level III	Comment
BP and oxygenation	Insufficient data	BP should be monitored and hypotension (systolic BP <90 mm Hg) avoided	Oxygenation should be monitored and hypoxia (oxygen saturation <92%) avoided.	Hypotension or hypoxia increases morbidity and mortality rates.
Hyperosmolar therapy	Insufficient data	Mannitol is effective for control of raised ICP. Arterial hypotension should be avoided	Restrict mannitol use before ICP monitoring; however, use mannitol in patients with signs of herniation or neurologic deterioration.	Studies suggest that hypertonic saline might be as good or better, but further evidence is needed.
Prophylactic hypothermia	Insufficient data	Insufficient data	Prophylactic hypothermia is not sufficiently associated with decreased mortality rates. It is associated with higher Glasgow Outcome Scale scores.	Mortality might be reduced if hypothermia is maintained for >48 hours.
Infection prophylaxis	Insufficient data	Periprocedural antibiotics for intubation should be administered. Early tracheostomy should be performed.	Routine ventricular catheter exchange or prophylactic antibiotic use for ventricular catheter placement is not recommended.	Ventriculostomies and other ICP monitors should be placed under sterile conditions to closed drainage systems.
Deep vein thrombosis prophylaxis	Insufficient data	Insufficient data	Graduated compression stockings or intermittent pneumatic compression stockings are recommended. Low-molecular-weight heparin or low-dose heparin should be used.	There are no data on when it is safe to start pharmacologic prophylaxis.
Indications for ICP monitoring	Insufficient data	ICP should be monitored in all salvageable patients with severe TBI and an abnormal CT scan.	ICP monitoring is indicated in patients with severe TBI with a normal CT scan if there is unilateral or bilateral motor posturing, and systolic BP <90 mm Hg.	ICP data are useful in predicting outcome and guiding therapy.
ICP thresholds	Insufficient data	Treatment should be initiated with ICP >20 mm Hg	A combination of ICP values and clinical and brain CT findings should be used to determine the need for treatment.	Current data support 20 to 25 mm Hg as an upper threshold, above which treatment to lower ICP should be started.
CPP thresholds	Insufficient data	Aggressive attempts to maintain CPP >70 mm Hg with fluids and pressors should be avoided because of the risk of ARDS.	CPP of <50 mm Hg should be avoided.	Optimal CPP is 60 to 70 mm Hg.

TABLE 6-9 Summary of Recommendations From *Guidelines for the Management of Severe Traumatic Brain Injury*, continued (These are not pediatric-specific guidelines, so they should be adjusted accordingly.)

Issue	Level I	Level II	Level III	Comment
Brain oxygen monitoring and thresholds	Insufficient data	Insufficient data	Jugular venous saturation <50% or brain tissue oxygen tension <15 mm Hg are treatment thresholds.	Current evidence suggests episodes of desaturation or low oxygen tension are associated with worse outcomes.
Anesthetics, analgesics, and sedatives	Insufficient data	Prophylactic administration of barbiturates to induce burst suppression. EEG is not recommended. High-dose barbiturate administration is recommended to control elevated ICP refractory to maximum standard treatment.		Analgesics and sedatives are a common management strategy for ICP control, although there is no evidence to support their efficacy.
Nutrition	Insufficient data	Patient should be fed to attain full caloric replacement by day 7 after injury.		It has not been established that any method of feeding is better than another or that early feeding before 7 days improves outcome.
Antiseizure prophylaxis	Insufficient data	Prophylactic phenytoin or valproate is not recommended for preventing late posttraumatic seizures. Anticonvulsants are indicated to decrease the incidence of early posttraumatic seizures, which are not associated with worse outcomes.		Routine seizure prophylaxis later than 1 week after TBI is not recommended.
Hyper-ventilation	Insufficient data	Prophylactic hyperventilation ($PaCO_2$ <25 mm Hg) is not recommended.	Hyperventilation is recommended as a temporizing measure to reduce ICP. Hyperventilation should be avoided for the first 24 hours after injury.	Cerebral blood flow can decrease dangerously low in the first hours after TBI; hyperventilation could further contribute to ischemia.
Steroids	The use of steroids is not recommended for improving outcome or reducing ICP.			Steroid use is associated with increased mortality and morbidity rates.

Abbreviations: ARDS, acute respiratory distress syndrome; BP, blood pressure; CPP, cerebral perfusion pressure; CT, computed tomography; EEG, electroencephalography; ICP, intracranial pressure; TBI, traumatic brain injury.

Adapted from: *Guidelines for the Management of Severe Traumatic Brain Injury.* New York, NY: Brain Trauma Foundation; 2007.

injury, dural laceration, and intracranial hemorrhage are factors that determine whether late-onset seizures occur. Approximately 5% of hospitalized patients with head trauma develop late posttraumatic seizures. The long-term prognosis is worse in these patients because as many as 75% will develop a chronic seizure disorder.

Initial therapy for seizures can include a short-acting anticonvulsant (0.1 to 0.3 mg/kg of diazepam or 0.05 to 0.1 mg/kg of lorazepam), followed by a long-acting anticonvulsant (20 mg/kg of phenytoin). Phenytoin should be infused at a rate no faster than 1 mg/kg per minute or 50 mg/min, whichever is the slower rate. Fosphenytoin can be infused much faster, at rates up to 150 mg of phenytoin equivalents per minute. Prophylactic anticonvulsant therapy might also be indicated if extensive cortical lesions are evident on examination or CT scan. One week of therapy is common practice with focal lesions or blood on CT scan.

Extracranial Head Injuries

Scalp Injuries

Scalp injuries are fairly common. The scalp is vascular, and scalp lacerations can be a source of major hemorrhage. If direct pressure does not control the hemorrhage, either infiltration of lidocaine (lignocaine) with epinephrine (adrenaline; maximum of 7 mg/kg) or hemostat application to the galea with external reflection will temporarily control most bleeding areas. The wound then should be explored with a gloved finger. Evidence of bone fragments or open or depressed fractures necessitate neurosurgical consultation before closure. A running, locked suture closure can help with hemostasis. Pressure applied directly to the repaired wound also enhances hemostasis.

Subgaleal Hematoma

Subgaleal and cephalohematomas are blood clots beneath the galea and pericranium, respectively. The latter is limited by suture lines so that it involves only one skull bone. These injuries occur frequently in children younger than 1 year. The child might have a lump that is not noticed for several days. Children with subgaleal hematomas commonly present with a soft, boggy swelling, occasionally in association with a linear fracture.

Because of the fluctuant nature of these lesions, they often are diagnosed as a CSF collection that has leaked through the fracture. However, these swellings usually are liquefied subgaleal blood that can spread circumferentially around the entire skull. These lesions should be followed expectantly because attempts at surgical treatment, including aspiration, can predispose the patient to infection. Sufficient blood leakage can occur into the subgaleal space in an infant to produce anemia.

Spinal Injuries

Spinal injuries are relatively uncommon in children. It should be assumed that all children who have sustained multiple trauma or head or neck trauma (blunt or penetrating), have a high-risk mechanism of injury (eg, motor vehicle crash, ejection from vehicle, lap belt injury, sports injury, fall, or dive), or have been shaken vigorously have a spinal injury until proved otherwise.[17] Most spinal injuries occur in boys and are secondary to blunt trauma, most often motor vehicle crashes. As many as 20% are secondary to penetrating injury from knives and bullets

Signs and symptoms suggestive of spine or spinal cord damage include:

- Altered level of consciousness
- Abnormal neuromotor or neurosensory examination
- Report of neurologic abnormality at any time after injury
- Neck or back tenderness
- Crepitus or pain on palpation or movement
- Limitation of neck or back motion
- Unexplained hypotension

Most spine injuries in children are to the cervical spine. Patel et al[5] reviewed the NPTR data for a 10-year period and found 1,098 patients (1.5%) with cervical spine injury of 75,172 injured children. Of the children with neurologic defects, 59% had no radiologic abnormality (SCIWORA) and 75% had incomplete injuries. Upper cervical spine injuries were associated with higher mortality rates and were just as likely to occur in children older than 8 years. Table 6-10 summarizes the signs and symptoms of cervical spine injury. Occasionally, bradycardia also can occur because of unopposed parasympathetic tone in a cervical spine injury. In this situation, accompanying signs are those of neurogenic shock (hypotension with warm, flushed skin) and spinal shock (decreased deep tendon reflexes, decreased sensory level, flaccid sphincters, and hypotonia).

Goals in the care of children with spinal trauma include effective stabilization of the primary spinal injury and prevention of progression to a more severe or significant injury. Management involves recognition of the possibility of spinal injury and taking steps to prevent secondary injury by adherence to the ABC (airway, breathing, circulation) approach of resuscitation, along with steps to prevent further movement or displacement of a potentially unstable spine. The devastating nature of a

---

TABLE 6-10 Signs and Symptoms of Cervical Spine Injury

- Abnormal motor examination (paresis, paralysis, flaccidity, ataxia, spasticity, abnormal rectal tone)
- Abnormal sensory examination (pain, sensation, temperature, paresthesias, anal wink)
- Altered mental status
- Neck pain
- Torticollis
- Limitation of motion
- Neck muscle spasm
- Neck ecchymosis or swelling
- Abnormal or absent reflexes
- Clonus without rigidity
- Diaphragmatic breathing without retractions
- Neurogenic shock (hypotension with bradycardia)
- Priapism
- Decreased bladder function
- Fecal retention
- Unexplained ileus
- Autonomic hyperreflexia
- Blood pressure variability with flushing and sweating
- Poikilothermia
- Hypothermia or hyperthermia

Adapted from: Woodward G. Neck trauma. In: Fleisher GR, Ludwig S, eds. *Textbook of Pediatric Emergency Medicine.* 6th ed. Baltimore, MD: Williams & Wilkins; 2010.

---

cervical cord injury with paralysis or death makes it imperative that a potentially unstable cervical spine injury not be missed.

Cervical spine and cord injury can present anywhere along the continuum of severity. The cervical column can incur a fracture that is stable and not a neurologic threat, or a patient can have no evidence of bony injury with a complete cervical cord transection. There is a subset of children (eg, those with Down syndrome) whose underlying medical problems make them more susceptible to cervical cord injuries as a result of atlantoaxial instability with relatively trivial trauma. It is estimated that 3.8% of pediatric patients with multiple trauma have a spine and/or spinal cord injury.[3] Many, if not most, patients with spinal column injuries present without overt neurologic deficits. In several studies, most patients with spinal injuries had evidence of concurrent head injury.

Neurologic damage from spinal injuries can be caused by many different anatomical problems. The spinal canal might be impinged on by fracture fragments, blood, or a herniated disk. The spinal cord can be compromised directly by edema, hypoperfusion, contusion, laceration, or transection. The effects of a head injury can make the diagnosis of concurrent spine injury difficult if not impossible in the early stages of evaluation. Although spinal injury must always be assumed, it is helpful when possible to distinguish between neurologic deficits that result from brain trauma and those that result from spinal cord trauma. Brain-injured patients often have diffuse or regional deficits (one side of the body) and intact bulbocavernosus and anal reflexes, whereas patients with spinal cord injuries often present with neurologic deficits in a myotome distribution, neuromotor disparity between arms and legs, flaccidity, absent reflexes, and loss of sphincter tone (spinal shock).

Immobilization

If a protective helmet is still in place after a sports-related injury, this should be removed slowly and carefully, with lateral expansion of the helmet, rotation of the helmet to clear the occiput, neck support, and stabilization during the removal process. A second rescuer should be available to maintain immobilization from below during this maneuver, using pressure on the jaw and occiput. After helmet removal, inline immobilization is reestablished from above.[18]

For immediate transfer, soft cervical collars offer no protection for an unstable spine, and semirigid collars alone might still allow flexion, extension, and lateral movement of the cervical spine. Ideal immobilization for transport includes a semirigid cervical collar (eg, Stifneck) in conjunction with a full spine board and soft spacing devices between the head and securing straps. For more information on C-spine immobilization, see Online Chapter 26, Critical Procedures.

The child's head is disproportionately large compared with an adult's head. Fifty percent of the postnatal head circumferential growth occurs by the age of 18 months, whereas 50% of the postnatal growth of the chest does not occur until the age of 8 years. The relatively large occiput flexes the neck when a child is placed on a hard surface.[19] Recommendations include using a spine board with a recess in the head area to accommodate a child's large occiput or placing a 2.5-cm (1-in) blanket under the torso to allow the neck to rest in a neutral position.[20] Cervical spine alignment can be greatly improved by these techniques, with avoidance of inadvertent flexion and anterior displacement of a potentially unstable spine. These amendments to spinal immobilization can be discontinued for patients 8 years or older, in whom skull and body proportions approximate those of an adult.

Inline manual neck immobilization (performed by a caretaker whose sole responsibility is to ensure there is no neck motion) is used to assist with airway maneuvers. Care should be taken to avoid traction (ie, pulling) on the cervical spine to prevent longitudinal stress and secondary cord injury.

Management

Orotracheal intubation with manual inline cervical stabilization is the preferred method of airway control in children with suspected or proven spine injury. A surgical airway or fiberoptic-assisted intubation performed by skilled personnel can be considered in patients with unstable spinal injury.

A study by Bracken et al[21,22] suggests that methylprednisolone in a dose of 30 mg/kg for 15 minutes, followed by infusion of 5 to 6 mg/kg per hour for 23 hours, started within 8 hours after acute spinal cord injury (ASCI), improves functional outcome in some patients. Although these studies specifically excluded children younger than 13 years, the poor functional outcome of patients with documented spinal cord injury has led many experts to recommend use of this still controversial protocol in children and adults. Alternatively, Prendergast et al[23] found that methylprednisolone therapy for penetrating ASCI might impair recovery of neurologic function. The evidence evaluation by Short[24] of all clinical studies determined that high-dose methylprednisolone use in ASCI cannot be justified. High-dose corticosteroids increase the complication rate without proven benefit.

Clinical Features

Many clues can aid in the diagnosis of a spinal cord injury (Table 6-10).[25,26] The signs and symptoms can be obvious or masked by other injuries, such as altered level of consciousness resulting from hypovolemic shock, a concurrent head injury, or the ingestion of alcohol, drugs, or toxic substances. Head and spinal cord injuries can present with overlapping abnormal neurologic signs, and differentiation can be difficult. A complete history is imperative to assess whether abnormal neurologic function, such as paresthesias, paralysis, or paresis, was present at any time after injury. These symptoms might have been transient and might not be present at the time of examination or volunteered by the patient during the history taking but still suggest an underlying spinal cord injury. The physical examination should include assessment of the patient for neck or paraspinal back tenderness, pain, limitation of motion, and muscle spasm, as well as for neurologic signs, particularly those of neurogenic shock (ie, hypotension, bradycardia, peripheral flush) and spinal shock (ie, flaccidity, areflexia, loss of anal sphincter control).

A catastrophic cervical spinal cord injury should be strongly suspected in any child who has sustained cardiac arrest shortly after trauma. After successful cardiopulmonary resuscitation, vigorous isotonic crystalloid resuscitation and pressor support might be needed. A careful assessment of the cervical spine will address three issues: fracture identification, determination of subluxation/malalignment, and suspicion of ligamentous laxity. In the acute setting, begin with a lateral cervical spine film and a CT scan of the cervical spine. Spinal cord injury without radiographic abnormality is possible, and an MRI of the cervical spine might also be needed.[27] If in doubt, prolonged immobilization is essential until an injury is unequivocally recognized or ruled out, a process that might take a week or longer.

Diagnostic Studies

Pediatric versus Adult Anatomy

The anatomy and evaluation of the pediatric spine differ in many ways from those of the adult spine. The fulcrum of the cervical spine of an infant is at approximately C2-3. By 5 to 6 years of age it is located at C3-4, and by 8 years of age it is at the same level as adults at C5-6. This is in part the result of the relatively large head size of a child compared with that of an adult. The higher fulcrum of a child's spine, along with relatively weak neck muscles and poor protective reflexes, accounts for fractures in younger children that involve the upper cervical spine. Older children and adults have fractures that more often involve the lower cervical spine.

The large amount of cartilage in the pediatric spine can cushion forces distributed to the spine but can make radiographic evaluation challenging. The pediatric cervical spine appears to have more anterior and posterior movement than its adult counterpart due to ligamentous laxity and relatively horizontal facet joints. These differences in part account for the anterior pseudosubluxation (physiologic subluxation) that can be seen between C2-3 and C3-4 up to the age of 16 years. These factors also allow the apparent predental space (between the dens and anterior ring of C1) to be increased to a maximum of 5 mm (adult maximum is 3 mm). Moreover,

cartilaginous growth centers (synchondroses) can look like fractures to the untrained eye.

The pediatric cervical spine also has the ability to revert to a relatively normal appearance after a significant distortion, which can hinder the radiographic search for abnormalities. Neurologic symptoms from spinal cord compression, including compression by epidural hematomas, can be slower to manifest in a young child than in an adult due to increased room around the spinal cord within the spinal column in a young child.

Plain Radiography, CT, and Magnetic Resonance Imaging

Radiographic evaluation of the cervical spine is an essential step in the assessment. Options include plain radiography, CT, and magnetic resonance imaging (MRI). The CT scan demonstrates fractures clearly. A CT scan often is used as a secondary screen when adequate plain radiographs cannot be obtained or to confirm suspected fractures. A CT scan provides good soft tissue detail and allows for the possibility of reconstruction images but does not provide the intrathecal, ligamentous, disk, or vascular detail that can be obtained with MRI. An MRI scan is more appropriate for evaluation of the subacute or chronic stages of injury or an acute problem with cord impingement by blood or soft tissues. MRI does not image cortical bone and other modalities and should not be used to evaluate the cervical spine for fractures.

The plain radiograph remains the initial test of choice in the acutely traumatized patient. Several authors have attempted to devise criteria to limit the number of patients who receive cervical spine radiographs. The perception of unnecessary tests must be balanced against the severity of consequences that can occur with a missed cervical spine injury. The literature suggests that if the patient does not have a high-risk mechanism of injury (eg, motor vehicle crash, sports injury, fall, dive, or penetrating neck injury), is awake and alert, is not under the influence of drugs or alcohol, is age appropriate, does not have cervical spine pain, has no tenderness or muscle spasm on palpation (especially in the midline), has normal neck mobility without limitation of motion, has a completely normal neurologic examination without history of abnormal neurologic signs or symptoms at any time after the injury, and has no painful distracting injuries that can mask neck pain, the cervical spine can be clinically cleared.

In a substudy of the National Emergency X-Radiology Utilization Study, 3,065 children younger than 18 years were evaluated for cervical spine injury. Only 30 patients (0.98%) had a cervical spine injury. These investigators showed that five criteria (midline cervical tenderness, altered level of alertness, evidence of intoxication, neurologic abnormality, and tenderness and distracting injury) had a sensitivity of 100% (95% confidence interval, 87.8% to 100%), a specificity of 19.9%, and a negative predictive value of 100% (95% confidence interval, 99.2% to 100%) in identification of children who required spinal radiographs. Only 88 patients (3%) were younger than 2 years, and none had cervical spine injury, so caution must be used in translating these criteria for cervical spine immobilization to this age group.[28]

In a PECARN study, Leonard et al[29] analyzed 540 children with cervical spine injury using a case-control study design for signs and symptoms predictive of injury. They identified eight factors: altered mental status, focal neurologic findings, neck pain, torticollis, substantial torso injury, predisposing conditions, diving injury, and high-risk motor vehicle crash. Having one or more of these factors was 94% sensitive and 32% specific for cervical spine injury. Adding information from out-of-hospital and transferring hospital sources improve the sensitivity but decreased the specificity.

When radiographs are obtained, a normal lateral radiograph does not clear the cervical spine but allows assessment of gross malalignment or distraction. The sensitivity of a single lateral cervical spine radiograph for fracture has been reported to vary between 82% and 98%.

A lateral cervical spine radiograph should include C1-7 and the C-7/T-1 junction. Additional films, including an anteroposterior view of C3-7 and an open-mouth anteroposterior view of C1-2 (odontoid view) in an age-appropriate child, will increase the sensitivity of the initial radiographic evaluation to greater than 95%. If at any point during the radiographic evaluation a fracture is identified, further plain radiographs often are not necessary. At that point, CT might be more useful in delineating the extent of the injury. An algorithm for considering radiographic evaluation is presented in **Figure 6.19**.

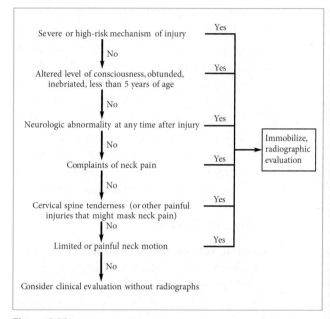

Figure 6.19 Radiographic versus clinical evaluation of the cervical spine in the traumatized patient.

Adapted from Woodward G. Neck trauma. In: Fleisher GR, Ludwig S, eds. *Textbook of Pediatric Emergency Medicine.* 6th ed. Baltimore, MD: Williams & Wilkins; 2010. Reprinted with permission.

The cervical spine has anterior elements (vertebral bodies, intervertebral disks, ligaments) and posterior elements (lamina, pedicles, neural foramen, facet joints, spinous processes, ligaments). The initial three-view series can provide a good evaluation of the anterior cervical spine, but it is not ideal for evaluation of the posterior cervical spine. Oblique (pillar) views are helpful to evaluate the posterior elements. Flexion and extension films for assessment of ligamentous stability can be obtained in an awake patient by having the patient flex and extend the neck as far as able without discomfort. These films can be inadequate because the neck muscles have splinted the cervical column in a position of comfort or stability and subsequent alignment will not change with flexion or extension. If questions remain concerning the integrity of the cervical spine after obtaining these radiographs, CT should be considered.

Evaluation of Radiographs

When evaluating radiographs of the cervical spine, use a systematic approach. The ABC (alignment, bones, cartilage, soft tissues) method of evaluating the lateral cervical radiograph is useful. Alignment is assessed, as demonstrated in **Figure 6.20**. The spinal cord lies between the posterior spinal line and the spinolaminal line. The usual lordotic curve of these lines might not be present in children younger than 6 years, in those on hard spine boards (the large occiput forces the neck in a flexed direction), in those with cervical collars, or in those with cervical neck muscle spasm. As mentioned, pseudosubluxation or physiologic subluxation can be seen in the upper cervical spine until the age of 16 years. Gross abnormalities should be detectable through assessment of alignment (**Figures 6.20 and 6.21**).

When evaluating the bones, look for typical abnormalities, which can be subtle. Compression fractures are suggested by differences in the heights of adjacent vertebral bodies. Structures, including the skull, teeth, and cartilage growth centers, can simulate fractures (Table 6-11).

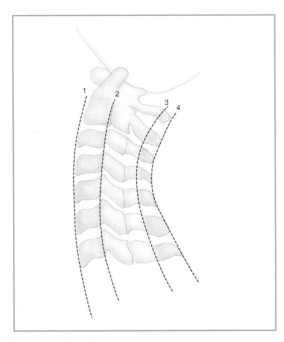

Figure 6.20 Lordotic curves seen with normal cervical spine alignment. Line 1: Anterior spinal line (also called anterior vertebral line). Line 2: Posterior spinal line (also called posterior vertebral line). Line 3: Spinolaminar line. Line 4: Line connecting the tips of the spinous processes.

TABLE 6-11   Radiographic Characteristics of the Pediatric Cervical Spine

• Cartilage artifact
  – Tapered anterior vertebrae
  – Apparently absent anterior ring of C1
  – Atlas (C1) body not ossified at birth and might fail to close
  – Axis (C2) four ossification centers
  – Apex of odontoid ossifies between ages of 12 and 15 years
  – Spinous process ossification centers
• Increased mobility
  – Pseudosubluxation
  – C1 override on dens
  – Increased predens space (5 mm maximum)
  – Ligament laxity
  – Facet joints shallow
• Growth plates (synchondrosis)
  – Dens ossifies between the ages of 3 and 8 years (can persist into adulthood)
  – Posterior arch of C1 ossifies at the age of 3 years
  – Anterior arch of C1 ossifies at the age of 6 to 9 years
• C1 internal diameter reaches adult size at the age of 3 to 4 years
• C2 through C7 internal diameter reaches adult size at the age of 5 to 6 years
• Lack of cervical lordosis
• Fulcrum varies with age (see text)
• Soft tissue variability with respiration
• Congenital clefts or other bony abnormalities (os odontoideum), spondylolisthesis, spina bifida, ossiculum terminale
• Rare compression fractures
• Approaches adult characteristics by the age of 8 years

Assess radiolucent cartilage after bone. Cartilaginous areas include the synchondroses, or growth plates, and intervertebral disk spaces. The growth plates can mimic fractures. Growth plates can be differentiated from fractures by their location and regular, smooth, sharp borders compared with the irregular appearance and often different locations of fractures. Growth centers in the anterior-superior vertebral bodies cause a sloped appearance that can look like anterior compression fractures to the untrained eye. The vertebral disk space also should be

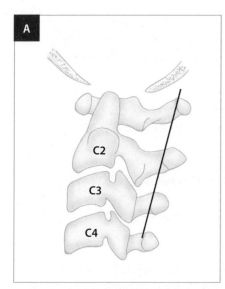 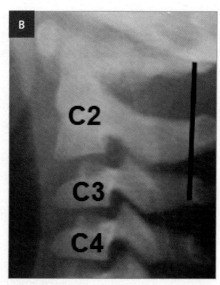 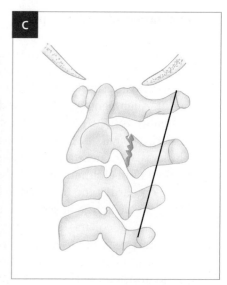

Figure 6.21 Distinguish true subluxation from pseudosubluxation of the cervical spine. A. The Swischuk ine is drawn from the anterior cortical margin of the spinous process of C1 through the anterior cortical margin of the spinous process of C3; in healthy patients without true subluxation, the Swischuk line passes through the anterior cortical margin of the spinous process of C2 or within 2 mm of it. B. Pseudosubluxation as the Swischuk line drawn passes through the anterior cortical margins of the spinous process of C2 even though the body of the C2 vertebrae is forward on C3 (pseudosubluxation). C. True subluxation of C2 on C3 and the Swischuk line drawn does not pass through the anterior cortical margin of C2.

evaluated because abnormalities can suggest specific mechanisms of injury. A vertebral disk space that is narrowed anteriorly can indicate disk extrusion from compression, whereas a widened space suggests a hyperextension injury with posterior ligamentous disruption.

Evaluation of soft tissue is extremely important. Abnormal soft tissue spaces might be the only clue to an underlying ligament, cartilage, or subtle bone injury that is not overt on a plain radiograph. Soft tissue thickening can represent blood or edema, which suggests an underlying injury. A rule of thumb is that the prevertebral (retropharyngeal) soft tissue anterior to C3 (see Figure 6.21B) should be less than two-thirds the width of the adjacent vertebral body. This space will approximately double below C4 (the level of the glottis) because the usually non–air-filled esophagus is included in this area. Crying, neck flexion, or the expiratory phase of respiration can produce a pseudothickening in the prevertebral space. Soft tissue abnormality should be reproducible on repeated radiographs if there is an underlying injury.

Multiple types of neck injury can be seen in the child, ranging from minor muscular strains with torticollis, to stable bony injuries, to unstable cervical injuries, with and without neurologic damage. Five percent or more of patients with a cervical spine injury will have an additional spinal injury at another level, and these injuries should be actively sought.

Specific Injuries

Jefferson Fracture

The Jefferson fracture is a bursting fracture of the ring of C1 secondary to an axial load as might be sustained in a diving injury (**Figure 6.22**). Although the fracture can be unstable, neurologic impairment often is not present initially because the fracture fragments splay outward and do not physically impinge on the spinal cord. The fracture usually is seen best on the open-mouth odontoid view; the radiographic criterion for diagnosis of a Jefferson fracture is lateral offset of the lateral mass of C1 of greater than 1 mm from the vertebral body of C2. Neck rotation can produce a false-positive result.

Approximately one-third of Jefferson fractures are associated with other fractures, most often involving C2. The pseudo-Jefferson fracture of childhood is present in 90% of children at the age of 2 years and usually normalizes by 4 to 6 years. The pseudo-Jefferson fracture has the radiographic appearance of a Jefferson

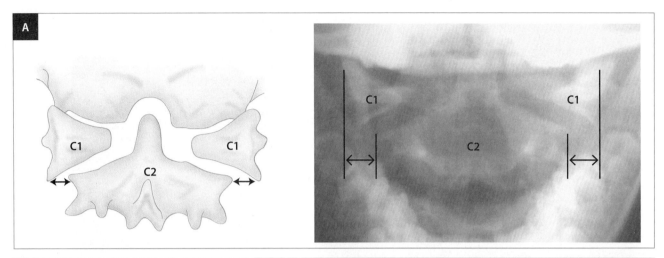

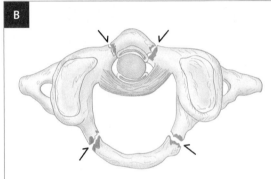

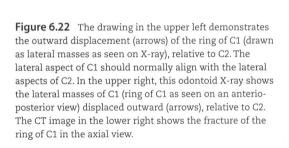

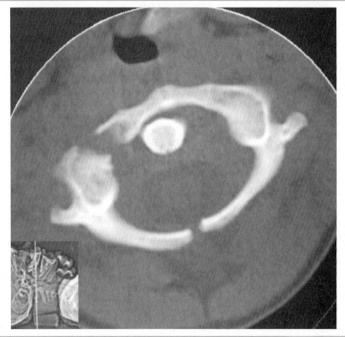

Figure 6.22 The drawing in the upper left demonstrates the outward displacement (arrows) of the ring of C1 (drawn as lateral masses as seen on X-ray), relative to C2. The lateral aspect of C1 should normally align with the lateral aspects of C2. In the upper right, this odontoid X-ray shows the lateral masses of C1 (ring of C1 as seen on an anterio-posterior view) displaced outward (arrows), relative to C2. The CT image in the lower right shows the fracture of the ring of C1 in the axial view.

fracture due to increased growth of the atlas (C1) compared with the axis (C2) and radiolucent cartilage artifact. If a Jefferson fracture is suspected in a child younger than 4 years, a CT scan is usually needed to further elucidate the injury. The CT scan is helpful in the evaluation of suspected injuries in the C1-2 area. Odontoid views are difficult to obtain in children younger than 3 years because they are unable to cooperate with the open-mouth view.

Hangman Fracture

The hangman fracture is a traumatic spondylolisthesis of C2 (**Figure 6.23**). This injury occurs as a result of hyperextension that fractures the posterior elements of C2 as can occur with diving injuries, falls, and frontal motor vehicle crashes. Hyperflexion after the hyperextension leads to anterior subluxation of C2 on C3 and subsequent cervical cord damage. The subluxation seen with a hangman fracture can sometimes be mistaken for the pseudosubluxation or physiologic subluxation seen in the C2-3 or C3-4 region in approximately 25% of children younger than 8 years. The posterior cervical line of Swischuk can help to distinguish a subtle hangman fracture from pseudosubluxation as depicted in Figure 6.21, but this is not always reliable, as depicted in Figure 6.23. The arch of C2 should be within 1.5 to 2 mm of this line, and if it is greater than this, it indicates an

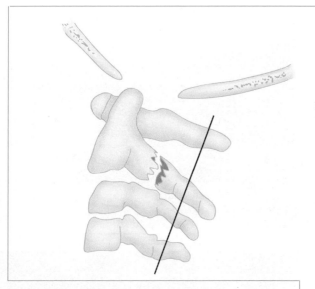

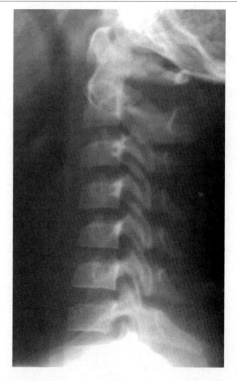

Figure 6.23 Diagram of hangman fracture (above) in which the posterior arch of C2 is not close enough to the Swischuk line. However, note the radiograph (right) that demonstrates a hangman fracture in which the posterior arch of C2 is close to the Swischuk line demonstrating that the Swischuk line alignment can be unreliable.

THE CLASSICS

Radiographic Features Suggestive of Cervical Spine Injury/Fractures

- Loss of normal lordosis
- Vertebral disk space narrowed anteriorly (disk extrusion from compression) or widened (hyperextension injury with posterior ligamentous disruption)
- Prevertebral (retropharyngeal) space at C3, more than two-thirds the anteroposterior width of the adjacent vertebral body
- Lateral mass offset by greater than 1 mm (Jefferson fracture)
- Spondylolisthesis of C2 (Hangman fracture)
- Widened predental space (>5 mm)
- Increased space between the occiput and C1 and/or widened predens space (atlantoaxial dislocation)
- Widening of an intervertebral disk space (distraction injury)
- Odontoid view showing one lateral mass of C1 forward and closer to the midline and other lateral mass appearing narrow and away from the midline (rotatory subluxation)

occult hangman fracture as the source of the anterior subluxation of C2 on C3. This line should be used only for evaluation of anterior subluxation of C2 on C3.

Atlantoaxial Subluxation

Atlantoaxial subluxation is the result of movement between C1 and C2 secondary to transverse ligament rupture or a fractured dens (**Figure 6.24A**, **Figure 6.24B**, and **Figure 6.24C**). Ligament instability precipitated by tonsillitis, cervical adenitis, pharyngitis, arthritis, connective tissue disorders, or Down syndrome can allow minor trauma to result in ligamentous damage. Subluxation due to transverse ligament disruption will be evidenced by a widened predens (preodontoid) space on a lateral radiograph. The normal predens measurement in children is less than 5 mm compared with less than 3 mm in adults. Steel's rule of three states that the area within the ring of C1 is composed of one-third odontoid, one-third spinal cord, and one-third connective tissue. Space therefore is available for limited dens movement or predens space widening without neurologic compromise. Neurologic symptoms often are not seen until the predens space exceeds 7 to 10 mm. Dens

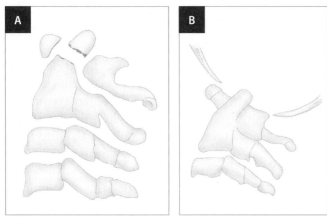

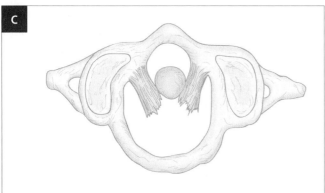

Figure 6.24 A. Dens fracture. B. Widened predental space secondary to transverse ligament rupture. C. Transverse ligament rupture.

fractures cause atlantoaxial subluxation more often than ligamentous disruption in a young child because the weakest part of the child's musculoskeletal system is the osseous component. These fractures are seen in young infants secondary to a rapid deceleration while in improperly positioned forward-facing car seats.

Distraction Injury

Distraction injuries result from a longitudinal stress to the cervical column. The most dangerous of these is occipitoatlantal dissociation. These injuries can contribute to a significant percentage of deaths in pediatric acute trauma. Although severe distraction injuries are incompatible with long-term survival, initial cardiopulmonary resuscitation might be possible. These injuries can be obvious or subtle on the lateral radiograph. Increased space between the occiput and C1 or widening of an intervertebral disk space without an obvious adjacent compression fracture indicates the possibility of a distraction injury. Distraction injuries also can be seen with difficult newborn deliveries. The spinal cord can distract only 6.4 mm (¼ in) before there is permanent neurologic damage. An MRI scan is useful in assessing an infant or other stable patient with diminished motor activity who is suspected of having a distraction injury.

Rotary Subluxation

Rotary subluxation is a cervical spine injury that often is missed or undiagnosed due to difficulty in interpreting the radiographs. Rotary subluxation or displacement can follow minor or major trauma or be spontaneous. These patients rarely present with abnormal neurologic findings. They present in the typical (cock-robin) position, with muscle spasm of the sternocleidomastoid muscle on the same side to which the chin points. In contrast, in patients with muscular torticollis, the chin points to the side opposite that involved. This is logical considering that the action of the sternocleidomastoid is an attempt to reestablish normal neck position.

The CT scan appears to be the most useful diagnostic tool in rotary subluxation. Patients with mild rotary subluxation should be treated with a cervical collar and analgesia for comfort; those with moderate rotary displacement need immobilization and occasionally traction. If there is anterior displacement of C2 on C1, a longer period of immobilization might be necessary to allow injured ligaments to heal.

Spinal Epidural Hematoma

Spinal epidural hematomas also are seen in the pediatric population. These are venous bleeds that compress the adjacent spinal cord and present with ascending neurologic symptoms hours or days after often apparently minor trauma. An MRI scan is helpful in the evaluation of these patients. Rapid evaluation and surgical decompression are mandatory to prevent further neurologic compromise.

SCIWORA

Spinal cord injury without radiologic abnormality (SCIWORA) occurs mainly in children younger than 8 years who present with or develop symptoms consistent with cervical cord injuries, without radiographic evidence of bone abnormality. In children, much of the strength of the spinal column is derived from cartilage and ligaments, although the ligaments are not as strong as in adults. This difference in tensile strength increases the potential for isolated ligamentous injury.[27,30] These injuries are usually partial and are associated with sports-related injuries and child abuse.[31] There is a subset of patients who have initial transient neurologic symptoms, who apparently recover and then return an average of 1 day (but up to 4 days) later with significant neurologic abnormalities. For this reason, many recommend hospitalization and immobilization for young patients who have experienced transient neurologic symptoms. Magnetic resonance imaging is helpful in this situation.

Chest Injuries

Blunt thoracic trauma is commonly encountered in children and can cause injuries that require immediate attention to establish adequate ventilation. A child's chest wall is compliant and allows energy transfer to the intrathoracic structures, frequently without evidence of injury to the external chest wall. The elasticity of the chest wall increases the likelihood of pulmonary contusions and direct intrapulmonary hemorrhage, usually without overlying rib fractures. Significant thoracic injuries rarely occur alone and usually are a component of major multisystem injury. Analysis of the NPTR data indicates that mortality from chest injury diagnoses is exceeded only by mortality from central nervous system injury. In most cases, both organ systems are injured, resulting in more severe disease.

Specific Injuries and Management

Children with pulmonary contusion can initially manifest few physical findings. Early radiographs might show minimal changes that can be confused with evidence of aspiration, which commonly occurs in children with multisystem injury. A child receiving bag-mask ventilation might accumulate air in the stomach. As the airway is further manipulated, the likelihood of acute gastric dilation associated with vomiting of gastric acid and stomach contents is increasingly likely. Thus, every child with a significant mechanism of injury should be assumed to be at risk of aspiration at the moment of injury and during initial management.

Children with any possibility of pulmonary injury require careful monitoring and serial evaluations of ventilation and oxygenation. The child receiving mechanical ventilation can experience desaturation, increasing PCO_2, and/or decreasing pulmonary compliance. Children who are not intubated can develop increasing tachycardia, rales, hemoptysis, and a decreasing arterial oxygen saturation. Early recognition is critical for effective therapy. Once a child with pulmonary contusion and/or potential aspiration deteriorates to a point that mechanical ventilation is required, a prolonged ventilator course, nosocomial pneumonia, and possibly acute respiratory distress syndrome become increasingly likely.

Pneumothorax can occur with blunt or penetrating trauma and consists of air in the pleural space from lung, tracheobronchial, or penetrating injury. Minimal collections of air in the pleural space might be undetected on examination and are seen best on an expiratory chest radiograph or CT scan. Small air collections can be obscured if a plain radiograph is taken with the patient in the supine position. Mediastinal, pericardial, and subcutaneous emphysema are the result of air tracking along the bronchi or pulmonary vessels.

Collapse of one lung can produce signs of hypoxia, hyperresonance to percussion, asymmetry of chest wall movement, and decreased breath sounds on the affected side. Treatment involves tube thoracostomy with underwater seal drainage. Bilateral pneumothoraces and tension pneumothorax are life-threatening injuries. With bilateral pneumothoraces and severe tension pneumothorax, the patient is hypoxic, has minimal or absent breath sounds bilaterally, and is typically hypotensive. A needle or an over-the-needle catheter placed in the second intercostal space anteriorly or in the fourth to fifth intercostal space laterally in the axillary line (at the level of the nipple) can be lifesaving until chest tubes can be placed. Remember to administer oxygen to all patients who sustain significant blunt chest trauma.

An open pneumothorax can be sucking or not, depending on size and other factors. Fortunately, gunshot and stab wounds are infrequent in childhood, and open pneumothoraces usually occur as the result of extensive animal attack or injuries involving farm or industrial machinery. The presenting injury is usually associated with significant soft tissue loss that can mask the presence of the sucking chest wound. These children need immediate sedation and analgesia so that a thorough evaluation of the chest injury can be accomplished. If the opening is larger than the airway, spontaneous ventilation will become ineffective. Place an occlusive dressing (gauze impregnated with petroleum jelly) over the wound and tape it on three sides. Insert a chest tube immediately. If the patient exhibits sudden respiratory deterioration after the closure, tension pneumothorax should be suspected. Remove the dressing briefly to let any air under pressure escape until the chest tube is placed or repositioned.

Tension pneumothorax is commonly a lethal chest injury. It frequently develops after the patient's arrival in the hospital and can especially occur in patients receiving mechanical ventilation who receive high inspiratory volumes under positive pressure to aerate injured lung parenchyma. The picture is that of sudden cardiorespiratory failure. The pleural pressure rises and the lung collapses. The mediastinum shifts, compressing the opposite lung. The superior vena cava kinks, leading to decreased venous return. The resulting decreased cardiac output is the immediate threat to life (**Figure 6.25**).

The diagnosis must be established by physical examination prompted by a high index of suspicion. Classically, the neck veins are distended and the trachea is deviated; however, these findings are not apparent in smaller children with a short neck or one who is wearing a cervical collar to immobilize the cervical spine. There are decreased breath sounds with

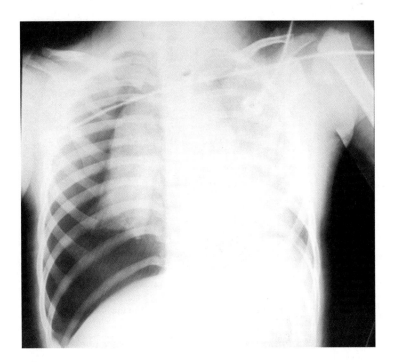

Figure 6.25 Tension pneumothorax in a 4-year-old boy with blunt chest trauma.

tympany and hypotension. Immediate treatment is required to improve cardiac output, including needle thoracostomy to convert the tension pneumothorax to a simple pneumothorax, followed by placement of a thoracostomy tube. Needle thoracentesis can be performed within seconds and will provide several minutes of stability while a chest tube is inserted. Do not wait for radiologic confirmation.

Traumatic hemothorax is treated with chest tube insertion and concomitant volume replacement. If massive bleeding is noted, the chest tube should be clamped and the patient prepared for immediate thoracotomy. Continued bleeding after chest tube placement (>2 to 4 mL/kg per hour) indicates major vascular injury and the need for open thoracotomy.

Traumatic asphyxia occurs with sudden massive compression of the chest. The pressure is transmitted up the superior vena cava to the head and neck. Clinical signs include petechiae of the head and neck, subconjunctival hemorrhages, hemoptysis, and occasional depressed level of consciousness (**Figure 6.26**). Pulmonary contusion and great vessel injury might be present. Upper abdominal injuries might also be found. Treatment consists of management of component

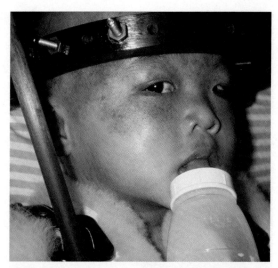

Figure 6.26 Traumatic asphyxia in a child after being pinned against a garage door by a car. Note the petechiae and subconjunctival hemorrhages in the head and neck area.

injuries. Administer oxygen, place chest tubes as needed, limit fluids, and elevate the head of the bed. If Pa_{O_2} decreases, the use of positive end-expiratory pressure might be indicated.

Cardiac tamponade more commonly occurs as an iatrogenic injury after cardiac catheterization, postoperative open heart surgery, or placement of a central venous catheter. It also can occur with a penetrating or crush injury. Blood accumulates in the pericardial sac so the heart cannot fill during diastole, causing low cardiac output. The diagnostic triad includes shock (associated with narrowed pulse pressure), distended neck veins, and muffled heart sounds. Massive hepatomegaly can be present. Treatment consists of a large fluid bolus and pericardiocentesis. The aspiration of a small volume of fluid from the pericardial space can be lifesaving. If there is time, echocardiography can be helpful in confirming the diagnosis.

Abdominal Injuries

The onset of symptoms of abdominal injury can be rapid due to massive hemorrhage or more gradual from an organizing clot or evolving bacterial or chemical peritonitis. Children with suspected abdominal injuries might need only careful observation, with judicious fluid and blood replacement. The decision to observe injuries of this type should be made only by the surgeon who will be responsible for emergency surgical intervention and perioperative care. If the abdominal injury results in such significant blood loss that resuscitation requires more than 40 mL/kg, immediate surgical exploration might be necessary.

Diagnostic Studies

Initially, the abdominal examination results might be normal despite significant disease. Sequential reexamination is essential to rule out an evolving abdominal problem. Focused Assessment with Sonography for Trauma (FAST) is an excellent way to evaluate for intraperitoneal fluid. New technology has produced small portable devices that are becoming available in every ED. The examination in children is not intended to replace detailed studies performed in radiology departments because up to one-third of solid organ injuries in children are intraparenchymal. The FAST examination has one simple mission: the identification of fluid in the pericardium, subhepatic or perisplenic spaces, or the pelvis. The FAST examination can be performed quickly and noninvasively on any trauma patient and can often demonstrate significant changes as fluid resuscitation proceeds.

Computed tomography, serial abdominal examination, and monitoring are used in children more often than diagnostic peritoneal lavage (DPL). Even in centers in which radionuclide scanning, CT, and ultrasonography are used to evaluate the intra-abdominal contents, DPL still can occasionally be helpful to rule out intra-abdominal hemorrhage in the child with a depressed level of consciousness and injuries requiring immediate surgical intervention on another organ system **(Figure 6.27)**. This situation might include a child who requires urgent neurosurgical or orthopedic surgical care. Using DPL to determine abdominal injury is not appropriate in a lucid child who does not require immediate surgery.

Management

Accurate assessment of abdominal injury remains one of the most challenging aspects of treatment of the injured child. Although it is rare that a child will require an operation for abdominal trauma,

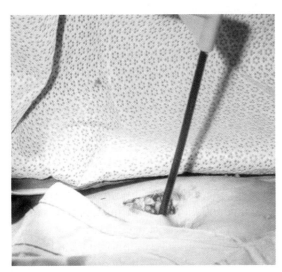

Figure 6.27 Positive peritoneal lavage in a 16-year-old girl with a ruptured spleen.

KEY POINTS

Management of Abdominal Trauma: Indications for Surgery

- Hemodynamic instability despite maximal resuscitative efforts
- Transfusion of greater than 50% of total blood volume
- Radiographic evidence of pneumoperitoneum
- Intraperitoneal bladder rupture
- Grade 5 renovascular injury
- Gunshot wound to the abdomen
- Evisceration of intraperitoneal or stomach contents
- Peritonitis—fecal or bowel contamination on DPL

indications for surgery include hemodynamic instability despite maximal resuscitative efforts, need of a transfusion of greater than 50% of total blood volume, radiographic evidence of pneumoperitoneum, intraperitoneal bladder rupture, grade 5 renovascular injury, gunshot wound to the abdomen, evisceration of intraperitoneal or stomach contents, signs of peritonitis, or evidence of fecal or bowel contamination on DPL. A DPL is rarely performed on children because even if frank blood is aspirated, a child would not require surgery unless he or she becomes hemodynamically unstable after appropriate fluid resuscitation. A DPL also confounds any subsequent abdominal examination.

Less obvious injuries can emerge gradually as significant threats if not accurately and rapidly identified. These include such things as intestinal perforation that stimulates a localized inflammatory process rather than general peritonitis, pancreatic contusion or ductular injury, urinoma, and obstructing duodenal hematoma. As stated earlier, the absence of external injury does not exclude significant internal injury. Clinical suspicion and an understanding of the mechanism of injury are critically important. Treatment of the child with a suspected abdominal injury consists of the following steps: establishing the presence of the injury, determining the need for surgical intervention, setting the priority of surgical intervention in relation to

other lifesaving maneuvers, and understanding the expected natural history of the lesion and those objective findings that confirm that the expected natural history is, in fact, occurring. The primary tools used to arrive at this therapeutic decision include thorough and repeated physical examinations, FAST examination, and abdominal CT. If time and treatment priority will allow, these should be accomplished in every child at risk within an hour of arrival in the ED.

Liver and Spleen Injuries

The liver and spleen are organs commonly injured from blunt trauma in the child. These injuries can be sufficiently extensive to require immediate exploration, but recent experience indicates that they are frequently self-limited in children. This has stimulated the evolution of protocols in which stable children are treated expectantly with bed rest, frequent examinations, serial hemoglobin determinations, and monitoring all under surgical supervision. The option of immediate surgical intervention must be available at all times. The decision to treat nonoperatively is solely the responsibility of the surgeon and must be based on physical examination and evaluation.

Essentially, hepatic injuries fall into one of three categories. Those with massive disruption presenting with intractable bleeding are now treated with immediate damage control laparotomy intended to stop bleeding and pack injuries before exsanguination, hypocoagulation, and hypothermia lead to inevitable fatality. These children are then resuscitated in the pediatric intensive care unit and returned to the operating room for further care under more controlled circumstances.

Children with evidence of intraperitoneal hemorrhage documented by CT to be hepatic in origin will usually have spontaneous healing of the organ. These injuries occasionally result in abscesses or hematobilia. As long as the child remains hemodynamically stable, no emergent surgical intervention is necessary. Between these two extremes are those children with significant hepatic disruption that require careful management of fluid volume and red blood cell mass. These are the patients at risk of sudden exsanguination, and they require scrupulous monitoring in a unit prepared for immediate surgical intervention if so indicated.

Pancreatic/Duodenal Injuries

High-speed deceleration (such as ejection from a vehicle or a seatbelt injury) or direct blows to the upper abdomen can produce pancreatic or duodenal trauma. The most commonly reported pancreatic lesions are fractures and severe contusions, usually in the midportion of the gland where it overlies the lumbar spine. This can present as relatively acute-onset peritonitis, or it can produce a posttraumatic pseudocyst that develops within days to weeks of injury. Duodenal injury can produce retroperitoneal leak as well as frank duodenal disruption. It should be considered in any abused child. Intramural duodenal hematoma is a lesion frequently seen in children who sustain blunt abdominal trauma. It commonly causes signs and symptoms of upper intestinal obstruction. As with pancreatic injuries, a high index of suspicion is the key to expedient and accurate recognition.

Intestinal Injuries

The intestine can be perforated by deceleration trauma. This is commonly associated with lap belt injuries and can present with evidence of abdominal wall contusion or lumbar vertebral blowout (Chance) fracture. Intestinal perforation can present immediately with free air, notable on abdominal radiographs, or it can emerge with the evolution of bacterial peritonitis during a period of 12 to 24 hours.

Careful clinical evaluation for at least 24 hours is critical for accurate and timely diagnosis of these injuries in any child considered to be at risk. Because there is no absolutely reliable imaging modality for confirmation of this diagnosis, every child considered at risk for gastrointestinal injury must be monitored for at least 24 hours. Abdominal pain that worsens or persists beyond this period must be explained before the child can be cleared for release. This might require repeat CT with enteric contrast, laparoscopy, or laparotomy based on interpretation of physical findings. Such a progression of clinical evaluation requires that the surgeon responsible for the patient's trauma care evaluate the child on arrival to establish the baseline to which subsequent examinations will be compared.

Genitourinary Injuries

Potential damage to the genitourinary system must be considered in the evaluation of every child with abdominal or multiple trauma injuries. Like hepatic and splenic injuries, most renal lesions will heal without surgical intervention (**Figure 6.28**). Those that require emergent surgery usually involve major renal pedicle disruptions with perinephric hematomas (grade 5) and complete loss of renal function (**Figure 6.29**).

The challenge facing the physician responsible for initial assessment and stabilization is the clinical determination of significant genitourinary injury and the most efficacious method for evaluation. Because most renal injuries involve minor, self-limited contusions, extensive and expensive evaluations can be clinically irrelevant. The combination of significant flank trauma, abdominal injury, and hematuria (even microscopic) in an injured child is an indication for a CT scan with IV contrast to assess bilateral function and absence of extravasation. Lower urinary tract disruption occurs primarily in association with severe pelvic trauma, the prototype of which

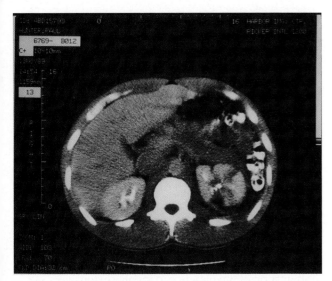

Figure 6.28 Computed tomographic scan of the abdomen showing a large left renal laceration (right side of image) with a urinoma. Although large, this laceration healed without surgical intervention.

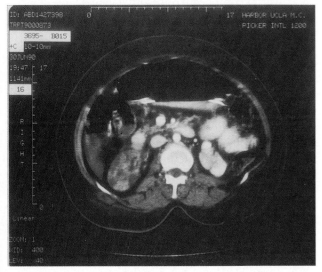

Figure 6.29 Computed tomographic scan of the abdomen showing a devascularized right kidney (left side of image) from blunt trauma to the abdomen. Immediate surgical intervention to revascularize the kidney is indicated.

is the straddle (bicycle) injury. A child who has blood at the urethral meatus requires retrograde urethrography to determine whether a lower urinary tract injury is present. Potential bladder injuries should be assessed with a CT cystogram or formal cystogram after a urethrogram.

Burns

According to the Burn Foundation, an estimated 250,000 children sustain burn-related injuries annually. Scald injuries are more commonly seen in young children and can be a result of intentional injury. Flame-related injuries more often occur in older children, including those playing with lighters or matches or stoking fires with flammable liquids.

Thermal injuries can be stratified as first, second, third, or fourth degree or, more preferably, as partial thickness and full thickness. First-degree burns (eg, sunburn) are characterized by erythema and pain with no loss of epidermal integrity. Although first-degree burns generally do not require IV fluid replacement, the presence of extensive body surface sunburn in an infant or toddler might require hospitalization for fluid replacement.

Second-degree or partial-thickness burns are characterized by a red or mottled appearance. They are recognized by blister formation or a moist, weeping appearance if the epidermis has already sloughed. Because both first-degree and second-degree burns involve partial-thickness destruction, they are painful, especially when exposed to air because of tissue desiccation.

Third-degree or full-thickness burns are dark and leathery, mottled, or white and waxy. If the surface is red, it will not blanch with pressure. These full-thickness burns are dry and lack sensation. Fourth-degree burns are rare and most common with high-voltage electrical injuries. These burns involve tissues deep into the skin.

Burn depth determines whether epithelialization will occur. Partial-thickness burns are capable of healing, but deep partial-thickness burns can take up to 6 weeks to heal and are more inclined to form hypertrophic scars. Determining burn depth can be difficult, even for experienced burn care practitioners. Burns that appear shallow immediately after injury can ultimately prove to be deeper. Burns that tend to convert to deeper injuries include scald burns, grease burns, and burns that become infected.[32]

Partial-thickness burns heal through the regeneration of the epidermis by the epidermal appendages (hair follicles, sweat glands). Superficial partial-thickness burns do not require grafting but might benefit from the placement of biologic dressings (eg, TransCyte).[33,34] Healing is often complete in 2 weeks or less. Deep partial-thickness burns will take more than 2 weeks to heal and generally benefit from the placement of either biologic dressings or skin grafting. Full-thickness injuries will not regenerate because the epidermal appendages are destroyed. Skin grafting is required unless the injury is minor.

Temperature and duration of contact determine the depth of tissue injury. This is demonstrated best in scald injuries. At 44°C (111°F), cellular destruction will not occur for approximately 6 hours of contact in adults and older children. A typical setting in the United States for a hot water heater is 60°C to 65°C (140°F to 149°F), and water at this temperature will produce a full-thickness burn in as little as 2 to 5 seconds. Lowering the temperature to 54°C (130°F) will prolong exposure time to 30 seconds to produce a full-thickness burn, and lowering it further to 49°C (120°F) prolongs this time to 5 minutes.[35]

Different types of thermal exposure have different effects. Flash injuries dissipate a large amount of heat for a short duration. They usually are partial-thickness burns. Flame burns can produce high temperature with prolonged contact and are associated with the highest risk of serious full-thickness injury. Contact burns from hot metal, including radiators, floor heating grates, oven racks, and irons, often produce full-thickness burns with a cutaneous pattern corresponding to the agent of injury.

Smoke inhalation, carbon monoxide poisoning, and airway edema with respiratory compromise are the most common causes of early death after a burn injury. After the first few hours, shock is usually the most common cause of death. Burns involving more than 30% of the body surface area result in a generalized increased capillary permeability. The extravasation of large amounts of fluid into the extravascular space results in hypovolemia, hypoperfusion, and diffuse peripheral edema that affects both burned and unburned tissues. Thermal effects can also result in the destruction of red blood cells. Electrical injuries, burns associated with soft tissue trauma, and those associated with prolonged immobilization of the patient can involve extensive destruction of muscle tissues potentially resulting in myoglobinuria and renal failure. Gastrointestinal ileus can complicate burns involving a large body surface area.

Diagnostic Studies

Laboratory

Children suspected of having an inhalation injury should have arterial blood gases and carboxyhemoglobin level measured. Carboxyhemoglobin levels elevate with significant inhalation injuries. Indications for intubation include persistent or worsening respiratory distress, a Pa_{O_2} less than 60 mm Hg, or a Pa_{CO_2} greater than 50 mm Hg in the face of optimal conservative management.

Radiology

Children suspected of having inhalation injury should receive an initial chest radiograph, although this will usually be normal in the first few hours after injury. If the child was injured in a car crash, jumped from a burning building, or was involved in an explosion, there is a chance of coexisting multiple injuries; additional screening radiographs might be indicated to rule out specific injuries.

Management

The upper airway is susceptible to obstruction as a result of exposure to superheated air. Except in severe cases, the subglottic airway is usually protected from direct thermal injury by the larynx. Facial burns, singed nasal hairs and eyebrows, carbonaceous deposits in the oral pharynx, carbonaceous sputum, oropharyngeal edema, history of impaired mentation, confinement in a burning environment, voice change, hoarseness, or persistent coughing can indicate inhalation injury or burns.[36]

Initial signs can be subtle. However, progressive airway edema can occur with fluid resuscitation, requiring ongoing evaluation. The small diameter of an infant's and child's airway requires ongoing vigilance and lowers the threshold for intubation. Oxygen should be administered via a nonrebreather mask for any suspected inhalation injury and to treat carbon monoxide inhalation.

Estimating burn depth is classified as previously described by degree or by partial or full thickness. First-degree burns are not included in standard resuscitation formulas. The Lund and Browder chart divides the body surface into areas by percentage (**Figure 6.30**). In adults, the rule of nines is an easy way to determine body surface area (**Figure 6.31**). However, this formula is modified in children because of the disproportionate size of the child's head and neck relative to lower extremities. The Lund and Browder chart is typically used for children 10 years and younger. The palm of the patient's hand (including the fingers) represents approximately 1% of the child's body surface.

The Parkland formula is the most common method of determining fluid resuscitation after a burn. It is intended only as a guide to initiate fluid resuscitation. Continued fluid requirements are dictated by the physiologic status of the patient.

On the basis of this formula, the patient receives 2 to 4 mL of LR solution per percentage of burn multiplied by the child's weight in kilograms. The Parkland formula does not include maintenance fluid requirements in a child, so these must be added. Half of the resuscitation fluid is administered during the first 8 hours, with the remainder given during the next 16 hours. Colloid and blood are not routinely given in the first 24 hours after a burn, but in severe burns the judicious use of albumin might be worthwhile. A dose of 1 g/kg can be administered as a bolus over 30 to 90 minutes.

Nasogastric tubes are indicated in patients with burns involving more than 25% of total body surface area. In burns less than 25% of the total body surface area, a nasogastric tube should be inserted if the child experiences nausea, vomiting, or abdominal distention. If possible, nasogastric or nasojejunal tube feeding should be initiated once the child has stabilized within hours of admission.

Children with burns exceeding 15% of estimated body surface area require IV fluid resuscitation. Intravenous lines should be established peripherally, preferably in an unburned upper extremity. If the burns are extensive, the catheter can be placed in any accessible vein. Burn patients are more prone to phlebitis and septic phlebitis in saphenous veins. Fluid replacement is based on an accurate body weight, and the child should be weighed without dressings or clothing as soon as feasible.

Consideration should be given to insertion of a Foley catheter if fluid resuscitation is needed. In thermal, scald, or contact burns, a urine output of 1 to 2 mL/kg per hour is desired, up to a maximum of 30 to 40 mL per hour. If a patient sustains an electrical burn, a urine output of twice that goal is desired because of the increased incidence of myoglobinuria and subsequent renal failure. Resuscitation fluids can be titrated up or down, depending on the ongoing physiologic status of the patient and the adequacy of urine output. If urine output becomes excessive, the rate of fluid infusion should be decreased.

Initial Burn Wound Care

The first principle in burn wound management is to "stop the fire." All clothing should be

Region	%
Head	
Neck	
Ant. Trunk	
Post. Trunk	
Right arm	
Left arm	
Buttocks	
Genitalia	
Right leg	
Left leg	
Total burn	

Relative percentages of body surface area affected by growth

Age (years)	A (half of head)	B (half of one thigh)	C (half of one leg)
0	9.5	2.75	2.5
1	8.5	3.25	2.5
5	6.5	4	2.75
10	5.5	4.25	3
15	4.5	4.5	3.25
Adult	3.5	4.75	3.5

Figure 6.30 The Lund and Browder chart.

Adapted from Lund, CC and Browder, NC. *Surg. Gynecol. Obstet.* 1944;79:352–358.

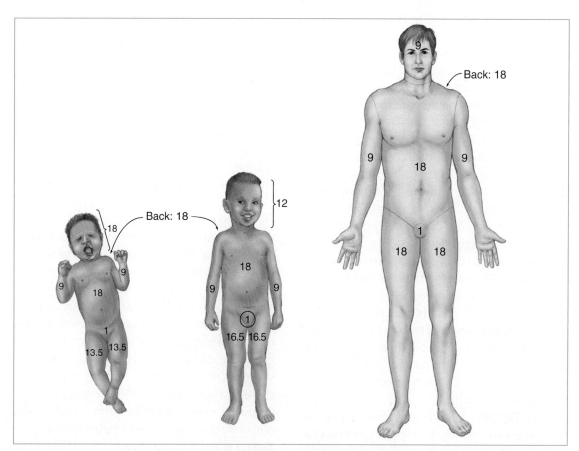

Figure 6.31 The rule of nines is a quick way to estimate the amount of surface area that has been burned. It divides the body into sections, each representing approximately 9% of the total body surface area. The proportions differ for infants, children, and adults.

removed in the resuscitation area. Some synthetic fabrics can melt into hot plastic residue and continue to burn the patient. Because undue exposure can result in hypothermia, heat lamps should be used to maintain optimal temperature. Rings and jewelry should be removed and retained to give to the child's family.

History taking must elicit information and details regarding the circumstances of the injury, specifically where it occurred and whether the patient was using alcohol or drugs at the time. Two historical points that are especially relevant are whether the patient was inside or outside a building and whether potential additional injury might have occurred as a result of attempts at escape or rescue. Illnesses, medications, allergies, and immunization status are also critical factors that can influence initial care.

The wound should be cleansed with saline. Blisters should be left intact because they serve as a biologic sterile dressing. Dead skin can be débrided with moist gauze or surgical instruments.

Analgesia and sedation can be administered after resuscitation is begun. Large wounds might require large doses of narcotics to comfort the patient. Initial dosing should be in small increments with careful monitoring of heart rate, respiration, and blood pressure. Guidelines are presented in Table 6-12.

TABLE 6-12 Commonly Used Sedatives and Analgesics for Burn Patients	
Drug	Dosage
Fentanyl	1 to 2 mcg/kg IV
Morphine	0.1 to 0.2 mg/kg IV/IM
Midazolam (Versed)	0.05 to 0.2 mg/kg IV/IM
Lorazepam (Ativan)	0.1 mg/kg IV
Ketamine	1 to 2 mg/kg per dose IV 3 to 5 mg/kg IM
Abbreviations: IM, intramuscularly; IV, intravenously.	

After débridement and initial cleansing, further care will be dictated by whether the child is at the final destination. Children who will be transferred to another institution might simply have their wounds dressed with saline, sterile gauze, and bulky dressings. Covering the wounds reduces the pain. Children who are already at a center prepared to care for burn wounds will require a topical antimicrobial agent. Bacitracin ointment can be used on facial burns, whereas silver sulfadiazine is the topical agent of choice for partial-thickness and full-thickness wounds elsewhere on the body. Burns to the ears that are partial thickness or full thickness and might involve cartilage are treated with mafenide acetate (Sulfamylon). However, both silver sulfadiazine and mafenide acetate contain sulfa and should be avoided in patients with sulfa allergy or glucose-6-phosphate dehydrogenase deficiency. Pillows should be avoided in favor of elevating the head of the bed.

The use of systemic antibiotics rarely is indicated in the initial management of the burn wound. Tetanus immunization should be brought up to date.

Circumferential Full-Thickness Burns

Circumferential burns can pose a unique problem. With fluid resuscitation, edema develops beneath the unyielding burn eschar and pressure builds. Decreased or absent distal perfusion of the extremity can occur within the first 12 to 24 hours after the injury. Signs include cyanosis, impaired capillary refill, paresthesias, and pain. If the torso is circumferentially burned, respiratory compromise can be profound. Early escharotomy should be considered. This usually is a problem only with full-thickness burns, but deep partial-thickness burns can occasionally cause distal ischemia.

Escharotomy and Fasciotomy

It is important to evaluate the overall status of perfusion serially with Doppler ultrasonography. When signs of decreasing flow are present, longitudinal incisions (escharotomies) should be made on the medial and lateral aspects of the extremity. Incisions must be carried across involved joints. Incise to a depth that allows separation of the cut edges of eschar. This often will decrease the elevated compartment pressure and enhance peripheral circulation. The eschar of a third-degree burn is insensate and does not require local or general anesthesia for escharotomy. This can be done at the bedside. The thorax and abdomen also can sustain extensive full-thickness injury, resulting in respiratory insufficiency. Escharotomies on the chest, back, and abdomen can facilitate more adequate ventilation. Fasciotomy might be necessary with electrical burns to salvage an extremity because of the incidence of deep muscle damage and edema within a fascial compartment. Fasciotomy should be performed in an operating room.

Pitfalls in Burn Care

Failure to recognize a respiratory or inhalation component of a burn that occurred in an enclosed space, or any associated multiple trauma, can result in a major catastrophe. Avoid underestimation of burn size and depth by approaching the assessment in a disciplined manner. The Parkland formula and others are just the starting point. Ongoing fluid therapy must be titrated to effect. The extent of the burn depth or the possibility of later grafting is not predictable at the time of initial assessment. It is best to be cautious about prognosis.

Nonrecognition of myoglobinuria or hemoglobinuria and the need for alkalinization of the urine can lead to renal failure. Failure to perform escharotomy and fasciotomy when appropriate can lead to respiratory compromise or loss of an extremity.

Guidelines for Triage and Disposition

The guidelines in Table 6-13 determine transfer to a burn center. If there is any doubt, admit a burned child to the hospital. Apply these guidelines based on the circumstances of each patient, including age, preexisting medical conditions, extent and nature of thermal injury, and social circumstances involved.

Transfer to a major burn center can be facilitated through direct telephone communication between the referring and receiving physicians. Preexisting transfer plans are helpful. Maintain adequate records to provide continuity in observation and care. Before a patient leaves the primary facility, prepare him or her for transport with a secure airway, functioning IV catheter, nasogastric tube, urinary catheter, proper burn dressing, and adequate analgesia. All pertinent information regarding tests, temperature, pulse,

fluid administration, and urine output should be recorded and sent with the patient. Radiographs taken during assessment should also be sent.

Electrical Trauma

A number of factors determine the effect of electrical current on the body, including the following:

- Resistance: wet skin or water immersion decreases resistance precipitously, thereby increasing current delivered to tissue but resulting in few surface burns.

TABLE 6-13 Criteria for the Transfer of Patients With Burn Injuries

1. Partial-thickness and full-thickness burns >10% of the total body surface area (BSA) in patients <10 years or >50 years of age
2. Partial-thickness and full-thickness burns >20% BSA in other age groups
3. Partial-thickness and full-thickness burns involving the face, eyes, ears, hands, feet, genitalia, or perineum or those that involve skin overlying major joints
4. Full-thickness burns >5% BSA in any age group
5. Significant electrical burns, including lightning injury (significant volumes of tissue beneath the surface might be injured and result in acute renal failure and other complications)
6. Significant chemical burn
7. Inhalation injury
8. Burn injury in patients with preexisting illness that could complicate management, prolong recovery, or affect mortality
9. Any burn patient in whom concomitant trauma poses an increased risk of morbidity or mortality can be treated initially in a trauma center until stable before transfer
10. Children with burns seen in hospitals without qualified personnel or equipment for their care should be transferred to a burn center with these capabilities
11. Burn injury in patients who will require special social and emotional or long-term rehabilitative support, including cases involving suspected child abuse and neglect

Adapted from: Committee on Trauma American College of Surgeons. *Resources for Optimal Care of the Injured Patient.* Chicago, IL: American College of Surgeons; 2008.

In contrast, in and around tissue with high resistance, such as calluses, more heat will evolve, resulting in cellular necrosis and worse surface burns.

- Current type: alternating current is much more dangerous at lower voltage than direct current and can result in ventricular fibrillation at very low voltage. Alternating current also causes tetanic muscle contractions that make many electrical injury patients unable to "let go" after contact with a circuit.
- Current pathway: current follows the pathway of least resistance from contact point to the ground. Current that crosses the heart or brain is most dangerous.

The most frequent and serious problems involved in electrical injury include third-degree or fourth-degree cutaneous burns, cardiopulmonary arrest or injury, associated physical trauma, infection of burned tissue, myoglobinuria, and third-space loss with renal injury, neurologic injury, tympanic membrane rupture, cataracts, and peripheral vessel occlusion.

Four types of electrical burn injury can occur, as follows:

- Direct injury from contact with the electrical source
- Flash burn (similar to a gas flame flash burn)
- Arc burn (measured at 2,500°C [4,532°F])
- Flame injury from ignition of clothing

In addition, blunt injury can occur if a person is thrown by the intense muscle spasm that can be triggered by the electrical current or from falls

Prolonged hypotension and massive muscle necrosis predispose the electrical burn patient to severe infections, which are the most common causes of death among those who are successfully resuscitated. Although electrical injury patients can have minimal external manifestations, extensive underlying tissue damage and occult trauma often exist and should be presumed to be present until proved otherwise.[37] In patients injured by generated electrical power sources, care must be taken by rescuers to avoid injury to themselves

Lightning injuries, which follow the same laws of physics as other electrical injuries, usually present somewhat differently.[37,38] Patients struck by lightning rarely have external or deep internal burn injuries. Cardiac arrest is the main cause of death, although permanent neurologic sequelae often occur in those who survive the initial incident. Lightning injuries rarely have associated myoglobinuria, and fluid resuscitation might not be necessary unless there are massive burns.

Management

In addition to the standard protocols described in earlier sections of this chapter, there are special characteristics of initial care of the child with an electrical burn. Hypotension is usually secondary to hypovolemia and is treated with a crystalloid fluid challenge of 20 mL/kg, which can be repeated as necessary. If a pressor agent is needed to achieve adequate perfusion, low-dose dopamine is the agent of choice because of its beneficial effect on renal perfusion

Pay special attention to potential intracranial injury; entrance and exit burn wounds; signs of intra-abdominal hemorrhage, peritonitis, or ileus; evidence of fractures or dislocations; and diminished or absent pulses. Assess the patient for signs of blunt injury that can occur as a result of a fall or being thrown by intense muscle spasm. Traditional burn formulas frequently underestimate crystalloid requirements because they do not take into account the deep muscle injury typical of electrical burns and the massive third-space shift that can occur. Fasciotomies, not just escharotomies, will be necessary to treat a compartment syndrome.

An indwelling urinary catheter to monitor urine output and a central venous catheter can be useful. Blood transfusion usually is not required within the first 24 hours of care unless there is ongoing occult hemorrhage. Cardiac dysrhythmias, acidosis secondary to muscle necrosis, renal injury, and gastric dilation might be encountered. If myoglobinuria is present, the goal of fluid resuscitation should be a urine output of 1 to 1.5 mL/kg per hour while the urine is pigmented and 0.5 to 1 mL/kg per hour after the urine clears. Sodium bicarbonate can be added to half NS (or more dilute crystalloid solutions) to promote alkalinization of the blood to pH 7.35 to 7.40, which will help prevent the precipitation of myoglobin in the renal tubules. Mannitol (0.25 to 0.5 g/kg IV bolus followed by continuous infusion at 0.25 to 0.5 g/kg per hour) might be indicated to enhance renal perfusion and avoid myoglobinuric renal failure, one of the main causes of death in the past

Because lightning injuries seldom involve deep injuries or myoglobinuria, fluid loading, osmotic diuresis, and fasciotomies rarely are needed.

Disposition

Electrical burns are considered major burns according to the American Burn Association classification system. Transfer to a burn center is appropriate for all seriously injured patients

Admission to the hospital is recommended for severe electrical burns. However, for the stable patient with relatively isolated burns, including lip burns, studies have shown that the patient can be safely released after 4 hours of observation in the ED, provided caretakers are instructed regarding proper methods for controlling late hemorrhage, which can occur from the labial artery.[35]

Cardiac monitoring is controversial. Those with low-voltage electrical injuries probably can be safely discharged if they display no mental status changes or cardiac dysrhythmias. Creatinine phosphokinase level has no relationship to the amount of burn or to the overall prognosis of the electrically injured patient.

Surgical consultation or follow-up is necessary for electrical injury patients. For cases of arc burns to the lip, consultation or follow-up with an experienced oral or plastic surgeon is necessary because severe bleeding can occur when the burn eschar separates from the underlying labial artery (usually 5 to 9 days after the injury) and because long-term splinting, particularly when the burn involves the commissure, might be necessary to avoid microstomia. Growth retardation of the mandible, maxilla, or dentition can occur.

Patients struck by lightning can present more as cardiac or neurologic emergencies than as burn or trauma patients. A baseline electrocardiogram is indicated. Changes include nonspecific ST-T wave changes, T-wave changes, axis shift, QT prolongation, and ST-segment elevation. Admission usually is indicated, but children with completely normal examination, laboratory test, and electrocardiography results can be discharged if there is adequate home observation and close follow-up.

> ### KEY POINTS
>
> **Management of Electrical Injury**
> - Begin crystalloid fluid challenge of 20 mL/kg; a central catheter might be useful.
> - Place an indwelling urinary catheter to monitor urine output.
> - Alkalize urine and force diuresis if myoglobinuria develops.
> - Consider pressor agents after adequate fluid resuscitation (dopamine).
> - Perform fasciotomies for deep muscle injury and compartment syndrome.
> - Perform ongoing assessments for intracranial injury, intra-abdominal injury, cardiac dysrhythmias, and compartment syndrome.

Other Burns

Abuse

An alarming number of children are subjected to maltreatment.[39] Intentional injury should be suspected and thoroughly investigated if there is evidence of any unusual pattern of the burn wound or if the history given does not explain the nature of the injury. A clenched fist and "gloved" forearm burn distribution and "stocking" or bilateral lower extremity and buttocks injuries suggest involuntary submersion (**Figure 6.32**). Cigarette and steam iron pattern burns are findings that warrant a social services investigation. See Chapter 7, Child Maltreatment.

Chemical Burns

Early management of most chemical burns, particularly strong acid and alkali burns, must include irrigation with copious amounts of water or saline to dilute any chemical substance. Alkali burns usually are more significant than acid injuries because they penetrate deep into the tissue, and they will require longer surface irrigation. Avoid self-injury by wearing gloves and protective clothing. After removal of all the chemical substance, the burn wound can be managed with débridement, applications of topical antibiotic creams, and dressings.

Summary

The continued development of increasingly sophisticated emergency medical systems has improved the quality of care for all pediatric injury patients by establishing evidence-based protocols of care, well-defined primary and

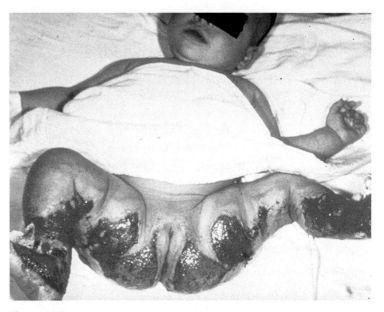

Figure 6.32 Lower extremity and buttock burn suggesting immersion injury from child abuse.

definitive care centers, and effective procedures for expeditious transfer. Predetermined referral patterns and transfer agreements facilitate, standardize, and regionalize optimal care for the injured child. The process is complex and relies on accurate clinical assessment, effective initial management, efficient communication, and complete integration of all components. No system will be better than its weakest part. In addition, no system will be effective if its various components are not applied in an orderly and timely manner. The key to success is a complete understanding of the nature of pediatric injury. Although this will not eliminate the injury, it will significantly enhance the likelihood that the patient will not just survive but will also enjoy a quality of life that is the birthright of every child.

Check Your Knowledge

1. Which of the following statements regarding secondary brain injury is correct?
   A. Begins to occur 6 hours after a primary traumatic brain insult
   B. Has no long-term consequences once corrected
   C. Most commonly due to respiratory failure and shock
   D. Occurs on the opposite side of the brain after a blow to the head
   E. Occurs rarely in children

2. Proper initial airway management of an agitated 6 year old rescued from a burning house who is noted to have singed nasal hairs and facial burns and responds to verbal stimulation by flailing all four extremities should be:
   A. humidified oxygen by nonrebreather mask until his agitation resolves.
   B. positive pressure ventilation by mask to avoid the need for intubation.
   C. nasal-tracheal intubation.
   D. oral tracheal intubation using sedation and paralysis after preoxygenation.
   E. immediate surgical airway.

3. The target Pa_{CO_2} for initial management of pediatric traumatic brain injury is:
   A. 15 mm Hg
   B. 25 mm Hg
   C. 35 mm Hg
   D. 45 mm Hg
   E. Does not matter

4. The fastest means to obtain emergency vascular access for volume replacement if a peripheral intravenous catheter is not promptly successful in a hypovolemic and hypotensive patient is:
   A. intraosseous needle insertion.
   B. saphenous venous cutdown.
   C. internal jugular central venous access under ultrasonography guidance.
   D. femoral vein central venous access.
   E. nasogastric tube insertion.

5. Surgical evaluation is necessary for which of the following trauma patients?
   A. Child who has evidence of visceral disruption
   B. Child who is not hemodynamically stable
   C. Child who needs surgical treatment
   D. One whose injury mechanism or initial clinical findings suggest internal organ system derangement
   E. All of the above

References

1. Inon AE, Haller JA. Caring for the injured children of our world: A global perspective. *Surg Clin North Am.* 2002;82:435–445.
2. Carrico CJ, Holcomb JB, Chaudry IH. Scientific priorities and strategic planning for resuscitation research and life saving therapy following traumatic injury: Report of the PULSE trauma workgroup. *Ann Emerg Med.* 2002;9:621–626.
3. *National Pediatric Trauma Registry.* Boston, MA: New England Medical Center; 2000.
4. Rifkinson-Mann S. Head injuries in infants and young children. *Cont Neurosurgery.* 1993;15:1–6.
5. Patel JC, Tepas JJ, Mollitt DL, Pieper P. Pediatric cervical spine injuries: Defining the disease. *J Pediatr Surg.* 2001;36:373–376.
6. Stafford PW, Blinman TA, Nance ML. Practical points in evaluation and resuscitation of the injured child. *Surg Clin North Am.* 2002;82:273–301.

7. Rossaint R, Bouillon B, Cerny V, et al. Management of bleeding following major trauma: An updated European guideline. *Crit Care.* 2010;14:R52.

8. Bruce DA, Alavi A, Bilaniuk L, Dolinskas C, Obrist W, Uzzell B. Diffuse cerebral swelling following head injuries in children: The syndrome of "malignant brain edema." *J Neurosurgery.* 1981;54:170–178.

9. Pigula FA, Wald SL, Shackford SR, Vane DW. The effect of hypotension and hypoxia on children with severe head injuries. *J Pediatr Surg.* 1993;28:310–314.

10. Muizelaar JP, Marmarou A, DeSallesa AAF, et al. Cerebral blood flow and metabolism in severelyhead-injured children, Part I: Relationship with GCS score, outcome, ICP and PVI. *J Neurosurgery.* 1989;71:63–71.

11. Kitchens J, Groff DB, Nagaraj HS, Fallat ME. Basilar skull fractures in childhood with cranial nerve involvement. *J Pediatr Surg.* 1991;26:992–994.

12. Schutzman SA, Greenes DS. Pediatric minor trauma. *Ann Emerg Med.* 2001;37:65–74.

13. Halstead ME, Walter KD, American Academy of Pediatrics Council on Sports Medicine and Fitness. Clinical report sport-related concussion in children and adolescents. *Pediatrics.* 2010;126:597–615.

14. Kuppermann N, Holmes JF, Dayan PS, et al. Identification of children at very low risk of clinically-important brain injuries after head trauma: A prospective cohort study. *The Lancet.* 2009;374:1160–1170.

15. Duhaime AC, Alario AJ, Lewander WJ, et al. Head injury in very young children: Mechanisms, injury types, and opthalmologic findings in 100 hospitalized patients younger than 2 years of age. *Pediatrics.* 1992;90:179–185.

16. Brain Trauma Foundation. *Guidelines for the Management of Severe Traumatic Brain Injury.* 3rd ed. New York, NY: Brain Trauma Foundation; 2007.

17. Bonadio WA. Cervical spine trauma in children: Part II. Mechanisms and manifestations of injury, therapeutic considerations. *Am J Emerg Med.* 1993;11:256–278.

18. McSwain ME Jr, Gamelli RL. *Helmet Removal From Injured Patients* [poster]. Chicago, IL: American College of Surgeons, Committee on Trauma; 1997.

19. Curran C, Dietrich AM, Bowman MJ, Ginn-Pease ME, King DR, Kosnik E. Pediatric cervical-spine immobilization: Achieving neutral position? *J Trauma.* 1995;39:729–732.

20. Nypaver M, Treloar D. Neutral cervical spine positioning in children. *Ann Emerg Med.* 1994;23:208–211.

21. Bracken MB, Shepard MJ, Collins WF, et al. A randomized, controlled trial of methylprednisolone or naloxone in the treatment of acute spinal-cord injury. Results of the Second National Acute Spinal-Cord Injury Study. *N Engl J Med.* 1990;322:1405–1411.

22. Bracken MB, Shepard MJ, Holford T, et al. Administration of methylprednisolone for 24 or 48 hours or tirilazad mesylate for 48 hours in the treatment of acute spinal cord injury. *JAMA.* 1997;277:1597–1604.

23. Prendergast MR, Sake JM, Ledgerwood AM, Lucas CE, Lucas WF. Massive steroids do not reduce the zone of injury after penetrating spinal cord injury. *J Trauma.* 1994;37:576–580.

24. Short D. Is the role of steroids in acute spinal cord injury now resolved? *Curr Opin Neurol.* 2001;14:759–763.

25. Bonadio WA. Cervical spine trauma in children: Part I. General concepts, normal anatomy, radiographic evaluation. *Am J Emerg Med.* 1993;11:158–165.

26. Laham JL, Cotcamp DH, Gibbons PA, Kahana MD, Crone KR. Isolated head injuries versus multiple trauma in pediatric patients: Do the same indications for cervical spine evaluation apply? *Pediatr Neurosurg.* 1994;21:221–226.

27. Pang D, Pollack IF. Spinal cord injury without radiographic abnormality in children—the SCIWORA syndrome. *J Trauma.* 1989;29:654–664.

28. Panacek EA, Mower WR, Holmes JF, Hoffman JR, for the NEXUS Group. Test performance of the individual NEXUS low-risk clinical screening criteria for cervical spine injury. *Ann Emerg Med.* 2001;38:22–25.

29. Leonard JC, Kuppermann N, Olsen C, et al. Factors associated with cervical spine injury in children after blunt trauma. *Ann Emerg Med.* In press. 2010 Oct 28.

30. Ruge JR, Sinson GP, McLone DG, Cerullo LJ. Pediatric spinal injury: The very young. *J Neurosurg.* 1988;68:25–31.

31. Brown RL, Brunn MA, Garcia VF. Cervical spine injuries in children: A review of 103 patients treated consecutively at a level 1 pediatric trauma center. *J Pediatr Surg.* 2001;36:1107–1114.

32. Gibran NS, Heimbach DM. Current status of burn wound pathophysiology. *Clin Plast Surg.* 2000;27:11–22.

33. Lukish JR, Eichelberger MR, Newman KD, et al. The use of a bioactive skin substitute decreases length of stay for pediatric burn patients. *J Pediatr Surg.* 2001;36:1118–1121.

34. Jones I, Currie L, Martin R. A guide to biological skin substitutes. *Br J Plast Surg.* 2002;55:185–193.

35. Fallat ME, Rengers SJ. The effect of education and safety devices on scald burn prevention. *J Trauma.* 1993;34:560–564.

36. Monafo WW. Initial management of burns. *N Engl J Med.* 1996;335:1581–1586.

37. Andrews CJ, Cooper MA, ten Duis HJ, et al. The pathology of electrical and lightning injuries. In: Wecht CJ, ed. *Forensic Sciences.* New York, NY: Matthew Bender and Co; 1995.

38. Cooper MA, Andrews CJ. Lightning injuries. In: Auerbach P, ed. *Wilderness Medicine: Management of Wilderness and Environmental Emergencies.* 3rd ed. St. Louis, MO: Mosby-Year Book; 1995:261–289.

39. Lenoski EF, Hunter KA. Specific problems of inflicted burn injuries. *J Trauma.* 1977;17:842–846.

A 5-year-old boy is struck by a car while crossing the street. Paramedics find the boy unconscious and lying in the middle of the street approximately 5 m from the vehicle. They begin an initial assessment using the Pediatric Assessment Triangle: Appearance: unconscious, not responsive to surroundings; work of Breathing: tachypneic, with no retractions; and Circulation: pale color and delayed capillary refill time. The paramedics stabilize the cervical spine, administer 100% oxygen by face mask, obtain intravenous access in the right antecubital fossa en route to the hospital, and infuse 500 mL of normal saline.

On arrival in the emergency department, the patient's airway is open, there are increased secretions, and the trachea is midline. There is symmetric chest wall motion and poor tidal volume with no retractions, and breath sounds are equal. The child's color is pale, and the skin is diaphoretic. There is no jugular venous distention, and capillary refill time is 4 seconds. The heart rate is 160/min with a thready peripheral pulse quality. Blood pressure is 75 by palpation. The abdomen is distended and tense on palpation, and the pelvis is stable. The anal sphincter is intact, and results of the stool test are negative for occult blood. The patient remains unconscious. There is no spontaneous eye opening. He responds to painful stimuli with flexor posturing. Pupils are midposition, 4 mm bilaterally, and sluggishly reactive to light. He has a contusion on the forehead, an abrasion on the left arm with swelling at the level of the elbow, an abrasion on the left flank, and deformity on the left femur.

1. *What is the physiologic status of this child?*
2. *What are your initial management priorities?*
3. *Does this patient meet an indication for surgery?*

What is the physiologic status of this child?
- Hypovolemic shock—decompensated

What are your initial management priorities?
- Contact surgeon (nurse or clerk to call with critical information based on primary [initial] survey).
- Suction airway.
- Begin rapid sequence intubation (indications of decompensated shock and need for neurologic resuscitation, low Glasgow Coma Scale Score).
- Administer etomidate, lidocaine (lignocaine), succinylcholine (suxamethonium) or rocuronium, followed by lorazepam for continued sedation.
- Etomidate is the sedative of choice in the hypotensive pediatric trauma patient.
- Obtain vascular access in at least two sites (prefer antecubital fossa).

- Resuscitate with normal saline, 40 mL/kg, followed by packed red blood cells (PRBCs) at 10 mL/kg.
- Perform radiography:
  - Chest: normal
  - Anteroposterior pelvis: normal
  - C-spine series: normal
- Obtain blood for type and cross-match (priority) if able, then measure hemoglobin, electrolytes, amylase, and glucose levels, prothrombin time, and partial thromboplastin time; perform renal and liver function tests.
- Initial hemoglobin level of 10 g/dL decreases to 7 g/dL after initial resuscitation and then increases to 9 g/dL after 200 mL of PRBCs.
- Alanine aminotransferase level is 100 IU/L and aspartate aminotransferase level is 80 IU/L.
- Perform trauma examination.
- Place urinary catheter—dipstick positive for blood, microscopic evaluation with 50 RBC/hpf.
- Place nasogastric tube—drains gastric contents and air, no blood noted.
- Perform additional radiography:
  - Computed tomography (CT) of the head: normal
  - CT of the abdomen: liver and spleen lacerations (grade II); moderate blood in the peritoneal cavity; renal contusion but bilaterally functioning kidneys
  - Reassessment after two units of PRBCs and 800 mL of saline; heart rate, 120/min; patient more responsive
  - Family informed of patient's condition

Does this patient meet an indication for surgery?

Although the patient presented in decompensated shock, initial resuscitation stabilized the patient. This patient now requires further care in a pediatric intensive care unit.

chapter 7

Child Maltreatment

Carol D. Berkowitz, MD, FAAP, FACEP
Meta L. Carroll, MD, FAAP, FACEP

Objectives

1 Describe common presentations of all forms of child maltreatment, including physical abuse, sexual abuse, child neglect, and Münchausen Syndrome by Proxy (MSBP).

2 Describe the clinical care and diagnostic studies that should be performed in suspected child maltreatment cases.

3 Explain the practitioner's responsibility in notifying authorities of suspected child maltreatment.

Chapter Outline

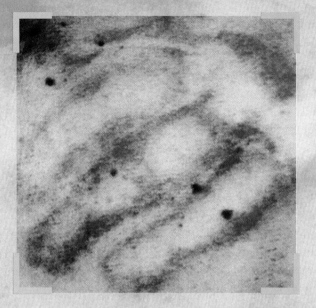

CASE SCENARIO 1

A 3-year-old boy is referred to the emergency department (ED) from his preschool because he has bruises on his face, left pinna, and lower back. The parents say the child is very active and frequently falls.

1. *What bruises commonly result from unintentional injury, and what bruises suggest inflicted trauma?*
2. *What are the appropriate diagnostic studies to evaluate suspected child physical abuse? How does the child's age affect what studies are obtained?*
3. *If inflicted trauma is suspected, what agencies must be notified to assist in the investigation?*

Introduction

Child maltreatment is defined by the Child Abuse Prevention and Treatment Act as "…any recent act or failure to act on the part of a parent or caretaker, which results in death, serious physical or emotional harm, sexual abuse or exploitation, or an act or failure to act which presents an imminent risk of serious harm."[1] Child maltreatment results from inappropriate or abnormal child-rearing practices and includes physical abuse, sexual abuse, emotional abuse, neglect, and Münchausen syndrome by proxy (MSBP).

Data from the US Department of Health and Human Services reveals approximately 3.3 million cases of child abuse and neglect annually, including 6 million cases reported to child protective services in 2006 through the National Child Abuse and Neglect Data System.[2] Of those, 905,000 children were determined to have been abused or neglected. The highest prevalence, in infants from birth to 1 year, was 24.4 cases per 1,000.[2] An estimated 1,530 children died of abuse or neglect. For each case of child maltreatment reported, it is estimated that there are one to two cases that go unrecognized.

The most vulnerable populations are infants, preverbal young children, children with chronic disease, and children with disabilities.

Factors that increase the risk of physical abuse to a child include social isolation, lack of family supports, chemical dependency, domestic violence, and poverty. However, physical abuse occurs within families of all cultural backgrounds and socioeconomic strata.

For many children, the ED is the point of entry into the health care system. Because some children with minor abuse injuries might be subsequently severely injured or killed, the practitioner working in this area must have a high level of suspicion for signs and symptoms associated with inflicted trauma. A classic report noted that nearly one-third of infants diagnosed as having abusive head trauma had been evaluated previously in an ED for symptoms unrecognized as being related to abuse.[3] The possibility of abuse should be considered with every traumatic injury treated. The practitioner should be alert to the possibility of maltreatment by any unexplained or poorly explained injury, evidence of neglect, delay in seeking appropriate medical care, or contradictory histories.

A multidisciplinary approach in which the practitioner works in cooperation with hospital-based medical staff, social workers, community-based child protective service workers and law enforcement personnel has become the model for the evaluation process. In a cooperative multidisciplinary milieu, the child benefits from the knowledge of a broad range of experts, the elimination of unnecessary duplicate interviews and examinations, and the avoidance of oversights that result when agencies work in isolation. Critical decisions affecting the child and the family are better made by a multidisciplinary team.

This chapter reviews in detail the major categories of child maltreatment: physical abuse, sexual abuse (including acute sexual assault), child neglect, and MSBP. In the ED, it is difficult to diagnose MSBP, a condition frequently associated with multiple hospitalizations and that requires the interaction of a multidisciplinary team for diagnosis.

Psychological or emotional abuse is also difficult to diagnose. Although psychological abuse can occur by itself, it is frequently associated with intentional physical injury and sexual abuse. Psychological injury is often responsible for the most serious long-term conditions and the cyclic intergenerational pattern of abuse.

Physical Abuse

Clinical Features and Assessment

Recognition of physical abuse is important for two reasons: (1) to accurately diagnose and manage the inflicted trauma and (2) to prevent further injury or death. Abuse occurs in all segments of the population. A careful history and a comprehensive physical examination is needed to detect the signs and symptoms of inflicted injuries.

To adequately evaluate abuse, the physician should follow the guidelines of listen, look, explain, evaluate, record, and report. Obtain a careful, complete history, including the precise details of how the injury occurred from both the caregiver and the child. Conflicting, vague, or evasive answers, and changing histories suggest abuse. Was the event witnessed? Does the child accuse the caregiver, or does the caregiver inappropriately blame the child, a sibling, or a third party for causing the injury? Does the caregiver protect his or her companion rather than the child? Is the child unusually fearful or withdrawn or overly friendly or trusting? Such patterns of behavior often suggest abuse. Does the child engage in pseudomature or seductive behavior, or does he or she voice age-inappropriate sexual verbalizations? This should raise suspicion of sexual abuse. Most importantly, is the history consistent with the injuries?

What are the circumstances surrounding the injury? When did the injury occur? And when did the caregiver seek medical help? Who brought the child to the hospital? Has the child been examined by his or her regular physician? Often, an abused child has been seen by different physicians to avoid raising suspicion about abuse. Is there a history of previous injuries or ingestions? Multiple prior injuries or a history of being "accident prone" can also be a marker of child abuse.

What is the behavior of the caregiver? Does this person seem under the influence of drugs or alcohol or bizarre in affect? Does the caregiver show appropriate concern for the condition of the child? Both lack of concern and excessive concern for a minor injury should raise suspicion. Does this person seem overly aggressive, unusually hostile, or excessively critical or demanding of the child or the practitioner? Does this person admit to being abused as a child? Individuals who were abused as children might be caught up in a pattern of intergenerational violence.

The goal of history taking is to create a detailed timeline, from the time the child last appeared well, to the onset of symptoms, until the present, noting all childcare settings and caretakers involved. In summary, key concerns in the medical history are as follows:

- Unusual aspects of the medical history, including a history from the child or parent inconsistent with the physical examination, a discrepancy between stories, injuries attributed to a young sibling, or a story that just does not make sense
- History describing a minor mishap that is inconsistent with a major injury
- History inconsistent with the developmental capability of the child (infants younger than 6 months rarely injure themselves, and even bruising in an infant is a red flag) (**Figure 7.1**)
- Delay in obtaining medical care or prior sporadic or inconsistent routine health care

There is a literature-based adage, "Those who don't cruise, don't bruise."[4] Common sense and a basic knowledge of motor milestones for infants and children will help in determining the likelihood that the injury occurred in the stated manner.

A complete medical history is essential and should include the following:

- General medical history, including past medical and surgical history, prior injuries and hospitalizations, current medications, allergies, complete review of systems, and current symptoms
- Social history, including identifying household members, domestic violence, substance abuse in the household, prior or current involvement with child protective services and/or police, and prior child maltreatment in the household

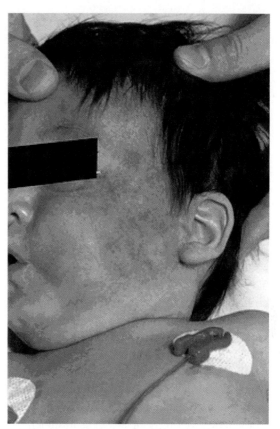

Figure 7.1 Even bruising in an infant should be a red flag.

- Behavioral history, including the description of any change in emotional status, learning problems, school problems, or other behavioral changes
- Developmental history to assess the child's achievement of milestones, current motor skills, and dexterity and to detect significant developmental delay

YOUR FIRST CLUE

Signs and Symptoms of Physical Abuse
- Historical features suggestive of physical abuse
- Inconsistent history
- Delay in seeking medical care
- History of mechanism of injury inconsistent with developmental age

Finally, for the injured child accompanied by a caregiver who has specific knowledge of the child maltreatment, obtain the name, address, and telephone number of the alleged perpetrator and his or her relationship to the child, information that will prove valuable to the investigation and help ensure the child's future safety.

Physical Examination

When obtaining the history or examining the injured child, note the child's interaction with the parent or caregiver. Is the child comfortable and happy in the caregiver's lap, or does the child avoid the caregiver and seek out each stranger who enters the room? Is the caregiver affectionate, concerned, and warm toward the child, or does he or she demonstrate no bonding or regard for the child?

The complete physical examination includes the child's general appearance and vital signs; height, weight, and head circumference in the infant or child who appears small for age, developmentally delayed, or neglected; head and neck examination, noting scalp swelling, fontanel fullness, bruising and petechiae on the face and ears, drainage from ears or nose, hemotympanum, bleeding around the nares, retinal hemorrhages, and abrasions or bruises on the neck; oropharynx examination, noting frenulum tears in the infant, as well as tongue bruising or bite marks, buccal mucosal bruising, and dental trauma; chest examination, identifying chest wall deformities and bruising; abdominal examination, noting distention, tenderness, bowel activity, and skin bruising or marks; genital examination, noting scars, bruises, lesions, abrasions, blood or discharge, and perianal tags, fissures, and bruising; back examination, noting tenderness and bruising; buttocks inspection, noting bruises, scars, patterned marks; examination of the extremities, noting deformity, neurovascular compromise, and bruising; and complete neurologic examination.

Bruises and Bites

The physically abused child might have injuries of the skin, soft tissue, bones, central nervous system, or internal organs. Ninety percent of such children have only superficial injuries, such as bruises, bites, lacerations, puncture marks, burns, or signs of strangulation. Common locations for bruises caused by abuse include the buttocks and lower back (from paddling, whipping, or spanking), genitalia and inner thighs (from punishment for masturbation or toilet training mishaps), cheeks (from slapping or grabbing), upper lip and frenulum of the tongue (from forced feeding or jamming the bottle in the mouth), neck (from strangulation), and ear lobes and pinnae (from boxing, pinching, and slapping). Injuries sustained from pinching, blows by a hand, or forceful grabbing of a child can appear as oval bruises, linear bruising, petechiae, or outlines of digits (**Figure 7.2**).

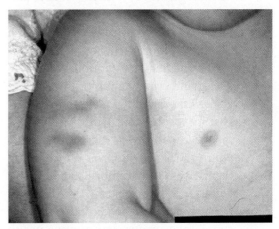

Figure 7.2 Human hand and fingertip marks can appear as oval bruises.

The dating of bruises is at best an inexact science. Although traditional teaching has described a predictable progression of bruise coloration (from red to blue, then green, yellow, and brown), the time required for the evolution of the bruise to ultimate healing is dependent on multiple factors. These factors include the depth and location of the injury, the nature of the particular tissue area and its blood supply, the skin complexion, and the presence of repetitively injured tissue. A superficial bruise can appear and heal more quickly, whereas a deep injury can take days to surface. A blow to an area of loose areolar tissue, around the eyes or genitals, can also bruise and heal more quickly than an area of dense tissue with well-supported blood vessels (eg, thigh or buttocks). A child whose skin is repetitively injured can also heal more quickly. The dark complexion of some children can hide bruising.[5–7]

Therefore, dating of bruises remains imprecise.[8]

Although analysis of bruise aging has great limitations, a physician should examine the abused child carefully, note the location, size, shape, and color of each bruise; include a written description of the bruises with an accompanying drawing or body diagram; and consider photography with a ruler and color wheel (for color standardization) in the frame.

A bruising clinical decision rule was recently developed to help discriminate physical child abuse from unintentional trauma. This rule demonstrated that bruises on the torso, ear, or neck for children 4 years or younger and bruises in any region for an infant younger than 4 months was 97% sensitive and 84% specific for predicting abuse.[9] The torso includes the chest, abdomen, back, buttocks, hip, and genitourinary region. A way to remember the areas of concerning bruising and ages for this rule is TEN-4.[9]

It is important to distinguish inflicted trauma from birthmarks, unintentional injuries, and bruises caused by coagulopathies. Unintentional bruises usually occur over bony prominences, especially the knees, shins, and foreheads of toddlers. Mongolian spots occur on the buttocks, back, and extremities in many infants, particularly black, Asian, Native American, and Hispanic infants (**Figure 7.3**). They are normal birthmarks and not bruises.

In addition, people of certain cultures, such as Southeast Asian, might use folk remedies that produce lesions that appear abusive (referred to as Caio gao, they can resemble ecchymoses or hematomas) but are well intentioned and are not fundamentally harmful.

Occasionally, excessive bruising might be due to bleeding dyscrasias, such as idiopathic thrombocytopenia or von Willebrand disease. Coagulation studies (prothrombin time, partial thromboplastin time, and platelet count) must be performed on all children with extensive bruises. Although a bleeding time was recommended in the past, this has been replaced by a platelet function analyzer test. Additional studies can be suggested as part of a forensic workup to eliminate rare disorders such as factor XIII (fibrin-stabilizing factor) deficiency, which might be associated with fatal intracranial hemorrhage.

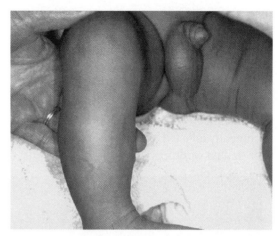

Figure 7.3 Mongolian spots appear on the buttocks, back, and extremities of many infants.

Bites inflicted by an adult on a child are always abusive and can be identified by the short linear patterned marks of an incomplete bite and oval or elliptical outlines with central bruising of a complete bite. When evaluating such a bite wound, seek the assistance of a forensic dentist, who will measure and document the bite and provide valuable assistance in matching the wound with an imprint of the perpetrator's teeth. A quick measurement that can help the emergency physician distinguish a bite inflicted by a child versus an adult is the width of the imprint left by the maxillary canine teeth. A measured width greater than 3 cm corresponds to an adult bite and, as such, constitutes abuse and should prompt reporting and investigation.[10]

Burns

Burns due to abuse are most commonly immersion burns, patterned contact burns, and cigarette burns. Burns that are deep and involve large areas of skin must be evaluated in the context of the history provided by the caregiver. Most concerning for abuse are immersion burns that characteristically have clearly demarcated edges. They can involve bilateral extremities or buttocks or demonstrate a stocking or glove distribution (**Figure 7.4**). Such injuries require communication with law enforcement officials, who will investigate the home and evaluate the tub, sink, taps, and water temperatures (Table 7-1). The multidisciplinary team then evaluates this information in light of the child's motor skills, the parent's history, and the distribution of burns on the child. The estimation of the severity and involved total body surface area of the burn will determine the need for patient transfer to a burn center for subspecialty care. Although uncommon, multisystem injury (eg, skeletal, head, abdominal) can accompany inflicted burn injury, warranting further trauma workup.

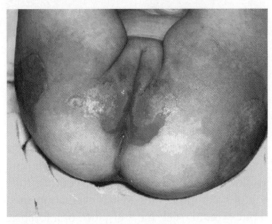

Figure 7.4 Immersion burn of the buttocks.

TABLE 7-1 Time and Temperature Required to Produce a Partial-Thickness and/or Full-Thickness Thermal Burn	
Temperature, °C (°F)	Time, seconds
54.4 (130)	10
57 (135)	4
60 (140)	1
64.9 (149)	0.5

Adapted from: Jenny C. Cutaneous manifestations of child abuse. In: Reece RM, Christian CW, eds. *Child Abuse: Medical Diagnosis and Management*. Elk Grove Village, IL: American Academy of Pediatrics; 2009:19–51.

Ambulatory young children might unintentionally come in contact with hot objects, such as steam irons or curling irons, particularly when left on floors or low tables within easy reach. The resultant burn involves a single site, causes immediate pain and withdrawal of the body part by the child, elicits a rapid response from the caregiver, and usually results in a more superficial injury. More concerning are deep or multiple patterned burns from such household objects—injuries that must be evaluated with caution because they are more likely to be inflicted by someone else.

Inflicted cigarette burns are usually deep, 8 to 10 mm in diameter, circular, multiple, and found on the hands and feet. When a child unintentionally comes into contact with the burning tip of a cigarette, the injury is single, more ovoid in shape (as the child brushes the cigarette tip), and superficial.

The most common burn scenario in children is injury due to the splash or spilling of hot liquids. Typically, young children will attempt to grasp a cup or container from a counter, table, or stovetop, splashing the hot liquid down onto the front of themselves, resulting in burns of the face, chest, and upper extremities. The area most severely burned is the site the liquid comes in contact with first. As the liquid runs down and heat dissipates, the resultant burn is less severe and leaves a pattern on the skin that demarcates the flow.[7]

Head Injuries

The most frequent cause of death in children who have been physically abused is head injury. In a series of patients admitted to the neurosurgical service at Children's Hospital of Philadelphia, at least 80% of the deaths due to head trauma in children younger than 2 years were the result of abuse. The average age of children with abusive head trauma is between 5 and 10 months.[11] One retrospective series found that one-third of all the children younger than 3 years with head injury were abused.[12] The abused infant or child with a head injury might be difficult to recognize because he or she might be brought into the ED for care of respiratory symptoms, poor feeding, lethargy, irritability, seizures, vomiting, listlessness, or reports of minor trauma. This absence of accurate history and lack of obvious external signs of injury can result in initial misdiagnosis (eg, viral syndrome or colic). In an analysis of missed cases of abusive head trauma, 31% of 173 abused children were initially seen by physicians who failed to make the correct diagnosis. More concerning, 15 of the patients were reinjured before identification of abusive head trauma.[3] Thus, in all infants and young children with head trauma, careful evaluation of the history, the caregiver, the child's motor development, and the child's examination is critical. Particular care must be taken with the head-injured infant not yet "cruising" or walking. This young group of patients, although under appropriate supervision, will rarely sustain severe brain injury due to nonintentional trauma.

The mechanisms of injury that have been described in abusive head trauma include (1) violent shaking of the infant, causing a "whiplash" movement of the head and delivering shearing forces to the brain and intracranial vessels that bridge the subdural space; (2) a violent impact as the infant's head is slammed against a firm surface (eg, crib, wall), delivering tremendous force with the abrupt deceleration of the head but providing no external physical evidence of the impact; and (3) a combination of the two.[11]

The presence of diffuse, multiple, and multi-layered retinal hemorrhages in the infant with head injury is highly associated with an abusive mechanism (**Figure 7.5**). Examination of the retinas using a traditional ophthalmoscope and performed by a nonophthalmologist can identify more than 75% of retinal hemorrhages when present. The use of mydriatic drops can greatly facilitate viewing the retina. However, consultation with a pediatric ophthalmologist is essential in obtaining the best possible examination of the retina (through dilated indirect ophthalmoscopy) that allows complete viewing of the retina to its edge (ora serrata) and detailed description of the extent, depth, number, and severity of hemorrhages. The ophthalmologist can also provide essential photographic documentation of retinal findings using a specialized retinal camera. Although the term retinal hemorrhage is nonspecific and nondiagnostic, an ophthalmologist's description of multiple hemorrhages throughout the retina that extend to the ora serrata in the presence of preretinal, vitreous, or subretinal hemorrhage is virtually pathognomonic of abusive head trauma (in the absence of a severe obvious nonintentional mechanism of injury or life-threatening central nervous system disease). Without pupillary dilatation, retinal viewing can be difficult and hemorrhages can go undetected. Thus, the emergency physician should remember to document that the examination is "limited" or "preliminary" to prevent confusion about the presence of hemorrhages that are later identified by an ophthalmologist.[13]

For the child who presents with severe brain injury and a history of a short fall, the medical literature provides good evidence of the benign nature of injuries that result from minor mechanisms, such as rolling off a bed or tumbling down stairs.[14–16] Thus, an alternative explanation is more likely, and further evaluation of the child is essential (eg, head computed tomography [CT], skeletal survey, retinal examination). Short falls can produce local deformation of the skull or a short linear skull fracture (particularly temporal or parietal areas) with small underlying subdural or epidural blood collections or contusions. Such mechanisms, however, do not result in complex skull fractures or severe or diffuse brain injury or death.[14–16] A meta-analysis by Chadwick et al[17] of short falls in children reported a 0.48 per million chance of death after a short fall.

Diagnostic Studies

The most common CT finding in abusive head trauma is subdural hematoma, particularly along the falx in the parietal and occipital regions. Other findings include mass effect due to subdural hematomas or parenchymal injury, subarachnoid hemorrhage, intraparenchymal hemorrhage, parenchymal tears, loss of gray

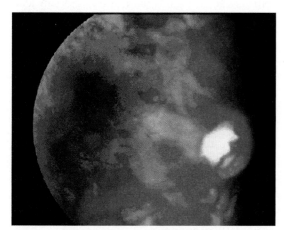

Figure 7.5 The presence of diffuse and multiple retinal hemorrhages in an infant with head injury is highly associated with an abusive mechanism.

or white matter differentiation, hemorrhagic contusions, and a "brighter" appearance to the cerebellum relative to the cerebral hemispheres, signaling severe anoxic brain injury and swelling (reversal sign). In some cases, despite the infant's abnormal neurologic examination results, the initial head CT can appear normal. Magnetic resonance imaging (MRI) will detect parenchymal injuries missed on CT and is frequently used in dating the abnormal findings, as well as identifying cervical spine injuries that can also result from violent shaking.

Management

In the injured infant with head trauma and suspected abuse, approach treatment as you would for a child with multisystem trauma, including assessment of the patient's airway, breathing, and circulation; spine immobilization; Glasgow Coma Score and identification of focal neurologic deficits; vital signs; and completion of a detailed secondary survey. Evaluate the child for occult skeletal and abdominal trauma even in the absence of cutaneous injury or bruising. Proceed with a skeletal survey, laboratory studies of the blood and urine, and abdominal imaging as appropriate.

Abdominal Injuries

Injuries due to inflicted abdominal trauma can present in young children with mild symptoms, such as poor feeding or listlessness; symptoms specific to the abdomen, such as pain and vomiting; or in the child with peritonitis or shock due to bleeding or sepsis. The caregiver might

---

THE CLASSICS

CT Findings in Infants With Intentional Head Injury
- Subdural hematoma
- Subarachnoid hemorrhage
- Intraparenchymal hemorrhage or contusion
- Cerebellar injury

---

describe a minor event (eg, short fall or tumble down stairs) but often no traumatic mechanism is provided. Stairway falls are well documented to result in superficial soft tissue and minor bony injuries but not abdominal visceral injuries.[16] Most inflicted abdominal injuries are not identified by abdominal bruising. Nonetheless, examine the child carefully for tenderness or bruising of the abdomen, flank, inguinal and perineal areas, and back.

Any injury to the liver, spleen, pancreas, stomach, or bowel that is unexplained by major unintentional trauma must be investigated as an abusive injury. Although these injuries are uncommon, abdominal trauma is the second most common cause of fatal child abuse, with an estimated mortality rate of 40% to 50%.[18] This high rate can be attributed to significant delay in making the diagnosis, requiring that the physician maintain a high index of suspicion in the face of no obvious external injury and an inaccurate history.[19]

Liver injury, including laceration and contusion, can result in bleeding into the peritoneal cavity, or it might be contained by the surrounding liver capsule. Liver enzymes are good markers for injury; aspartate aminotransferase levels greater than 450 IU/dL and alanine aminotransferase levels greater than 250 IU/dL are highly sensitive for liver injury seen on abdominal CT, although any value over 80 IU/dL warrants further imaging.[20]

Splenic injury must be suspected in a child with chest or abdominal trauma and can lead to significant blood loss and shock. Suspected splenic injury should also prompt rapid imaging with CT.

The most common cause of pancreatitis in the infant and young child is trauma. The young patient with any symptoms referable to the abdomen or who presents septic or in shock should have amylase and lipase levels checked—excellent markers of injury to the pancreas. Pancreatic contusion, laceration, or ductal injury is best imaged by CT as well. Ultrasonography is useful in identification of a pancreatic pseudocyst.

Stomach or bowel perforation and bowel hematomas without perforation have been reported in cases of physical abuse. The child might present early with peritonitis or hemorrhagic shock, or symptoms can evolve over time, with medical attention sought hours or days after the inflicted injury. The most common site of bowel perforation is the duodenum due to its relatively fixed location in the retroperitoneum. Plain radiography of the abdomen can reveal free intraperitoneal air, bedside ultrasonography can detect free fluid, and CT might identify the specific injury (**Figure 7.6**). However, bowel perforations can be difficult to identify by imaging and should prompt early laparotomy to localize and repair the injury.[19]

For all infants and young children with abdominal injury, optimal treatment requires early recognition of clinical findings inconsistent with history, rapid assessment and stabilization, early consultation with surgery, detailed abdominal imaging and appropriate laboratory testing, reporting to child protective services and police, and transfer to the appropriate trauma or tertiary care center if necessary. Particular clinical patterns and vital signs are associated with certain types of injuries.[18] Once the abdominal injury is identified and definitive care provided, continued evaluation for evidence of multisystem trauma is necessary, which includes radiographic skeletal and head imaging.

Skeletal Injury

Although young and school-aged children commonly sustain fractures, all skeletal injuries must necessitate a thoughtful assessment in the ED. Nonintentional fractures generally found in active, ambulatory children are isolated fractures and usually involve certain common anatomical locations. These locations include the distal radius and ulna, supracondylar area of the humerus, mid to lateral portion of the clavicle, mid or distal tibia, distal fibula, and in older, preschool, and school-aged children, the area involving the growth plates near joints (ie, Salter-Harris fractures).

In contrast, inflicted skeletal trauma found in younger children and infants usually cannot be explained by simple episodes because of their small body mass and early motor skills. In the infant not yet pulling to stand, any fracture should be concerning, and the history and mechanism of injury provided by the caregiver should be evaluated with care. Any concern about abusive fractures in an infant should prompt further radiographic study (ie, skeletal survey) and protective services investigation.[21,22]

Fractures at sites that are infrequently fractured, in the absence of a major mechanism of injury (eg, pedestrian hit by a car), should raise an immediate concern about physical abuse. These fractures include the scapulae, ribs, pelvis, and vertebrae. So too, multiple fractures of varying stages of healing in an infant or otherwise healthy child with normal bones are highly suggestive of physical abuse (**Figure 7.7**). Dating of long-bone fractures can be determined with identification of certain radiographic findings, as summarized in Table 7-2. Certain long-bone fractures, including humerus and femur, although not pathognomonic for abuse, certainly raise serious concern for abuse if no appropriate unintentional mechanism is provided. Again, such long-bone injuries in a young infant who

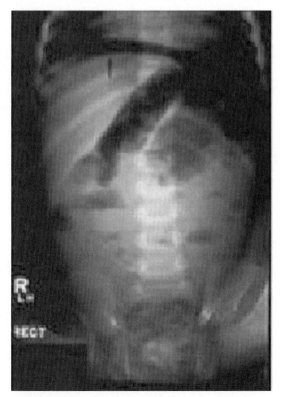

Figure 7.6 Plain radiograph with free air under the diaphragm from jejunal rupture.

is not yet standing or cruising require immediate workup with a skeletal survey and protective services investigation.

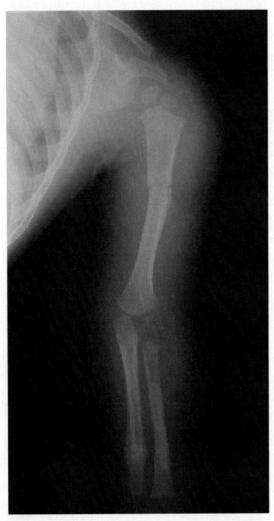

Figure 7.7 Acute transverse fracture of the humerus, healing transverse fracture of the distal radius, and nearly healed fracture of the ulna.

TABLE 7-2 **Dating of Bone Injuries**	
Age of Injury	Radiographic Bone Appearance
0–2 days	Fracture, soft tissue swelling
0–5 days	Visible fragments
10–14 days	Callus, periosteal new bone
8 weeks	Dense callus after fracture

Radiographic Findings Suggestive of Physical Abuse

- Metaphyseal chip (bucket-handle) fractures
- Rib fractures
- Multiple fractures in different stages of healing

Fractures highly specific for abuse include the injuries of the metaphyses in infants and young children, described as corner, bucket-handle, or classic metaphyseal lesions. Forces that twist and shear this immature, weak, and vulnerable area of the infant's bone are the result of two common abuse mechanisms: a violent grasp or twist of the limb, using the arm or leg as a handle, or violent shaking of the infant with resultant flailing limbs.

Rib fractures in infants and toddlers, whether identified incidentally on chest radiograph or in a patient with serious multisystem injury, are commonly associated with physical abuse. It takes great force to break the ribs of an infant or child; the flexibility and compliance of the young chest wall and ribs make noninflicted mechanisms most unlikely, even secondary to stress such as chest compressions during vigorous resuscitation. One common abuse mechanism of injury is an adult grasping an infant's chest with both hands, and squeezing and compressing the chest while violently shaking the infant. This front-to-back compression of the chest wall fractures the ribs in two areas: near their articulations with vertebrae posteriorly and along the lateral surfaces. All cases involving rib fractures should be investigated and should prompt careful history taking, physical examination, skeletal survey, strong consideration for head CT imaging, evaluation for other chest and abdominal trauma, reporting, and hospital admission.

Diagnostic Studies

Laboratory

A complete blood cell (CBC) count, including a smear, differential, and platelet count, and coagulation studies (partial thromboplastin time and prothrombin time) are indicated in patients with multiple bruises to rule out coagulopathy. These studies are also critical evidence in any subsequent trial. Cultures of the base of burns are helpful because bullous impetigo can resemble scald lesions. However, common skin pathogens frequently grow in culture from these sites. Liver enzymes, amylase, and lipase levels are indicated in cases of suspected abdominal injuries or when screening for occult abdominal trauma. Preliminary evidence suggests that the differential rate of rise in the alanine aminotransferase and aspartate aminotransferase levels might help in the timing of hepatic trauma.[20]

Radiology

Skeletal trauma in an infant or young child thought to be inflicted warrants at least two radiographic views of the injured extremity, being sure to include the joint above and below the area of suspected fracture. When the child is stable, proceed with a skeletal survey in all infants and toddlers with a fracture that might be from abuse. Also, a skeletal survey is indicated in all patients younger than 2 to 3 years if there is a concern for any abusive injury, including cutaneous, abdominal, or head trauma. The routine screening skeletal survey, which consists of 19 separate radiologic images, includes frontal views of the chest, humeri, forearms, hands, pelvis, femurs, legs, and feet, as well as a lateral thoracolumbar view and frontal and lateral views of the skull. Additional views (eg, oblique projections) might help delineate suspicious findings. A nuclear medicine bone scan is sometimes used to augment the skeletal survey because of its high sensitivity in identifying acute fractures, particularly those that might not appear on initial skeletal survey (eg, acute nondisplaced rib fractures) or when the findings on skeletal survey are equivocal. For such equivocal findings, an alternative approach is the use of "coned-down" radiographic views of the skeletal area in question.

When a child's presentation raises concern about head injury due to symptoms, neurologic findings, concerning mechanism, or visible trauma to the head, immediately obtain a noncontrast head CT scan. Magnetic resonance imaging of the brain is ordered in the inpatient setting in two clinical scenarios: to accurately date the ages of hematomas in infants who have been repetitively injured and to detect subtle inflicted brain injury not detected by CT. Also, when stable, always consider an urgent skeletal survey in the infant or young child to identify occult skeletal trauma.

Management

Part of the appropriate management includes the careful recording of the appearance and location of all bruises, bites, lacerations, punctures, burns, sores, and signs of choking (eg, strangulation marks) or restraint (eg, rope burns) (Table 7-3).[23] Use legible handwriting, and create appropriate diagrams as necessary. Suspicious skin lesions should be photographed using a good color-balanced photographic technique. Law enforcement can assist with photographic documentation. Forensic photography by police provides not only documentation of injuries but ensures the chain of custody of important photographic evidence. Also record the verbatim statement of the child and parents. Exact recordkeeping will become very important if the case comes under scrutiny of the legal system.

Reporting suspected abuse to the appropriate child welfare authorities and law enforcement agencies, as mandated by all states and US territories, should be done immediately, not deferred to the staff at a referral children's hospital or trauma center. The final determination of abuse is informed by medical opinion but requires the expertise and investigative

---

KEY POINTS

Documenting and Reporting Physical Abuse

- Document all injuries.
- Obtain photographs of physical findings.
- Record verbatim statement from child and/or parent.
- Report incident to child protective services.

TABLE 7-3 Differential Diagnosis of Abuse and Neglect

Findings	Differential Diagnosis	Diagnostic Assessment
Bruises	Trauma; nonintentional and intentional	PT, PTT, platelet count, CBC count
	Henoch-Schönlein purpura	
	Leukemia	Blood culture, fibrinogen, FSP, D-dimer
	Sepsis	
Burns	Nonintentional/intentional	Culture of base of lesion
	Infection	
	Bullous impetigo	
Head injury	Trauma: intentional/ nonintentional	CT scan, ophthalmoscopic examination
	Aneurysm	MRI
	Tumor	
	Infection	
Abdominal findings	Trauma: intentional/ nonintentional	Imaging studies (CT scan)
Pain/tenderness		Abdominal ultrasonography urinalysis, liver enzymes, amylase, cultures
Perforations	Tumor	
Hematomas	Infection	
Skeletal findings	Trauma: birth/intentional/ nonintentional	Radiographs, skeletal scurvy, bone scan, calcium, phosphorus, alkaline phosphatase, 25-hydroxy vitamin D, skin biopsy, genetic consult, soft tissue swelling, CBC, VMA, bone marrow, cultures, ESR, bone biopsy
Fractures		
Metaphyseal/epiphyseal	Osteogenesis imperfecta	
	Rickets	
	Hypophosphatasia	
	Leukemia	
	Tumor: primary and metastatic	
	Scurvy	
	Menkes syndrome	
Growth impairment	Organic	As suggested by history, physical examination, and PE (eg, electrolytes, BUN, organic acids, chromosomes)
	Nonorganic	
	Mixed type	

Abbreviations: BUN, blood urea nitrogen; CBC, complete blood cell; CT, computed tomography; ESR, erythrocyte sedimentation rate; FSP, fibrin split products; MRI, magnetic resonance imaging; PE, physical examination; PT, prothrombin time; PTT, partial thromboplastin time; VMA, vanillylmandelic acid.

skills of child protection specialists and/or law enforcement officers who are specially trained for this task. Remember, filing a report of suspected child abuse is required by law. Admission of the child to the hospital might be required for care of traumatic injuries, further inpatient workup, or the safety of the child until a suitable caretaker is identified by social services. Manage acute problems, such as head, abdominal, and skeletal injuries, in an expeditious manner, paying careful attention to the ABCs (airway, breathing, and circulation) of initial assessment and resuscitation. Many infants with such injuries require hospitalization in an intensive care unit. Seek appropriate medical and surgical consultation. Notify the appropriate children's protective services. Law enforcement agencies can also be notified in appropriate cases.

A 5-year-old girl presents to the ED with blood on her panties. There is no history of trauma, but the mother states that the daughter often has a yellow stain on her panties. The mother denies any concern about sexual abuse. You are unable to question the girl independently because she is frightened and will not separate from her mother. She will allow an examination if her mother stays with her. The results of the physical examination are normal except for findings in the anogenital area. She is sexual maturity rating 1. The hymen is irregular with fleshy lesions that appear friable on its edge. There is blood on the panties but no frank bleeding. The results of the anal examination are normal.

1. *What are the common causes of anogenital bleeding in children?*
2. *What are the pitfalls in obtaining a history from a child related to sexual abuse?*
3. *What physical findings are associated with acute and prior sexual abuse?*
4. *What is the significance of a sexually transmitted infection in a prepubescent child?*

Sexual Abuse

Background and Epidemiology

Child sexual abuse is the involvement of a child in sexual activities that he or she does not understand, for which he or she cannot give informed consent, or that violate social taboos. Such abuse includes oral, vaginal, or rectal contact or penetration; digital contact or penetration; fondling and/or caressing; sexual exploitation; or psychological sexual stress. Although exact prevalence rates are unknown, estimates indicate that 25% of girls and 10% of boys have been sexually abused. Although rates of sexual abuse can be higher for girls, boys are less likely to disclose the abuse. Children are abused at all ages but are most likely to be abused between the ages of 8 and 12 years.

Perpetrators of sexual abuse are most often known and trusted acquaintances, relatives, or household members. The children are befriended and then manipulated or coerced and can endure long periods of abuse before disclosing it.

Sexual abuse must be differentiated from sexual play, which occurs between children of the same age or developmental stage and can represent normal activity in young children. Sexual play involves no coercion, force, or injury to the participants.[1] However, sexual play can occur when there is inappropriate involve-

ment of one of the children in adult sexual activity. For example, it is neither normal nor age-appropriate sexual behavior for a 5-year-old child to put his mouth around the penis of another 5-year-old child.

Clinical Features

History

A sexually abused child can present for medical evaluation with a clear disclosure of the abuse or with a variety of behavioral or medical issues. Behavioral changes might be the only manifestation of abuse and include temper tantrums, clinging to caregivers, sexual acting out, sexual victimization of others, aggression, nightmares, developmental regression, disturbances in appetite, withdrawal, self-injurious behavior, phobias, school problems, and depression.

Medical symptoms might be nonspecific, as in the child with recurrent abdominal pain or headaches. More specific medical indicators of sexual abuse include genital pain, bleeding, irritation, and itching; sexually transmitted infections; pregnancy; recurrent urinary tract infections; foreign body in the vagina or rectum; anogenital bruising; and dysuria and/or painful defecation.

History taking in cases of child sexual abuse must proceed in a manner unlike other pediatric evaluations. The history should be conducted in a quiet, private setting, allowing adequate time for interviewing the parent without interruption. The physician should interview the parent or caregiver alone while the child stays with someone else. Allow the parent to express his or her specific concerns with regard to sexual abuse. If a child's disclosure of abuse prompted the ED visit, obtain information on the circumstances surrounding the disclosure, details of the child's disclosure, and the specifics of the caregiver's questioning of the child. Ask the parent about behavioral changes or any medical concerns or symptoms.

For the caregiver who describes genital symptoms with no expressed concern of abuse, feel free to introduce the topic of sexual abuse, proceeding in a professional, nonjudgmental manner. Alternatively, a parent can present to the ED wanting the physician to "Tell me if my child was molested." Explore the parent's specific concerns about behavioral changes, physical symptoms, and household members or other caregivers.

Next, obtain a thorough medical history, including past illnesses, operations, chronic conditions, developmental history, medications, and allergies. Ask about current symptoms, including abdominal, urinary, and genital symptoms that will help direct the ensuing medical evaluation. If possible, pinpoint the time and place of the most recent contact between the child and the presumed perpetrator. Also, obtain a detailed social history, including household occupants, child care arrangements, substance abuse, violence within the household, and the mother's history of sexual or physical abuse.

The history provided by a child is the most important aspect of the medical evaluation and diagnosis of child sexual abuse. As such, once the emergency physician has obtained essential information from the parent, he or she must make a determination about the appropriate timing and location of the child interview. For many children, repeated interviewing—by emergency personnel, police, protective services workers, and social workers—might prove deleterious to the child and to the case investigation. With repeated interviewing, a child might feel threatened, intimidated, and doubted. Also, for the physician unaccustomed to asking a young child questions about sexual abuse, the interview might include

leading questions or suggest answers and thus contaminate the information subsequently obtained from the child by investigators.

Remember that all investigative interviews have civil and criminal ramifications; they can have an impact on custodial arrangements and criminal prosecution. Thus, local protocols that identify children best served by a child advocacy center or sexual abuse specialty clinic should be used and the complete medical evaluation deferred to the appropriate setting. Such procedures require a multidisciplinary approach that incorporates the expertise of medical, social services, law enforcement, and child advocacy personnel.

Deferral of the complete examination and forensic interview of the child requires that the following criteria are met in the ED:

- Careful screening of the home situation and all caregivers
- Complete medical history
- Child is without medical symptoms that suggest genital injury or infection (eg, no bleeding, discharge, or pain)
- Caregiver compliance with referral plan is ensured
- Child advocacy center or child abuse specialist contacted and follow-up arrangements made
- Clear safety plan established, ensuring no contact with the presumed perpetrator
- Report made to local child protective services and police
- Child has undergone a medical screening examination in compliance with the federal Emergency Medical Treatment and Labor Act

However, an emergency medical evaluation should proceed in all cases in which there is reasonable suspicion that a child has been sexually abused within the preceding 72 hours, the child has medical issues that raise concern about genital injury or infection, or in all cases in which a child's safety cannot be ensured without a complete medical and psychosocial evaluation. Referral to a Sexual Assault Response Team should be considered if such teams are readily available for immediate consultation and are skilled in the examination of children and adolescents.

If indicated and the child is willing to talk

about the abuse, the interview of the child should be conducted in privacy, in an unrushed manner, and without the presence of the parent. The physician first establishes rapport with the child by discussing nonthreatening topics, such as birthdays, playmates, pets, or school. Such conversation also helps determine the child's vocabulary and verbal skills. The topic of sexual abuse can be introduced with an open-ended question such as, "Do you know why your mommy brought you to the doctor today?" or "Your mommy told me that someone might have hurt you. Can you talk to me about it?" This allows the child to provide the history in his or her own words, with open-ended prompts such as, "Can you tell me what else happened?" In general, questions that elicit a yes or no answer should be avoided; for example, if a child who acknowledges being touched could be asked to elaborate on the experience with questions such as, "How did it feel?" and "Who have you told about this?" For younger children, a more specific question would be, "Did it hurt you?" or "Did you tell anyone about it?" Throughout the interview, be sure to reassure the child, offer support, and provide positive statements such as, "You're very brave to talk about this." Such support starts the long process of psychological and emotional healing.

Physical Examination

Record the stage of development of secondary sexual characteristics (sexual maturity rating) in all children. Record the child's height and weight in the medical record. Perform a general physical examination with special attention to the genital findings. Those findings can differ in acute and chronic molestation. In both instances, note abnormalities in the genital and anal areas.

Examine the genital area of the young girl by having her lie supine on the examination table or sitting in her caregiver's lap, with her legs in a frog-leg position. After initial external inspection, gently hold the labia majora with gloved hands and provide lateral and posterior traction to reveal the labia minora, clitoris, urethra, hymen, hymenal orifice, fossa navicularis, and posterior fourchette. The anus can be viewed with the child in a lateral decubitus position with her knees drawn up to her chest or lying

supine and hugging her knees. In general, all girls should also be examined in the knee-chest position where the full contour of the hymen is more easily evaluated. Contrary to initial concerns that children would find this position anxiety provoking (ie, represent an attack from behind), this has not proven to be the case. Have the child assume an "up on all fours" position, with her head and chest lowered to the bed and her bottom in the air (**Figure 7.8**). Consider demonstrating this position to the patient to help them understand what you'd like them to do.

The young boy is best examined lying supine on the bed, with inspection of penis, glans, urethral meatus, scrotum, and perineum and gentle palpation of the testes. Again, the anus can be inspected with the boy lying either supine or on his side, with his knees drawn up, or in the prone knee-chest position. Take note of abrasions, bruises, petechiae, lacerations, scars, sores, ulcers, or other lesions. Carefully document all findings, both normal and abnormal, and use a body diagram with genital detail to draw and describe findings.

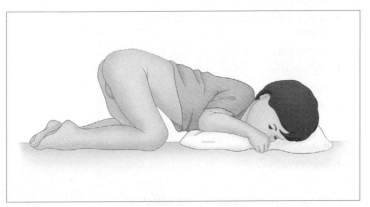

Figure 7.8 Have the child assume an "up on all fours" position, with the head and chest lowered to the bed and the bottom in the air.

Acute Injury

In general, there is no need to perform an internal pelvic examination on any prepubescent girl unless there is concern about penetrating vaginal or rectal injuries. If there is vaginal bleeding and no external source can be identified, then the child must be referred urgently to a pediatric gynecologist or surgeon for an examination while under anesthesia. Careful external inspection often reveals any acute injury or the abnormal findings of chronic abuse as described below. There might be extragenital bruises and injuries, especially in cases of acute molestation. These can involve grip marks on the forearms where the child was held or lacerations on the inner lip if the child was struck on the face in an effort to quiet her or him. Look for bruising around the upper thighs and genital and anal areas. There might be abrasions, lacerations, edema, and petechiae. The vagina and rectum might be in spasm after acute trauma. In approximately 50% of cases, there might be no physical signs after acute anal penetration.

Chronic or Prior Molestation

Physical findings in a child who has been previously or continually molested also might be absent or subtle. Changes in the genital or anal area will depend on the activity engaged in by the child or perpetrator. Exposure, fondling, and oral-genital contact might not produce changes. Chronic or recurrent penile or digital penetration can disrupt the hymen. There might be healed tears (transections) that appear as irregularities in the hymen. The hymen itself will lose its thin, fine appearance and will appear thickened. The edge of the hymen might be rounded, and there might be rounded hymenal remnants that resemble the hymenal tags seen in the neonatal period. Note the coloring of the genital tissues; blood vessels in areas of previous trauma can appear distorted. An introitus (vaginal opening) that appears to be gaping, allowing easy visualization of the vaginal wall rugae, also might be a sign of chronic penetration if the amount of hymenal tissue is reduced. There is, however, great variation, depending on the child's age, size, relaxation state, and method of examination (eg, supine with traction or separation or prone knee-chest position) and measurement.[24] There might also be findings suggestive of a sexually transmitted infection, such as the presence of a vaginal discharge, ulcers, or polyplike lesions. Condyloma acuminatum, or venereal warts, can appear as friable, fleshy lesions in the anogenital area. Condyloma latum is an eruption of flat, broad warts secondary to syphilis. Studies, however, have consistently shown that most children who have been sexually abused have normal anogenital examination results.[25]

Chronic anal penetration leads to scarring and observable changes in the anal area in a small percentage of patients. The skin in the perianal area might be thickened, hyperpigmented, and lichenified from chronic frictional irritation. The adiposity in the perianal area can be lost, leading to a funneled appearance, although this finding is infrequent. Anal fissures can be noted with ongoing abuse. Such fissures can have a characteristic wedge-shaped appearance, being external to the external sphincter and wider distally than proximally. As fissures heal, they can form scars or tags of hypertrophied tissue. The appearance of the rugae in the perianal area can change; rugae become fewer in number, thickened, and more prominent, extending a greater distance from the anus. The anal tone can also change with chronic anal penetration. Observe relaxation and gaping of the external sphincter with separation of the buttocks. In addition, the anal wink, a normal protective reflex, might be lost or diminished. These findings are not significant if there is stool in the rectal ampulla.

Colposcopy is a useful adjunct to the evaluation of a child for chronic sexual abuse. The instrument allows for 5 to 20 times magnification of the area being examined and might reveal evidence of scars or disruptions in the vascular pattern that are not visible to the naked eye. Colposcopy is usually accompanied by video or photographic documentation of the examination findings.

Carefully record normal and abnormal findings. Diagrams and photographs are helpful in documenting the findings.

Differential Diagnosis

For children who present with medical symptoms, consideration must be given for other conditions. In the young girl who presents with vaginal or genital bleeding, consider unintentional injury, infection (*Shigella,* pinworms, group A β-hemolytic streptococcus), condyloma acuminatum, foreign body, polyps, tumor, precocious puberty, hemangioma, urethral prolapse, and urinary tract infection. In the neonate with vaginal bleeding, maternal estrogen withdrawal is the likely cause. The differential for vulvovaginal symptoms is described in Table 7-4.

Diagnostic Studies

The laboratory assessment is especially important in cases of acute molestation; collect specimens that will serve as evidence. Several studies have demonstrated that clothing worn by the abused patient retains forensic evidence even after 24 hours. Details for the proper collection of specimens are usually included in the sexual assault kits kept in EDs or supplied by the police who accompany a sexual assault patient to the hospital. In general, collect any loose pubic hairs and, if the patient has entered puberty, samples of the patient's pubic and scalp hair. A medicine

dropper or nonbacteriostatic saline–moistened (not dry) cotton-tipped applicator can be used for specimen collection. Obtain specimens of semen if present; place on a glass slide and air-dry for DNA or other forensic determinations. A blue (Wood's) light is useful for locating bodily fluids, which can be swabbed for evaluation, including detecting amylase. Place permanent smears in Papanicolaou fixative. Semen will fluoresce under a Wood's light, as will urine until it dries and other substances, including some lotions and skin care products.[26] When semen is detected on a nongenital body area, remove dried semen samples with cotton swabs using nonbacteriostatic saline. Perform a pregnancy test on any sexual abuse patient who is at risk.

Obtain specimens to detect sexually transmitted infections from the body areas listed in Table 7-5 in abused children when signs and symptoms suggest the need. Not all prepubertal children need to be tested. Obtain serologic testing as listed in Table 7-5.[27] Once a child is out of the newborn period, gonorrhea, *Chlamydia,* and syphilis are presumed evidence of intimate sexual contact. In addition, test any patient with a vaginal discharge for bacterial vaginosis and *Trichomonas vaginalis.* With proper consent, try to establish the human immunodeficiency virus (HIV) status of both the patient and perpetrator. The prevalence of HIV in one's community is also important in determining the need for HIV testing and postexposure prophylaxis (PEP).

For some children, there will be tremendous fear generated by the examination and the collection of laboratory specimens. Try to gain the child's cooperation by having the child be aware of what is happening and about to happen. The child often can be instructed to obtain his or her own cultures under direct supervision.

If the child is uncooperative or out of control, suspend the evaluation. In this way, the practitioner avoids the "second sexual assault," when a physical or genital examination in the ED frightens the patient or causes more psychological trauma than the sexual assault itself. It is always better to suspend the evaluation and try again the next day, perhaps in the quieter setting of an advocacy center or specialty clinic. However, if the child is completely uncooperative and a serious injury is suspected (as evidenced by vaginal bleeding or severe bruising), then an examination with the child under anesthesia should be performed.

On completion of the evaluation, summarize the findings. Table 7-6 presents a scheme for summarizing the information and setting a course of action. The California Office of Criminal Justice Planning has many useful forms designed to set a course of action.[28] These forms are used to synthesize the physical findings with the history and are particularly helpful for the forensic assessment of the case.

TABLE 7-4 Vulvovaginal Symptoms: Differential Diagnosis

Nonspecific Vulvovaginitis
- Poor hygiene, local irritation, tight-fitting clothing, obesity, lack of estrogenization

Infection
- Respiratory flora (group A β-hemolytic streptococcus, *Streptococcus pneumoniae*, *Neisseria meningitidis*)
- Enteric flora (*Shigella, Yersinia*)
- Pinworms
- *Candida*
- Sexually transmitted infections (*Neisseria gonorrhoeae, Chlamydia trachomatis, Trichomonas, vaginalis, Gardnerella vaginalis*, herpes simplex, human papillomavirus)

Vaginal foreign bodies (eg, toilet paper)
Polyps, tumors
Systemic illness
- Crohn disease, Kawasaki disease, scarlet fever

Congenital anomalies
- Ectopic ureter, double vagina, pelvic fistula

Urethral prolapse
Skin diseases
- Psoriasis, seborrhea, lichen sclerosus et atrophicus

Adapted from: Vandeven AM, Emans SJ. Vulvovaginitis in the child and adolescent. *Pediatr Rev.* 1993;14:141–147.

TABLE 7-5 Sexually Transmitted Disease Testing

Female Child
- *Neisseria gonorrhoeae* culture: pharynx, vagina, anus
- *Chlamydia* culture: vagina, anus
- Wet prep, Gram stain, culture if vaginal discharge present
- Hepatitis B and C serologic tests, human immunodeficiency virus test, rapid plasma reagin test for syphilis
- Urinalysis for *Trichomonas*, sperm

(Note: In the prepubertal girl, cervical cultures are not obtained.)
For adolescents, urine can be obtained for nucleic acid amplification tests

Male Child
- *N gonorrhoeae* culture: pharynx, urethra, anus
- *Chlamydia* culture: urethra, anus
- Wet prep, Gram stain, culture if penile discharge present
- Hepatitis B and C serologic tests, human immunodeficiency virus test, rapid plasma reagin test for syphilis
- Urinalysis

For adolescents, urine can be obtained for nucleic acid amplification tests

Adapted from: Finkel MA, Giardino AP, eds. *Medical Evaluation of Child Sexual Abuse: A Practical Guide.* 3rd ed. Elk Grove Village, IL: American Academy of Pediatrics; 2009.

TABLE 7-6 Findings and Interpretation: Child Sexual Abuse

Anogenital Findings
- Normal anogenital examination
- Abnormal anogenital examination
- Indeterminate anogenital examination

Assessment of Anogenital Findings
- Consistent with history
- Inconsistent with history
- Limited or insufficient history

Interpretation of Anogenital Findings
- Normal examination result: can neither confirm nor negate sexual abuse
- Nonspecific examination result: might be caused by sexual abuse or other mechanisms
- Sexual abuse highly suspected
- Definite evidence of sexual abuse and/or sexual contact

Need Further Consultation or Investigation

Laboratory results or photographic review pending (can alter assessment)

Source: State of California Office of Criminal Justice Planning. *Findings and Interpretation: Child Sexual Abuse.* Sacramento: State of California Office of Criminal Justice Planning; July 1, 2001:6. OCJP 925.

Management

Both prepubertal and postpubertal children who have been molested might have sexually transmitted infections (STIs) and need appropriate diagnostic evaluations and therapy, unless the patient or family objects (Table 7-7). If an adolescent has a negative pregnancy test result in the ED, the possibility of pregnancy still should be discussed, as should the use of an emergency contraceptive drug ("morning-after pill"). Levonorgestrel (Plan B), a totally synthetic progestogen, is associated with less nausea and vomiting and is a currently preferred treatment strategy. If not available, treatment with ethinyl estradiol and norgestrel (Ovral) should be offered to patients at risk. The dose is two tablets in the ED and two additional tablets in 12 hours. An antiemetic before use is recommended. Withdrawal bleeding can occur within the subsequent 21 days.

Disposition, Reporting, and Follow-up Care

If the child presents with severe symptoms or a serious or life-threatening condition, make immediate arrangements for hospital admission or

TABLE 7-7 STD Treatment of Child Sexual Abuse (Prepubertal or Weight <45 kg)

Neisseria gonorrhoeae	Ceftriaxone, 125 mg IM × 1 dose
Chlamydia trachomatis	Azithromycin, 20 mg/kg (maximum, 1 g) PO × 1 dose Erythromycin base, 50-mg/kg dose PO four times daily × 10–14 days
Gardnerella	Metronidazole, 5-mg/kg dose PO three times daily × 7 days, or clindamycin, 10-mg/kg dose PO three times daily × 7 days, or amoxicillin/clavulanic acid, 20-mg/kg dose PO twice daily × 7 days
Trichomonas	Metronidazole, 15-mg/kg dose PO three times daily × 7 days
Syphilis	Ceftriaxone, 50 mg/kg IM/IV × 1 dose
HSV (first clinical episode)	Acyclovir, 400 mg PO three times daily × 7–10 days
Hepatitis B*	HBIG, 0.06 mg/kg IM, + vaccine series
HIV (PEP)	Contact infectious disease specialist before starting zidovudine, 160 mg/m² PO every 6 hours × 28 days, and lamivudine, 4 mg/kg PO twice daily × 28 days, and nelfinavir, 20–30 mg/kg PO three times daily × 28 days

Abbreviations: HBIG, hepatitis B immune globulin; HIV, human immunodeficiency virus; HSV, herpes simplex virus; IM, intramuscularly; IV, intravenously; PEP, postexposure prophylaxis; PO, orally.

*Unimmunized child and perpetrator with acute hepatitis B infection.

Adapted from: Workowski KA, Levine WC. Sexually transmitted diseases treatment guidelines-2006. *MMWR Recomm Rep.* 2006; 51(RR11):1–94; *Red Book 2009 Report of the Committee on Infectious Diseases.* 28th ed. Elk Grove Village, IL: American Academy of Pediatrics; 2009; and Havens PL and the Committee on Pediatric AIDS. Postexposure prophylaxis in children and adolescents for nonoccupational exposure to human immunodeficiency virus. *Pediatrics.* 2003;111:1475–1489.

transfer to a tertiary care facility. In cases in which the perpetrator is unknown but there is significant concern that he or she lives in the child's home, proceed with arrangements for hospital admission or placement into an alternative safe home environment with child protective or social service assistance. When the child identifies the presumed perpetrator, discharging the child requires careful formation of a safety plan that ensures the child's protection. The child's parent or primary caregiver must understand that it is mandatory that there be no contact between the child and the presumed perpetrator and that failure to protect the child will result in removal of the child from the home to safety.

Reassure children who have been molested that they are all right and that their bodies have not been damaged in any way. Most hospitals and counties have patient advocates available on call to support rape survivors during the initial emergency department assessment.

Referral to counseling agencies is recommended for all acute and chronic sexual abuse patients. Notify law enforcement and children's services of the physical findings of sexual abuse.

The practitioner is obligated by law to report all cases of suspected child abuse. Although the specifics of reporting differ from state to state, in general, practitioners must make a report by telephone immediately to law enforcement and child protective services. Follow this oral report with a timely written report, preferably within hours, but always within 3 days.

Confronting a family about child abuse can be difficult. It is important to keep in mind the vital role of the reporting practitioner as an advocate for the child who is being evaluated. In addition, the abusive parent often is seeking help for himself or herself when bringing in the injured child. The practitioner thus might be able to help not only the child but also the troubled parent.

Consultation with other professionals (eg, social workers or psychologists) is helpful in completing the evaluation and disposition planning, especially when evaluating sexually abused children and adolescents.

KEY POINTS

Management of Sexual Abuse

- Perform complete history and physical examination.
- Obtain STI cultures if history or signs and symptoms warrant.
- Obtain blood for serologic testing.
- Contact child protective services and law enforcement.
- Inform family.
- Offer pregnancy and sexually transmitted infection prophylaxis as appropriate.
- Arrange hospital admission for children at further risk of abuse or those with significant injury; closely follow for all others.
- Contact the primary care physician.
- Document your findings.

Police bring a 14-year-old girl to the ED. She reports that she was walking home from school when a car pulled up and two men grabbed her and pulled her into the car. She states that they took her to a house and dragged her up a flight of stairs. One man pointed a gun at her and stood laughing and talking while the second one pulled off her pants and raped her. Then, the first man raped her while the second stood holding the gun. She reports no oral or anal penetration and no condom use. She states that, some time later, the men left the house, allowing her to escape and call the police. When her mother arrives, she states that her daughter is always lying and made up this story to avoid getting into trouble for having sex.

1. What are the medical treatment priorities for this patient?
2. When should HIV prophylaxis be considered?
3. The mother refuses to provide consent for the emergency care of her daughter. How should the emergency physician proceed?

Acute Sexual Assault

Sexual assault is the sexual contact of one person with another without appropriate legal consent. Legal definitions of rape also include the use of force or threat of force by the perpetrator. An acute assault is one that occurs within 72 hours of presenting for medical evaluation and care. Those most vulnerable to sexual assault include young children, female adolescents, the disabled or developmentally delayed, and those under the influence of drugs or alcohol. In the United States, the incidence of rape peaks in female adolescents between 16 to 19 years of age. Of the 700,000 women who are raped each year, an estimated 61% are younger than 18 years.[29] An anonymous survey of high school students in the United States revealed that almost 20% reported one episode of forced sexual contact, with approximately half never reporting the assault.[29] Another survey of female adolescents revealed that most knew the perpetrator and that 57% of these assaults occurred during a date.[30] Of the few sexual assault patients who seek medical care, more than half might present to the physician with another symptom, further limiting the physician's ability to provide much-needed therapies and making accurate estimates of disease incidence impossible. In cases of drug-facilitated sexual assault, the substance most commonly identified is alcohol.[29] The reported incidence of sexually assaulted boys in the high school population is 5%.[31]

For the child or adolescent who presents to the ED after a sexual assault, the following should be accomplished: identify and treat all physical injuries; reduce or eliminate the risk of sequelae of the assault, including genital injury, pregnancy, and STIs; carefully document the history provided, physical examination findings, and laboratory test results, providing a permanent record of the evaluation; collect forensic evidence and maintain the chain of custody of evidentiary materials; provide referral for follow-up medical care and psychological counseling; and establish communication with law enforcement for crime investigation and prosecution of the perpetrator.

For the minor child assaulted by a parent or adult in a caregiver role, emergent reporting to local child protective services is critical for the child's future safety and well-being, as well as the safety of other children in contact with the perpetrator.

Medical Assessment of Acute Sexual Assault

For the child or adolescent in the ED after a sexual assault, provide a quiet room where the history and physical examination can be conducted in private. The medical assessment can be facilitated by the presence of a patient advocate or hospital social worker who serves to support the child and ensure that he or she is not left alone. Essential history obtained by the emergency physician includes a general medical history, gynecologic history (including information about menstruation, pregnancies, sexual activity, contraceptive use, and recent surgery or infections), social and developmental history (particularly important in the young child), and a history of the assault.

For the very young child or the child who is too traumatized to provide detailed information, interview the accompanying caregiver alone; the caregiver will provide much-needed medical information and might be able to provide details concerning the child's initial disclosure of the assault. A child who is unwilling to discuss the assault should not be forced to do so but might disclose at a later time in a forensic interview or therapeutic setting.

For the adolescent who is able to provide details of the assault, obtain the following information: identifying information about the perpetrator or perpetrators; the date, time, and specific location of the assault; the circumstances and details of the assault; the threats, use of restraints, use of drugs or alcohol, and use of weapons; the physical injuries inflicted before, during, or after the assault; the patient's symptoms; and the patient's activities after the assault (eg, showering, urinating, douching, changing clothes, eating or drinking, brushing teeth).

For the adolescent who is unable to provide such details, focus the history on three main areas: the nature of the sexual contact, the use of force or threats, and the patient's symptoms. Later interviewing by police personnel will likely uncover details of the assault necessary for the investigation and criminal prosecution. In the ED, medical care and psychological support should take top priority.

In the acute sexual assault case involving a young child, take time to establish rapport, assess verbal skills, and determine developmental stage by conversing on nonthreatening topics. Introduce the topic of the assault with a question that is gentle and open-ended. For example, "Do you know why you came to see the doctor today?" or "Your mommy told me that something happened to you that made you feel bad. Can you talk to me about it?" This provides the child an opportunity to explain what happened in his or her own words. Information provided by the child's disclosure leads to more specific questions, which should not be leading or suggest answers. Again, a child who is unwilling or unable to describe details of the assault should not be forced to do so. Reassure the child and turn the focus to physical symptoms, which will assist in the medical evaluation. A forensic interview, also described as a "patient-sensitive interview," can be deferred to a time and place best suited to the young child's needs.

For assaulted patients of all ages, be sure to include a therapeutic message throughout the interview. Such statements as "This was not your fault," "This has happened to other girls and boys," "I'm here to help you get better," and "You are very brave to talk about it" must be said and repeated. Follow-up counseling for the psychological trauma is essential to recovery, but emotional support and the process of healing should begin in the ED.

Physical Examination

Physical examination includes careful inspection and documentation of the patient's general physical appearance and demeanor, height and weight, vital signs, and evidence of injury to the head and neck, chest, abdomen, extremities, back, buttocks, and anus. Pay careful attention to skin findings, including bruises, ligature marks, and other injuries, as well as stains, areas of dried secretions, or areas that fluoresce under a Wood's lamp. Examination of the genitalia requires external inspection noting bruising, bleeding, bite marks, petechiae, secretions, stains, or any sign of trauma. For the female adolescent, external inspection, speculum examination, and bimanual examination are needed. In contrast, no speculum examination should be performed on a prepubertal female patient. Rather, assist her in lying supine on the examining table (or sitting in her caregiver's lap) and assuming a frog-leg position for gentle inspection only. Any abnormal or concerning findings on examination should be confirmed by inspecting the child in a second position (ie, the knee-chest position, in which the child is on all fours on the table with head and chest on the table and bottom in the air). In cases of vaginal bleeding with no visible external trauma or when there is concern about a foreign body in the anogenital area, prepare the patient for an examination under anesthesia after obtaining the appropriate surgical or gynecologic consultation.

Although physical findings on genital examination of the sexually assaulted child can be absent, minimal, or nonspecific, care should be taken to complete a thorough examination under good lighting and with magnification, if available. Most EDs are not equipped for colposcopy, but such magnification can improve the identification of injuries. A study of sexually assaulted females examined with a colposcope (ages ranged from 11 years to adulthood) identified important genital areas most frequently injured, including the posterior fourchette, labia minora, hymen, and fossa navicularis. The injuries included tears (most often found on the posterior fourchette and fossa), abrasions, and bruising. However, in this series, more than one-third of the patients had no visible trauma, which in part demonstrates the rapid healing of highly vascular structures and emphasizes that the history of the assault remains the most important data provided by a patient.[32]

Diagnostic Testing

While performing the physical examination, be mindful of the requirements of forensic evidence collection. The adolescent or child wearing the same clothing worn at the crime scene or clothing put on immediately after the assault should disrobe in the ED on a sheet from the forensic evidence collection kit. Important forensic material can be retrieved from a patient's clothing even after time has elapsed. This careful collection of debris from the clothing captures material that places the patient and/or perpetrator at the crime scene. Any areas of staining on the skin or stains that fluoresce under a blue or Wood's lamp might be the perpetrator's semen or other secretions and should be swabbed with nonbacteriostatic saline on cotton-tipped swabs. The completed forensic kit includes the patient's clothing, debris collection from clothing, skin swabs, hair combings from the patient's head and pubic area, swabs from the female patient's mouth, vagina and perianal areas, swabs from the male patient's mouth, urethra, and perianal areas, fingernail scrapings, and a sample of blood. Also, collect and package any item that was in or near the vagina during or after the assault (eg, the speculum, sanitary napkin, tampon, or other foreign body).

Swabs from the mouth, urethra, vagina, perianal areas, and skin surface areas should be collected for the forensic kit. Subsequent swabs should be collected for culture testing; these are not placed in the forensic kit but rather sent to the appropriate hospital laboratory. For the child who is unable to tolerate evidence collection or culture testing, remember that the first priority during this examination is the patient's comfort and health. Proceed only with those procedures and interventions that are medically necessary.

Toxicologic testing should be considered in all cases in which there is reasonable cause to suspect the patient has been drugged. The patient can provide a history of altered mental status or memory deficit or describe "waking up" in an unfamiliar location. The patient might present to the ED unconscious or with an altered mental status. Obtain urine and blood samples as promptly as possible, and follow the local forensic laboratory protocols for obtaining consent, specimen collection and labeling, and transfer of specimens to the laboratory.

Table 7-8 summarizes the appropriate diagnostic testing for the sexual assault patient who presents within 72 hours of the attack. Table 7-5 provides the diagnostic testing for the prepubertal female. Table 7-9 summarizes the appropriate 2-week follow-up testing for the sexual assault patient.

Treatment

Table 7-10 reviews the appropriate dosing of antibiotics used in sexually transmitted infection (STI) prophylaxis for adolescents. Table 7-7 is for children <45 kg.

Significant controversy exists about the risk of HIV transmission after a sexual assault and the appropriate indications for the use of PEP

TABLE 7-8 Diagnostic Testing After Acute Sexual Assault

Adolescent Female

Oral	Gonorrhea culture
Cervical	Gonorrhea and *Chlamydia* cultures
Vaginal	Wet prep, Gram stain, bacterial culture
Rectal	Gonorrhea culture, *Chlamydia* culture
Blood	Hepatitis B and C serologic tests, RPR test, HIV test
Urine	Urinalysis (and culture as indicated) and urine hCG Nucleic acid amplification for gonorrhea and *Chlamydia*
Imaging/laboratory tests	As indicated for suspected skeletal, head, chest, abdominal injuries

Male

Oral	Gonorrhea culture
Urethral	Gonorrhea and *Chlamydia* cultures
Rectal	Gonorrhea and *Chlamydia* cultures
Blood	Hepatitis B and C serologic tests, RPR test, HIV test
Urine	Urinalysis (and culture as indicated) Nucleic acid amplification for gonorrhea and *Chlamydia*
Imaging/laboratory tests	As indicated for suspected skeletal, head, chest, abdominal injuries (prepubertal female, see Table 7-5)

Abbreviations: hCG, human chorionic gonadotropin; HIV, human immunodeficiency virus; RPR, recurrent respiratory papillomatosis.

Adapted from: Bechtel K, Podrazik M. Evaluation of the adolescent rape victim. *Pediatr Clin North Am.* 1999;46:809–823.

TABLE 7-9 Follow-up Testing in Sexual Assault

Follow-up Testing at 2 Weeks:
- If no antibiotics are received at first encounter, consider repeat culture testing.
- If testing and treatment are performed at first encounter, review results and discuss current symptoms of patient.

Follow-up Testing at 4–6 Weeks:
- Obtain blood for rapid plasma reagin test for syphilis.

Follow-up Testing at 12 Weeks:
- Obtain blood for hepatitis B serologic tests and human immunodeficiency virus tests.

Follow-up Testing at 6 Months:
- Obtain blood for human immunodeficiency virus tests.

Adapted from: Bechtel K, Podrazik M. Evaluation of the adolescent rape victim. *Pediatr Clin North Am.* 1999;46:809–823.

against HIV. The largest body of human and animal data has prompted recommendations for the use of therapy in the occupational setting (eg, needlestick injuries in health care workers) and perinatal settings. In 2003, the American Academy of Pediatrics, Committee on AIDS published guidelines for nonoccupational HIV PEP in children and adolescents.[33] The presumption is that there is the existence of a brief window after exposure in which the HIV viral load is small and therapy might be efficacious; therefore, consideration should be given to offering PEP to those who have been sexually assaulted. Those patients at highest risk should be counseled and offered PEP. High-risk patients include those attacked by a perpetrator with known HIV or at high risk for HIV (eg, intravenous drug user), the patient attacked by multiple perpetrators, the patient with anal findings consistent with penetration, or an assault that occurred in a high prevalence area for HIV. Provision of the first dose within 1 hour of the assault is ideal but often impossible. Consider providing the medication necessary for the first 72 hours of the PEP regimen, within which time the patient can be seen by a local HIV or infectious disease specialist who will reconsider the risk of HIV and the risk-benefit ratio of treatment, provide patient counseling, and establish a follow-up testing and care plan.[33]

TABLE 7-10 Sexually Transmitted Disease Prophylaxis and Treatment After Sexual Assault (Adolescent or Weight >45 kg)

Neisseria gonorrhoeae	Ceftriaxone, 250 mg IM, or cefixime, 400 mg PO × 1 dose
Chlamydia trachomatis	Azithromycin, 1 g PO, or doxycycline, 100 mg PO twice daily × 7 days (for those >8 years and not pregnant)
Gardnerella	Metronidazole, 2 g PO (or 500 mg PO twice daily × 7 days), or clindamycin, 300 mg PO twice daily × 7 days
Trichomonas	Metronidazole, 2 g PO (or 500 mg PO twice daily × 7 days)
Syphilis	Ceftriaxone, 250 mg IM × 1 dose
HSV (first clinical episode)	Acyclovir, 400 mg PO three times daily × episode 7–10 days, or famciclovir, 250 mg PO three times daily × 7–10 days, or valacyclovir, 1 g PO twice daily × 7–10 days
Hepatitis B*	HBIG, 0.06 mg/kg IM, + vaccine series
HIV	Contact local infectious disease specialist before starting zidovudine and lamivudine (Combivir), 1 tablet PO twice daily × 28 days, and indinavir, 800 mg PO every 8 hours × 28 days

Abbreviations: HBIG, hepatitis B immune globulin; HIV, human immunodeficiency virus; HSV, herpes simplex virus; IM, intramuscularly; IV, intravenously; PEP, postexposure prophylaxis; PO, orally.

*Unimmunized teen and perpetrator with acute hepatitis B infection.

Adapted from: Workowski KA, Levine WC. Sexually transmitted diseases treatment guidelines-2006. *MMWR Recommen Rep.* 2006;55(RR11):1–94; *Red Book 2009 Report of the Committee on Infectious Diseases.* 28th ed. Elk Grove Village, IL: American Academy of Pediatrics; 2006; and Havens PL and the Committee on Pediatric AIDS. Postexposure prophylaxis in children and adolescents for nonoccupational exposure to human immunodeficiency virus. *Pediatrics.* 2003;111:1475–1489.

CASE SCENARIO 4

A 3-month-old boy with a fever for 1 day is brought to the ED by his mother. The mother reports that he is a good eater, taking six to seven 240-mL (8-oz) bottles of formula a day. The infant is the mother's fourth child. A review of the past medical history reveals that the infant was at the 50th percentile for weight and length at birth and was full term. On physical examination, the infant is now below the fifth percentile for weight and at the 50th percentile for height and head circumference. The temperature is 37.4°C (99.3°F). The infant is apathetic, appears hypertonic, and avoids eye contact. There is mild rhinorrhea, but the throat, ears, and lungs are clear. There is a moderate diaper rash and caked stool in the diaper area. The infant is also dirty and smells like stale milk.

1. *What physical findings are noted with failure to thrive (FTT)?*
2. *What are the interactional characteristics of infants with environmental (nonorganic) FTT?*
3. *What, if any, laboratory studies should be part of the routine evaluation of FTT?*

Neglect

The most common form of child abuse is neglect; more than 1 million cases of child neglect are reported annually. Neglect can be categorized as physical neglect, which includes medical neglect and failure to provide for common needs such as food, clothing, and shelter; emotional neglect; and educational neglect. Neglect of children is often insidious. It has many profoundly negative consequences and often goes unreported for months or years because of the lack of either positive physical findings or a specific crisis point. The forms of neglect seen most often in the ED are abandonment, medical neglect, and nonorganic FTT.

Abandonment

Abandonment is leaving a child without proper care or supervision in a situation in which harm can come to the child. There are no specific lengths of time or conditions dictated by society; thus, there must be value judgments made by the health care team in deciding when to initiate a report. Children who are abandoned must be thoroughly examined and assessed for signs of neglect such as malnutrition and dehydration, and such cases must be reported to child welfare authorities. If there are no provisions for community-based emergency foster care, the child should be admitted to the hospital for protective care.

Some cases of abandonment involve newborn infants whose mothers might not have disclosed their pregnancies. Such infants might be rescued alive from trash receptacles and brought to the ED. In recent years, attention has focused on the enactment of safe haven laws, which allow a mother to surrender her newborn infant to hospital personnel or other designated individuals without the risk of criminal prosecution for abandonment.

Medical Neglect

Medical neglect is a term indicating that, despite appropriate instructions from a health care professional, a parent fails to provide or obtain health services for a child. Because of this parental neglect, the child sustains injury, develops an illness, or has worsening of a medical condition. An example would involve the failure of parents to comply with recommendations for the care of a child's asthma. Such noncompliance can involve failed medical appointments, frequent visits to the ED, preventable hospitalizations, and even intensive care unit admissions. Cases of medical neglect can be difficult to document, especially when parents change care physicians. When medical neglect is encountered, the physician must file a report with a child protection agency.

Failure to Thrive

Failure to thrive is a disorder characterized by impairment of physical, emotional, and intellectual growth that occurs because of disturbances in the manner in which an infant or child is nourished and nurtured. The hallmark of the disorder is impairment of growth, with height or weight below the fifth percentile or normal height with low weight (low body mass index). Because many chronic medical disorders lead to impairment of physical growth, differentiate the child whose growth is related to environmental factors from the child with a medical problem, although the two conditions are not mutually exclusive.

Clinical Features

Patients with FTT often present to the ED with symptoms unrelated to the growth retardation. They also might have been physically or sexually abused. They frequently have concurrent illnesses related to malnutrition, particularly gastroenteritis. An astute practitioner will recognize that a child is malnourished or too small for chronologic age. In all cases, refer to the growth chart, and plot the child's weight, length, height, and head circumference.

Physical Examination

The physical examination of an infant might reveal findings of malnutrition, such as diminished subcutaneous tissue, thin extremities, and prominent ribs. A child's head might appear disproportionately large because weight and length are more greatly affected than head circumference. The examination might also reveal signs of dehydration. Infants with nonorganic FTT exhibit distinct behavioral characteristics. They often have a watchful, wary, wide-eyed gaze and avoid eye contact. They are hypertonic and dislike close interpersonal interactions, pulling away from the examiner. Observe mother-infant interactions to determine whether these are disturbed. Little vocalization occurs between such a mother and a nonthriving infant. Vocalization that does occur might be negative. A mother frequently will hold an infant at arm's length or leave the child unattended in an infant seat, on the floor, or on the examining table.

Diagnostic Studies

There are no routine studies in the evaluation of the infant with FTT.[34] Perform studies as suggested by the history and physical examination findings. Routine health maintenance laboratory studies, such as a hemoglobin or lead level, are appropriate if these have not been obtained.

Differential Diagnosis

The differential diagnosis of growth impairment is long and includes medical conditions such as genetic, cardiac, gastrointestinal, metabolic, endocrine, and infectious disorders, in addition to growth impairment attributable to a nonnurturing environment. The history and physical examination will suggest whether the condition is related to an in utero insult (maternal infection, drug or alcohol abuse), malnutrition, familial short stature, a specific medical condition, or environmental FTT.

Management

Infants and children suspected of having FTT might require admission to the hospital. Alternatively, appropriate management and investigative procedures can proceed in an outpatient setting. From 90% to 95% of infants and children with nonorganic FTT gain weight as expected after intervention. Some cases of nonorganic FTT can be reportable under state child abuse reporting laws.

YOUR FIRST CLUE

Nonorganic Failure to Thrive
- Weight less than the fifth percentile
- Hypertonic
- Dislikes personal contact
- Does not freely make eye contact
- Signs of malnutrition
- Head appears large
- Signs of dehydration

CASE SCENARIO 5

A 7-year-old girl presents to the ED with hematuria. The mother, who works as a medical assistant in a physician's office, reports that her daughter has a history of recurrent hematuria and has been worked up extensively in the past at different hospitals in different states. The cause of the hematuria is unclear, although the daughter is usually treated with antibiotics. The mother has brought in a specimen of urine that appears pink-tinged. She states that if another urine specimen is needed, it should be obtained by catheterization, which the mother volunteers to do, stating she has done it multiple times in the past. The mother voices her concern that the daughter has a rare condition and she hopes that the physicians at your institution will finally be able to determine her problem.

1. *What are the various forms of MSBP?*
2. *What approach is necessary to diagnose the condition?*

Münchausen Syndrome By Proxy

Münchausen syndrome by proxy is the least common form of child abuse and was initially referred to as the "hinterland of child abuse." The condition was first reported in 1977 by Meadows.[35] Alterative terms have been proposed for the condition, including induced or factitious illness or disorders, factitious disorder by proxy, pediatric condition falsification, and medical child abuse.[36,37] Some evidence suggests that the condition is more common than previously suspected. One report estimated 600 new cases of MSBP involving suffocation and intentional poisoning each year in the United States.[38]

There are, in fact, three different manifestations of MSBP, and these are not mutually exclusive. The types include fabricated, simulated, and induced illness. In the fabricated disorder, the caregiver simply lies about the symptoms. For example, a mother states that her infant has episodes when he stops breathing. In the simulated form, the mother alters laboratory specimens to simulate the findings that would be present if her child had the disease. For example, the mother adds blood (her own or from packaged meat from a butcher) to her child's urine specimen to simulate hematuria. The most dangerous form of MSBP occurs when a parent induces the symptoms in the child. For example, a parent claims that the child has recurrent fevers, and the parent injects the child with a pyrogenic agent, such as diphtheria and tetanus toxoids and acellular pertussis. The parent, usually the mother, has access to material because of her job in a medical setting.

Clinical Features

There are multiple conditions that can present as a manifestation of MSBP. As noted in the case scenario, a bleeding disorder is a common form of presentation. Other symptoms might include apnea, seizures, fever, electrolyte disturbances, allergies, gastrointestinal problems (pain, vomiting, diarrhea, constipation), and educational disabilities.

There are unifying aspects to the history in children with MSBP. Abnormal events such as

seizures are usually not witnessed. Physicians have been unable to determine the cause of the child's problem. The family has moved from one health care professional to another in search of answers. The parent is eager for more diagnostic studies, even ones that are invasive. In addition, the parent is a good historian, medically very knowledgeable, and eager to help.

Münchausen syndrome by proxy should be differentiated from cases in which the parent represents the "worried well." These are parents whose children might have had minor illnesses, such as ear infections or colds, but then appear repeatedly at the physician's office for every minor illness or low-grade fever. Sometimes such parents became concerned during a single illness when the child was subjected to a more extensive diagnostic evaluation such as a lumbar puncture. The parents then became concerned that other febrile illnesses might be indicative of a serious problem. Such parents benefit from an educational approach by an empathetic health care professional.

Physical Examination

Findings on physical examination will vary with the alleged symptoms. Often, the child appears completely well despite the parent's comments to the contrary. If the child's symptoms have been induced or if the child has been subjected to invasive procedures, such as the insertion of a gastrostomy tube or Broviac catheter, the presence of these devices will be apparent.

Diagnostic Studies

The results of diagnostic studies are usually

normal. For example, electroencephalogram results are normal in the face of MSBP and a history of seizures. Study results can be abnormal when disorders have been induced by the administration of certain agents, such as warfarin to induce a coagulopathy or insulin to induce hypoglycemia.

Differential Diagnosis

The differential diagnosis includes all medical conditions that present with similar signs and symptoms of the factitious condition.

Management

Diagnosing MSBP takes a skilled physician and a support team that involves psychologists, social workers, lawyers, law enforcement, and judges. Some institutions have installed covert video surveillance cameras to ensure the safety of the child and intervene if harm is imminent. The use of such cameras has revealed attempts by parents to suffocate infants hospitalized with a history of apnea.[39]

Establishing the diagnosis of MSBP is difficult. In addition, multiple physicians are often involved in the care of the child, including subspecialists and intensivists. Not infrequently, one member of the health care team remains skeptical that the child's problem is simulated, fabricated, or induced. This individual might align with the family and prevent the intervention necessary to ensure the safety of the child and the appropriate psychological services for the parents. The offending parent in a case of MSBP usually does

not have a psychosis but rather a personality disorder. The parent is narcissistic and relishes the attention he or she receives when serving as the historian about the child's illness.

There are multiple risks to the child from MSBP. Symptoms induced by the caregiver can cause permanent damage, disability, or even death. Likewise, invasive diagnostic tests ordered by the health care team might be traumatic. In addition, the psychological damage to the child is serious and potentially debilitating. Sometimes these children grow up believing they are invalids, or are unable to trust those closest to them, or both.

Summary

The problems of child abuse and neglect are complex multifactorial issues of individual behavior, family function, and societal stresses. The physician cannot be expected to treat child abuse in the same way as an infectious illness. The management of abuse more closely resembles the treatment of a chronic disease, one that often requires many different therapists from different professional backgrounds and varied hospital-based and community agencies. However, no therapy can begin without recognition and reporting of the problem. In these tasks, the emergency physician is unique and bears a heavy responsibility for being a vigilant and consistent child advocate. Failure to do so unwittingly condones the abuse and positions the child for further injury, both physically and psychologically. The overriding principle is that suspicion requires reporting and investigation; investigation can lead to safety for the child.

THE BOTTOM LINE

- Problems of child maltreatment are complex and multifactorial.
- Treatment of the child requires multiple disciplines.
- Suspicion of child maltreatment must be reported.
- Reporting prevents further injury or death.

Check Your Knowledge

1. When assessing the history of a traumatic injury, which of the following factors should raise concern about inflicted trauma?
   A. History is inconsistent with the development level of the child
   B. Injury is alleged to have been inflicted by a young sibling
   C. Minor mishap has resulted in a major injury
   D. All of the above

2. Which of the following events is the most common cause of death from inflicted trauma?
   A. Abusive head injury
   B. Burns
   C. Inflicted abdominal trauma
   D. Suffocation or strangulation

3. An infant with environmental failure to thrive (FTT) will manifest any of the following findings except:
   A. Growth impairment
   B. Impaired mother-infant interaction
   C. Skeletal dysplasia
   D. Watchful, wary gaze

4. Which of the following cases would be consistent with Münchausen syndrome by proxy (MSBP)?
   A. Mother who administers *Echinacea* and goldenseal to her child for upper respiratory tract symptoms
   B. Mother who administers ipecac to her healthy child and complains about intractable vomiting
   C. Parents who refuse a blood transfusion for their hemorrhaging child because to do so conflicts with their religious beliefs
   D. Parents who refuse to administer insulin to their child with diabetes because to do so conflicts with their religious beliefs

References

1. US Department of Health and Human Services, Administration for Children & Families, Administration on Children, Youth and Families, Children's Bureau, Office on Child Abuse and Neglect. The Child Abuse Prevention and Treatment Act, June 2003: p 44.

2. US Department of Health and Human Services Administration for Children & Families. *Child Maltreatment 2006*. Washington, DC: US Dept of Health and Human Services: 2008. http://www.acf.hhs.gov/programs/cb/pubs/cm06/.

3. Jenny C, Hymel KP, Ritzen A, Reinert SE, Hay TC. Analysis of missed cases of abusive head trauma. *JAMA*. 1999;281:621–626.

4. Sugar NF, Taylor JA, Feldman KW. Bruises in infants and toddlers: those who don't cruise don't bruise. *Arch Pediatr Adolesc Med*. 1999;153:399–403.

5. Schwartz AJ, Ricci LR. How accurately can bruises be aged in abused children? Literature review and synthesis. *Pediatrics*. 1996;97:254–257.

6. Labbe J, Caouette G. Recent skin injuries in normal children. *Pediatrics*. 2001;108:271–276.

7. Jenny C, Reece RM. Cutaneous manifestations of child abuse. In: Reece RM, Christian CW, eds. *Child Abuse Medical Diagnosis and Management*. 3rd ed. Elk Grove Village, IL: American Academy of Pediatrics; 2009:19–51.

8. Maguire S, Mann MK, Sibert J, Kemp A. Can you age bruises accurately in children? A systematic review. *Arch Dis Child*. 2005;90;187–189.

9. Pierce MC, Kaczor K, Aldridge S, O'Flynn J, Lorenz DJ. Bruising characteristics discriminating physical child abuse from accidental trauma. *Pediatrics*. 2010;125:67–74.

10. Hyden PW, Gallagher YA. Child abuse intervention in the emergency room. *Pediatr Clin North Am*. 1992;39:1053–1081.

11. Bruce DA, Zimmerman RA. Shaken impact syndrome. *Pediatr Annals*. 1989;18:482–494.

12. Reece RM, Sege R. Childhood head injuries—accidental or inflicted? *Arch Pediatr Adolesc Med*. 2000;154:11–15.

13. Levin AV. Retinal hemorrhages: advances in understanding. *Pediatr Clin North Am*. 2009;56:333–344.

14. Tarantino CA, Dowd D, Murdock TC. Short vertical falls in infants. *Pediatr Emerg Care*. 1999;15:5–8.

15. Lyons TJ, Oates RK. Falling out of bed: a relatively benign occurrence. *Pediatrics*. 1993;92:125–127.

16. Joffe M, Ludwig S. Stairway injuries in children. *Pediatrics*. 1988;82:457–461.

17. Chadwick DL, Bertocci G, Castillo E, et al. Annual risk of death resulting from short falls among young children: Less than 1 in 1 million. *Pediatrics*. 2008;121:1213–1224.

18. Cooper A, Floyd T, Barlow B, et al. Fifteen years experience with major blunt abdominal trauma due to child abuse. *J Trauma*. 1988;28:1483.

19. Nance ML, Cooper A. Visceral manifestations of child physical abuse. In: Reece RM, Christian CW, eds. *Child Abuse Medical Diagnosis and Management*. Elk Grove Village, IL: American Academy of Pediatrics; 2009:167–187.

20. Lindberg D, Markoroff K, Harper N, et al, for the ULTRA Investigators. Utility of hepatic transaminases to recognize abuse in children. *Pediatrics*. 2009;124:509–516.

21. Thomas SA, Rosenfield NS, Leventhal JM, Markowitz RI. Long-bone fractures in young children: distinguishing accidental injuries from child abuse. *Pediatrics*. 1991;88:471–476.

22. Bullock B, Schubert CJ, Brophy PD, Johnson N, Reed MH, Shapiro RA. Cause and clinical characteristics of rib fractures in infants. *Pediatrics*. 2000;105:e48.

23. Limbos MA, Berkowitz CD. Documentation of child physical abuse: how far have we come? *Pediatrics*. 1998;102:53–58.

24. Heger AH, Ticson L Guerra L, et al. Appearance of the genitalia in girls selected for nonabuse: Review of hymenal morphology and nonspecific findings. *J Pediatr Adolesc Gynecol.* 2002;15:27–35.

25. Adams JA, Harper K, Knudson S, Revilla J. Examination findings in legally confirmed child sexual abuse: It's normal to be normal. *Pediatrics.* 1994;94:310–317.

26. Santucci KA, Nelson DG, McQuillen KK, et al. Wood's lamp utility in the identification of semen. *Pediatrics.* 1999;104:1342–1344.

27. Finkel MA, Giardino AP, eds. *Medical Evaluation of Child Sexual Abuse: A Practical Guide.* 3rd ed. Elk Grove Village, IL: American Academy of Pediatrics; 2009.

28. State of California Office of Criminal Justice Planning. *Findings and Interpretation: Child Sexual Abuse.* (Sacramento, CA: State of California Office of Criminal Justice Planning) July 1, 2001:6. OCJP 925.

29. Poirier MP. CME review article: Care of the female adolescent rape victim. *Pediatr Emerg Care.* 2002;18:53–59.

30. Koss, MP, Gidycz CA, Wisinewski N. The scope of rape: Incidence and prevalence of sexual aggression and victimization in a national sample of higher education students. *J Consult Clin Psychol.* 1987;55:162–170.

31. Davis TC, Peck GQ, Storment JM. Acquaintance rape and the high school student. *J Adolesc Health.* 1993;14:220–224.

32. Slaughter L, Brown CR, Crowley S, Peck R. Patterns of genital injury in female sexual assault victims. *Am J Obstet Gynecol.* 1997;176:609–616.

33. Havens PL, Committee on Pediatric AIDS. Postexposure prophylaxis in children and adolescents for nonoccupational exposure to human immunodeficiency virus. *Pediatrics.* 2003;111:1475–1489.

34. Berkowitz CD. Failure to thrive. In: *Berkowitz, CD, ed. Berkowitz's Pediatrics: A Primary Care Approach.* 3rd ed. Elk Grove Village, IL: American Academy of Pediatrics; 2008:717–721.

35. Meadows R. Münchausen syndrome by proxy: The hinterland of child abuse. *Lancet.* 1977;2:343–345.

36. Ayoub CC, Alexander R, Beck D, et al; APSAC Taskforce on Münchausen by Proxy, Definitions Working Group. Position paper: Definitional issues in Münchausen by proxy. *Child Maltreat.* 2002;7:105–111.

37. Roesslerr TA, Jenny C. *Medical Child Abuse: Beyond Münchausen Syndrome by Proxy.* Elk Grove Village, IL: American Academy of Pediatrics; 2008.

38. McClure RJ, Davis PM, Meadow SR, Sibert JR. Epidemiology of Münchausen syndrome by proxy on non-accidental suffocation and non-accidental poisoning. *Arch Dis Child.* 1996;75:57–61.

39. Southall DP, Plunkett MC, Banks MW, Falkov AF, Samuels MP. Covert video recordings of life-threatening child abuse: Lessons for child protection. *Pediatrics.* 1997;100:735–760.

A 3-year-old boy is referred to the emergency department (ED) from his preschool because he has bruises on his face, left pinna, and lower back. The parents say the child is very active and frequently falls.

1. *What bruises commonly result from unintentional injury, and what bruises suggest inflicted trauma?*
2. *What are the appropriate diagnostic studies to evaluate suspected child physical abuse? How does the child's age affect what studies are obtained?*
3. *If inflicted trauma is suspected, what agencies must be notified to assist in the investigation?*

On further evaluation, this 3-year-old has a large purple hematoma on his left pinna, four red linear oval marks on his left cheek that appear consistent with a handprint, and a yellow green hematoma measuring 5 × 5 cm on the upper part of the left buttock. There is also a circumferential bruise on the glans of the penis. When questioned while alone with you, the child states, "Daddy say me bad boy. Me make peepee. Daddy very mad. Me very bad." The complete blood cell (CBC) count, prothrombin time, partial thromboplastin time, and platelet counts are all normal. The child also undergoes a skeletal survey, which does not reveal any fractures.

This child's injuries involve the ears and nonbony areas and are all consistent with inflicted trauma. The circumferential injury on the glans of the penis suggests a pinchmark, not an uncommon injury associated with inappropriate punishment for toilet-training mishaps. The child's statements would corroborate this conclusion.

Law enforcement and child protective services should be notified about the findings. In addition, the parents need to be advised about the physician's concerns and obligation as a mandated reporter to notify the appropriate agencies.

A 5-year-old girl presents to the ED with blood on her panties. There is no history of trauma, but the mother states that the daughter often has a yellow stain on her panties. The mother denies any concern about sexual abuse. You are unable to question the girl independently because she is frightened and will not separate from her mother. She will allow an examination if her mother stays with her. The results of the physical examination are normal except for findings in the anogenital area. She is sexual maturity rating 1. The hymen is irregular with fleshy lesions that appear friable on its edge. There is blood on the panties but no frank bleeding. The anal examination results are normal.

1. *What are the common causes of anogenital bleeding in children?*
2. *What are the pitfalls in obtaining a history from a child related to sexual abuse?*

CASE SUMMARY 2 CONT.

3. *What physical findings are associated with acute and prior sexual abuse?*
4. *What is the significance of a sexually transmitted infection in a prepubescent child?*

There are a number of causes of anogenital bleeding in children. In this case the presence of fleshy lesions suggests venereal warts. The lesions in the child's genital area are most consistent with condyloma acuminatum. You order additional studies for other sexually transmitted infections (gonorrhea, Chlamydia, syphilis, and human immunodeficiency virus [HIV]), which all produce negative results. The case is reported as suspected child sexual abuse to child protective services.

Pitfalls center around the child's age and lack of maturity and also that the child might not understand that the molestation is wrong. Children also want to please and might answer yes to specific questions; this is why it is best to ask open-ended questions so the child must respond without being prompted. The child subsequently undergoes a forensic interview and discloses that she has been molested by her father for 1 year.

Children have a great capacity to heal injuries in the anogenital area. Signs of chronic abuse, depending on the type of abuse, can be subtle and include paucity of hymenal tissue, scarring, deep notches, and loss of the normal rugal pattern to the anus, or examination results can be normal.

The presence of a sexually transmitted infection beyond the neonatal period should be presumed secondary to sexual abuse, and a report should be made.

CASE SUMMARY 3

Police bring a 14-year-old girl to the ED. She reports that she was walking home from school when a car pulled up and two men grabbed her and pulled her into the car. She states that they took her to a house and dragged her up a flight of stairs. One man pointed a gun at her and stood laughing and talking while the second one pulled off her pants and raped her. Then, the first man raped her while the second stood holding the gun. She reports no oral or anal penetration and no condom use. She states that, some time later, the men left the house, allowing her to escape and call the police. When her mother arrives, she states that her daughter is always lying and made up this story to avoid getting into trouble for having sex.

1. *What are the medical treatment priorities for this patient?*
2. *When should HIV prophylaxis be considered?*
3. *The mother refuses to provide consent for the emergency care of her daughter. How should the emergency physician proceed?*

The 14-year-old girl was forcibly raped against her will and able to describe genital contact made by two male perpetrators. The ED management priorities include

CASE SUMMARY 3 CONT.

reassurance and support for the patient, a complete physical examination, careful inspection of the genital area (which revealed acute abrasions of the fossa and posterior fourchette), thorough documentation of the history provided and examination findings, completion of the forensic kit and transfer of the kit to the crime laboratory, sexually transmitted disease and pregnancy prophylaxis, and reporting to law enforcement. The mother provides no consent for the emergency care, but in the state where this assault occurred, state statutes support the adolescent's desire to seek medical care after a sexual assault, without parental consent.

This patient also presents a difficult problem with postexposure prophylaxis (PEP) against HIV. Assaulted by multiple perpetrators, strong consideration is given to starting therapy. The biggest challenge to proceeding with the 30-day PEP regimen, however, is a frequent failure of adolescent rape survivors to comply with the therapy. Given the mother's lack of support demonstrated in the ED, the patient is unlikely to find the parental support for necessary follow-up medical care. Careful assessment of the maturity of the patient and her capacity to understand the treatment, its benefits and ill effects, and communication with an alternative supportive adult in the teen's life will prove valuable in the care of this patient. Additional consideration is usually given to the background rate of HIV in the community in which the assault occurred.

CASE SUMMARY 4

A 3-month-old boy with a fever for 1 day is brought to the ED by his mother. The mother reports that he is a good eater, taking six to seven 240-mL (8-oz) bottles of formula a day. The infant is the mother's fourth child. A review of the past medical history reveals that the infant was at the 50th percentile for weight and length at birth and was full term. On physical examination, the infant is now below the fifth percentile for weight and at the 50th percentile for height and head circumference. The temperature is 37.4°C (99.3°F). The infant is apathetic, appears hypertonic, and avoids eye contact. There is mild rhinorrhea, but the throat, ears, and lungs are clear. There is a moderate diaper rash and caked stool in the diaper area. The infant is also dirty and smells like stale milk.

1. *What physical findings are noted with FTT?*
2. *What are the interactional characteristics of infants with environmental (nonorganic) FTT?*
3. *What, if any, laboratory studies should be part of the routine evaluation of FTT?*

The infant's length and head circumference are normal at the 50th percentile, but the weight is less than fifth percentile. The infant is apathetic and avoids eye contact. Laboratory studies reveal a normal CBC count, chemical test results, and urinalysis results. A home assessment reveals there are limited financial resources and inadequate food. The family is living in an apartment without heat or hot water.

The mother feels completely overwhelmed by the situation. Her husband has been unemployed and drinks heavily. She has no one to help her with the children.

Protective services is contacted. They institute a program geared toward family preservation. The family is placed on a waiting list for adequate housing. The three oldest children are enrolled in Head Start. Formula is obtained for the infant, and the family is referred to the food stamp program.

A 7-year-old girl presents to the ED with hematuria. The mother, who works as a medical assistant in a physician's office, reports that her daughter has a history of recurrent hematuria and has been worked up extensively in the past at different hospitals in different states. The cause of the hematuria is unclear, although the daughter is usually treated with antibiotics. The mother has brought in a specimen of urine that appears pink-tinged. She states that if another urine specimen is needed, it should be obtained by catheterization, which the mother volunteers to do, stating she has done it multiple times in the past. The mother voices her concern that the daughter has a rare condition and she hopes that the physicians at your institution will finally be able to determine her problem.

1. *What are the various forms of MSBP?*
2. *What approach is necessary to diagnose the condition?*

There are three types of MSBP, which include fabricated, simulated, and induced illness. In this case, the illness is fabricated by the mother. The urine sample brought in by the mother tests positive for blood. The medical staff requests a fresh specimen. The child is allowed to void into a cup under the direct observation of the nursing staff. The mother is asked to wait outside the restroom. The urine specimen is free of blood. The daughter denies any urine symptoms.

In this case, the approach to establish the diagnosis begins with suspicion of the syndrome. Asking the mother to wait outside the restroom was critical to establish that the child indeed has no hematuria. Social service is consulted and prior medical records are requested. The case is referred to child protective services once the records are received and reveal that the child has been seen on 58 different occasions at 32 different hospitals. She has undergone three renal biopsies and multiple different diagnostic studies, all of which have been negative for a cause of hematuria or an underlying medical disorder.

chapter 8

Nontraumatic Surgical Emergencies

Pamela J. Okada, MD, FAAP
Barry A. Hicks, MD, FAAP, FACS

Objectives

1 Describe the common causes of rectal bleeding in infants with abdominal distention.

2 Recognize that bilious emesis in an infant is a surgical emergency and that malrotation with midgut volvulus must be evaluated and treated immediately.

3 Describe the classic triad of intussusception and recognize that intussusception can present with lethargy.

4 Describe the common causes of testicular pain.

5 Describe the common causes of inguinal or scrotal masses.

6 Establish and discuss the clinical features and emergency management of several important acute surgical disorders in children.

Chapter Outline

Necrotizing Enterocolitis
Malrotation and Midgut Volvulus
Pyloric Stenosis
Intussusception
Meckel Diverticulum
Testicular Torsion
Pediatric Inguinal Hernia
Appendicitis

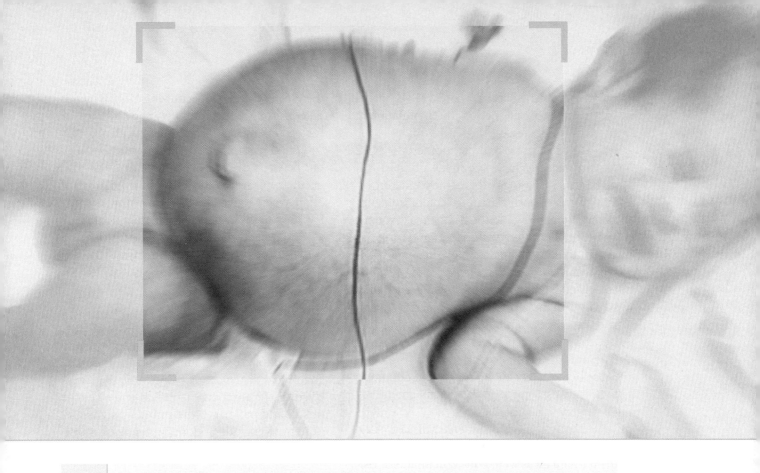

CASE SCENARIO 1

A 4-day-old girl presents to the emergency department (ED) after an episode of bloody stools and increasing abdominal distention. She has not been feeding well and is sleeping between feedings. She was born at 34 weeks' gestation by emergency cesarean delivery because the mother had pregnancy-induced hypertension. The infant did well after delivery and was discharged to home. She had been taking commercial formula every 3 hours but during the past 6 hours has not been feeding at all and has been more lethargic.

On physical examination, the infant is afebrile, with a respiratory rate of 45/min and a heart rate of 180/min. Head, neck, lung, and heart examinations are normal except for tachycardia. The abdomen is distended; the overlying skin is mildly shiny and erythematous, and bowel sounds are hypoactive. Femoral pulses are present, but capillary refill to the lower extremities is delayed. A stool sample obtained from the diaper is positive for blood.

1. *What could be the cause of rectal bleeding and abdominal distention in this neonate?*
2. *What diagnostic tests could be helpful?*

Necrotizing Enterocolitis

Necrotizing enterocolitis (NEC) is an acquired neonatal disorder characterized by necrosis of the mucosal and submucosal layers of the gastrointestinal (GI) tract. The pathologic hallmarks of NEC are coagulation necrosis, inflammation, and hemorrhage in the involved segment of intestine.

NEC is primarily a disease of premature, very low-birth-weight (VLBW) infants and usually presents in the immediate newborn period. During the 1960s, the incidence of NEC increased significantly, reflecting the advent of neonatal intensive care units. Advances in obstetric and neonatal care have improved survival rates for premature infants, and as more VLBW infants survive the neonatal period, the population at risk for NEC increases.[1–3]

The exact cause and pathogenesis of NEC remain unclear; NEC is a complex multifactorial disease. Predisposing factors of the premature infant include abnormal bacterial colonization, intestinal immaturity, intestinal ischemia, hypoxia, and formula feeding with hypertonic formulas or rapid feeding regimens.[4,5] Recent studies suggest that there might be genetic polymorphisms associated with the development and severity of NEC. All of these promote mucosal destruction and stimulate proinflammatory mediators that lead to bowel infarction and necrosis. Necrotizing enterocolitis is still recognized as an important cause of morbidity and mortality and continues to be the most common indication for emergency GI surgery in neonates.

Although NEC is considered a disease of the premature, VLBW infant, it occasionally affects the term infant as well. Full-term infants at risk are those with a history of intrauterine growth retardation, congenital heart disease, perinatal asphyxia, hypoglycemia, polycythemia, respiratory distress, maternal cocaine use, maternal pregnancy-induced hypertension, or umbilical artery catheters. Recently, high-dose intravenous immunoglobulin for severe isoimmune hemolytic jaundice was found to be associated with higher incidence of NEC.[6–13]

In 1978, Bell et al[14] developed a system for the diagnosis of NEC and grading severity of disease. The three-part staging system classified infants as having stage I (suspect), stage II (definite), or stage III (advanced) disease. The staging system was later modified to include clinical, GI, and radiographic findings and treatment recommendations based on staging of disease.[15]

Epidemiology

Necrotizing enterocolitis is the most common GI emergency seen in the neonatal intensive care unit, occurring in 1% to 5% of all admitted infants or in 1 to 3 per 1,000 live births. With an incidence in VLBW infants of 7% to 14% and a mortality rate approaching 15% to 50%, NEC continues to represent a serious clinical problem.[1,2,4] The more immature the infant at birth,

the greater the risk of acquiring NEC. There is no consistent association between sex, race, or socioeconomic status and NEC incidence.

Full-term infants are at low risk for NEC, but between 5% and 25% of all cases of NEC occur in term infants.[4,8,10–13] In this group of infants, NEC typically develops within the first few days of life, whereas premature infants are at a prolonged risk and usually develop NEC between the seventh and 14th days of life and occasionally as late as the third week of life.[1,11,12]

Clinical Features

The clinical presentation of a full-term infant with NEC is similar to the preterm neonate and can resemble sepsis. Subtle signs can include abdominal distention, feeding intolerance, delayed gastric emptying, jaundice, and a change in stooling pattern. More ominous signs and symptoms include abdominal tenderness, bilious emesis, grossly bloody stools, oliguria,

---

YOUR FIRST CLUE

Signs and Symptoms of NEC

Early

- Appearance: subdued
- Work of breathing: normal
- Circulation: normal

Late

- Appearance: lethargic, poorly responsive
- Work of breathing: effortless tachypnea (compensatory for metabolic acidosis)
- Circulation: delayed capillary refill, cool, pallor, mottled extremities, rapid pulse, poor skin turgor, abdominal wall erythema

Other clinical findings

- Abdominal distention
- Feeding intolerance
- Delayed gastric emptying
- Bloody stools
- Lethargy
- Temperature instability

hypotension, lethargy, temperature instability, apneic episodes, and respiratory distress.[1,4,16,17]

Complications

A delay in the diagnosis of NEC can lead to bowel perforation, sepsis, profound metabolic acidosis, disseminated intravascular coagulopathy, respiratory failure, cardiovascular collapse, and death. Unfortunately, with the sudden-onset form of NEC, these complications can occur despite rapid diagnosis and intervention.[18]

The mortality rate from NEC in the full-term infant is 5% compared with 15% to 50% in preterm infants.[1,4,19–21] Smaller infants, infants with more severe disease, and those requiring surgery all have higher case fatality rates. Infants who survive surgery are at risk for long-term complications, such as intra-abdominal abscesses, intestinal strictures, and adhesions (10% to 35%), which can result in bowel obstruction, short bowel syndrome (malabsorption syndrome), bacterial overgrowth and life-threatening sepsis, electrolyte and water loss from the ileostomy, or cholestasis secondary to prolonged total parenteral nutrition (TPN) administration.[21–25] Furthermore, survivors of NEC are at risk for worse neurodevelopmental outcome than those with prematurity alone. Infants who require surgery for NEC have an even higher risk of poor neurologic outcome than those who receive only medical treatment.[26–30]

Diagnostic Studies

Laboratory

Laboratory studies are nonspecific. Stool samples can show occult blood or be grossly bloody. There are numerous causes of GI bleeding in the newly born infant.[18–20] However, most of the causes are not associated with abdominal distention (Table 8-1).

In more severe illnesses, blood analysis can show respiratory and metabolic acidosis, neutropenia, thrombocytopenia, and evidence of disseminated intravascular coagulopathy.[1,31] The full-term infant might even show a leukocytosis with a polymorphonuclear predominance. The clinical picture of NEC is similar to the sepsis syndrome, and laboratory studies might help differentiate the two (Table 8-2).

Many serologic markers have been suggested for the diagnosis of NEC. A recent systematic review of the literature combined data from studies that used C-reactive protein, intestinal folic acid-binding protein, and platelet-activating

TABLE 8-1 Causes of Gastrointestinal Bleeding and Abdominal Distention in the Newborn Infant		
	Abdominal Distention	Rectal Bleeding
• Swallowed maternal blood		+
• Hemorrhagic disease of the newborn		+
• Malrotation with volvulus	+	+
• Intestinal infection	+	+
• Neonatal pseudomembranous colitis		+
• Necrotizing enterocolitis	+	+
• Hirschsprung disease and associated enterocolitis	+	+
• Cow's milk or soy protein intolerance	+/–	+
• Anal fissure		+
–Intentional trauma		+
–Sepsis with intestinal ileus	+	+

TABLE 8-2 **Laboratory Studies to Consider in an Infant With Necrotizing Enterocolitis**
• Complete blood cell count with differential
• Blood culture
• Electrolytes
• Blood urea nitrogen
• Creatinine
• Glucose
• Cerebrospinal fluid analysis and culture
• Stool for occult blood
• Stool for culture
• Prothrombin time/partial thromboplastin time
• Fibrin split products
• Fibrinogen
• Arterial blood gas
• Urinalysis, urine culture

factor.[32–36] Of these, C-reactive protein was sensitive but not specific for NEC; platelet-activating factor and intestinal folic acid-binding protein were both sensitive and specific for NEC. Serial CRP can help distinguish Bell stage I NEC from ileus or benign pneumatosis. However, to date there is no consensus on the utility of serologic markers. Clinical judgment is still the most sensitive and specific indicator of disease.

Radiography

Plain abdominal radiographs might reveal an ileus, a persistent loop of bowel, pneumatosis intestinalis, portal venous gas (PVG), or a gasless abdomen (**Figure 8.1A** and **8.1B**). Two pathognomonic diagnostic radiographic signs are pneumatosis intestinalis (the formation of intramural intestinal gas) and intrahepatic PVG. Portal venous gas can be a fleeting radiographic finding but when present signifies serious disease (Bell stage II) (**Figure 8.2**). Although PVG can be seen on plain abdominal radiographs as in Figure 8.2, it can be more easily seen using hepatic ultrasonography.

Pneumoperitoneum is seen in advanced disease (Bell stage III) and signifies bowel perforation (**Figure 8.3**). On a supine radiograph, free air is seen centrally and appears as a vertically aligned ellipse, called the football sign. On a left lateral decubitus radiograph, free air is seen between the liver and the abdominal wall.

On a cross-table lateral radiograph, free air is seen anteriorly and is distributed evenly over the entire abdomen. All of these findings occur less frequently in full-term infants.[21,37]

Magnetic Resonance Imaging

Magnetic resonance imaging (MRI) has come under study for its use in the diagnosis of intestinal necrosis in the premature infant with symptoms suggestive of NEC.[36,38] Areas of intestinal necrosis found at laparotomy corresponded to bubblelike formations in the intestinal segments on MRI. From a logistic standpoint, obtaining an MRI in a premature infant can be prohibitively difficult. Detection of NEC by MRI in the full-term infant might be more feasible but is rarely necessary.

Ultrasonography

Recently, bedside ultrasonography has become useful in the evaluation for NEC in neonates with a gasless distended abdomen.[39–42] Ultrasonographic findings aid in the decision to perform surgical treatment. Doppler ultrasonography is used to evaluate mesenteric blood flow in the superior mesenteric artery and to predict the subsequent risk of dysmotility. Color Doppler ultrasonography can also be useful in following the progression of NEC from initial hyperemia of the bowel wall to ischemia and finally to bowel wall thinning.

Differential Diagnosis

The differential diagnosis of NEC includes sepsis with intestinal ileus, intestinal infection, spontaneous bowel perforation (colon, ileum, or stomach),

---

THE CLASSICS

Classic Laboratory and Radiographic Findings of NEC
- Metabolic acidosis
- Neutropenia
- Thrombocytopenia
- Pneumatosis intestinalis
- Intrahepatic PVG
- Pneumoperitoneum

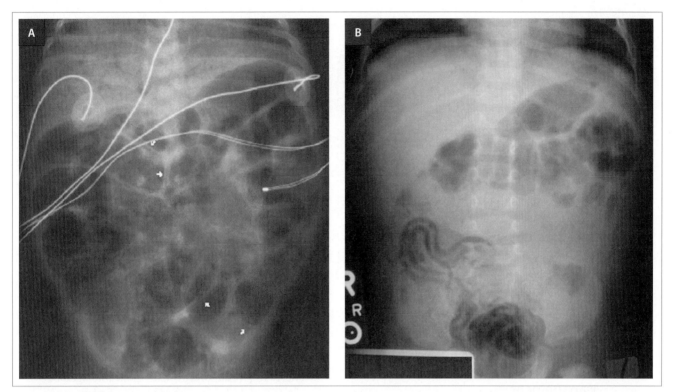

Figure 8.1 Examples of pneumatosis intestinalis. In these abdominal radiographs of different patients with necrotizing enterocolitis, note the gas bubbles located within the bowel wall. This is known as intramural air and is sometimes described as railroad tracks because the inner and outer mucosal walls are separated by the air, giving it an appearance of two parallel lines. The white arrows point this out in 8.1A; 8.1B shows a term infant with impressive pneumatosis intestinalis.

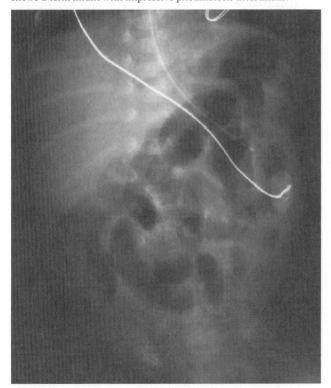

Figure 8.2 Portal venous gas. Note the tiny air densities superimposed over the liver. These air densities are gas bubbles within the portal venous system or the biliary tree.

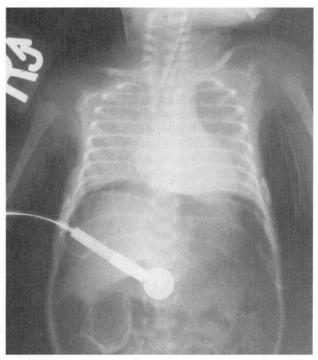

Figure 8.3 Pneumoperitoneum in an infant with necrotizing enterocolitis. The amount of intraperitoneal air is extensive in this radiograph. Small amounts of free air can be difficult to identify on plain radiographs, especially if taken as a flat plate. Small amounts of free intra-abdominal air can be best seen on an upright, lateral decubitus or a cross-table lateral view.

Differential Diagnosis of NEC
- Sepsis with intestinal ileus
- Intestinal infection
- Spontaneous bowel perforation
- Intestinal obstruction
- Malrotation with volvulus
- Hirschsprung disease
- Neonatal appendicitis
- Neonatal pseudomembranous colitis
- Intentional trauma

malrotation with volvulus, Hirschsprung disease, neonatal appendicitis, neonatal pseudomembranous colitis, and intentional trauma.

Management

Emergency Department and Follow-up Care

The treatment for uncomplicated NEC (no stricture or perforation) is medical management. Current treatment recommendations are to place an orogastric tube for low intermittent suction, administer broad-spectrum antibiotics (gram-positive, gram-negative, and anaerobic coverage is recommended), and stop oral feedings for 10 to 14 days. Hypotension is treated with crystalloid, blood products, and pressors. Ventilation should be assisted if abdominal distention impairs ventilation and oxygenation or for evidence of sepsis (hypotension or metabolic acidosis). Nutritional support is provided by TPN. This nonsurgical management is successful in 75% of patients.[20] Surgical intervention is indicated if there is evidence of perforation or intestinal necrosis. Relative indications for surgery include clinical deterioration, refractory acidosis, oliguria, hypotension, persistent thrombocytopenia, ventilatory failure, portal venous gas (PVG), a fixed dilated loop of bowel, or erythema of the abdominal wall. Surgical interventions include laparotomy with resection and proximal end ostomy or laparotomy with resection and primary anastomosis and, rarely, peritoneal drainage.[20,43–46]

What to Avoid and Why

Failure to recognize that full-term infants can develop NEC is the first problem to avoid. Aggressive early intervention in the term infant has offered a favorable prognosis, with survival rates exceeding 90%.[11]

Avoid relying on systemic findings (such as temperature or hemodynamic instability) or metabolic derangements (such as metabolic acidosis) as determining factors for early surgical intervention. These findings are not reliable early indicators of the extent of disease in the term infant. A number of term infants with pneumoperitoneum or obstruction are otherwise stable but have extensive and advanced disease at laparotomy. It is thought that the term infant has a greater physiologic reserve than the preterm infant, and a low threshold for early laparotomy will improve prognosis.[11]

Controversies in Management

There are several controversies in the management of NEC, including type and length of intravenous antibiotic coverage, surgical indications (relative versus absolute[14,15]), type of surgical intervention (laparotomy with resection and proximal stoma formation versus laparotomy with resection and primary anastomosis[21]), peritoneal drainage,[20,45] timing of feeding once the infant is clinically well (10 versus 14 days of nothing by mouth), and even refeeding formulas (electrolyte solutions versus diluted or full-strength formulas) and regimens (bolus versus continuous feedings).

Although data are limited, current research supporting the use of probiotics and prebiotics is emerging. Probiotics are living microorganisms, which when ingested, colonize the GI tract. Beneficial effects of probiotics include increased

Necrotizing enterocolitis should be considered as a potential diagnosis in term infants who present with signs of sepsis syndrome. Begin resuscitation with fluids and contact a surgeon early.

intestinal permeability and enhanced mucosal IgA response and might aid in the prevention of NEC. Other areas of recent study include prebiotics (nondigestible dietary supplements such as long chain carbohydrates or mucins), argi-nine supplementation, free radical scavengers, acidification of gastric contents, polyunsaturated fatty acids, and oral immunoglobulins. These treatments are not recommended for clinical use until further trials are completed.[4,47–50]

CASE SCENARIO 2

A 4-week-old boy arrives in the ED with a 1-day history of decreased activity and vomiting. The infant is breastfed and has had no difficulty nursing but has vomited intermittently. During the past 3 hours, the infant has vomited frequently. The last few episodes of vomiting produced green vomitus. The birth history was uncomplicated. The infant was born full term by spontaneous vaginal delivery.

On physical examination, the infant is lethargic, pale, and grunting. His respiratory rate is 60/min, heart rate is 190/min, blood pressure is 80/60 mm Hg, and rectal temperature is 36°C (96.8°F). The anterior fontanel is sunken. The lungs are clear to auscultation, but occasional grunting sounds are noted. Abdominal examination reveals decreased bowel sounds, and the abdomen is distended and tender to palpation. The genital examination results are normal. The extremities are mottled with poor perfusion.

1. *What important cause of bilious emesis in an infant must be excluded immediately?*
2. *What is the radiographic study of choice in the evaluation of an infant with bilious emesis?*
3. *Why must the evaluation of an infant with bilious emesis be performed emergently?*

Malrotation and Midgut Volvulus

Malrotation of the midgut occurs when the normal rotational process and fixation of the intestine fail to occur during gestation. Lack of fixation of the small bowel results in obstructing peritoneal adhesive bands (Ladd bands) forming between the cecum and the right abdominal wall. These Ladd bands cause compression of the duodenum and mechanical obstruction (**Figure 8.4**).[51,52]

A second and far more serious cause of bowel obstruction is malrotation complicated by midgut volvulus (**Figure 8.5**). The small bowel is suspended on a narrow pedicle (containing the superior mesenteric artery), and the small bowel can twist around this narrow axis, resulting in torsion of the entire midgut. This is a surgical emergency because small bowel necrosis can occur within hours.[53] Midgut volvulus occurs in 70% of infants with malrotation.[54]

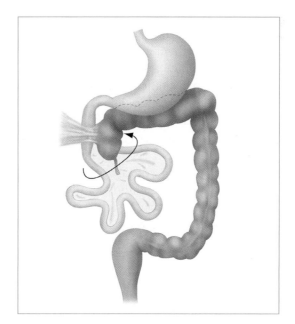

Figure 8.4 Ladd bands compression of the duodenum. This diagram shows the mesenteric stalklike attachment of the cecum (Ladd bands) in the malrotation malformation, which can cause a bowel obstruction by compressing the duodenum.

The term malrotation focuses attention on the embryology of the defect instead of the anatomical malformation itself. In a healthy patient, the small bowel is suspended by mesentery, which is attached to the abdominal wall as a broad fan, and is too broad to twist (**Figure 8.6**). In malrotation, this attachment is a narrow stalk, making it prone to twisting (Figures 8.4 and 8.5). A twist of this stalk results in catastrophic bowel ischemia, which results in infarction unless surgical detorsion is immediately performed. This midgut volvulus should be distinguished from sigmoid volvulus, which largely occurs in elderly adults. Malrotation might more accurately be called "guts on a stalk" to stress the anatomy of the malformation and its consequence rather than its embryology.

Malrotation is associated with a number of conditions and syndromes. Malrotation is invariably present in children with gastroschisis, omphalocele, and congenital diaphragmatic hernia, is commonly present in heterotaxy syndromes, and is occasionally associated with intestinal atresias, cloacal extrophy, Hirschsprung disease, prune belly syndrome, and trisomies 13, 18, and 21. The incidence of malrotation is 45 times greater in children with trisomy 21 than those without.[51]

Epidemiology

The incidence of malrotation is 1 in 500 live births. Between 25% and 40% of patients with symptomatic malrotation present within the first week of life, an additional 10% (50% total) present within the first month, 75% to 90% present before 1 year of age, and the remaining present after 1 year of age. The identification of malrotation after 1 year of age is evenly distributed throughout childhood and is found incidentally in adulthood. There is a 2:1 male predominance in cases presenting in the neonatal period. Mortality from malrotation ranges from 4% to 8%.[55,56]

Clinical Features

Malrotation typically presents in the first month of life with feeding intolerance, bilious vomiting, and, less consistently, sudden onset of abdominal pain (crying). Bilious emesis is usually the first sign of volvulus and is present in 77% to

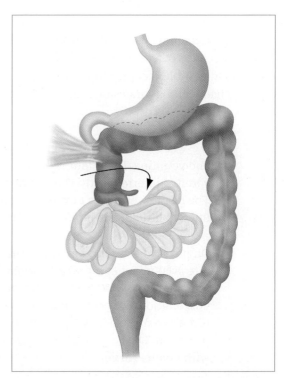

Figure 8.5 Midgut volvulus. This diagram depicts the catastrophic nature of a midgut volvulus, which results in ischemia and subsequent infarction of most of the small bowel as it twists around its stalklike mesenteric attachment in the malrotation malformation.

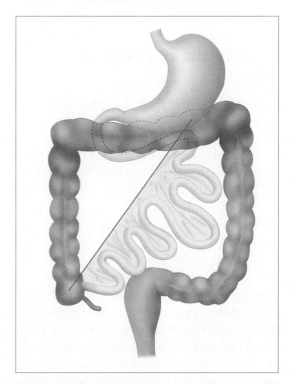

Figure 8.6 Representation of the normal mesenteric bowel suspension; note that its attachment is broad, preventing the bowel from twisting on itself.

100% of cases.[54] Older infants and children can present with vague, nonspecific symptoms, such as chronic, intermittent vomiting and cramping abdominal pain, failure to thrive, constipation, bloody diarrhea, and hematemesis.[51,55–58]

Physical examination results might include a normal abdominal examination in 50% to 60% of patients.[54,59] One-third of patients present with abdominal distention without tenderness. As intestinal ischemia progresses to necrosis, bowel distention, abdominal pain, and evidence of peritonitis develop. As ischemia progresses to infarction, fever, erythema, and edema of the abdominal wall, peritonitis and abdominal distention worsen, and profound dehydration and vascular collapse occur.

Complications

In the neonate, volvulus can rapidly result in significant bowel ischemia with abdominal distention, bloody stools, and eventually hypovolemia, shock, and peritonitis. Short of death, intestinal infarction of the entire midgut (nearly all of the small bowel) is the most serious complication of this condition, which is not compatible with survival without lifelong parenteral hyperalimentation or small bowel transplantation.[56]

Diagnostic Studies

Laboratory

Laboratory studies are not particularly helpful in the diagnosis of malrotation and midgut volvulus.

Radiology

Plain films of the abdomen can be normal or can reveal proximal gastric or duodenal distention with or without distal intraluminal air. On an upright film, triangular gas shadows in the right upper quadrant are produced as the liver edge overlies the air-filled duodenum. This pattern, called the duodenal triangle, has been reported as a plain film sign of midgut volvulus in the neonate.[60]

Malrotation with or without midgut volvulus cannot be excluded by a normal plain radiograph. A limited upper GI contrast study, designed to visualize the duodenum and proximal jejunum, is the most reliable method to diagnose malrotation. The malrotated duodenum is often coiled (as in a midgut volvulus) to the right of the midline, giving a corkscrew appearance as seen in **Figure 8.7**. A cutoff appearance of the contrast ("beak") suggests obstruction from the volvulus.[61]

It is important to identify a malrotation even in the absence of a midgut volvulus. Patients with malrotation are at risk of midgut volvulus later in life. The hallmark radiographic criterion for malrotation is failure of the ligament of Treitz, or the duodenal-jejunal flexure, to cross to the left of the midline. The normal position of the duodenal-jejunal flexure is left of the left-sided pedicles of the vertebral body at the level of the duodenal bulb on frontal view and posterior (retroperitoneal) on lateral view. Barium enema and ultrasonography might identify anomalous anatomical findings, such as a nonfixed cecum or an abnormally oriented superior mesenteric artery, but these findings are not as reliable as the abnormally fixed ligament of Treitz on contrast study.[61–63]

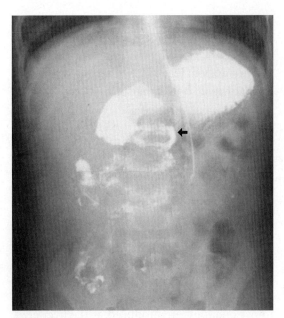

Figure 8.7 Corkscrew appearance of midgut volvulus on X-ray. The diagram in Figure 8.5 depicts the midgut volvulus. Thin barium permits the coil of the volvulus to be visualized. In other instances, the upper gastrointestinal tract contrast study will reveal a simple obstruction, and the coil will not be visualized.

Differential Diagnosis

The differential diagnosis for the infant with bilious emesis includes duodenal webs, duodenal stenosis, duodenal atresia, and any intestinal obstruction distal to the ampulla of Vater. Such obstructions include incarcerated inguinal hernia, Hirschsprung disease, meconium ileus, intestinal atresias, and imperforate anus in the young infant and intussusception in the older infant. However, an infant with bilious emesis could have a malrotation with midgut volvulus until proved otherwise.[62] Also note that a mid-

---

THE CLASSICS

Diagnostic Studies for Evaluation of Midgut Volvulus

Limited upper GI contrast study: the duodenum is coiled (midgut volvulus) or the duodenal-jejunal junction is malpositioned (malrotation).

WHAT ELSE?

Differential Diagnosis of Midgut Volvulus

- Duodenal web, stenosis, atresia
- Hirschsprung disease
- Meconium ileus
- Imperforate anus
- Intussusception
- Incarcerated inguinal hernia

---

gut volvulus almost always presents with bilious emesis (as opposed to non-bilious emesis).

The phenomenon known as intermittent volvulus occurs when the midgut twists and then untwists on its own. Such patients can present with a history of one or more previous episodes suggestive of an early midgut volvulus, which resolves. Identifying a malrotation in such patients is challenging but beneficial in that it can be corrected before a catastrophic midgut bowel infarction occurs.

Management

Emergency Department

Evaluation, resuscitation, surgical consultation, and preoperative preparation proceed simultaneously in patients with suspected malrotation with volvulus. In the ED, volume resuscitation, gastric decompression, and broad-spectrum antibiotics are administered. The surgical procedure for the correction of malrotation, called the Ladd procedure, includes detorsion of the volvulus, division of Ladd bands, separation of the duodenojejunal mesentery from the cecocolic mesentery, and appendectomy. An appendectomy is performed because the colon is positioned on the left side of the abdomen during a Ladd procedure. Subsequent diagnosis of appendicitis could be difficult. A gastrostomy is seldom indicated.

The incidence and type of complications that occur reflect the extent of ischemic bowel and intestinal necrosis found during surgery. With a viable intestine, postoperative care is straightforward and prognosis is excellent. The lifetime risk of adhesive small bowel obstruction is 1% to 10%. Volvulus should not recur once the malrotation is corrected.

With extensive ischemic bowel and intestinal necrosis, the bowel is untwisted and reduced into the abdominal cavity, and 12 to 24 hours later, a "second look" procedure can be performed to assess bowel viability. This allows the surgeon to resect the necrotic bowel and to create an enterostomy at the distal end of the proximal normal bowel. Bowel reconstruction is performed at a later operation. With extensive bowel resection, patients can develop short gut syndrome and might become dependent on TPN.

What to Avoid and Why

In the treatment of an otherwise healthy infant with bilious vomiting, a delay in diagnosis must be avoided. Delay can lead to the most serious complication: volvulus with necrosis of the entire midgut. In an acutely ill infant suspected to have malrotation with volvulus, time-consuming studies might be best replaced by laparotomy itself. In an otherwise stable infant, an emergency limited upper GI tract contrast study should be performed quickly.

Controversies in Management

Malrotation found incidentally in asymptomatic children should be repaired, but the timing of surgery remains controversial.[64,65] The role of laparoscopy in the pediatric patient with malrotation is also controversial. Laparoscopy allows benefits of early return to oral intake, shorter length of hospitalization, and less postoperative pain.[66–69] However, in circumstances involving ischemic volvulus or bowel resection, data are lacking.

KEY POINTS

Management of Suspected Midgut Volvulus

- ABCs (airway, breathing, circulation)
- Fluid resuscitation
- Gastric decompression
- Early surgical consultation

THE BOTTOM LINE

Important Concepts in the Evaluation and Management of Midgut Volvulus

- Bilious emesis in the neonate represents a true surgical emergency
- Bilious emesis in a neonate should be considered malrotation with midgut volvulus until proved otherwise
- A limited upper GI tract contrast study is the most reliable method to diagnose malrotation
- Any delay in treatment of malrotation with midgut volvulus could result in necrosis of the entire midgut

A 3-week-old, female infant presents with a 4-day history of projectile vomiting. She is a full-term product of a vaginal delivery. There were no complications at birth. For the first 2 weeks of life, the infant would occasionally spit up (normal for age). Currently, the vomiting is very forceful, as if it will "hit the wall." The infant is breastfed, and the vomit appears to be breast milk. There is no history of blood or green emesis, diarrhea, or fever. The mother is frustrated because the infant is losing weight and appears hungry.

On physical examination, the infant is dehydrated, with a sunken fontanelle and poor skin turgor. Her respiratory rate is 24/min, heart rate is 165/min, and temperature is 36.3°C (97°F). Cardiac and pulmonary examination results are normal except for tachycardia. Abdominal examination is difficult due to crying and tensing of the abdominal muscles. The infant's genitourinary examination results are normal. There is loss of subcutaneous fat of the thighs and buttocks.

1. *What maneuver can be done to help facilitate the abdominal examination?*
2. *What clinical signs can the physician look for during the examination?*
3. *What ancillary studies could help determine the diagnosis?*

Pyloric Stenosis

Hypertrophic pyloric stenosis (HPS) is the most common surgical cause of vomiting in infants. It is the result of hypertrophy of the circular musculature surrounding the pylorus, leading to compression of the longitudinal folds of mucosa and causing obstruction of the gastric outlet. The hypertrophied pylorus measures the size of an olive and is approximately 2 by 1 cm.

Infants with HPS typically present with nonbilious projectile vomiting in the second to fourth weeks of life. Symptoms rarely occur before 2 weeks or later than 4 to 6 months of age.[70]

Hypertrophic pyloric stenosis is primarily a disease of full-term infants. However, cases in the premature infant have been reported. Hypertrophic pyloric stenosis in the premature infant poses a difficult diagnostic challenge. Premature infants, on average, present later (fifth week of life), feed less vigorously, and vomit less forcefully.[71]

The cause of HPS remains unknown, but both genetic and environmental influences have been implicated. Hypertrophic pyloric stenosis tends to run in families.[72,73] Siblings of patients with HPS are 15 times more likely to develop the condition than children without a family history of the condition.

Research shows that 5% to 20% of sons and 2.5% to 7% of daughters of affected parents are at risk of developing HPS. The risk to children of affected mothers is three times greater than to those of affected fathers.[74,75]

Factors that have been implicated in the development of HPS are abnormalities in hormonal control (gastrin, cholecystokinin, secretin, somatostatin, and prostaglandins), abnormalities in pyloric innervation (ganglion cells, peptidergic and nitrergic innervation, nitric oxide synthase deficiency, reduced synapse formation, or reduced nerve-supporting cells), abnormalities of extracellular matrix proteins, abnormalities of smooth muscle cells, and abnormalities in growth factors.[76–86]

Environmental causes have also been implicated in the development of HPS. These include maternal anxiety, maternal smoking and drug use, infant feeding practices, and oral erythromycin use in neonates.[87–91] Evidence to date suggests that erythromycin exposure in pregnant women and breastfeeding infants is not associated with increased risk of HPS in infants.[92,93]

Epidemiology

The incidence of pyloric stenosis is approximately 1.5 to 4.0 per 1,000 live births.[94–102] Recently, a decrease in HPS incidence has been reported in a number of countries, such as Sweden, Denmark, and Scotland.[103–105] Male infants are consistently affected more often than female infants, with a 2:1 to 5:1 male-female ratio. Although rare, HPS can present in premature infants.

Clinical Features

The classic patient with HPS is a male infant between 2 and 6 weeks of age with forceful projectile emesis. The emesis is always nonbilious and occurs 10 to 30 minutes after feeding. The infant appears hungry and will usually feed vigorously if given the chance. After 60 to 90 mL (2 to 3 oz) of feeding, the infant will stop eating and play with the nipple, with eyes open wide. Reverse peristaltic waves traveling upward across the abdomen might be visualized because the gastric contents cannot pass the hypertrophied pyloric sphincter. The ensuing emesis vomit will be expelled with force, as if it is "hitting the wall." Thus it might be more effective to ask parents if the vomitus can hit the wall, rather than asking them if it is projectile (because to a layperson, all vomit projects). The vomitus contains milk and gastric juices; sometimes it might be "coffee ground" in appearance due to gastritis and/or esophagitis.

The overall appearance of the infant presenting with HPS varies. Infants can be generally well appearing (normal Pediatric Assessment Triangle) or present with prolonged vomiting, severe dehydration, and lethargy (abnormal Pediatric Assessment Triangle). Physical examination findings of dehydration are seen with altered level of consciousness, sunken fontanel, sunken eyes, skin tenting, delayed capillary refill, or mottled and cool extremities. Abdominal findings can include abdominal distention, visible gastric peristaltic waves traveling across the abdomen, and a small mobile mass ("olive") palpable in the right upper quadrant region. This olive-sized and shaped pylorus is difficult to feel. It is best felt by experienced hands while the child is feeding (ie, when the abdominal musculature is most relaxed).

Complications

If the vomiting is allowed to continue for days, dehydration, weight loss, lethargy, and evidence of shock will occur. Caregivers might give a history of decreased urine output and activity.

YOUR FIRST CLUE

Signs and Symptoms of Pyloric Stenosis

Early

- Normal Pediatric Assessment Triangle

Late:

- Appearance: decreased level of consciousness, decreased activity
- Work of breathing: effortless tachypnea
- Circulation: delayed capillary refill, cool, mottled extremities, rapid pulse

Other findings

- More common in males
- Nonbilious, forceful emesis that can "hit the wall"
- Appears hungry
- Visible peristaltic waves
- Palpable olive-shaped pylorus in the right upper quadrant

Diagnostic Studies

Laboratory

Characteristic electrolyte findings are a hypochloremic, hypokalemic metabolic alkalosis. Infants might also exhibit an increased indirect bilirubin level, which might be due to increased enterohepatic recirculation, a relative deficiency of hepatic glucuronyltransferase activity, and/or poor caloric intake.[106,107]

Radiology

Plain radiographs might reveal a large dilated stomach with no air in the small bowel or colon. These findings are consistent with a gastric outlet obstruction (**Figure 8.8**).

Until recently, the upper GI tract contrast study was the "gold standard" for diagnosis of pyloric stenosis. Positive upper GI tract signs of HPS are the string sign (a single streak of barium in the lumen of the elongated pylorus), the beak sign (the beginning of the elongated pyloric channel), and the double track sign (double streaks of barium passing through the narrow pylorus) (**Figure 8.9**).[108] Currently, abdominal ultrasonography is the imaging modality of choice

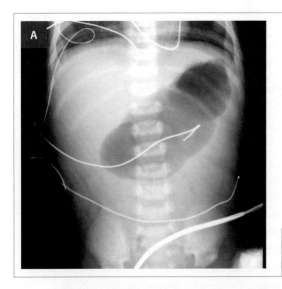

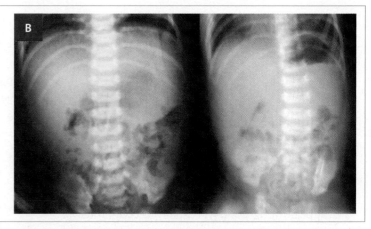

Figure 8.8 Pyloric stenosis. The first image (A) shows a large dilated stomach with no distal air. The second pair of images (B) shows a dilated fluid-filled stomach with a small amount of air in the small bowel and colon.

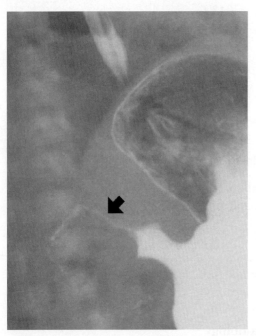

Figure 8.9 String sign of pyloric stenosis seen on barium upper GI tract series. The "string" represents the thin pyloric lumen.

used to visualize the muscle hypertrophy and measure the pyloric canal length diagnostic of HPS. A muscle thickness of 4 mm or more and a channel length of 15 mm or more is confirming (**Figure 8.10A** and **8.10B**).[109–112] Ultrasonography is advantageous because it is noninvasive, free of ionizing radiation, and without risk of aspiration of contrast material. Recent literature describes the feasibility and high accuracy of bedside ultrasonography performed by emergency physicians and surgeons in the diagnosis

of HPS.[113–116] Disadvantages of ultrasonography are that it is operator dependent and, in a negative or equivocal study, an upper GI tract contrast study might be necessary.

Differential Diagnosis

Although most symptoms are benign and self-limiting, the differential diagnosis of vomiting in an infant is broad. Disorders to consider with HPS include gastroesophageal reflux, overfeeding technique, and cow's milk intolerance. Other primary GI conditions include gastric or proximal duodenal web, obstructions, malrotation with midgut volvulus, and gastric volvulus. Vomiting can also be secondary to extraintestinal disorders involving the central nervous system (eg, increased intracranial pressure, intracranial hemorrhage, cerebral edema, or space-occupying lesions), renal system (eg,

THE CLASSICS

Classic Diagnostic Findings in Pyloric Stenosis

- Hyponatremic, hypochloremic, hypokalemic metabolic alkalosis
- Sonogram showing thickened and elongated pylorus
- Upper GI tract contrast study showing the string, beak, or double track signs

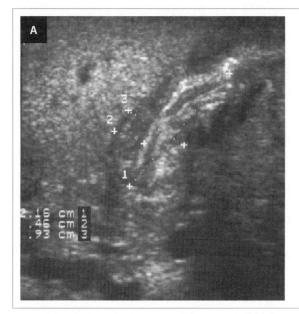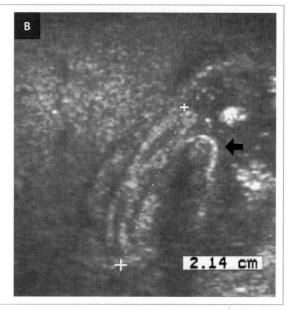

Figure 8.10 Sonographic imaging in pyloric stenosis. Figure 8.10A shows the measurements of the pylorus. The pyloric length measures 2.16 cm (line 1). The pyloric wall thickness measures 0.46 cm (line 2). The pyloric diameter measures 0.93 cm (line 3). These exceed the measurements of 1.6 cm (length) and 0.4 cm (wall thickness), respectively, which are indicative of pyloric stenosis. Figure 8.10B shows another view of the pylorus. The pyloric length measures 2.14 cm in this view. The black arrow points to a prominent indentation of the pylorus into the stomach, which is also indicative of pyloric stenosis.

obstructive uropathy and renal insufficiency), systemic infection (eg, meningitis, urinary tract infections, or sepsis), or metabolic abnormalities (eg, congenital adrenal hyperplasia or inborn error of metabolism).

Management

Emergency Department

Hypertrophic pyloric stenosis recognition is important, but surgical correction is not required immediately. Surgical intervention is performed after correction of electrolyte abnormalities, normalization of acid base status, and replenishment of fluid deficit. Provide a bolus of 20 mL/kg of normal saline at the time intravenous access is established. Follow the bolus with an infusion of 5% dextrose with half normal saline at 1.5 times the maintenance volume. Correct fluid and electrolyte abnormalities during 24 to 48 hours. Establish good urine output greater than 1 mL/kg per hour and then add 20 to 40 mEq/L of potassium chloride to the maintenance fluids. Place an orogastric or nasogastric tube to low intermittent suction to decompress the stomach. Provide oxygen and respiratory support as indicated. Surgical intervention is the Fredet-Ramstedt pyloromy-

otomy, which consists of a longitudinal incision through the hypertrophied muscle down to, but not through, the underlying mucosa.

WHAT ELSE?

Differential Diagnosis of Pyloric Stenosis

- Gastroesophageal reflux
- Overfeeding
- Cow's milk intolerance
- Malrotation with midgut volvulus
- NEC
- Central nervous system disease (eg, increased intracranial pressure, intracranial hemorrhage, cerebral edema, or mass-occupying lesions)
- Renal disease (eg, obstructive uropathy or renal insufficiency)
- Infection (eg, meningitis, urinary tract infection, or sepsis)
- Metabolic disease (eg, congenital adrenal hyperplasia or inborn error of metabolism)

Between 6 and 18 hours after surgical correction, infants are allowed to start feedings. Great variability in formula type, feeding regimens, and advancement exists, some advocate unrestricted on-demand feedings, while others prefer standardized feedings. Postoperative emesis is common and occurs in 65% to 90% of patients regardless of the regimen or protocol used.[117–119]

What to Avoid and Why

Avoid surgical intervention until metabolic alkalosis is resolved. Uncorrected alkalosis can delay recovery from anesthetic agents or cause postanesthetic apnea.

Controversies in Management

One area of controversy in management is the approach to repairing the hypertrophied pylorus. Pediatric surgeons might use the traditional abdominal approach, a laparoscopic technique, or an umbilical fold incision.[102,120–126] Laparoscopy and the umbilical fold incision provide smaller incisions and better cosmetic results. Laparoscopy results in less postoperative pain, reduced emesis, and time to full feedings and reduced wound complications. Recent research shows no difference in operating time or length of recovery when comparing the traditional abdominal approach and laparoscopy. However, the learning curve is steep, and the risk of incomplete pyloromyotomy after laparoscopy occurs 1.4% to 5.6% of the time and is rare with the traditional approach. The supraumbilical fold approach is not used in infants with a large pylorus and is associated with an increased wound infection and fascial dehiscence rate. The infraumbilical approach results in excellent cosmetic results, allows easy access to the pylorus, and is associated with minimal complications.[126]

Another area of controversy is the use of nonsurgical approaches to the treatment of HPS. Pyloric stenosis will spontaneously resolve within weeks to months. During this time, the infant can be maintained with parenteral nutrition. Intravenous and subsequent oral atropine sulfate administration has been shown to reduce the resolution time of pyloric stenosis and reduce the overall costs involved when compared with surgery.[102,127–129] Success rates range from 40% to 90%, depending on the study. Because surgical intervention is 95% successful and the complication risk is low, nonsurgical management is not generally accepted in the United States, but practices in other countries might differ.

A 6-month-old boy presents to a pediatrician's office with 1 day of crying and poor feeding. His mother states that during the past few hours he has had two episodes of vomiting breast milk. There is no fever, diarrhea, or cold symptoms. His mother states that the pain seems so intense that he draws his knees to his chest and "crawls" up her arms and shoulders. Between bouts of pain, he is calm and at times quite sleepy.

On physical examination, the infant is resting in his mother's arms. His respiratory rate is 18/min, heart rate is 130/min, and rectal temperature is 37.9°C (100.2°F). The anterior fontanelle is flat and soft. His lips are pink but dry. His lungs are clear to auscultation without increased work of breathing. The abdominal examination reveals normal bowel sounds, mild tenderness, and a soft mass in the right upper quadrant below the liver border. The genital examination results are normal. Soft stool obtained on rectal examination is positive for occult blood. While you discuss further management plans with the mother, the infant begins crying inconsolably.

1. *What could be the cause of this infant's abdominal pain?*

The mother of a 9-month-old boy calls you because the infant is sleeping too much. Earlier in the morning he had two episodes of vomiting. The vomit was not green or bloody. The infant passed a stool with mucus and urinated without difficulty.

On physical examination, the infant is lethargic. His respiratory rate is 20/min, heart rate is 120/min, and rectal temperature is 37.5°C (100°F). The anterior fontanelle is small and flat. Pupils are 4 mm and reactive. His lungs are clear to auscultation without increased work of breathing, and cardiovascular examination results are normal. The abdominal and genital examination results are also normal. The stool is positive for occult blood. The skin examination reveals no evidence of trauma.

1. *What surgical emergency could cause lethargy in this infant?*
2. *What diagnostic test could be performed to diagnose and treat this entity?*
3. *What is an important complication of an air enema, and how should the physician specifically intervene if respiratory difficulty occurs?*

Intussusception

Intussusception is an invagination of the proximal portion of the bowel into an adjacent distal bowel segment. It is second only to an incarcerated inguinal hernia as the most common cause of intestinal obstruction in infants.

Intussusception is classified according to the site of the inner intussusceptum and the outer intussuscipiens. Approximately 80% to 90% involve invagination of the ileum into the colon (ileocolic). The remainder are ileoileal, cecocolic, colocolic, and jejuno-jejunal, in decreasing order of frequency.[130,131]

Epidemiology

The peak age of occurrence is between 5 and 9 months, with most cases occurring in patients ages 3 months to 2 years. Research shows 10% to 25% of cases occur in children older than 2 years. Although rare, intussusception has been reported in preterm infants.[132–134] There is a male predominance of 2:1.[130,131,135–138] In children younger than 2 years, no pathologic lead point is found in more than 90% of patients. These cases are termed primary idiopathic but can be caused by lymphoid hyperplasia of Peyer patches, stimulated by an antecedent bacterial enteritis or viral infection.[139] There is a higher incidence in spring and autumn, suggesting a preceding viral infection. Adenovirus, human herpesvirus 6, and rotavirus have been reported to be associated with intussusception. Pathologic lead points are more commonly found in older children, with Meckel diverticulum being the most common. Other causes of lead points are intestinal duplications, hemorrhagic congestion, and vasculitis of the intestinal mucosa as seen in Henoch-Schönlein purpura, inspissated intestinal secretions as seen in cystic fibrosis, lymphomas, intestinal polyps, foreign bodies, and *Ascaris lumbricoides* infestation.[140–145] There was an association between rotavirus vaccine (Rotashield; Wyeth Lederle Vaccines, Philadelphia, Pennsylvania) and intussusception that led to the voluntary withdrawal of the vaccine in 1999. Currently, two new rotavirus vaccines (RV1 and RV5) are available (Rotateq; Merck & Co, Whitehouse Station, New Jersey; and Rotarix; Glaxo Smith Kline, Rixensart, Belgium). Results of phase 3 randomized controlled clinical trials have shown both RV1 and RV5 are well tolerated and not associated with intussusception.[146–149]

Clinical Features

The classic triad of intussusception is intermittent colicky abdominal pain, vomiting, and bloody mucoid ("currant jelly") stools. Most infants, however, present with only two symptoms. The most frequent symptom is colicky abdominal pain (85% to 90%) that lasts 2 to 10 minutes followed by a period of relief when the infant appears calm. In between episodes the infant/child sometimes can be seen playing and acting rather normal. This behavior can mislead the examiner into thinking the child has mild gastroenteritis rather than intussusception. This pattern usually repeats every 20 to 30 minutes. Classically, the young infant manifests abdominal pain by forcefully drawing up the legs onto the abdomen and crying. The paroxysmal nature of these painful attacks suggests small bowel obstruction. The second most common symptom is vomiting (65% to 80%). Initially, emesis can be nonbilious but can become bilious or feculent. Stools might initially be negative for blood or positive for occult blood. It is not until significant bowel ischemia occurs that stools become grossly bloody, which is why the presence of "currant jelly" stools is usually a late finding.[130,131,137,138] Patients with intussusception can also have fever and can occasionally present without abdominal pain.

Lethargy, hypotonia, and pallor are other symptoms seen in intussusception. In a review of patients with lethargy due to intussusception, all had either melena or a palpable abdominal mass on physical examination. The exact mechanism for lethargy in intussusception is unclear. Several mechanisms have been postulated. One hypothesis is that the breakdown of intestinal mucosa and release of endotoxin or other mediators from the bowel enter the bloodstream and then affect the central nervous system. Another mechanism suggests that a release of endogenous opioid from the ischemic bowel contributes to profound lethargy.[150–156] Dehydration can be a contributing factor.

On physical examination, 15% to 30% of infants with intussusception can have normal examination results. Classically, abdominal examination reveals emptiness in the right lower quadrant; in more than half of the cases, a soft sausage-shaped mass is palpable in the right upper quadrant extending along the transverse colon.[130,131,138] In patients with extensive involvement of the bowel, the mass might be palpable only on rectal examination. Rarely, protrusion of the intussuscepted intestine occurs through the rectum. Differentiating between a simple prolapsed rectum and intussusception is important and is easily accomplished. Ability to insert a finger between the mass (intussusceptum) and the rectal lining indicates an intussusception.

Complications

With undiagnosed or misdiagnosed intussusception, ischemic bowel will become necrotic and can perforate. Late signs include progressive dehydration, abdominal distention, peritonitis, and hypovolemic shock.

Diagnostic Studies

Laboratory

Laboratory tests are nonspecific and generally not helpful. Testing the stool for occult blood can be helpful if positive. Occult blood has been found in 43% of patients with intussusception, and its presence might help increase the index of suspicion for intussusception.[157,158]

Radiology

Abdominal plain radiographs can be helpful in the diagnosis of intussusception but, if normal, do not exclude the disease.[159] Radiographic findings suggestive of intussusception include a soft tissue mass (**Figure 8.11**), target sign (**Figure 8.12A** and **8.12B**), absence of cecal gas and stool (**Figure**

8.13; see also Figure 8.11), meniscus sign (also called the crescent sign) (**Figure 8.14A**, **8.14B**, and **8.14C**), paucity of bowel gas (**Figure 8.15**), and a bowel obstruction (**Figure 8.16**). Radiographic evidence of small bowel obstruction can be more apparent if the presentation is delayed. A soft tissue mass can be seen in the right upper quadrant in up to 50% of the cases (this includes the target sign). A left-side-down decubitus view can improve the radiographic diagnosis of intussusception. An upright or decubitus plain film is helpful to identify intestinal perforation if present.[160,161] Although the barium enema is considered the "gold standard" study in the diagnosis of intussusception (**Figure 8.17**), air contrast enemas have been used and have been shown to be as effective in the diagnosis and treatment of intussusception when used by radiologists skilled in this procedure (**Figure 8.18** and **Figure 8.19A** and **8.19B**).[162–169] Radiologists who have not been trained in air contrast enemas often prefer barium or water-soluble contrast enemas.

Barium and air contrast enemas are contraindicated in cases involving intestinal perforation, peritonitis, or decompensated shock.

More recently, ultrasonography has been used to diagnose intussusception with up to 100% accuracy (98% to 100% sensitivity, 88% to 100% specificity) when interpreted by a radiologist skilled in the sonographic diagnosis of intussusception.[170–174] Sonographic screening in children reduces radiation exposure and

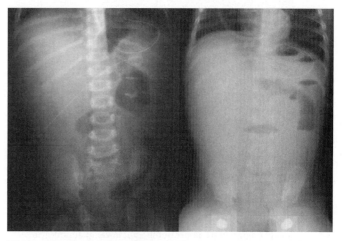

Figure 8.11 Right upper quadrant soft tissue mass in intussusception. There is a fullness in the right upper quadrant with a soft tissue mass (absence of gas). Note that the liver edge (subhepatic angle) is obscured by the mass. This is suggestive of intussusception.

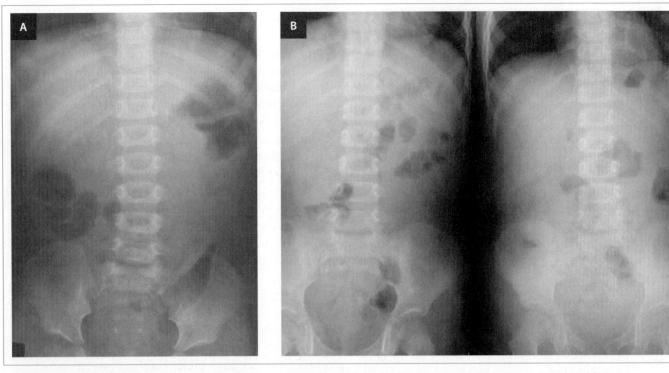

Figure 8.12 Target sign in intussusception. This sign is more specific for intussusception. This right upper quadrant soft tissue mass has a target appearance (similar to a faint doughnut). The target signs are not obvious, but they can be clearly identified in these two radiographs. Note that 8.12A demonstrates a crescent sign in the left upper quadrant.

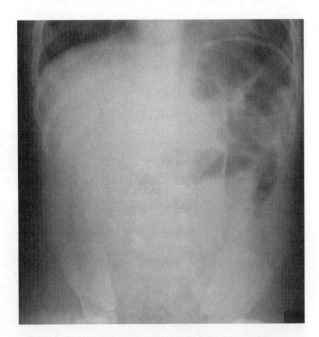

Figure 8.13 Absence of cecal stool and gas. Note the solid homogeneous nature in the right lower quadrant. The same appearance can be seen in Figure 8.11. This is nonspecific but suggestive of intussusception. Identification of definite gas and stool in the cecum makes it unlikely that an ileocecal intussusception is protruding through this area.

can reduce costs and patient discomfort when compared with air contrast or barium enema. Characteristic sonographic findings are the target sign or doughnut sign on transverse view (**Figure 8.20**) and the sandwich sign on longitudinal view. The quality of the study and its interpretation are operator dependent. However, when used appropriately, a negative sonogram (that is reliably negative) obviates unnecessary diagnostic enemas. Ultrasonography also can be used to obtain other information, including detection of lead points. If the skill of the available radiologist provides the physician with only modest certainty, then ultrasonography should not be performed because a negative sonogram will still require a contrast enema to definitively rule out intussusception and a positive sonogram will require a contrast enema for confirmation and reduction.

Differential Diagnosis

The differential diagnosis for intussusception includes conditions that cause intestinal

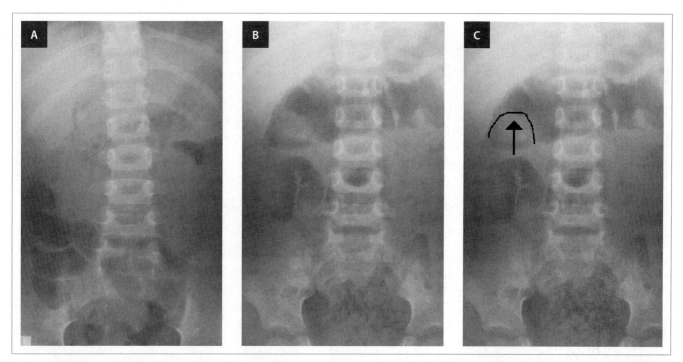

Figure 8.14 Meniscus sign (crescent sign). The crescent sign (left upper quadrant in 8.14A) is formed by the intussusceptum protruding into a gas-filled pocket. This makes the air pocket resemble a crescent as in the left image. However, in 8.14B, the intussusceptum is traveling superiorly in the right upper quadrant as it approaches the hepatic flexure. Note that the gas-filled pocket is very large, so even though the intussusceptum can be visualized within this gas-filled pocket (pointing superiorly), as in 8.14C, the resultant shape is not a crescent. Thus, the crescent sign is not always crescent shaped. It should be more accurately called "the intussusceptum protruding into a gas-filled pocket sign," but that is too long to say.

obstruction, abdominal pain, and blood in the stool. These symptoms include malrotation with midgut volvulus, Meckel diverticulum, incarcerated inguinal hernia, intentional trauma, and infectious enteritis of the alimentary tract.

Management

Emergency Department and Follow-up Care

Once intussusception is suspected, obtain surgical consultation, withhold oral intake, establish intravenous access, and resuscitate the infant with intravenous fluids. Once free peritoneal air is excluded by plain radiography or sonography, nonsurgical reduction by air contrast enema or barium enema is attempted first. It is successful in 60% to 90% of cases. Contraindications to nonsurgical reduction are signs of peritonitis, hypovolemic shock, or demonstration of a

---

THE CLASSICS

Diagnostic Studies for Intussusception

- Soft tissue mass, target sign, crescent sign on plain radiograph
- Target sign by sonography
- Intussusception on air or barium contrast enema

WHAT ELSE?

Differential Diagnosis of Intussusception

- Meckel diverticulum
- Incarcerated inguinal hernia
- Intentional trauma
- Gastroenteritis
- Cow's milk or soy protein allergy or other benign processes

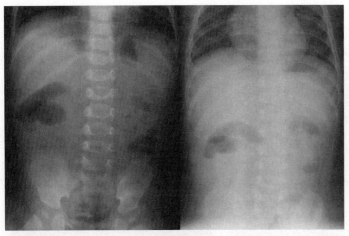

Figure 8.15 Paucity of bowel gas. This radiograph demonstrates a general paucity of gas. There are only a few bowel loops that are faint on the upright view (right image), and these are actually air-fluid levels, suggesting that this is actually a bowel obstruction that is most likely due to intussusception.

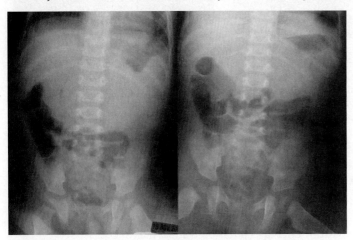

Figure 8.16 Bowel obstruction. Note the poor distribution of gas on the flat view (left image) and the dilated (smooth) bowel loops on the upright view (right image), which indicate the presence of a bowel obstruction that is most likely due to intussusception. A possible target sign is visible in the right upper quadrant. Figure 8.15 also demonstrates a bowel obstruction due to intussusception.

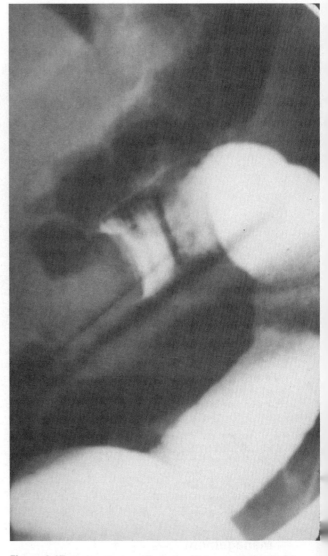

Figure 8.17 Barium enema diagnosis of intussusception. In this image, barium fills the ascending colon and part of the transverse colon. The barium column encounters a mass within the transverse colon (the intussusceptum).

pathologic lead point on a sonogram. Complications of hydrostatic reduction are intestinal perforation and nonreduction. Surgical reduction is necessary when contrast enema reduction is contraindicated or unsuccessful. Laparotomy is performed through a right transverse incision at the level of the umbilicus. The intussusceptum is gently milked out of the intussuscipiens. Nonviable bowel and any lead points are resected. Intussuscepted bowel segments are examined for adequate reperfusion. Routine use of antibiotics is controversial.

The risk of recurrence of intussusception after surgical reduction is less than 4%. The risk of recurrence of intussusception after enema reduction is 10%. Most first recurrences develop within the first 8 months. Most are not due to pathologic lead points and thus can be managed by hydrostatic reduction.[175,176]

What to Avoid and Why

Complete physical examination and normal plain radiographs are seldom sufficient to eliminate the diagnosis of intussusception with

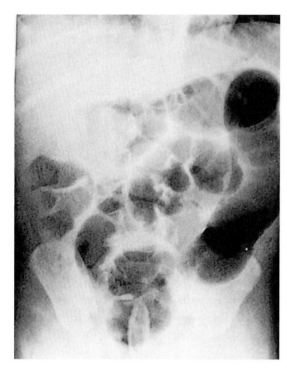

Figure 8.18 Air contrast enema diagnosis of intussusceptions. In this image, air contrast distends the descending colon. As the air contrast enters the transverse colon, it encounters a mass (the intussusceptum) just to the right of the midline. This is not as obvious as in the barium enema; because air is normally present in the small bowel as well, the air contrast does not stand out as much.

certainty. Consider ultrasonography of the abdomen or an air or barium contrast study to aid in the diagnosis.

Hydrostatic reduction of an intussusception is contraindicated in toxic, ill-appearing patients and patients with evidence of peritonitis. These findings indicate the presence of gangrenous intestine, for which emergency surgery is necessary.

In the patient with profound lethargy, do not forget intussusception as a potential cause. Intussusception is easily treatable, and development of gangrenous bowel can be avoided.

Controversies in Management

For infants without evidence of peritonitis but with a history of symptoms that exceeds 24 hours and an obstructive pattern on abdominal plain radiographs, management controversies exist. These infants are believed to be at an increased risk of perforation. Some radiologists attempt reduction with gentle hydrostatic

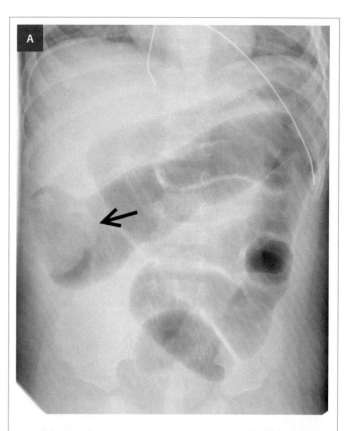

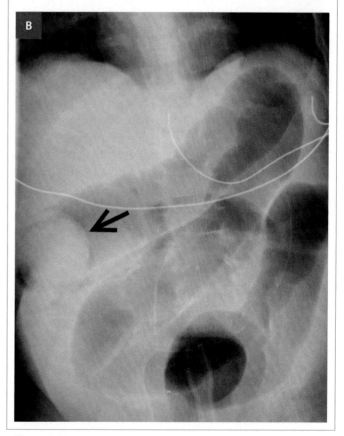

Figure 8.19 Air contrast enemas revealing diagnosis of intussusception.

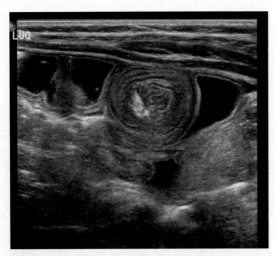

Figure 8.20 Sonographic image of doughnut sign. Similar to the target sign on plain film radiography, this sonographic doughnut sign is indicative of intussusception.

pressure, whereas others recommend surgical correction as first-line therapy.

In an effort to reduce postreduction recurrence due to lymphoid hyperplasia, intramuscular dexamethasone as premedication before air contrast enema has been used. In one clinical trial, 1 child of 122 treated with dexamethasone had a recurrence in the 6-month follow-up period.[177] This is in contrast to the 117 nontreated children who had eight episodes of recurrence during the same period. Dexamethasone appears to be beneficial, but larger clinical trials need to be conducted before widespread use is advocated.

Postreduction management is also controversial. Patients can be observed in the ED for 4 to 6 hours or admitted to the hospital for up to 24 hours after uncomplicated hydrostatic reduction of the intussusception. Patients are observed for evidence of recurrent intussusception, feeding intolerance, peritonitis, and other complications. Recent literature supports that a select population can be safely treated as outpatients.[178,179]

> ### KEY POINTS
>
> **Management of Intussusception**
> - Resuscitate with fluids
> - Stop oral intake
> - Consult pediatric surgeon early
> - Obtain appropriate radiographic studies

> ### THE BOTTOM LINE
>
> - Consider intussusception in all infants with abdominal pain and vomiting
> - A normal plain radiograph does not exclude intussusception, so a second study (air/barium enema or ultrasonography) is needed
> - An infant with intussusception can present with profound lethargy

A 2-year-old boy presents to the ED by ambulance. His mother had called 911 because she discovered that his diaper was full of bright red blood. The child has had previous bowel movements with streaks of blood. He does not seem to be in pain but is less active than normal. There is no history of mucus in the stools, fever, or vomiting. He is feeding well.

On physical examination, the child is alert and appropriately fearful. His respiratory rate is 24/min and nonlabored, heart rate is 140/min, blood pressure is 100/60 mm Hg, and temperature is 37°C (98.6°F). Head and neck examination reveals pale conjunctivae and mucous membranes. Cardiovascular examination reveals mild tachycardia with a soft 2/6 systolic ejection murmur at the left lower sternal border. Abdominal and genitourinary examination results are normal. Examination of the anus reveals no evidence of trauma, fissures, or tags. Stool is grossly bloody. The skin is without bruising or petechiae.

1. *What are the priorities of treatment in this child?*
2. *How can the physician differentiate upper GI tract bleeding from lower GI tract bleeding?*
3. *What could be the cause of painless rectal bleeding in this previously healthy child?*
4. *In a child who is actively bleeding from the rectum, would radiographs be helpful or indicated?*

Meckel Diverticulum

Meckel diverticulum is a congenital true diverticulum of the distal ileum that contains all layers of the intestinal wall. It forms as a result of incomplete obliteration of the omphalomesenteric (vitelline) duct during the ninth gestational week.[180] Normally, the omphalomesenteric duct disappears just before the midgut returns to the abdomen. Persistence of some portion of this omphalomesenteric duct results in a constellation of congenital anomalies; Meckel diverticulum is the most common.[181]

Meckel diverticulum is clinically significant because it can contain gastric or pancreatic tissue. Gastric tissue produces acid, which results in ulceration and bleeding. Meckel diverticulum can also remain attached to the abdominal wall by a fibrous cord that forms from incomplete obliteration of the distal portion of the omphalomesenteric duct. This fibrous cord acts as a focus around which the intestines can twist, forming a volvulus and resulting in intestinal obstruction.

More than 60% of children with symptomatic Meckel diverticula are younger than 2 years.

Signs and symptoms are typically related to bleeding, inflammation, or intestinal obstruction.[181]

The rule of twos is often quoted as an easy way to remember some facts about Meckel diverticulum: 2% prevalence, two types of heterotopic mucosa (gastric and pancreatic), located within 2 ft (61 cm) of the ileocecal valve, approximately 2 in (5 cm) in length, and 2 cm in diameter, with symptoms usually occurring before a child is 2 years old (**Figure 8.21**).

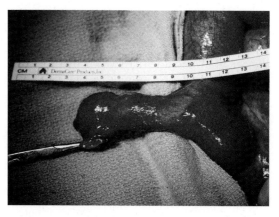

Figure 8.21 Meckel diverticulum found at laparotomy measuring approximately 5 cm (2 in) long.

Epidemiology

Meckel diverticulum is the most common congenital anomaly of the GI tract and is found in approximately 2% of the population.[182] It occurs in equal frequency between males and females when diverticula are incidentally discovered. However, in symptomatic cases, males are three to four times more commonly affected than females. An increased incidence of Meckel diverticulum is found in children with esophageal atresia, imperforate anus,[183] small omphaloceles,[184] and Crohn disease.[185]

Clinical Features

The most common clinical presentations of Meckel diverticulum are lower GI tract bleeding, intestinal obstruction (due to intussusception or volvulus), and inflammatory complications (diverticulitis, similar to appendicitis).[186–189]

Lower GI tract bleeding presents as melena (black, tarry stools) or hematochezia (bright red blood from the rectum). The bleeding from a Meckel diverticulum is generally painless, episodic, and, at times, massive. Bowel obstruction can occur due to an intussusception with the diverticulum as the lead point, herniation of the bowel through a patent omphalomesenteric fistula, or volvulus of the distal small bowel. Clinical signs include vomiting, abdominal pain, bloody stools, and a palpable abdominal mass. If symptoms are allowed to progress, signs of dehydration, peritonitis, and shock will develop. Inflammation of a Meckel diverticulum can mimic the clinical picture of appendicitis. The symptoms of Meckel diverticulitis include periumbilical, right lower quadrant, and lower midline pain, vomiting, and diffuse peritoneal irritation.

Complications of unrecognized Meckel diverticulum include massive GI hemorrhage, obstruction due to volvulus, intussusception with potential for the development of peritonitis, bowel ischemia, and shock.

Other complications of Meckel diverticulum are rare but have been reported in the literature. These complications include impaction of foreign bodies (eg, stones, pins, or parasites) and future development of primary GI cancer, such as carcinoid, sarcoma, lymphoma, adenocarcinoma, and leiomyoma.

YOUR FIRST CLUE

Signs and Symptoms of Meckel Diverticulum

Early

- Appearance: normal depending on the presentation type
- Work of breathing: normal
- Circulation: normal

Late

- Appearance: weak
- Work of breathing: effortless tachypnea (compensatory for metabolic acidosis)
- Circulation: delayed capillary refill, cool, pallor, poor skin turgor, mottled extremities, rapid pulse

Other findings

- Painless, rectal bleeding
- Black, tarry stools

Diagnostic Studies

Laboratory

Laboratory study results are nonspecific. Occult bleeding with anemia is an infrequent presentation of Meckel diverticulum. A complete blood cell count and prothrombin time/partial thromboplastin time help differentiate a coagulopathy as the cause of bleeding.

Radiology

Technetium Tc 99m pertechnetate scintigraphy, or Meckel scan, is the diagnostic procedure of choice in children with GI bleeding suggestive of Meckel diverticulum.[190] Bleeding Meckel diverticula contain ectopic gastric mucosa in 95% of cases. Technetium Tc 99m pertechnetate isotope concentrates in the gastric mucosa of the stomach and Meckel diverticulum. As the isotope is excreted, it collects in the urinary bladder. The use of pentagastrin, histamine$_2$ blockers, and glucagon enhances the accuracy of the scan.[189] Fasting, nasogastric suctioning, and bladder catheterization also increase the diagnostic yield of the scan. A 10-year review of technetium Tc 99m scans of Meckel diverticula found 1.7% of scans were false negative and

0.05% were false positive. The sensitivity was 85%, specificity was 95%, and accuracy was 90%.[191,192] If bleeding persists after a negative scan and Meckel diverticulum is still suspected, an additional scan is indicated. If the scan remains negative despite enhancing measures, other studies, such as isotope-labeled red blood cell scan or angiography, can be considered.[193]

Differential Diagnosis

The differential diagnosis of Meckel diverticulum presenting as lower GI tract bleeding in a child includes gastroenteritis (bacterial), inflammatory bowel disease, polyps, duplications, arteriovenous malformations, intussusception, Henoch-Schönlein purpura, and pseudomembranous colitis. Brisk upper GI tract bleeding caused by peptic ulcer disease and variceal bleeding can also present in a similar manner; however, these usually can be distinguished from Meckel diverticulum by the presence of bloody gastric aspirates, which would indicate an upper GI tract bleed. In children with massive, painless rectal bleeding, the differential diagnosis is more defined and includes polyps, duplications, hemangiomas, arteriovenous malformations, coagulopathy, and inflammatory bowel disease.

Management

Emergency Department

Protection of the airway, respiratory support, and administration of oxygen are clinically indicated. Resuscitate with crystalloid fluid (normal saline or lactated Ringer solution) in boluses of 20 mL/kg. Transfuse with packed red blood cells (10 mL/kg) for significant hemorrhage. For children with obstructive symptoms, place an orogastric tube for intestinal decompres-sion, give broad-spectrum antibiotics (gram-positive, gram-negative, and anaerobic coverage), resuscitate with crystalloid fluid, and consult a pediatric surgeon emergently for exploratory laparotomy. Rapid relief of the obstruction reduces the risk of ischemic bowel involvement. Patients without obstruction and risk of intestinal ischemia can undergo surgical resection once hemodynamically stable and the hematocrit approaches near normal values.

Surgical resection of the diverticulum is performed through a transverse right lower quadrant incision or by laparoscopy. Depending on the extent of involvement, surgical resection will include placement of linear staples at the base of the diverticulum with subsequent amputation, a V-shaped incision at the base of the diverticulum with resection and enteroplasty, or sleeve resection of the involved portion of the ileum with an end-to-end anastomosis of the intestines.[194–196] Appendectomy is also performed.

What to Avoid and Why

Patients without obstruction should not undergo operation until hemodynamically stable. Bleeding from a Meckel diverticulum is usually episodic and typically stops spontaneously. Surgery can usually be deferred until the patient is stabilized with intravenous fluids and blood products.

Controversies in Management

Controversy exists over the management of a Meckel diverticulum discovered incidentally at laparotomy. The risk of future complications from an incidentally discovered Meckel diverticulum is estimated to be 4% to 6%.[197,198] Younger age has been associated with an increased risk of complications. Thus, pediatric surgeons will generally remove a Meckel diverticulum found in an infant or young child. Resection is also considered if the diverticulum contains palpable ectopic gastric mucosa, in the presence of omphalomesenteric remnants with abdominal wall attachments, or if there is a history of unexplained abdominal pain. Resection of Meckel diverticulum in an older child and adult without symptoms is controversial. Risks and benefits must be evaluated on an individual basis.[199]

KEY POINTS

Management of Meckel Diverticulum
- ABCs
- Gastric decompression
- Fluid resuscitation
- Correct severe anemia

THE BOTTOM LINE

- Determine site of bleeding within the GI tract (upper versus lower)
- Consult a pediatric surgeon emergently for evidence of hemorrhagic obstruction or peritonitis
- Correct hypovolemia and anemia before surgery of nonobstructed diverticula

---

CASE SCENARIO 7

A 13-year-old boy is brought into the ED by his parents at 4:00 AM after he was awakened by a sudden onset of left scrotal pain. The previous day, he was in his usual state of good health and played in his school's football game. He has had several brief, less intense but similar episodes in the past. He now has a tender, swollen left hemiscrotum, and the testis appears to ride higher in the scrotum. There is absence of cremasteric reflex on the left. He experiences pain with any movement and is nauseated.

1. What is your differential diagnosis?
2. Are any imaging modalities available or indicated?
3. Is there an indication for surgical intervention?
4. Is the contralateral testis at risk?

Testicular Torsion

Scrotal pain and swelling in the male pediatric population are common presenting symptoms in the ED. The so-called acute scrotum can include several diagnoses that afflict the male population, but distinguishing those boys with acute testicular torsion in a rapid manner is vital for testicular salvage. Tissue loss is directly proportional to the duration of testicular ischemia, and salvage rates decrease markedly when repair is delayed more than 8 hours after the acute event. Even though only some patients with an acute scrotum are found to have acute testicular torsion, it is the working diagnosis until proved otherwise.[200–202]

Testicular torsion has been estimated to occur in 1 of every 4,000 males before the age of 25 years.[203] The estimated incidence of testicular torsion for males ages 1 to 25 years in the United States is 4.5 cases per 100,000 per year. The estimated incidence of testicular torsion in males aged 10 to 19 years is 8.6 cases per 100,000 per year.[204] The peak incidence occurs around the age of 13 years, coinciding with the onset of puberty. Another age peak occurs in the perinatal period, and newborns present with a discolored or hard scrotum due to a necrotic testis that is beyond salvage. The occurrence is rare after the age of 30 years.[205,206]

The cause of testicular torsion in a child appears to be movement of a testis that is abnormally fixed or suspended within its investment by the tunica vaginalis. In the infant, it appears to be lack of fixation of the testicular tunics in the scrotum. If the tunica vaginalis, the portion of the processus vaginalis that normally invests (surrounds) the lower portion of the testis, has an abnormally high attachment to the spermatic cord, the testis is not fixed, and intravaginal torsion can occur. This bell clapper deformity allows the testis to lie transversely and to rotate due to poor fixation. Prenatal torsion and torsion of cryptorchid testes are usually due to lack of fixation of the testicular tunics in the scrotum, and hence the entire cord might twist, which is known as extravaginal torsion. Outside the neonatal period, the bell clapper deformity is the abnormality found in most cases of testicular torsion, and it is commonly bilateral.

Clinical Features

The typical patient presents with sudden onset of severe pain in the groin or scrotum. Nausea and vomiting are commonly associated symptoms. The patient might have had similar episodes in the past that resolved, suggesting intermittent torsion, or a brief period of torsion that detorsed spontaneously.

Early in testicular torsion, the landmarks and physical features are most easily examined. As the time of torsion is prolonged, these findings became much less reliable due to pain, inflammation, and swelling. Early signs suggestive of testis torsion include a high-riding testis with a transverse lie, diffuse testicular tenderness, absence of the cremasteric reflex, and a palpable twist of the spermatic cord above the testis (**Figure 8.22**).

Complications

Delay in reestablishing blood flow to the torsed testis results in the loss of testicular function. Delays can occur both in the patient presenting for evaluation and by the physician recognizing torsion as the cause of the acute scrotum. Adolescents can be reluctant to bring testicular

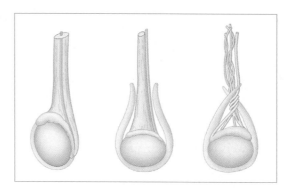

Figure 8.22 Testicular lie. The diagram on the left shows the normal testicular lie. The middle diagram shows a horizontal lie (the bell clapper deformity), which is prone to torsion. The diagram on the right depicts testicular torsion.

Gausche M. Genitourinary surgical emergencies. *Pediatr Ann.* 1996;25: 458–464. Printed with permission from Strange et al. *Pediatric Emergency Medicine: A Comprehensive Study Guide.* New York, NY: McGraw-Hill; 1996.

discomfort to the attention of a parent or physician, increasing the risk of delay in presentation. Testicular salvage rates of 80% to 96% are possible if surgical intervention is initiated within 6 to 8 hours of the acute onset of pain. This salvage rate decreases to less than 20% if surgical care is delayed by 12 hours or more.[207,208] Beyond 48 hours, the salvage rate is uniformly poor. Bilateral testicular loss, though uncommon, can occur in either a synchronous (at the same time) or metachronous (at different times) manner.

Diagnostic Studies

Laboratory studies are not sufficient for making a definitive diagnosis in the evaluation of the acute scrotum. Imaging studies might, on the other hand, be extremely useful when the diagnosis cannot be made solely based on the history and examination. The two modalities most helpful are testicular scintigraphy and real-time color Doppler sonography.

Testicular scintigraphy uses a radionuclide to analyze testicular perfusion. In most cases, the scan is performed quickly and has a reported positive predictive value of 95%. However, not all centers have immediate access to the technetium Tc 99m pertechnetate at all hours of the day.

Currently, the "gold standard" for imaging the acute testicle is color Doppler sonography. Real-time color Doppler sonography allows visualization not only of intratesticular arterial flow but also of testicular anatomy.[209,210] Color Doppler imaging is readily available, noninvasive, and highly accurate. When normal or increased flow to the testis in question is confirmed, torsion is rapidly excluded. If there is any uncertainty with a technically equivocal study, urgent surgical exploration is indicated.[211] No child with a high clinical index of suspicion for torsion should have a surgical procedure delayed to confirm clinical suspicion with a diagnostic study.

Differential Diagnosis

The three most common causes of the acute scrotum in the pediatric population are testicular torsion, torsion of a testicular appendage, and epididymo-orchitis.[200,212] Other processes

include scrotal trauma, hernias, hydroceles, varicoceles, Henoch-Schönlein purpura, and testicular tumors.[209,213] Testicular torsion must be ruled out urgently to prevent testicular loss.

Torsion of a testicular appendage, either an appendix testis or an appendix epididymis, occurs on average at 10 years of age. Sudden onset of pain limited to the scrotum without abdominal or urinary symptoms is most common. Fever is uncommon. Point tenderness at the superior aspect of the testis is sometimes found early in the process, and the "blue dot" sign of a visible tender nodule can be found in one-fifth of cases.[200,202] Most boys with torsion of a testicular appendage have never had a similar episode in the past, and most have a slightly more gradual onset of severity of pain, presenting to a physician more than 12 hours into the illness. Testicular scans and sonograms show increased flow and inflammation in the superior aspect of the testicle. If documented by clinical grounds or confirmed by imaging, treatment is expectant with analgesics alone. However, if there remains any doubt about the diagnosis, emergency scrotal exploration should be performed.

Epididymo-orchitis is the most common cause of the acute scrotum in sexually active males but is actually overestimated in most pediatric centers.[214,215] One can elicit a history of dysuria, recent fever, mumps, dysfunctional voiding, or even a recent sudden increase in abdominal pressure, such as with lifting or trauma.[200] The sudden increase in abdominal pressure can lead to a reflux of sterile urine down into the ejaculatory duct and vas deferens, causing epididymal inflammation. When a child is found to have documented epididymitis, an underlying anatomical urinary tract anomaly must be sought. The scrotal pain is usually slow in onset, less intense in nature, and associated with pyuria and a leukocytosis. Testicular scintigraphy and sonograms will document normal to increased flow to the affected testis. Treatment is with antibiotics and analgesics after cultures of the urine in all and urethral swabs for those who are sexually active.[212] Urine cultures are obtained for antibiotic sensitivity studies, but in many cases, cultures are falsely negative. Positive cultures show that coliforms are usually the cause in prepubertal males;

venereal organisms, such as *Neisseria gonorrhoeae* and *Chlamydia trachomatis*, are often found after puberty. Viral causes, including mumps, coxsackievirus, echovirus, and adenovirus, have also been implicated.

Scrotal trauma is a relatively common problem in active boys. Trauma can lead to torsion, scrotal hematoma, or impressive ecchymosis. Examination can be difficult, especially if the hematoma obscures the normal anatomy. Doppler sonography is useful in defining flow to the testes and demonstrating an intact tunica albuginea.[209,213] If the testicle is not clearly identified to be intact, concerns of testicular rupture must be entertained, and immediate urologic referral is indicated for surgical repair.

Management

Emergency Department

Analgesia with an intravenous narcotic is indicated for patients in significant pain. However, treatment of the pain should not delay evaluation and definitive treatment of the child. If the cause of the acute scrotum has been determined to be testicular torsion or if torsion cannot be excluded in a rapid manner, emergency scrotal exploration is indicated (**Figure 8.23**). Detorsion of the affected side is performed, and viability is

ascertained. If clearly nonviable, the testis is removed. If viable, orchiopexy is performed with three-point or four-point fixation with nonabsorbable sutures. The contralateral testis is then explored to be sure the cause of the ipsilateral torsion is the bell clapper deformity or if the testis is oriented in an abnormal plane due to the high incidence of bilaterality associated with anomalies of testicular fixation.

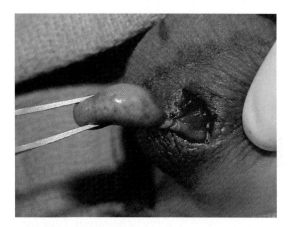

Figure 8.23 Torsion of the testis.

Manual detorsion can preserve testicular viability and provide time before irreversible necrosis occurs. Administer analgesia first. Because testes usually torse in a medial direction, perform manual detorsion by twisting the affected testis in an outward manner (ie, such that the anterior surface of the testis is rotated outward laterally). Twist the patient's right testis to the patient's right or twist the left testis to the patient's left until the pain is relieved. Successful detorsion can be evident by relief of painful symptoms along with a visible lengthening of the cord structures. More than a 360° twist might be required to fully detorse the affected testis. Manual detorsion is a temporizing procedure only. Definitive surgery to completely relieve the torsion is still indicated. In

---

WHAT ELSE?

Differential Diagnosis of Testicular Torsion
- Torsion of the appendix testis or appendix epididymis
- Epididymitis
- Orchitis
- Incarcerated inguinal hernia
- Scrotal trauma
- Hydrocele
- Varicocele
- Henoch-Schönlein purpura
- Scrotal cellulitis
- Kawasaki disease
- Testicular tumor
- Scrotal arthropod bites

KEY POINTS

Management of Testicular Torsion
- Obtain immediate surgical consultation
- Consider manual detorsion and analgesia

---

general, manual detorsion should be performed by the pediatric surgeon or pediatric urologist because it might otherwise confuse the diagnosis and delay needed surgery.

What to Avoid and Why

Avoid delay in surgical exploration of an acute scrotum if torsion is suspected. Testicular viability is directly related to the duration of torsion and is affected by patient and physician delay.

Controversies in Management

Color Doppler sonography can show misleading arterial flow in the early phase of torsion. Current investigations to increase the reliability of color Doppler sonography include analyzing the Doppler spectral wave form of blood flow and comparing it to the opposite testis and using high-resolution ultrasonography for direct visualization of the spermatic cord twist. Data from a multicenter trial support that high-resolution ultrasonography of the spermatic cord can identify torsion with 97.3% sensitivity and 99% specificity.[210,216,217]

THE BOTTOM LINE

- Testicular torsion is a surgical emergency
- Treatment is immediate surgery with detorsion and orchiopexy
- Diagnostic studies might be helpful in equivocal cases but must not delay surgical consultation

---

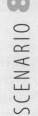

CASE SCENARIO 8

A 3-month-old boy born at 36 weeks of gestation presents to the ED with a 12-hour history of agitation, poor feeding, and right scrotal swelling. The parents have never noted this swelling before. The scrotal mass is tense and seems to transilluminate. It is difficult to palpate the testis on the right side. The left hemiscrotum is normal. Initial attempts at reducing the mass are met with a crying child and very anxious parents.

1. *Is this a hydrocele or a hernia?*
2. *Should further attempts be made to reduce the mass?*
3. *When should this lesion be repaired?*

Pediatric Inguinal Hernia

Inguinal hernias and hydroceles are common findings in the pediatric population. As more premature infants survive, the incidence of hernias and hydroceles is increasing, as are the number of pediatric surgical repairs performed. A hernia is the protrusion of a loop or portion of an organ or tissue through an abnormal opening. Inguinal hernias can be complicated by loss of bowel, testis, and ovary due to incarceration and strangulation.

Embryology

During the fifth week of gestation, the gonads develop as retroperitoneal structures. Near the 10th week, through a process of differentiated growth commonly called descent, the gonads can be found close to the groin and at the internal inguinal ring at 12 weeks. The peritoneum protrudes through the internal ring during the third month to form the processus vaginalis. At 28 weeks of gestation, the testes continue their descent, following the gubernaculum through the internal ring toward the scrotum, taking the processus vaginalis (which is attached to the anteromedial portion of the testis) with it. This external phase of descent appears to be dependent on release of testosterone from the fetal testis and from substances produced by the genitofemoral nerve.[218,219]

Incomplete obliteration of the proximal processus vaginalis, which normally occurs during the ninth month, results in the various types of inguinal hernias and hydroceles encountered in the pediatric population. Fusion of the distal processus with proximal patency results in an inguinal hernia. Complete failure of obliteration leaves a potential space for an inguinoscrotal hernia. Obliteration of the proximal processes with distal patency results in a noncommunicating scrotal hydrocele. If there is a very small proximal opening, a communicating hydrocele can result, with fluid moving between peritoneal and scrotal locations. If a small region along the middle portion of the processus is not obliterated while the distal and proximal portions are obliterated, a hydrocele of the cord, or canal of Nuck in the female, results.

The timing of obliteration of the processus vaginalis is highly variable. Approximately 40% of patent processus vaginalis close during the first few months of life, and an additional 20% close by 2 years of life. Up to 20% of asymptomatic adults have been shown to have a patent processus throughout a normal life.[218,219] In females, there is no external phase of gonadal descent. However, a peritoneal diverticulum (canal of Nuck) adherent to the round ligament, which corresponds to the processus vaginalis in males, does "descend" and, when patent through its attachment to the labia, predisposes females to formation of inguinal hernias.

The molecular mechanisms involved in closure of the patent processus vaginalis are not known. Failure of regression of smooth muscle, mediators of autonomic tone, and genes involved in testicular descent and closure of the patent processus vaginalis (eg, hepatic growth factor or calcitonin gene-related peptide) might play a role.[220–223]

Epidemiology

The anatomical congenital defect that leads to an inguinal hernia in later life occurs in 10 to 20 per 1,000 live births. Prematurity significantly increases the risk of hernias, with 7% to 10% of infants born at less than 36 weeks of gestation having hernias.[219,224,225] Hernias are more common on the right side in males due to later descent of the right testis. In term infants, hernias are present on the right side in 60%, are present on the left in 30%, and are bilateral in 10%.[226] The incidence of bilaterality approaches 50% in low-birth-weight premature infants[227]

(**Figure 8.24**). Males with hernias outnumber females 3:1 to 10:1 in most large series. Many associated conditions have been identified as risk factors for the development of inguinal hernias (Table 8-3).

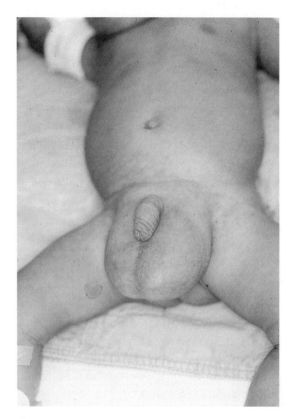

Figure 8.24 Bilateral inguinal hernias.

Clinical Features

Inguinal hernias and hydroceles in children usually present as an asymptomatic bulge or mass in the groin or scrotum. Most are documented in the first year of life, often when bathing or changing the diaper of a crying or straining child. The groin swelling usually spontaneously resolves when the child relaxes or with gentle manual pressure.

Complications

If a loop of intestine becomes entrapped (incarcerated) in a hernia, the child soon becomes very uncomfortable and irritable, develops intense pain, and soon has signs of bowel obstruction. If the hernia is not quickly reduced, strangulation occurs with ischemia of the bowel. This can occur in a 4-hour to 6-hour period. A tense incarcerated inguinal hernia can also

TABLE 8-3 Conditions Associated With Development of Inguinal Hernias

- Positive family history
- Cystic fibrosis
- Undescended testes
- Ambiguous genitalia
- Prematurity
- Exstrophy of bladder
- Low birth weight
- Hypospadias and epispadias
- Hydrops/neonatal ascites
- Peritoneal dialysis
- Ventriculoperitoneal shunt
- Mucopolysaccharidosis
- Connective tissue disorder
- Congenital abdominal wall defects
- Male sex

compromise the blood flow to the testis. Prompt reduction of the incarcerated hernia is essential to prevent tissue loss and associated complications.

The female with an incarcerated ovary in an inguinal hernia can be relatively asymptomatic until the ovarian blood supply is compromised by torsion or pressure-related ischemia. Although rare, this can occur in a short period, and repair of nonreducible hernias in female patients should not be unnecessarily delayed just because there does not appear to be bowel present within the hernia.

Diagnostic Studies

The physical examination of the child with a suspected inguinal hernia will document the anomaly in most cases. Having the child increase intra-abdominal pressure with straining, crying, or, in the older child, blowing into an occluded straw, or jumping will often assist with the demonstration of the inguinal bulge. Additional laboratory or radiographic studies are usually not indicated in the workup for a possible or known inguinal hernia or hydrocele. Although some surgeons will accept the diagnosis based on an accurate history and description by the parents or referring physician, it is not uncommon to require several examinations to document the defect definitively.

Differential Diagnosis

A scrotal hydrocele can often be differentiated from an inguinal hernia by the ability of the examiner to palpate a normal spermatic cord above the mass and feel no continuity of the lesion between the scrotum and the inguinal canal. For abdominal contents to reach the scrotum, they must traverse the inguinal canal. A tense inguinoscrotal hydrocele can be very difficult to differentiate from an incarcerated inguinal hernia by examination alone. However, the hydrocele will typically have caused no symptoms, whereas the hernia is usually tender and can cause obstructive symptoms. Caution must be used when decisions are made using transillumination of an inguinal or scrotal mass because both an incarcerated inguinal hernia and a hydrocele might transilluminate. The differential diagnosis of an inguinal or scrotal mass is listed in Table 8-4.

TABLE 8-4 Differential Diagnosis of an Inguinal or Scrotal Mass

- Inguinal hernia
- Cryptorchid testis
- Hydrocele
- Varicocele
- Retractile testis
- Torsion of testis
- Torsion of appendix testis
- Trauma
- Lymphadenitis
- Tumor

Management

Emergency Department

An inguinal hernia will not resolve spontaneously. The patient should be referred to a pediatric surgeon and repair performed shortly after diagnosis. This will reduce the risk of incarceration and its attendant complications, especially in the first year of life. Patients with hydroceles that do not enlarge, are not tense, and are not reducible with manual pressure can be observed because many will resolve in the first year of life.[228]

The child with an incarcerated hernia must be seen as soon as possible by a surgeon. Most incarcerated hernias have not yet strangulated and can be manually reduced. Reduction prevents the need for an emergency surgical procedure, which has significantly increased risks during the repair due to the associated edema and tissue friability. However, if the hernia is not reducible without undue pressure, strangulation could be present, and an emergency surgical reduction and repair are indicated. Children who have been vomiting due to incarcerated hernias require intravenous fluid resuscitation. Adjuncts to make the manual reduction easier include Trendelenburg positioning, sedation, and gentle pressure for a period of several minutes.

What to Avoid and Why

The child with a red, tender inguinal or scrotal mass who appears toxic and the child with a bowel obstruction or peritoneal signs should not undergo attempts at manual reduction. These children should undergo emergent surgical intervention once resuscitated.

KEY POINTS

Management of Inguinal Hernia
- ABCs
- Resuscitation with intravenous fluids
- Consideration of orogastric or nasogastric tube
- Surgical consultation
- Consideration of manual reduction with sedation, Trendelenburg position, and gentle upward pressure

Controversies in Management

The controversies in inguinal hernia management usually center around the indications for contralateral groin exploration and the timing of repair of hernias in the very premature neonate. Some surgeons recommend routine contralateral exploration for younger patients based on the high incidence of development of contralateral hernias. Other investigators recommend a unilateral operation because of the low risk of contralateral reoccurrence, as well as the potential risk of injury to the vas deferens or spermatic vessels.[229,230] Inguinal ultrasonography and transinguinal laparoscopy are two recent modalities used for the identification of a contralateral processus vaginalis. Surgeons must exercise appropriate judgment based on the age, sex, and comorbid conditions in the child with a hernia.

THE BOTTOM LINE

- Inguinal hernias will not spontaneously resolve
- Transillumination occurs with both hernias and hydroceles
- Manual reduction of an incarcerated hernia can be performed

An 8-year-old boy presents to the ED with a 24-hour history of abdominal pain. Initially, the pain was dull, vague, and located in the epigastric and periumbilical regions. This was followed by several hours of nausea and multiple episodes of vomiting. During the past 6 hours, the pain has become more pronounced in his right lower quadrant. His mother states that several family members have a viral illness. This young boy has a low-grade fever, normal urinalysis results, and a white blood cell count at the upper range of normal. He refuses to ambulate. He has reproducible tenderness in his right lower quadrant despite attempts at distraction.

1. Are other studies indicated before disposition?
2. Does the viral illness in the family sway your thinking?
3. Does a normal white blood cell count cloud the picture?

A 2-year-old boy presents to the ED with 2 days of nausea and vomiting, headache, and right leg pain. The vomitus is nonbilious and nonbloody and consists of stomach contents. The child was seen in the ED the previous day and was given a normal saline bolus and ondansetron. The results of cranial computed tomography (CT), electrolyte panel, and urinalysis were normal. The child was sent home with an oral rehydration solution. The child continued to vomit intermittently throughout the night and in the morning had five loose, green stools and right leg pain.

On physical examination, the child is febrile with a blood pressure of 90/60 mm Hg, a heart rate of 146/min, and a respiratory rate of 30/min. He appears dehydrated with sticky oral mucous membranes and delayed capillary refill. Head and neck examination reveal normal pupillary reflexes and a supple neck without meningismus. Heart and lung examination results are normal except for tachycardia. The abdomen is distended with normoactive bowel sounds, diffuse abdominal tenderness, and voluntary guarding of all quadrants. The genitourinary examination results are normal for a circumcised Tanner 1 male. Hips are without limitation of motion, effusion, warmth, or erythema. The child cries during the entire examination.

1. What are the priorities of care for this child?
2. What is your differential in a young child with undifferentiated abdominal pain?
3. Should pain medication be withheld until a definitive diagnosis is made?

Appendicitis

Acute appendicitis is the most common condition for which children require emergent abdominal surgery. Before 1886, the source of the inflammatory process in the right lower quadrant was thought to be the cecum itself, and descriptions used the term typhlitis, from the Greek typhlon or cecum. Reginald Fitz, in 1886, correctly identified the source of the process as the appendix.[231] As a practicing pathologist, he described the signs and symptoms of both acute and perforated appendicitis and theorized that obstruction of the appendiceal lumen was involved with the process. McBurney, in 1889, described the point of greatest tenderness that bears his name to this day.[232]

Epidemiology

Acute abdominal pain accounts for approximately 4% of office visits in children aged 5 to 14 years.[233] Of these children, acute appendicitis will be the ultimate diagnosis in 1% to 8%.[234] The lifetime risk of acute appendicitis is between 7% and 9%.[235] Although uncommon in children younger than 2 years, appendicitis occurs even in the neonatal period. The incidence increases from 1 to 2 cases per 10,000 children per year between birth and 4 years to approximately 25 cases per 10,000 children per year for children aged 10 to 17 years.[236,237]

A seasonal variation has been documented in the incidence of appendicitis, corresponding somewhat to outbreaks of enteric infections and viral illnesses.[235] A diet high in refined sugars and low in fiber appears to increase the risk of appendicitis. Countries with high dietary fiber intake have less than 10% the incidence of appendicitis compared with Europe and North America.[238,239] It is believed that a high-fiber diet speeds stool transit time and decreases the incidence of appendiceal luminal obstruction. Neonatal appendicitis is uncommon because the appendix is funnel shaped and is less likely to become obstructed. Furthermore, the soft diet, recumbent position, and decreased exposure to infectious diseases make appendicitis less frequent.[240]

Despite its relatively high occurrence, the diagnosis of appendicitis in a child can be difficult even with the most experienced physicians. Among children between 6 and 17 years of age, appendicitis is the second most common cause of malpractice litigation against emergency physicians.[241] The most challenging pediatric patients to diagnose as having appendicitis are the young, preverbal child, in whom the perforation rate is as high as 80% to 100%.

Clinical Features

The child with acute appendicitis can present with a wide variety of symptoms. This complex presentation in a child unable to relate a classic history contributes to the common misdiagnosis of appendicitis. The classic presentation of periumbilical pain followed by anorexia, nausea and vomiting, right lower quadrant pain, and then fever is present in less than half of the children with appendicitis.[242,243]

The initial vague periumbilical pain is due to distention of the appendiceal lumen. This referred pain corresponds to the T-10 dermatome shared by the entire midgut. Later, as the appendix becomes inflamed, the adjacent peritoneal irritation causes the pain to localize in the periappendiceal region.

The lack of a classic presentation of appendicitis often results in a delay in the diagnosis. The lack of anorexia is common in children. Small, frequent, loose stools are also a frequent finding in children with appendicitis, which can mislead physicians into believing that the child has gastroenteritis. Dysuria with or without mild hematuria and pyuria can be present if an inflamed appendix is lying on the ureter or bladder. Flank or back pain can be the predominant symptom in a child with an inflamed retrocecal appendix.

The older child with appendicitis typically appears ill and is hesitant to move. Children writhing in pain or vigorously trying to escape the examiner are unlikely to have appendicitis. However, the younger child often presents earlier in the clinical course and can have mild and nonspecific signs and symptoms. A low-grade fever is common. A high-grade fever is more common late in the course of perforated appendicitis. The presence of fever alone or in combination with rebound tenderness is significantly associated with pediatric appendicitis. Fever increases the likelihood of appendicitis by three-fold, whereas the absence of fever lowers the likelihood by two-thirds.[244] Rebound tenderness triples the odds of acute appendicitis and the absence decreases the odds by two-thirds. The physical examination in the child with acute appendicitis usually reveals right lower quadrant tenderness with evidence of localized peritoneal irritation. Peritonitis might be suspected if there is sharply increased pain when going over a bump in the road, bumping the stretcher, or on coughing and is confirmed when there is percussion tenderness or rebound tenderness.[245]

Complications

Delaying the diagnosis of acute appendicitis can lead to perforation, abscess formation, wound infection, sepsis, bowel obstruction, infertility in females, and death. The risk of appendicitis progressing to perforation is higher in children than in adults. The widely published rates of perforation in large series of children range from 20% to more than 70%.[246–249] This is especially common in younger children because they are not able to communicate as well as older children. Up to 50% of children with perforation can have one of the aforementioned complications after eventual diagnosis.

Diagnostic Studies

There is no single specific laboratory test that will diagnose appendicitis and rule out other causes for a child's illness.[250] In the child with a classic history and physical examination results consistent with acute appendicitis, there is no need for further laboratory or radiographic evaluation. An urgent appendectomy is indicat-

ed. However, because the classic symptoms are frequently absent, studies are often helpful. An elevated white blood cell count can be present in appendicitis but is not helpful in differentiating perforated from nonperforated appendicitis and will not exclude other diseases associated with an inflammatory process in the abdomen (enteritis, pelvic inflammatory disease, and other infectious diseases).[251,252] In addition, a normal white blood cell count in a child with reproducible right lower quadrant tenderness or peritonitis does not exclude the diagnosis of appendicitis.

In those patients with a confusing or unusual presentation, several imaging studies are available. These include plain radiographs, ultrasonography, CT, and barium enema. Plain radiographs can be helpful in cases of a bowel obstruction or perforated viscus but will usually not be of assistance in uncomplicated appendicitis. A fecalith is visible on plain radiographs in only 10% of cases (**Figure 8.25A**, **8.25B**, **8.25C**, **8.25D**, and **8.25E**).

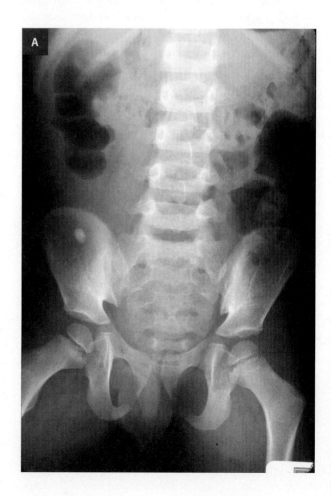

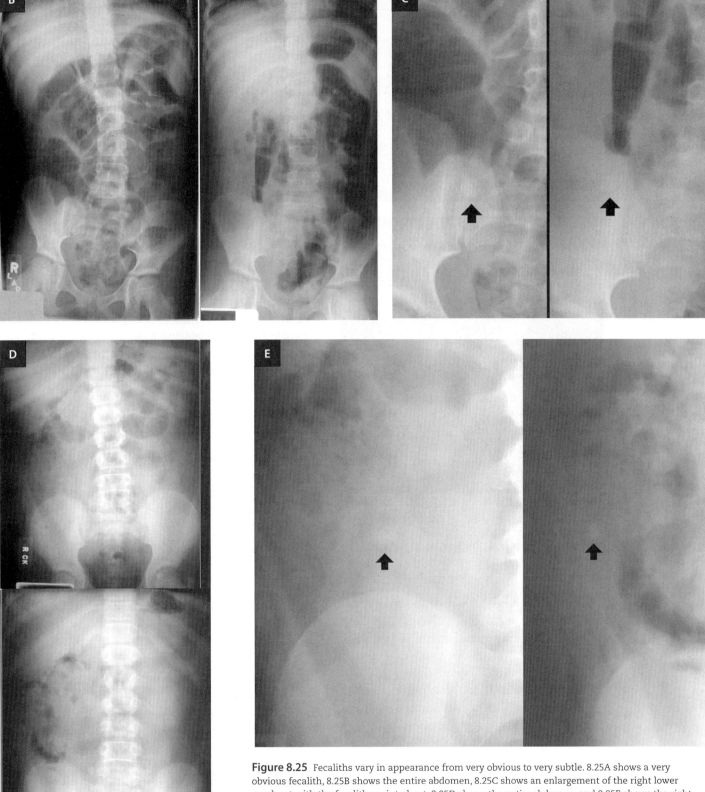

Figure 8.25 Fecaliths vary in appearance from very obvious to very subtle. 8.25A shows a very obvious fecalith, 8.25B shows the entire abdomen, 8.25C shows an enlargement of the right lower quadrant with the fecaliths pointed out, 8.25D shows the entire abdomen, and 8.25E shows the right lower quadrant enlarged. Fecaliths can have varying shapes and densities. Their location is in the right lower quadrant, but their exact location cannot be precisely defined.

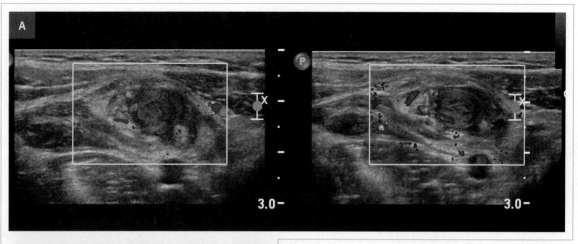

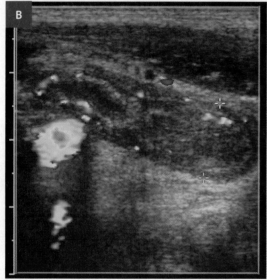

Figure 8.26 Sonogram views. 8.26A shows a graded compression sonogram and 8.26B shows sonogram, long view, measuring 1.14 cm in diameter, consistent with appendicitis.

Graded compression ultrasonography is particularly useful in the child with equivocal clinical signs and in the female with possible pelvic organ disease.[253,254] Ultrasonography is advocated because it is fast, well tolerated, noninvasive, and lacks ionizing radiation. A diagnostic criterion for acute appendicitis is a noncompressible, enlarged appendix measuring greater than 6 mm in maximal diameter.[255,256] Other findings of appendicitis include an appendicolith, pericecal, or periappendiceal fluid. On transverse imaging, a target sign is seen. The diagnostic accuracy of ultrasonography in the diagnosis of acute appendicitis varies and is operator dependent. Sensitiv-ity ranges from 78% to 99%, whereas specificity ranges from 88% to 98%.[251,257,258] Ultrasonography is helpful in identifying appendicitis, but a negative ultrasound scan does not exclude appendicitis unless a normal appendix is clearly visualized (**Figure 8.26A** and **8.26B**).

A focused abdominal CT might be useful in children with an atypical or delayed presentation. In many American hospitals, abdominal CT is the diagnostic study of choice. Performance of the abdominal CT is currently debated and dependent on use of contrast (oral, intravenous, or rectal). Sensitivities for a noncontrasted CT range from 66% to 97%, with specificities of 90% to 100%.[259–262] Addition of rectal or intravenous contrast increases sensitivities to 92% to 100%, with specificities of 87% to 99%.[263–265] An abdominal CT, however, requires more time, has risks and complications associated with contrast use, and results in radiation exposure. Ionizing

THE CLASSICS

Classic Diagnostic Studies for Appendicitis

- Leukocytosis, neutrophilia
- Calcified fecalith on abdominal radiograph
- Noncompressible appendix, appendicoliths, or peritoneal fluid/complex mass on sonography

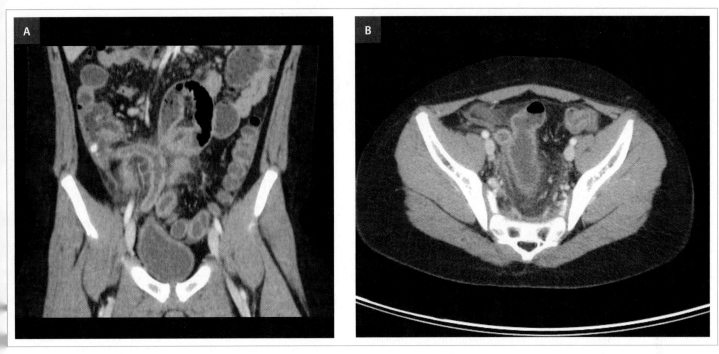

Figure 8.27 A. Coronal abdominal computed tomogram revealing appendicitis. B. Axial view at the level of the appendix, revealing appendicitis.

radiation exposure can increase a child's lifetime risk of developing cancer, and thus the decision to perform an abdominal CT should be considered carefully.[266–268] In the case of perforated appendicitis with abscess formation, an abdominal CT can identify those that can be drained percutaneously with an interval appendectomy that can be performed several weeks later (**Figure 8.27**). Barium enema has been used in the past but adds little to the focused abdominal CT using enteral and intravenous contrast agents.

Imaging and surgical consultation decisions for uncertain cases are evolving and are highly dependent on the expertise available in an institution. The accuracy of ultrasonography is highly dependent on the skill of the physician interpreting the results. Diagnostic accuracy rates published in studies from tertiary care centers are not necessarily achievable in general hospitals. Ultrasonography is often unable to reveal the appendix, making the study nondiagnostic. Computed tomography has a high sensitivity, specificity, and positive predictive value in most studies; however, it requires more time and intravenous and enteral contrast, and it results in radiation exposure. Surgical consul-

tation is not easily obtainable in many centers. Thus, in many centers, an imaging study (CT or ultrasonography) is performed first, and a surgeon is consulted only if a surgical condition is confirmed or if the possibility of a surgical condition still cannot be ruled out.

WHAT ELSE?

Differential Diagnosis of Appendicitis

- Gastroenteritis
- Mesenteric adenitis
- Constipation
- Ovarian disease (eg, cyst, teratoma, pelvic inflammatory disease, or torsion)
- Meckel diverticulitis
- Lower respiratory tract infection
- Urinary tract infection
- Pyelonephritis
- Musculoskeletal trauma
- Abdominal trauma

Laparoscopy has gained popularity both as an adjunct in the diagnosis of possible appendicitis and as a therapeutic modality.[269–272] The postpubertal female with lower abdominal pain is especially well suited for diagnostic laparoscopy and laparoscopic appendectomy if indicated. The pelvic organs are very well visualized, and specific ovarian disease can be treated with the laparoscope as well.

Differential Diagnosis

The differential diagnosis of abdominal pain is extensive. Most children presenting with abdominal pain do not undergo surgical intervention, so the final diagnosis is often based on presenting signs. The most common diagnoses after excluding appendicitis include gastroenteritis, respiratory infections, urinary tract infections, constipation, gynecologic disorders, and musculoskeletal or abdominal trauma. On initial presentation, children with missed appendicitis are more likely to be younger, have vomiting before pain, complain of dysuria or diarrhea, and have signs of respiratory infections compared with those with documented appendicitis at initial presentation.

Management

Emergency Department

Children with suspected appendicitis should be given nothing by mouth, and intravenous fluid resuscitation should be instituted. Prompt surgical therapy will reduce the complications and associated morbidity and mortality in children with appendicitis. Broad-spectrum antibiotics should be considered.[273]

> ## KEY POINTS
>
> **Management of Appendicitis**
> - Stop oral intake
> - Resuscitate with intravenous fluids
> - Obtain surgical consultation
> - Consider broad-spectrum antibiotics
> - Consider pain medications

For those who are discharged from the ED with a diagnostic impression of a nonsurgical cause, appendicitis and other serious abdominal conditions can be missed on initial evaluation. This is a high liability risk that can be reduced by providing parents with a standardized set of instructions describing the possibility of a serious condition for which they should return to the ED, including the signs and symptoms of appendicitis and other serious conditions.

Controversies in Management

Controversies exist in several areas in the management of suspected appendicitis. What antibiotic or combination of antibiotics is best suited for the child with simple vs perforated appendicitis? A recent Cochrane database analysis of 45 published studies of adults and children with appendicitis who were randomized to receive antibiotics versus placebo showed that antibiotic prophylaxis is effective in the prevention of postoperative infections.[273] However, no recommendations for the duration of antibiotic administration or antibiotic regimens were discussed. Does the child who presents in the middle of the night require an emergent appendectomy, or is it safe to wait until the next morning? How should the child with a perforated appendix and associated right lower quadrant mass be managed: with emergent appendectomy or with drainage and interval appendectomy?[274–278] Is laparoscopic appendectomy better than the traditional open approach? Laparoscopic appendectomy is now well accepted for the treatment of uncomplicated appendicitis in children. Laparoscopic appendectomy is associated with reduced postoperative pain, earlier recovery, shortened length of stay, and decreased intra-abdominal scarring. However, the benefit in children continues to be debated as it relates to increased surgical time and hospital costs when compared with open appendectomy. Although the benefits of laparoscopic appendectomy for the treatment of perforated appendicitis is similar to uncomplicated appendicitis, laparoscopic appendectomy has also been associated with an increase incidence of intra-abdominal abscesses when compared with open appendectomy in the pediatric population.[279–282]

Will pain control with narcotics interfere with the diagnosis and management of acute appendicitis in children? What impact on surgical decision making does pretreatment with narcotics have? Few studies involving pain control in children with suspected appendicitis have been performed. A single-center, randomized, double-blind, placebo-controlled trial confirmed that opiate use in children with undifferentiated abdominal pain did not impair the surgeon's ability to make a decision.[283] The answers to these questions have not been defined, and the emergency physician should consult a surgeon early in management to discuss these issues.

THE BOTTOM LINE

- Young children are at high risk for perforation
- Do not delay surgical consultation with ancillary studies if history and physical examination results are classic
- Children with appendicitis can have a normal white blood cell count
- Advanced imaging methods might be the only way to definitively diagnose or exclude appendicitis when classic findings are lacking

CHAPTER REVIEW

Check Your Knowledge

1. Which of the following causes of rectal bleeding in a full-term neonate is associated with abdominal distention?
   A. Anal fissure
   B. Hemorrhagic disease of the newborn
   C. Necrotizing enterocolitis
   D. Nodular lymphoid hyperplasia
   E. Swallowed maternal blood

2. Pneumatosis intestinalis and portal venous gas (PVG) can be viewed on all of the following imaging studies except:
   A. Abdominal computed tomography
   B. Magnetic resonance imaging
   C. Nuclear medicine scan
   D. Plain radiographs
   E. Ultrasonography

3. Which of the following complications of malrotation is the most serious?
   A. Bowel obstruction from compressing Ladd bands
   B. Hypochloremic metabolic alkalosis
   C. Intermittent volvulus
   D. Midgut volvulus
   E. Sigmoid volvulus

4. Which of the following statements regarding appendicitis in children is correct?
   A. Appendicitis can be definitively ruled out by physical examination.
   B. Discharge instruction sheets for patients with benign abdominal pain should not mention signs and symptoms of appendicitis because this would increase liability risk.
   C. A normal white blood cell count can be used to confidently rule out appendicitis.
   D. Roughly half of patients with appendicitis present in a nontypical manner.
   E. The value of ultrasonography in diagnosing appendicitis is not dependent on the skill of the individual performing the procedure.

References

1. Lin PW, Stoll BJ. Necrotising enterocolitis. *The Lancet*. 2006;368:1271–1283.
2. Kosloske AM. Epidemiology of necrotizing enterocolitis. *Acta Paediatr Suppl*. 1994;396:2–7.
3. Schwartz RM, Luby AM, Scanlon JW, Kellogg RJ. Effect of surfactant on morbidity, mortality, and resource use in newborn infants weighing 500 to 1500 g. *N Engl J Med*. 1994;330:1476–1480.
4. Schnabl KL, Van Aerde JE, Thomson AB, Clandinin MT. Necrotizing enterocolitis: A multifactorial disease with no cure. *World J Gastroenterol*. 2008;14:2142–2161.
5. Lin PW, Nasr TR, Stoll BJ. Necrotizing enterocolitis: Recent scientific advances in pathophysiology and prevention. *Semin Perinatol*. 2008;32:70–82.
6. Figueras-Aloy J, Rodriguez-Miguelez JM, Iriondo-Sanz M, Salvia-Roiges MD, Botet-Mussons F, Carbonell-Estrany X. Intravenous immunoglobulin and necrotizing enterocolitis in newborns with hemolytic disease. *Pediatrics*. 2010;125:139–144.
7. McElhinney DB, Hedrick HL, Bush DM, et al. Necrotizing enterocolitis in neonates with congenital heart disease: Risk factors and outcomes. *Pediatrics*. 2000;106:1080–1087.
8. Maayan-Metzger A, Itzchak A, Mazkereth R, Kuint J. Necrotizing enterocolitis in full-term infants: Case-control study and review of the literature. *J Perinatol*. 2004;24:494–499.
9. Ng S. Necrotizing enterocolitis in the full-term neonate. *J Paediatr Child Health*. 2001;37:1–4.
10. Martinez-Tallo E, Claure N, Bancalari E. Necrotizing enterocolitis in full-term or near-term infants: Risk factors. *Biol Neonate*. 1997;71:292–298.
11. Andrews DA, Sawin RS, Ledbetter DJ, Schaller RT, Hatch EI. Necrotizing enterocolitis in term neonates. *Am J Surg*. 1990;159:507–509.
12. Wiswell TE, Robertson CF, Jones TA, Tuttle DJ. Necrotizing enterocolitis in full-term infants. a case-control study. *Am J Dis Child*. 1988;142:532–535.
13. Polin RA, Pollack PF, Barlow B, et al. Necrotizing enterocolitis in term infants. *J Pediatr*. 1976;89:460–462.
14. Bell MJ, Ternberg JL, Feigin RD, et al. Neonatal necrotizing enterocolitis: Therapeutic decisions based upon clinical staging. *Ann Surg*. 1978;187:1–7.
15. Walsh MC, Kliegman RM. Necrotizing enterocolitis: Treatment based on staging criteria. *Pediatr Clin North Am*. 1986;33:179–201.
16. Yost CC. Neonatal necrotizing enterocolitis: Diagnosis, management, and pathogenesis. *J Infus Nurs*. 2005;28:130–134.
17. Horton KK. Pathophysiology and current management of necrotizing enterocolitis. *Neonatal Netw*. 2005;24:37–46.
18. Kanto WP Jr, Hunter JE, Stoll BJ. Recognition and medical management of necrotizing enterocolitis. *Clin Perinatol*. 1994;21:335–346.
19. Horwitz JR, Lally KP, Cheu HW, Vazquez WD, Grosfeld JL, Ziegler MM. Complications after surgical intervention for necrotizing enterocolitis: A multicenter review. *J Pediatr Surg*. 1995;30:994–998; discussion 998–999.
20. Chandler JC, Hebra A. Necrotizing enterocolitis in infants with very low birth weight. *Semin Pediatr Surg*. 2000;9:63–72.
21. Kabeer A, Gunnlaugsson S, Coren C. Neonatal necrotizing enterocolitis: A 12-year review at a county hospital. *Dis Colon Rectum*. 1995;38:866–872.
22. Duro D, Kalish LA, Johnston P, et al. Risk factors for intestinal failure in infants with necrotizing enterocolitis: A Glaser Pediatric Research Network Study. *J Pediatr*. 2010;157:203–208.
23. Petty JK, Ziegler MM. Operative strategies for necrotizing enterocolitis: The prevention and treatment of short-bowel syndrome. *Semin Pediatr Surg*. 2005;14:191–198.

24. Blakely ML, Lally KP, McDonald S, et al. Postoperative outcomes of extremely low birth-weight infants with necrotizing enterocolitis or isolated intestinal perforation: A prospective cohort study by the NICHD Neonatal Research Network. *Ann Surg.* 2005;241:984–994.

25. Simon NP. Follow-up for infants with necrotizing enterocolitis. *Clin Perinatol.* 1994;21:411–424.

26. Hintz SR, Kendrick DE, Stoll BJ, et al. Neurodevelopmental and growth outcomes of extremely low birth weight infants after necrotizing enterocolitis. *Pediatrics.* 2005;115:696–703.

27. Rees CM, Pierro A, Eaton S. Neurodevelopmental outcomes of neonates with medically and surgically treated necrotizing enterocolitis. *Arch Dis Child Fetal Neonatal Ed.* 2007;92:F193–198.

28. Schulzke SM, Deshpande GC, Patole SK. Neurodevelopmental outcomes of very low-birth-weight infants with necrotizing enterocolitis: A systematic review of observational studies. *Arch Pediatr Adolesc Med.* 2007;161:583–590.

29. Hall NJ, Hiorns M, Tighe H, et al. Is necrotizing enterocolitis associated with development or progression of intraventricular hemorrhage? *Am J Perinatol.* 2009;26:139–143.

30. Lodha A, Asztalos E, Moore AM. Cytokine levels in neonatal necrotizing enterocolitis and long-term growth and neurodevelopment. *Acta Paediatr.* 2010;99:338–343.

31. Ververidis M, Kiely EM, Spitz L, Drake DP, Eaton S, Pierro A. The clinical significance of thrombocytopenia in neonates with necrotizing enterocolitis. *J Pediatr Surg.* 2001;36:799–803.

32. Evennett N, Alexander N, Petrov M, Pierro A, Eaton S. A systematic review of serologic tests in the diagnosis of necrotizing enterocolitis. *J Pediatr Surg.* 2009;44:2192–2201.

33. Pourcyrous M, Korones SB, Yang W, Boulden TF, Bada HS. C-reactive protein in the diagnosis, management, and prognosis of neonatal necrotizing enterocolitis. *Pediatrics.* 2005;116:1064–1069.

34. Edelson MB, Sonnino RE, Bagwell CE, Lieberman JM, Marks WH, Rozycki HJ. Plasma intestinal fatty acid binding protein in neonates with necrotizing enterocolitis: A pilot study. *J Pediatr Surg.* 1999;34:1453–1457.

35. Thuijls G, Derikx JP, van Wijck K, et al. Non-invasive markers for early diagnosis and determination of the severity of necrotizing enterocolitis. *Ann Surg.* 2010;251:1174–1180.

36. Henry MC, Moss RL. Current issues in the management of necrotizing enterocolitis. *Semin Perinatol.* 2004;28:221–233.

37. Kliegman RM. Models of the pathogenesis of necrotizing enterocolitis. *J Pediatr.* 1990;117(1 pt 2):S2–S5.

38. Maalouf EF, Fagbemi A, Duggan PJ, et al. Magnetic resonance imaging of intestinal necrosis in preterm infants. *Pediatrics.* 2000;105(3 pt 1):510–514.

39. Miller SF, Seibert JJ, Kinder DL, Wilson AR. Use of ultrasound in the detection of occult bowel perforation in neonates. *J Ultrasound Med.* 1993;12:531–535.

40. Silva CT, Daneman A, Navarro OM, et al. Correlation of sonographic findings and outcome in necrotizing enterocolitis. *Pediatr Radiol.* 2007;37:274–282.

41. Epelman M, Daneman A, Navarro OM, et al. Necrotizing enterocolitis: Review of state-of-the-art imaging findings with pathologic correlation. *Radiographics.* 2007;27:285–305.

42. Faingold R, Daneman A, Tomlinson G, et al. Necrotizing enterocolitis: Assessment of bowel viability with color doppler US. *Radiology.* 2005;235:587–594.

43. Rescorla FJ. Surgical management of pediatric necrotizing enterocolitis. *Curr Opin Pediatr.* 1995;7:335–341.

44. Griffiths DM, Forbes DA, Pemberton PJ, Penn IA. Primary anastomosis for necrotising enterocolitis: A 12-year experience. *J Pediatr Surg.* 1989;24:515–518.

45. Moss RL, Dimmitt RA, Barnhart DC, et al. Laparotomy versus peritoneal drainage for necrotizing enterocolitis and perforation. *N Engl J Med.* 2006;354:2225–2234.

46. Moss RL, Dimmitt RA, Henry MC, Geraghty N, Efron B. A meta-analysis of peritoneal drainage versus laparotomy for perforated necrotizing enterocolitis. *J Pediatr Surg.* 2001;36:1210–1213.

47. Deshpande G, Rao S, Patole S, Bulsara M. Updated meta-analysis of probiotics for preventing necrotizing enterocolitis in preterm neonates. *Pediatrics.* 2010;125:921–930.

48. Claud EC, Walker WA. Bacterial colonization, probiotics, and necrotizing enterocolitis. *J Clin Gastroenterol.* 2008;42(suppl 2):S46–S52.

49. Martin CR, Walker WA. Probiotics: Role in pathophysiology and prevention in necrotizing enterocolitis. *Semin Perinatol.* 2008;32:127–137.

50. Mshvildadze M, Neu J. Probiotics and prevention of necrotizing enterocolitis. *Early Hum Dev.* 2009;85(10 suppl):S71–S74.

51. Strouse PJ. Disorders of intestinal rotation and fixation ("malrotation"). *Pediatr Radiol.* 2004;34:837–851.

52. Lampl B, Levin TL, Berdon WE, Cowles RA. Malrotation and midgut volvulus: A historical review and current controversies in diagnosis and management. *Pediatr Radiol.* 2009;39:359–366.

53. McCollough M, Sharieff GQ. Abdominal pain in children. *Pediatr Clin North Am.* 2006;53:107–137, vi.

54. Torres AM, Ziegler MM. Malrotation of the intestine. *World J Surg.* 1993;17:326–331.

55. Messineo A, MacMillan JH, Palder SB, Filler RM. Clinical factors affecting mortality in children with malrotation of the intestine. *J Pediatr Surg.* 1992;27:1343–1345.

56. Brandt ML, Pokorny WJ, McGill CW, Harberg FJ. Late presentations of midgut malrotation in children. *Am J Surg.* 1985;150:767–771.

57. Spigland N, Brandt ML, Yazbeck S. Malrotation presenting beyond the neonatal period. *J Pediatr Surg.* 1990;25:1139–1142.

58. Prasil P, Flageole H, Shaw KS, Nguyen LT, Youssef S, Laberge JM. Should malrotation in children be treated differently according to age? *J Pediatr Surg.* 2000;35:756–758.

59. Bonadio WA, Clarkson T, Naus J. The clinical features of children with malrotation of the intestine. *Pediatr Emerg Care.* 1991;7:348–349.

60. Potts SR, Thomas PS, Garstin WI, McGoldrick J. The duodenal triangle: A plain film sign of midgut malrotation and volvulus in the neonate. *Clin Radiol.* 1985;36:47–49.

61. Applegate KE, Anderson JM, Klatte EC. Intestinal malrotation in children: A problem-solving approach to the upper gastrointestinal series. *Radiographics.* 2006;26:1485–1500.

62. Williams H. Green for danger! Intestinal malrotation and volvulus. *Arch Dis Child Educ Pract Ed.* 2007;92:ep87–91.

63. Sizemore AW, Rabbani KZ, Ladd A, Applegate KE. Diagnostic performance of the upper gastrointestinal series in the evaluation of children with clinically suspected malrotation. *Pediatr Radiol.* 2008;38:518–528.

64. McVay MR, Kokoska ER, Jackson RJ, Smith SD. Jack Barney Award: The changing spectrum of intestinal malrotation: Diagnosis and management. *Am J Surg.* 2007;194:712–719.

65. Malek MM, Burd RS. The optimal management of malrotation diagnosed after infancy: A decision analysis. *Am J Surg.* 2006;191:45–51.

66. Matzke GM, Dozois EJ, Larson DW, Moir CR. Surgical management of intestinal malrotation in adults: Comparative results for open and laparoscopic Ladd procedures. *Surg Endosc.* 2005;19:1416–1419.

67. Palanivelu C, Rangarajan M, Shetty AR, Jani K. Intestinal malrotation with midgut volvulus presenting as acute abdomen in children: Value of diagnostic and therapeutic laparoscopy. *J Laparoendosc Adv Surg Tech A.* 2007;17:490–492.

68. Draus JM Jr, Foley DS, Bond SJ. Laparoscopic Ladd procedure: A minimally invasive approach to malrotation without midgut volvulus. *Am Surg.* 2007;73:693–696.

69. Fraser JD, Aguayo P, Sharp SW, Ostlie DJ, St Peter SD. The role of laparoscopy in the management of malrotation. *J Surg Res.* 2009;156:80–82.

70. Zenn MR, Redo SF. Hypertrophic pyloric stenosis in the newborn. *J Pediatr Surg.* 1993;28:1577–1578.

71. Janik JS, Wayne ER, Janik JP. Pyloric stenosis in premature infants. *Arch Pediatr Adolesc Med.* 1996;150:223–224.

72. MacMahon B. The continuing enigma of pyloric stenosis of infancy: A review. *Epidemiology.* 2006;17:195–201.

73. Panteli C. New insights into the pathogenesis of infantile pyloric stenosis. *Pediatr Surg Int.* 2009;25:1043–1052.

74. Finsen VR. Infantile hypertrophic pyloric stenosis—unusual familial incidence. *Arch Dis Child.* 1979;54:720–721.

75. Carter CO, Evans KA. Inheritance of congenital pyloric stenosis. *J Med Genet.* 1969;6:233–254.

76. Guarino N, Yoneda A, Shima H, Puri P. Selective neurotrophin deficiency in infantile hypertrophic pyloric stenosis. *J Pediatr Surg.* 2001;36:1280–1284.

77. Guarino N, Shima H, Oue T, Puri P. Glial-derived growth factor signaling pathway in infantile hypertrophic pyloric stenosis. *J Pediatr Surg.* 2000;35:835–839.

78. Shima H, Ohshiro K, Puri P. Increased local synthesis of epidermal growth factors in infantile hypertrophic pyloric stenosis. *Pediatr Res.* 2000;47:201–207.

79. Subramaniam R, Doig CM, Moore L. Nitric oxide synthase is absent in only a subset of cases of pyloric stenosis. *J Pediatr Surg.* 2001;36:616–619.

80. Abel RM. The ontogeny of the peptide innervation of the human pylorus, with special reference to understanding the aetiology and pathogenesis of infantile hypertrophic pyloric stenosis. *J Pediatr Surg.* 1996;31:490–497.

81. Vanderwinden JM, Mailleux P, Schiffmann SN, Vanderhaeghen JJ, De Laet MH. Nitric oxide synthase activity in infantile hypertrophic pyloric stenosis. *N Engl J Med.* 1992;327:511–515.

82. Huang PL, Dawson TM, Bredt DS, Snyder SH, Fishman MC. Targeted disruption of the neuronal nitric oxide synthase gene. *Cell.* 1993;75:1273–1286.

83. Dick AC, Ardill J, Potts SR, Dodge JA. Gastrin, somatostatin and infantile hypertrophic pyloric stenosis. *Acta Paediatr.* 2001;90:879–882.

84. Ohshiro K, Puri P. Pathogenesis of infantile hypertrophic pyloric stenosis: Recent progress. *Pediatr Surg Int.* 1998;13:243–252.

85. Huang LT, Tiao MM, Lee SY, Hsieh CS, Lin JW. Low plasma nitrite in infantile hypertrophic pyloric stenosis patients. *Dig Dis Sci.* 2006;51:869–872.

86. Jablonski J, Gawronska R, Gawlowska A, Kobos J, Andrzejewska E. Study of insulin-like growth factor-1 (IGF-1) and platelet-derived endothelial cell growth factor (PDEGF) expression in children with infantile hypertrophic pyloric stenosis. *Med Sci Monit.* 2006;12:CR27–30.

87. Sorensen HT, Norgard B, Pedersen L, Larsen H, Johnsen SP. Maternal smoking and risk of hypertrophic infantile pyloric stenosis: 10 year population based cohort study. *BMJ.* 2002;325:1011–1012.

88. Maheshwai N. Are young infants treated with erythromycin at risk for developing hypertrophic pyloric stenosis? *Arch Dis Child.* 2007;92:271–273.

89. Jedd MB, Melton LJ 3rd, Griffin MR, et al. Factors associated with infantile hypertrophic pyloric stenosis. *Am J Dis Child.* 1988;142:334–337.

90. Pisacane A, de Luca U, Criscuolo L, et al. Breast feeding and hypertrophic pyloric stenosis: Population based case-control study. *BMJ.* 1996;312:745–746.

91. Cooper WO, Griffin MR, Arbogast P, Hickson GB, Gautam S, Ray WA. Very early exposure to erythromycin and infantile hypertrophic pyloric stenosis. *Arch Pediatr Adolesc Med.* 2002;156:647–650.

92. Honein MA, Paulozzi LJ, Himelright IM, et al. Infantile hypertrophic pyloric stenosis after pertussis prophylaxis with erythromycin: A case review and cohort study. *The Lancet.* 1999;354:2101–2105.

93. Hypertrophic pyloric stenosis in infants following pertussis prophylaxis with erythromycin—Knoxville, Tennessee, 1999. *MMWR Morb Mortal Wkly Rep.* 1999;48:1117–1120.

94. Shim WK, Campbell A, Wright SW. Pyloric stenosis in the racial groups of Hawaii. *J Pediatr.* 1970;76:89–93.

95. Sule ST, Stone DH, Gilmour H. The epidemiology of infantile hypertrophic pyloric stenosis in Greater Glasgow area, 1980–96. *Paediatr Perinat Epidemiol.* 2001;15:379–380.

96. Dodge JA. Infantile hypertrophic pyloric stenosis in Belfast, 1957–1969. *Arch Dis Child.* 1975;50:171–178.

97. Hedback G, Abrahamsson K, Husberg B, Granholm T, Oden A. The epidemiology of infantile hypertrophic pyloric stenosis in Sweden 1987–96. *Arch Dis Child.* 2001;85:379–381.

98. Applegate MS, Druschel CM. The epidemiology of infantile hypertrophic pyloric stenosis in New York State, 1983 to 1990. *Arch Pediatr Adolesc Med.* 1995;149:1123–1129.

99. Tam PK, Chan J. Increasing incidence of hypertrophic pyloric stenosis. *Arch Dis Child.* 1991;66:530–531.

100. Schechter R, Torfs CP, Bateson TF. The epidemiology of infantile hypertrophic pyloric stenosis. *Paediatr Perinat Epidemiol.* 1997;11:407–427.

101. Mitchell LE, Risch N. The genetics of infantile hypertrophic pyloric stenosis: A reanalysis. *Am J Dis Child.* 1993;147:1203–1211.

102. Letton RW Jr. Pyloric stenosis. *Pediatr Ann.* 2001;30:745–750.

103. Nielsen JP, Haahr P, Haahr J. Infantile hypertrophic pyloric stenosis: Decreasing incidence. *Dan Med Bull.* 2000;47:223–225.

104. Persson S, Ekbom A, Granath F, Nordenskjold A. Parallel incidences of sudden infant death syndrome and infantile hypertrophic pyloric stenosis: A common cause? *Pediatrics.* 2001;108:E70.

105. Sommerfield T, Chalmers J, Youngson G, Heeley C, Fleming M, Thomson G. The changing epidemiology of infantile hypertrophic pyloric stenosis in Scotland. *Arch Dis Child.* 2008;93:1007–1011.

106. Woolley MM, Felsher BF, Asch J, Carpio N, Isaacs H. Jaundice, hypertrophic pyloric stenosis, and hepatic glucuronyl transferase. *J Pediatr Surg.* 1974;9:359–363.

107. Chaves-Carballo E, Harris LE, Lynn HB. Jaundice associated with pyloric stenosis and neonatal small-bowel obstructions. *Clin Pediatr (Phila).* 1968;7:198–202.

108. Shuman FI, Darling DB, Fisher JH. The radiographic diagnosis of congenital hypertrophic pyloric stenosis. *J Pediatr.* 1967;71:70–74.

109. Hernanz-Schulman M. Infantile hypertrophic pyloric stenosis. *Radiology.* 2003;227:319–331.

110. Ito S, Tamura K, Nagae I, et al. Ultrasonographic diagnosis criteria using scoring for hypertrophic pyloric stenosis. *J Pediatr Surg.* 2000;35:1714–1718.

111. Blumhagen JD, Noble HG. Muscle thickness in hypertrophic pyloric stenosis: Sonographic determination. *AJR Am J Roentgenol.* 1983;140:221–223.

112. Hernanz-Schulman M. Pyloric stenosis: Role of imaging. *Pediatr Radiol.* 2009;39(suppl 2):S134–S139.

113. Malcom GE 3rd, Raio CC, Del Rios M, Blaivas M, Tsung JW. Feasibility of emergency physician diagnosis of hypertrophic pyloric stenosis using point-of-care ultrasound: A multi-center case series. *J Emerg Med.* 2009;37:283–286.

114. Copeland DR, Cosper GH, McMahon LE, et al. Return of the surgeon in the diagnosis of pyloric stenosis. *J Pediatr Surg.* 2009;44:1189–1192.

115. McVay MR, Copeland DR, McMahon LE, et al. Surgeon-performed ultrasound for diagnosis of pyloric stenosis is accurate, reproducible, and clinically valuable. *J Pediatr Surg.* 2009;44:169–171.

116. Boneti C, McVay MR, Kokoska ER, Jackson RJ, Smith SD. Ultrasound as a diagnostic tool used by surgeons in pyloric stenosis. *J Pediatr Surg.* 2008;43:87–91.

117. Carpenter RO, Schaffer RL, Maeso CE, et al. Postoperative ad lib feeding for hypertrophic pyloric stenosis. *J Pediatr Surg.* 1999;34:959–961.

118. Leinwand MJ, Shaul DB, Anderson KD. A standardized feeding regimen for hypertrophic pyloric stenosis decreases length of hospitalization and hospital costs. *J Pediatr Surg.* 2000;35:1063–1065.

119. Georgeson KE, Corbin TJ, Griffen JW, Breaux CW Jr. An analysis of feeding regimens after pyloromyotomy for hypertrophic pyloric stenosis. *J Pediatr Surg.* 1993;28:1478–1480.

120. Perger L, Fuchs JR, Komidar L, Mooney DP. Impact of surgical approach on outcome in 622 consecutive pyloromyotomies at a pediatric teaching institution. *J Pediatr Surg.* 2009;44:2119–2125.

121. Haricharan RN, Aprahamian CJ, Morgan TL, Harmon CM, Georgeson KE, Barnhart DC. Smaller scars—what is the big deal: A survey of the perceived value of laparoscopic pyloromyotomy. *J Pediatr Surg.* 2008;43:92–96.

122. Hall NJ, Van Der Zee J, Tan HL, Pierro A. Meta-analysis of laparoscopic versus open pyloromyotomy. *Ann Surg.* 2004;240:774–778.

123. Fujimoto T, Lane GJ, Segawa O, Esaki S, Miyano T. Laparoscopic extramucosal pyloromyotomy versus open pyloromyotomy for infantile hypertrophic pyloric stenosis: Which is better? *J Pediatr Surg.* 1999;34:370–372.

124. St Peter SD, Holcomb GW 3rd, Calkins CM, et al. Open versus laparoscopic pyloromyotomy for pyloric stenosis: A prospective, randomized trial. *Ann Surg.* 2006;244:363–370.

125. Sola JE, Neville HL. Laparoscopic vs open pyloromyotomy: A systematic review and meta-analysis. *J Pediatr Surg.* 2009;44:1631–1637.

126. Emil S. Pyloromyotomy through an infra-umbilical incision: Open technique and superb cosmesis. *Eur J Pediatr Surg.* 2009;19:72–75.

127. Asai M, Katsube Y, Takita Y, et al. Intravenous atropine treatment in hypertrophic pyloric stenosis: Evaluation by clinical course and imaging. *J Nippon Med Sch.* 2007;74:50–54.

128. Meissner PE, Engelmann G, Troeger J, Linderkamp O, Nuetzenadel W. Conservative treatment of infantile hypertrophic pyloric stenosis with intravenous atropine sulfate does not replace pyloromyotomy. *Pediatr Surg Int.* 2006;22:1021–1024.

129. Yamataka A, Tsukada K, Yokoyama-Laws Y, et al. Pyloromyotomy versus atropine sulfate for infantile hypertrophic pyloric stenosis. *J Pediatr Surg.* 2000;35:338–342.

130. Gross RE, Ware PF. Intussusception in childhood; experiences from 610 cases. *N Engl J Med.* 1948;239:645–652.

131. Dennison WM, Shaker M. Intussusception in infancy and childhood. *Br J Surg.* 1970;57:679–684.

132. Margenthaler JA, Vogler C, Guerra OM, Limpert JN, Weber TR, Keller MS. Pediatric surgical images: Small bowel intussusception in a preterm infant. *J Pediatr Surg.* 2002;37:1515–1517.

133. Gorgen-Pauly U, Schultz C, Kohl M, Sigge W, Moller J, Gortner L. Intussusception in preterm infants: Case report and literature review. *Eur J Pediatr.* 1999;158:830–832.

134. Martinez Biarge M, Garcia-Alix A, Luisa del Hoyo M, et al. Intussusception in a preterm neonate; a very rare, major intestinal problem—systematic review of cases. *J Perinat Med.* 2004;32:190–194.

135. Stringer MD, Pablot SM, Brereton RJ. Paediatric intussusception. *Br J Surg.* 1992;79:867–876.

136. Hutchison IF, Olayiwola B, Young DG. Intussusception in infancy and childhood. *Br J Surg.* 1980;67:209–212.

137. Gierup J, Jorulf H, Livaditis A. Management of intussusception in infants and children: A survey based on 288 consecutive cases. *Pediatrics.* 1972;50:535–546.

138. Ein SH, Stephens CA. Intussusception: 354 cases in 10 years. *J Pediatr Surg.* 1971;6:16–27.

139. Nylund CM, Denson LA, Noel JM. Bacterial enteritis as a risk factor for childhood intussusception: A retrospective cohort study. *J Pediatr.* 2010;156:761–765.

140. Choong CK, Kimble RM, Pease P, Beasley SW. Colo-colic intussusception in Henoch-Schönlein purpura. *Pediatr Surg Int.* 1998;14:173–174.

141. Little KJ, Danzl DF. Intussusception associated with Henoch-Schönlein purpura. *J Emerg Med.* 1991;9(suppl 1):29–32.

142. Navarro O, Dugougeat F, Kornecki A, Shuckett B, Alton DJ, Daneman A. The impact of imaging in the management of intussusception owing to pathologic lead points in children: A review of 43 cases. *Pediatr Radiol.* 2000;30:594–603.

143. Ein SH, Stephens CA, Shandling B, Filler RM. Intussusception due to lymphoma. *J Pediatr Surg.* 1986;21:786–788.

144. Puri P, Guiney EJ. Small bowel tumours causing intussusception in childhood. *Br J Surg.* 1985;72:493–494.

145. Pollack CV Jr, Pender ES. Unusual cases of intussusception. *J Emerg Med.* 1991;9:347–355.

146. Belongia EA, Irving SA, Shui IM, et al. Real-time surveillance to assess risk of intussusception and other adverse events after pentavalent, bovine-derived rotavirus vaccine. *Pediatr Infect Dis J.* 2010;29:1–5.

147. Ciarlet M, Schodel F. Development of a rotavirus vaccine: Clinical safety, immunogenicity, and efficacy of the pentavalent rotavirus vaccine, RotaTeq. *Vaccine*. 2009;27(suppl 6):G72–G81.

148. Tate JE, Simonsen L, Viboud C, et al. Trends in intussusception hospitalizations among US infants, 1993-2004: Implications for monitoring the safety of the new rotavirus vaccination program. *Pediatrics*. 2008;121:e1125–1132.

149. Chen J, Heyse JF, Heaton P, Kuter BJ. Age dependence of the risk of intussusception following tetravalent rhesus-human reassortant rotavirus tetravalent vaccine: Is it beyond doubt? *Am J Epidemiol*. 2010;171:1046–1054.

150. Godbole A, Concannon P, Glasson M. Intussusception presenting as profound lethargy. *J Paediatr Child Health*. 2000;36:392–394.

151. Shaoul R, Gazit A, Weller B, Berman S, Jaffe M. Neurological manifestations of an acute abdomen in children. *Pediatr Emerg Care*. 2005;21:594–597.

152. Pumberger W, Dinhobl I, Dremsek P. Altered consciousness and lethargy from compromised intestinal blood flow in children. *Am J Emerg Med*. 2004;22:307–309.

153. Buettcher M, Baer G, Bonhoeffer J, Schaad UB, Heininger U. Three-year surveillance of intussusception in children in Switzerland. *Pediatrics*. 2007;120:473–480.

154. Conway EE Jr. Central nervous system findings and intussusception: How are they related? *Pediatr Emerg Care*. 1993;9:15–18.

155. Tenenbein M, Wiseman NE. Early coma in intussusception: Endogenous opioid induced? *Pediatr Emerg Care*. 1987;3:22–23.

156. Singer J. Altered consciousness as an early manifestation of intussusception. *Pediatrics*. 1979;64:93–95.

157. Losek JD. Intussusception: Don't miss the diagnosis! *Pediatr Emerg Care*. 1993;9:46–51.

158. Losek JD, Fiete RL. Intussusception and the diagnostic value of testing stool for occult blood. *Am J Emerg Med*. 1991;9:1–3.

159. Morrison J, Lucas N, Gravel J. The role of abdominal radiography in the diagnosis of intussusception when interpreted by pediatric emergency physicians. *J Pediatr*. 2009;155:556–559.

160. Hooker RL, Hernanz-Schulman M, Yu C, Kan JH. Radiographic evaluation of intussusception: Utility of left-side-down decubitus view. *Radiology*. 2008;248:987–994.

161. Littlewood Teele R, Vogel SA. Intussusception: The paediatric radiologist's perspective. *Pediatr Surg Int*. 1998;14:158–162.

162. Lui KW, Wong HF, Cheung YC, et al. Air enema for diagnosis and reduction of intussusception in children: Clinical experience and fluoroscopy time correlation. *J Pediatr Surg*. 2001;36:479–481.

163. Kirks DR. Air intussusception reduction: "The winds of change." *Pediatr Radiol*. 1995;25:89–91.

164. del-Pozo G, Albillos JC, Tejedor D, et al. Intussusception in children: Current concepts in diagnosis and enema reduction. *Radiographics*. 1999;19:299–319.

165. Palder SB, Ein SH, Stringer DA, Alton D. Intussusception: Barium or air? *J Pediatr Surg*. 1991;26:271–275.

166. Bonadio WA. Intussusception reduced by barium enema. Outcome and short-term follow-up. *Clin Pediatr* (Phila). 1988;27:601–604.

167. Hadidi AT, El Shal N. Childhood intussusception: A comparative study of nonsurgical management. *J Pediatr Surg*. 1999;34:304–307.

168. Heenan SD, Kyriou J, Fitzgerald M, Adam EJ. Effective dose at pneumatic reduction of paediatric intussusception. *Clin Radiol*. 2000;55(11):811–816.

169. Lai AH, Phua KB, Teo EL, Jacobsen AS. Intussusception: A three-year review. *Ann Acad Med Singapore*. 2002;31:81–85.

170. Henrikson S, Blane CE, Koujok K, Strouse PJ, DiPietro MA, Goodsitt MM. The effect of screening sonography on the positive rate of enemas for intussusception. *Pediatr Radiol*. 2003;33:190–193.

171. Harrington L, Connolly B, Hu X, Wesson DE, Babyn P, Schuh S. Ultrasonographic and clinical predictors of intussusception. *J Pediatr*. 1998;132:836–839.

172. Shanbhogue RL, Hussain SM, Meradji M, Robben SG, Vernooij JE, Molenaar JC. Ultrasonography is accurate enough for the diagnosis of intussusception. *J Pediatr Surg*. 1994;29:324–327; discussion 327–328.

173. Hryhorczuk AL, Strouse PJ. Validation of US as a first-line diagnostic test for assessment of pediatric ileocolic intussusception. *Pediatr Radiol*. 2009;39(10):1075–1079.

174. Ko HS, Schenk JP, Troger J, Rohrschneider WK. Current radiological management of intussusception in children. *Eur Radiol*. 2007;17:2411–2421.

175. Ein SH. Recurrent intussusception in children. *J Pediatr Surg*. 1975;10:751–755.

176. Beasley SW, Auldist AW, Stokes KB. Recurrent intussusception: Barium or surgery? *Aust N Z J Surg*. 1987;57:11–14.

177. Lin SL, Kong MS, Houng DS. Decreasing early recurrence rate of acute intussusception by the use of dexamethasone. *Eur J Pediatr*. 2000;159:551–552.

178. Bajaj L, Roback MG. Postreduction management of intussusception in a children's hospital emergency department. *Pediatrics*. 2003;112(6 pt 1):1302–1307.

179. Herwig K, Brenkert T, Losek JD. Enema-reduced intussusception management: Is hospitalization necessary? *Pediatr Emerg Care*. 2009;25:74–77.

180. Moore KL, Persaud, eds. *The Developing Human: Clinically Oriented Embryology*. 6th ed. Philadelphia, PA: WB Saunders Co; 1998.

181. Snyder C, ed. Meckel's diverticulum. In: Ashcroft KW, Murphy JP, Sharp RJ, et al, eds. *Pediatric Surgery*. 3rd ed. Philadelphia, PA: WB Saunders Co; 2000.

182. Matsagas MI, Fatouros M, Koulouras B, Giannoukas AD. Incidence, complications, and management of Meckel's diverticulum. *Arch Surg*. 1995;130:143–146.

183. Simms MH, Corkery JJ. Meckel's diverticulum: Its association with congenital malformation and the significance of atypical morphology. *Br J Surg*. 1980;67:216–219.

184. Nicol JW, MacKinlay GA. Meckel's diverticulum in exomphalos minor. *J R Coll Surg Edinb*. 1994;39:6–7.

185. Andreyev HJ, Owen RA, Thompson I, Forbes A. Association between Meckel's diverticulum and Crohn's disease: A retrospective review. *Gut*. 1994;35:788–790.

186. Yahchouchy EK, Marano AF, Etienne JC, Fingerhut AL. Meckel's diverticulum. *J Am Coll Surg*. 2001;192:658–662.

187. Brown RL, Azizkhan RG. Gastrointestinal bleeding in infants and children: Meckel's diverticulum and intestinal duplication. *Semin Pediatr Surg*. 1999;8:202–209.

188. St-Vil D, Brandt ML, Panic S, Bensoussan AL, Blanchard H. Meckel's diverticulum in children: A 20-year review. *J Pediatr Surg*. 1991;26:1289–1292.

189. Sagar J, KuV, Shah DK. Meckel's diverticulum: A systematic review. *J R Soc Med*. 2006;99:501–505.

190. Levy AD, Hobbs CM. From the archives of the AFIP. Meckel diverticulum: Radiologic features with pathologic Correlation. *Radiographics*. 2004;24:565–587.

191. Sfakianakis GN, Conway JJ. Detection of ectopic gastric mucosa in Meckel's diverticulum and in other aberrations by scintigraphy: ii. Indications and methods—a 10-year experience. *J Nucl Med*. 1981;22:732–738.

192. Cooney DR, Duszynski DO, Camboa E, Karp MP, Jewett TC Jr. The abdominal technetium scan (a decade of experience). *J Pediatr Surg*. 1982;17:611–619.

193. Ford PV, Bartold SP, Fink-Bennett DM, et al. Procedure guideline for gastrointestinal bleeding and Meckel's diverticulum scintigraphy. Society of Nuclear Medicine. *J Nucl Med*. 1999;40:1226–1232.

194. Stylianos S, Stein JE, Flanigan LM, Hechtman DH. Laparoscopy for diagnosis and treatment of recurrent abdominal pain in children. *J Pediatr Surg*. 1996;31:1158–1160.

195. Teitelbaum DH, Polley TZ Jr, Obeid F. Laparoscopic diagnosis and excision of Meckel's diverticulum. *J Pediatr Surg*. 1994;29:495–497.

196. Swaniker F, Soldes O, Hirschl RB. The utility of technetium 99m pertechnetate scintigraphy in the evaluation of patients with Meckel's diverticulum. *J Pediatr Surg*. 1999;34:760–765.

197. Gottlieb MM, Beart RW Jr. Surgical management of Meckel's diverticulum. *Ann Surg*. 1995;222:770.

198. Soltero MJ, Bill AH. The natural history of Meckel's diverticulum and its relation to incidental removal: A study of 202 cases of diseased Meckel's diverticulum found in King County, Washington, over a fifteen year period. *Am J Surg*. 1976;132:168–173.

199. Arnold JF, Pellicane JV. Meckel's diverticulum: A ten-year experience. *Am Surg*. 1997;63:354–355.

200. Leslie JA, Cain MP. Pediatric urologic emergencies and urgencies. *Pediatr Clin North Am*. 2006;53:513–527, viii.

201. Lewis AG, Bukowski TP, Jarvis PD, Wacksman J, Sheldon CA. Evaluation of acute scrotum in the emergency department. *J Pediatr Surg*. 1995;30:277–281.

202. Knight PJ, Vassy LE. The diagnosis and treatment of the acute scrotum in children and adolescents. *Ann Surg*. 1984;200:664–673.

203. Williamson RC. Torsion of the testis and allied conditions. *Br J Surg*. 1976;63:465–476.

204. Mansbach JM, Forbes P, Peters C. Testicular torsion and risk factors for orchiectomy. *Arch Pediatr Adolesc Med*. 2005;159:1167–1171.

205. Melekos MD, Asbach HW, Markou SA. Etiology of acute scrotum in 100 boys with regard to age distribution. *J Urol*. 1988;139:1023–1025.

206. Chiang MC, Chen HW, Fu RH, Lien R, Wang TM, Hsu JF. Clinical features of testicular torsion and epididymo-orchitis in infants younger than 3 months. *J Pediatr Surg*. 2007;42:1574–1577.

207. Lerner RM, Mevorach RA, Hulbert WC, Rabinowitz R. Color Doppler US in the evaluation of acute scrotal disease. *Radiology*. 1990;176:355–358.

208. Fenner MN, Roszhart DA, Texter JH Jr. Testicular scanning: Evaluating the acute scrotum in the clinical setting. *Urology*. 1991;38:237–241.

209. Swischuk LE. Swollen and painful left testicle. *Pediatr Emerg Care*. 2000;16:287–289.

210. Karmazyn B, Steinberg R, Kornreich L, et al. Clinical and sonographic criteria of acute scrotum in children: A retrospective study of 172 boys. *Pediatr Radiol*. 2005;35:302–310.

211. Kass EJ, Stone KT, Cacciarelli AA, Mitchell B. Do all children with an acute scrotum require exploration? *J Urol*. 1993;150(2 pt 2):667–669.

212. Haecker FM, Hauri-Hohl A, von Schweinitz D. Acute epididymitis in children: A 4-year retrospective study. *Eur J Pediatr Surg*. 2005;15:180–186.

213. Seng YJ, Moissinac K. Trauma induced testicular torsion: A reminder for the unwary. *J Accid Emerg Med*. 2000;17:381–382.

214. Caldamone AA, Valvo JR, Altebarmakian VK, Rabinowitz R. Acute scrotal swelling in children. *J Pediatr Surg*. 1984;19:581–584.

215. Anderson PA, Giacomantonio JM, Schwarz RD. Acute scrotal pain in children: Prospective study of diagnosis and management. *Can J Surg*. 1989;32:29–32.

216. Kalfa N, Veyrac C, Lopez M, et al. Multicenter assessment of ultrasound of the spermatic cord in children with acute scrotum. *J Urol*. 2007;177:297–301.

217. Dogra VS, Rubens DJ, Gottlieb RH, Bhatt S. Torsion and beyond: New twists in spectral Doppler evaluation of the scrotum. *J Ultrasound Med*. 2004;23:1077–1085.

218. Glick PL. *Inguinal Hernias and Hydroceles*. Philadelphia, PA: Elsevier; 2006.

219. Brandt ML. Pediatric hernias. *Surg Clin North Am*. 2008;88:27–43, vii–viii.

220. Tanyel FC, Okur HD. Autonomic nervous system appears to play a role in obliteration of processus vaginalis. *Hernia*. 2004;8:149–154.

221. Hosgor M, Karaca I, Ozer E, et al. The role of smooth muscle cell differentiation in the mechanism of obliteration of processus vaginalis. *J Pediatr Surg*. 2004;39:1018–1023.

222. Cook BJ, Hasthorpe S, Hutson JM. Fusion of childhood inguinal hernia induced by HGF and CGRP via an epithelial transition. *J Pediatr Surg*. 2000;35:77–81.

223. Ting AY, Huynh J, Farmer P, et al. The role of hepatocyte growth factor in the humoral regulation of inguinal hernia closure. *J Pediatr Surg*. 2005;40:1865–1868.

224. Rajput A, Gauderer MW, Hack M. Inguinal hernias in very low birth weight infants: Incidence and timing of repair. *J Pediatr Surg*. 1992;27:1322–1324.

225. Boocock GR, Todd PJ. Inguinal hernias are common in preterm infants. *Arch Dis Child*. 1985;60:669–670.

226. Rowe MI, Copelson LW, Clatworthy HW. The patent processus vaginalis and the inguinal hernia. *J Pediatr Surg*. 1969;4:102–107.

227. Rescorla FJ, Grosfeld JL. Inguinal hernia repair in the perinatal period and early infancy: Clinical considerations. *J Pediatr Surg.* 1984;19:832–837.

228. Rowe MI, Marchildon MB. Inguinal hernia and hydrocele in infants and children. *Surg Clin North Am.* 1981;61:1137–1145.

229. Mollen KP, Kane TD. Inguinal hernia: What we have learned from laparoscopic evaluation of the contralateral side. *Curr Opin Pediatr.* 2007;19:344–348.

230. Hata S, Takahashi Y, Nakamura T, Suzuki R, Kitada M, Shimano T. Preoperative sonographic evaluation is a useful method of detecting contralateral patent processus vaginalis in pediatric patients with unilateral inguinal hernia. *J Pediatr Surg.* 2004;39:1396–1399.

231. Fitz R. Perforating inflammation of the vermiform appendix. *Trans Assoc Am Physicians.* 1886:1.

232. McBurney C. Experience with early operative interference in cases of disease of the vermiform appendix. *NY Med J.* 1889;50.

233. Scholer SJ, Pituch K, Orr DP, Dittus RS. Clinical outcomes of children with acute abdominal pain. *Pediatrics.* 1996;98(4 pt 1):680–685.

234. Reynolds SL, Jaffe DM. Diagnosing abdominal pain in a pediatric emergency department. *Pediatr Emerg Care.* 1992;8:126–128.

235. Addiss DG, Shaffer N, Fowler BS, Tauxe RV. The epidemiology of appendicitis and appendectomy in the United States. *Am J Epidemiol.* 1990;132:910–925.

236. Brumer M. Appendicitis. Seasonal incidence and postoperative wound infection. *Br J Surg.* 1970;57:93–99.

237. Luckmann R. Incidence and case fatality rates for acute appendicitis in California. A population-based study of the effects of age. *Am J Epidemiol.* 1989;129:905–918.

238. Burkitt DP, Walker AR, Painter NS. Dietary fiber and disease. *JAMA.* 1974;229:1068–1074.

239. Burkitt DP. The aetiology of appendicitis. *Br J Surg.* 1971;58:695–699.

240. Karaman A, Cavusoglu YH, Karaman I, Cakmak O. Seven cases of neonatal appendicitis with a review of the English language literature of the last century. *Pediatr Surg Int.* 2003;19:707–709.

241. Selbst SM, Friedman MJ, Singh SB. Epidemiology and etiology of malpractice lawsuits involving children in US emergency departments and urgent care centers. *Pediatr Emerg Care.* 2005;21:165–169.

242. Golledge J, Toms AP, Franklin IJ, Scriven MW, Galland RB. Assessment of peritonism in appendicitis. *Ann R Coll Surg Engl.* 1996;78:11–14.

243. Rothrock SG, Skeoch G, Rush JJ, Johnson NE. Clinical features of misdiagnosed appendicitis in children. *Ann Emerg Med.* 1991;20:45–50.

244. Bundy DG, Byerley JS, Liles EA, Perrin EM, Katznelson J, Rice HE. Does this child have appendicitis? *JAMA.* 25 2007;298:438–451.

245. Rappaport WD, Peterson M, Stanton C. Factors responsible for the high perforation rate seen in early childhood appendicitis. *Am Surg.* 1989;55(10):602–605.

246. Pieper R, Kager L, Nasman P. Acute appendicitis: A clinical study of 1018 cases of emergency appendectomy. *Acta Chir Scand.* 1982;148:51–62.

247. Adolph VR, Falterman KW. Appendicitis in children in the managed care era. *J Pediatr Surg.* 1996;31:1035–1037.

248. Marchildon MB, Dudgeon DL. Perforated appendicitis: Current experience in a Childrens Hospital. *Ann Surg.* 1977;185:84–87.

249. Savrin RA, Clatworthy HW Jr. Appendiceal rupture: A continuing diagnostic problem. *Pediatrics.* 1979;63:36–43.

250. Andersson RE. Meta-analysis of the clinical and laboratory diagnosis of appendicitis. *Br J Surg.* 2004;91:28–37.

251. Sivit CJ, Siegel MJ, Applegate KE, Newman KD. When appendicitis is suspected in children. *Radiographics.* 2001;21:247–262, 288–294.

252. Wang LT, Prentiss KA, Simon JZ, Doody DP, Ryan DP. The use of white blood cell count and left shift in the diagnosis of appendicitis in children. *Pediatr Emerg Care.* 2007;23:69–76.

253. Rothrock SG, Green SM, Dobson M, Colucciello SA, Simmons CM. Misdiagnosis of appendicitis in nonpregnant women of childbearing age. *J Emerg Med.* 1995;13:1–8.

254. Barker AP, Davey RB. Appendicitis in the first three years of life. *Aust N Z J Surg.* 1988;58:491–494.

255. Sivit CJ. Imaging the child with right lower quadrant pain and suspected appendicitis: Current concepts. *Pediatr Radiol.* 2004;34:447–453.

256. Vasavada P. Ultrasound evaluation of acute abdominal emergencies in infants and children. *Radiol Clin North Am.* 2004;42:445–456.

257. Hahn HB, Hoepner FU, Kalle T, et al. Sonography of acute appendicitis in children: 7 years experience. *Pediatr Radiol.* 1998;28:147–151.

258. Baldisserotto M, Marchiori E. Accuracy of noncompressive sonography of children with appendicitis according to the potential positions of the appendix. *AJR Am J Roentgenol.* 2000;175:1387–1392.

259. Lowe LH, Penney MW, Stein SM, et al. Unenhanced limited CT of the abdomen in the diagnosis of appendicitis in children: Comparison with sonography. *AJR Am J Roentgenol.* 2001;176:31–35.

260. Lowe LH, Perez R Jr, Scheker LE, Stein SM, Heller RM, Hernanz-Schulman M. Appendicitis and alternate diagnoses in children: Findings on unenhanced limited helical CT. *Pediatr Radiol.* 2001;31:569–577.

261. Sivit CJ, Applegate KE, Stallion A, et al. Imaging evaluation of suspected appendicitis in a pediatric population: Effectiveness of sonography versus CT. *AJR Am J Roentgenol.* 2000;175:977–980.

262. Hoecker CC, Billman GF. The utility of unenhanced computed tomography in appendicitis in children. *J Emerg Med.* 2005;28:415–421.

263. Kaiser S, Finnbogason T, Jorulf HK, Soderman E, Frenckner B. Suspected appendicitis in children: Diagnosis with contrast-enhanced versus nonenhanced helical CT. *Radiology.* 2004;231:427–433.

264. Mullins ME, Kircher MF, Ryan DP, et al. Evaluation of suspected appendicitis in children using limited helical CT and colonic contrast material. *AJR Am J Roentgenol.* 2001;176:37–41.

265. Kharbanda AB, Taylor GA, Bachur RG. Suspected appendicitis in children: Rectal and intravenous contrast-enhanced versus intravenous contrast-enhanced CT. *Radiology.* 2007;243:520–526.

266. Brody AS, Frush DP, Huda W, Brent RL. Radiation risk to children from computed tomography. *Pediatrics*. 2007;120:677–682.

267. Brenner DJ, Hall EJ. Computed tomography—an increasing source of radiation exposure. *N Engl J Med*. 2007;357:2277–2284.

268. Frush DP, Donnelly LF, Rosen NS. Computed tomography and radiation risks: What pediatric health care providers should know. *Pediatrics*. 2003;112:951–957.

269. Vernon AH, Georgeson KE, Harmon CM. Pediatric laparoscopic appendectomy for acute appendicitis. *Surg Endosc*. 2004;18:75–79.

270. Lukish J, Powell D, Morrow S, Cruess D, Guzzetta P. Laparoscopic appendectomy in children: Use of the endoloop vs the endostapler. *Arch Surg*. 2007;142:58–62.

271. Jen HC, Shew SB. Laparoscopic versus open appendectomy in children: Outcomes comparison based on a statewide analysis. *J Surg Res*. 2010;161:13–17.

272. Wang X, Zhang W, Yang X, Shao J, Zhou X, Yuan J. Complicated appendicitis in children: Is laparoscopic appendectomy appropriate? A comparative study with the open appendectomy—our experience. *J Pediatr Surg*. 2009;44:1924–1927.

273. Andersen BR, Kallehave FL, Andersen HK. Antibiotics versus placebo for prevention of postoperative infection after appendicectomy. *Cochrane Database Syst Rev*. 2005;(3):CD001439.

274. St Peter SD, Aguayo P, Fraser JD, et al. Initial laparoscopic appendectomy versus initial nonoperative management and interval appendectomy for perforated appendicitis with abscess: A prospective, randomized trial. *J Pediatr Surg*. 2010;45:236–240.

275. McCann JW, Maroo S, Wales P, et al. Image-guided drainage of multiple intraabdominal abscesses in children with perforated appendicitis: An alternative to laparotomy. *Pediatr Radiol*. 2008;38:661–668.

276. Gillick J, Mohanan N, Das L, Puri P. Laparoscopic appendectomy after conservative management of appendix mass. *Pediatr Surg Int*. 2008;24:299–301.

277. Roach JP, Partrick DA, Bruny JL, Allshouse MJ, Karrer FM, Ziegler MM. Complicated appendicitis in children: A clear role for drainage and delayed appendectomy. *Am J Surg*. 2007;194:769–772.

278. Andersson RE, Petzold MG. Nonsurgical treatment of appendiceal abscess or phlegmon: A systematic review and meta-analysis. *Ann Surg*. 2007;246:741–748.

279. Taqi E, Al Hadher S, Ryckman J, et al. Outcome of laparoscopic appendectomy for perforated appendicitis in children. *J Pediatr Surg*. 2008;43:893–895.

280. Krisher SL, Browne A, Dibbins A, Tkacz N, Curci M. Intra-abdominal abscess after laparoscopic appendectomy for perforated appendicitis. *Arch Surg*. Apr 2001;136:438–441.

281. Ball CG, Kortbeek JB, Kirkpatrick AW, Mitchell P. Laparoscopic appendectomy for complicated appendicitis: An evaluation of postoperative factors. *Surg Endosc*. 2004;18:969–973.

282. Pham VA, Pham HN, Ho TH. Laparoscopic appendectomy: An efficacious alternative for complicated appendicitis in children. *Eur J Pediatr Surg*. 2009;19:157–159.

283. Bailey B, Bergeron S, Gravel J, Bussieres JF, Bensoussan A. Efficacy and impact of intravenous morphine before surgical consultation in children with right lower quadrant pain suggestive of appendicitis: A randomized controlled trial. *Ann Emerg Med*. 2007;50:371–378.

284. Dinkevich E, Ozuah PO. Pyloric stenosis. *Pediatr Rev*. 2000;21:249–250.

285. Senquiz AL. Use of decubitus position for finding the "olive" of pyloric stenosis. *Pediatrics*. 1991;87:266.

286. Gellis SS. Ancient technique of olive detection. *Pediatrics*. 1991;88:655–656.

A 4-day-old girl presents to the emergency department (ED) after an episode of bloody stools and increasing abdominal distention. She has not been feeding well and is sleeping between feedings. She was born at 34 weeks of gestation by emergency cesarean delivery because the mother had pregnancy-induced hypertension. The infant did well after delivery and was discharged to home. She had been taking commercial formula every 3 hours but during the past 6 hours has not been feeding at all and has been more lethargic.

On physical examination, the infant is afebrile, with a respiratory rate of 45/min and a heart rate of 180/min. The head, neck, lung, and heart examination results are normal except for tachycardia. The abdomen is distended; the overlying skin is mildly shiny and erythematous, and bowel sounds are hypoactive. Femoral pulses are present, but capillary refill to the lower extremities is delayed. A stool sample obtained from the diaper is positive for blood.

1. *What could be the cause of rectal bleeding and abdominal distention in this neonate?*
2. *What studies could help you decide the cause?*

The infant is fluid resuscitated, and an orogastric tube at low intermittent suction is placed to decompress the abdomen. Cultures are obtained. Supine and left lateral decubitus plain radiographs of the abdomen reveal pneumatosis intestinalis with PVG.

Ampicillin, gentamicin, and metronidazole are administered intravenously. Early surgical consultation is obtained. Enteral feedings are withheld for 10 to 14 days. Parenteral hyperalimentation is given during this time. Once the abdominal radiographs return to normal and 10 to 14 days of bowel rest are completed, feeding using an elemental formula is begun. Formula strength and volume are advanced very slowly. The infant tolerates slow advancement of feedings well without any signs or symptoms of obstruction due to stricture formation.

Laboratory studies are nonspecific. Preterm infants can show neutropenia, thrombocytopenia, or evidence of disseminated intravascular coagulopathy. Full-term infants can exhibit leukocytosis. Plain abdominal radiographs are helpful if positive and characteristically demonstrate an ileus, a persistent loop of bowel, intrahepatic PVG, pneumatosis intestinalis, or a gasless abdomen. Malrotation with midgut volvulus must also be considered and an upper gastrointestinal (GI) tract series might be warranted.

CASE SUMMARY 2

A 4-week-old boy arrives in the ED with a 1-day history of decreased activity and vomiting. The infant is breastfed and has had no difficulty nursing but has vomited intermittently. During the past 3 hours, the infant has vomited frequently. The last few episodes of vomiting produced green vomitus. The birth history was uncomplicated. The infant was full-term and born by spontaneous vaginal delivery.

On physical examination, the infant is lethargic, pale, and grunting. His respiratory rate is 60/min, heart rate is 190/min, blood pressure is 80/60 mm Hg, and rectal temperature is 36°C (96.8°F). The anterior fontanel is sunken. The lungs are clear to auscultation, but occasional grunting sounds are noted. Abdominal examination reveals decreased bowel sounds, and the abdomen is distended and tender to palpation. The genital examination results are normal. The extremities are mottled with poor perfusion.

1. *What important cause of bilious emesis in an infant must be excluded immediately?*
2. *What is the radiographic study of choice in the evaluation of an infant with bilious emesis?*
3. *Why must the evaluation of an infant with bilious emesis be performed emergently?*

Bilious emesis in an infant is considered diagnostic for malrotation with midgut volvulus until proven otherwise. The infant is given oxygen by face mask. Volume resuscitation and gastric decompression improve his circulatory status.

Plain abdominal radiographs reveal absence of free peritoneal air. A limited upper GI contrast study is the study of choice and confirms the presence of malrotation with midgut volvulus. The infant is immediately taken to the operating room to undergo the Ladd procedure with appendectomy.

The evaluation of an infant must be performed on an emergency basis because the infant with malrotation and midgut volvulus can infarct the entire midgut in 1 to 2 hours.

A 3-week-old, female infant presents with a 4-day history of projectile vomiting. She is a full-term product of a vaginal delivery. There were no complications at birth. For the first 2 weeks of life, the infant would occasionally spit up (normal for age). Currently, the vomiting is very forceful, as if it will "hit the wall." The infant is breastfed, and the vomitus appears to be breast milk. There is no history of blood or green emesis, diarrhea, or fever. The mother is frustrated because the infant is losing weight and appears hungry.

On physical examination, the infant is dehydrated, with a sunken fontanelle and poor skin turgor. Her respiratory rate is 24/min, heart rate is 165/min, and temperature is 36.3°C (97°F). Cardiac and pulmonary examination results are normal except for tachycardia. Abdominal examination is difficult due to crying and tensing of the abdominal muscles. The infant's genitourinary examination results are normal. There is loss of subcutaneous fat of the thighs and buttocks.

1. *What maneuver can be done to help facilitate the abdominal examination?*
2. *What clinical signs can the physician look for during the examination?*
3. *What ancillary studies could help determine the diagnosis?*

The infant is given a bottle of glucose water to facilitate examination of the abdomen. Feeding will allow the abdominal muscles to relax and facilitate palpation of the hypertrophied pyloric muscle in the upper pole of the epigastrium.

Flex the hips and knees to relax the abdominal muscles. Place an orogastric or nasogastric tube to empty the stomach of its contents to facilitate palpation of the hypertrophied pyloric muscle.[284]

The infant should be placed in the prone or lateral decubitus position. This allows the hypertrophied pyloric muscle to fall anteriorly in the abdominal cavity during gentle palpation and examination of the right epigastrium.[285,286] In this case, a small mass is palpated in the midepigastric area. The abdomen is soft and nontender.

After feeding, look for reverse peristaltic abdominal waves as the intestine moves from the infant's right to left. Peristalsis occurs in the opposite direction as the infant prepares to vomit. After feeding, reverse abdominal peristaltic waves are evident before an episode of projectile, nonbilious emesis.

The infant's electrolyte panel shows a hyponatremic, hypokalemic metabolic alkalosis. Intravenous fluids are given, starting with a 20-mL/kg normal saline infusion for 30 minutes followed by 5% dextrose in half normal saline, with a 20-mEq/L infusion of potassium chloride at 1.5 times maintenance requirement. Fluid and electrolyte losses are calculated and replenished for 48 hours. Once the metabolic abnormalities are corrected, the infant undergoes a pyloromyotomy without complications. She is currently tolerating breast milk and thriving.

CASE SUMMARY 4

A 6-month-old boy presents to a pediatrician's office with 1 day of crying and poor feeding. His mother states that during the past few hours he has had two episodes of vomiting breast milk. There is no fever, diarrhea, or cold symptoms. His mother states that the pain seems so intense that he draws his knees to his chest and "crawls" up her arms and shoulders. Between bouts of pain, he is calm and at times quite sleepy.

On physical examination, the infant is resting in his mother's arms. His respiratory rate is 18/min, heart rate is 130/min, and rectal temperature is 37.9°C (100.2°F). The anterior fontanelle is flat and soft. His lips are pink but dry. His lungs are clear to auscultation without increased work of breathing. The abdominal examination reveals normal bowel sounds, mild tenderness, and a soft mass in the right upper quadrant below the liver border. The genital examination results are normal. Soft stool obtained on rectal examination is positive for occult blood. While you discuss further management plans with the mother, the infant begins crying inconsolably.

1.   *What could be the cause of this infant's abdominal pain?*

The causes of abdominal pain and vomiting in an infant are numerous. These include intussusception, malrotation with midgut volvulus, Meckel diverticulum, incarcerated inguinal hernia, intentional trauma, gastrointestinal tract infections, and cow's milk or soy protein allergy. The infant is sent to the ED for fluid resuscitation and surgical consultation. Intravenous normal saline is given, and radiographs of the abdomen are obtained. Laboratory study results are nonspecific. A flat and upright abdominal plain radiograph reveals a paucity of gas in the area below the liver (hepatic flexure) with no free intra-abdominal air. An air contrast enema reveals an ileocecal intussusception, which is reduced without difficulty. He is hospitalized for overnight observation. He is discharged home after refeeding the following day without complications.

CASE SUMMARY 5

The mother of a 9-month-old boy calls you because the infant is sleeping too much. Earlier in the morning he had two episodes of vomiting. The vomit was not green or bloody. The infant passed a stool with mucus and urinated without difficulty.

On physical examination, the infant is lethargic. His respiratory rate 20/min, heart rate is 120/min, and rectal temperature is 37.5°C (100°F). The anterior fontanelle is small and flat. Pupils are 4 mm and reactive. His lungs are clear to auscultation without increased work of breathing, and cardiovascular examination results are normal. The abdominal and genital examination results are also normal. The stool is positive for occult blood. The skin examination reveals no evidence of trauma.

1. *What surgical emergency could cause lethargy in this infant?*
2. *What diagnostic test could be performed to diagnose and treat this entity?*
3. *What is an important complication of an air enema, and how should the physician specifically intervene if respiratory difficulty occurs?*

Intussusception in an infant can present as gastrointestinal symptoms or profound lethargy. An air contrast enema or a barium contrast enema can be used to diagnose and treat intussusception. An important complication of air contrast enema is perforation of the intestine with accumulation of free intraperitoneal air. An important complication of barium contrast enema is perforation of the intestine with accumulation of barium sulfate suspension, causing barium peritonitis. Management of perforation would include maintaining airway, breathing, and circulation. Emergency paracentesis for peritoneal aspiration of free air might be necessary if respiratory distress occurs. Urgent volume resuscitation with normal saline is mandatory if barium peritonitis occurs. Both would provide temporary relief until immediate surgical correction in the operating room is performed.

The infant is sent to the ED for evaluation of altered mental status. Intravenous normal saline is given. Laboratory studies reveal normal electrolyte and glucose levels, normal urinalysis results, negative urine toxicology screen results, and a normal blood gas analysis result. The complete blood cell count reveals a leukocytosis without a left shift and a normal hemoglobin level and hematocrit. Results of computed tomography of the head are normal. During the evaluation, the infant has three more episodes of vomiting and passes a bloody stool. Surgical consultation is obtained. Abdominal radiographs are normal. An air contrast enema reveals an ileocolic intussusception, which cannot be reduced by hydrostatic pressure. Surgical reduction is performed without complication, and the child does well postoperatively.

A 2-year-old boy presents to the ED by ambulance. His mother had called 911 because she discovered that his diaper was full of bright red blood. The child has had previous bowel movements with streaks of blood. He does not seem to be in pain but is less active than normal. There is no history of mucus in the stools, fever, or vomiting. He is feeding well.

On physical examination, the child is alert and appropriately fearful. His respiratory rate is 24/min and nonlabored, heart rate is 140/min, blood pressure is 100/60 mm Hg, and temperature is 37°C (98.6°F). Head and neck examination reveals pale conjunctivae and mucous membranes. Cardiovascular examination reveals mild tachycardia with a soft 2/6 systolic ejection murmur at the left lower sternal border. Abdominal and genitourinary examination results are normal. Examination of the anus reveals no evidence of trauma, fissures, or tags. Stool is grossly bloody. The skin is without bruising or petechiae.

1. *What are the priorities of treatment in this child?*
2. *How can the physician differentiate upper GI tract bleeding from lower GI tract bleeding?*
3. *What could be the cause of painless rectal bleeding in this previously healthy child?*
4. *In a child who is actively bleeding from the rectum, would radiographs be helpful or indicated?*

First, 100% oxygen by nonrebreathing mask is given. Second, intravenous access and laboratory tests, including a complete blood cell count with differential, prothrombin time/partial thromboplastin time, and type and crossmatch, are obtained. Despite a 20-mL/kg normal saline bolus, tachycardia and pallor continue. A bedside hemoglobin value of 8 mg/dL confirms suspicion of anemia and hypovolemia secondary to blood loss. A 10-mL/kg infusion of type-specific packed red blood cells is started. Technetium Tc 99m pertechnetate scan is inconclusive for a Meckel diverticulum, presumably because of active bleeding and pooling of blood in the intestines. The pediatric surgeon recommends exploratory laparotomy once the patient is hemodynamically stable and hemoglobin normalizes. At laparotomy, a 5-cm (2-in) diverticulum containing whitish-appearing heterotopic tissue is removed. The child does well postoperatively and has had no further occurrences of rectal bleeding.

To differentiate upper GI tract bleeding from lower GI tract bleeding, place an orogastric or nasogastric tube and lavage with saline. Blood-free aspirates indicate that bleeding is originating from the lower GI tract.

Painless rectal bleeding can be due to Meckel diverticulum, intestinal polyps, duplications, hemangiomas, arteriovenous malformations, coagulopathy, peptic ulcer disease, and inflammatory bowel disease. However, the latter two problems are typically associated with abdominal pain and discomfort.

In a child with lower GI tract bleeding, a technetium Tc 99m pertechnetate scan to search for a Meckel diverticulum is frequently obtained. However, if the scan is negative or if the child remains hemodynamically unstable despite volume resuscitation, most pediatric surgeons recommend exploratory laparotomy or laparoscopy for definitive treatment.[112] Some surgeons believe that regardless of scan results, children with brisk, painless lower GI tract bleeding require an exploratory laparotomy and omit the Meckel scan altogether. In a child with a few mild episodes of painless rectal bleeding and a negative Meckel scan, some physicians will obtain an esophagogastroduodenoscopy and a colonoscopy to rule out polyps or other mucosal lesions, but the endoscopy might not be able to directly view a Meckel diverticulum.

A 13-year-old boy is brought to the ED by his parents at 4:00 AM after he was awakened by a sudden onset of left scrotal pain. The previous day, he was in his usual state of good health and played in his school's football game. He has had several brief, less intense but similar episodes in the past. He now has a tender, swollen left hemiscrotum, and the testis appears to ride higher in the scrotum. There is absence of cremasteric reflex on the left. He experiences pain with any movement and is nauseated.

1. What is your differential diagnosis?
2. Are any imaging modalities available or indicated?
3. Is there an indication for surgical intervention?
4. Is the contralateral testis at risk?

The patient exhibits the classic history and physical findings of testicular torsion. He is given intravenous morphine for analgesia. No laboratory studies or imaging studies are performed. The patient is taken for emergency scrotal exploration. Detorsion produces a viable-appearing testis. A bell clapper deformity is noted, and bilateral orchiopexy is performed. The patient does well postoperatively.

The differential diagnosis of testicular torsion includes torsion of the appendix testis or appendix epididymis, epididymitis, orchitis, incarcerated inguinal hernia, trauma to the testis, Henoch-Schönlein purpura, scrotal cellulitis, Kawasaki disease, and testicular tumor.

Imaging modalities are available and include the technetium Tc 99m pertechnetate scan and color Doppler ultrasonography. Imaging studies are helpful in equivocal cases but should not delay surgical consultation. In cases of classic testicular torsion, imaging studies are not indicated. The patient has an acute testicular torsion for which detorsion and orchiopexy are clearly indicated.

The contralateral testis is at risk for future torsion. Testicular torsion in the peripubertal male is usually due to abnormal attachments of the tunica vaginalis and usually occurs bilaterally. The testes have a horizontal lie within the scrotal sac and are likely to become twisted. This abnormality is referred to as the bell clapper deformity. Bilateral orchiopexy is indicated.

CASE SUMMARY 8

A 3-month-old boy born at 36 weeks of gestation presents to the ED with a 12-hour history of agitation, poor feeding, and right scrotal swelling. The parents have never noted this swelling before. The scrotal mass is tense and seems to transilluminate. It is difficult to palpate the testis on the right side. The left hemiscrotum is normal. Initial attempts at reducing the mass are met with a crying child and very anxious parents.

1. *Is this a hydrocele or a hernia?*
2. *Should further attempts be made to reduce the mass?*
3. *When should this lesion be repaired?*

Although the scrotal mass transilluminates, there are several clues in the history that support the hypothesis that it is an incarcerated inguinal hernia. The mass is noticed for the first time, is associated with symptoms of agitation, poor feeding, and pain, and is unilateral. Most hydroceles are present since birth, are asymptomatic, and are more often bilateral. Further attempts at reduction by an experienced surgeon are warranted. Sedation and Trendelenburg positioning might facilitate successful reduction. Manual reduction involves squeezing gently the most dependent portion of the hernia in the direction of the inguinal canal. This is done while holding gentle pressure on the external inguinal ring with the thumb and forefinger of the other hand to "funnel" the incarcerated mass through the inguinal canal.

In this case, surgical consultation is obtained. A catheter and cardiac and pulse oximetry monitors are placed. The infant is given fentanyl (1 mcg/kg intravenously) and placed in the Trendelenburg position for manual reduction of the incarcerated inguinal hernia. The hernia is not reduced. Maintenance intravenous fluids are continued, and the infant is taken emergently for intraoperative repair.

In this scenario, the infant requires immediate surgical repair and reduction. If manual reduction is difficult but successful, elective repair can be scheduled. Patients with easily reducible inguinal hernias who are asymptomatic can be discharged from the ED to follow-up with their medical home, which can refer the patient to a surgeon for elective repair.

CASE SUMMARY 9

An 8-year-old boy presents to the ED with a 24-hour history of abdominal pain. Initially, the pain was dull, vague, and located in the epigastric and periumbilical regions. This was followed by several hours of nausea and multiple episodes of vomiting. During the past 6 hours, the pain has become more pronounced in his right lower quadrant. His mother states that several family members have a viral illness. This young boy has a low-grade fever, normal urinalysis results, and a white blood cell count at the upper range of normal. He refuses to ambulate. He has reproducible tenderness in his right lower quadrant despite attempts at distraction.

1. *Are other studies indicated before disposition?*
2. *Does the viral illness in the family sway your thinking?*
3. *Does a normal white blood cell count cloud the picture?*

No other studies are indicated for a classic case history as is presented here. A 20-mL/kg normal saline bolus is given intravenously. Surgical consultation is immediately obtained; the diagnosis of appendicitis is made, and morphine sulfate (0.1 mg/kg per dose) is given for pain control. The patient is taken to the operating room and is found to have a ruptured vermiform appendix.

An appendectomy is performed without further complications. Intravenous ampicillin, gentamicin, and clindamycin are given intraoperatively and continued until the child is afebrile, has a normal white blood cell count, and is tolerating a normal diet. This process in otherwise uncomplicated perforated appendicitis takes approximately 5 to 7 days.

The history of viral illness in family members is often present and does not predict the absence or presence of appendicitis.

A normal white blood cell count is seen in approximately 20% of patients with appendicitis; therefore, a normal count does not exclude appendicitis as a diagnosis.

A 2-year-old boy presents to the ED with 2 days of nausea and vomiting, headache, and right leg pain. The vomitus is nonbilious and nonbloody and consists of stomach contents. The child was seen in the ED the previous day and was given a normal saline bolus and ondansetron. The results of cranial computed tomography, an electrolyte panel, and urinalysis were normal. The child was sent home with an oral rehydration solution.

The child continued to vomit intermittently through the night and in the morning had five loose, green stools and right leg pain.

On physical examination, the child is febrile with a blood pressure of 90/60 mm Hg, a heart rate of 146/min, and a respiratory rate of 30/min. He appears dehydrated with dry oral mucous membranes and delayed capillary refill. Head and neck examination reveal normal pupillary reflexes and a supple neck without meningismus. Heart and lung examination results are normal except for tachycardia. The abdomen is distended with normoactive bowel sounds, diffuse abdominal tenderness, and voluntary guarding of all quadrants. The genitourinary examination results are normal for a circumcised Tanner 1 male. Hips are without limitation of motion, effusion, warmth, or erythema. The child cries during the entire examination.

1. *What are the priorities of care for this child?*
2. *What is your differential in a young child with undifferentiated abdominal pain?*
3. *Should pain medication be withheld until a definitive diagnosis is made?*

Ensure airway, breathing, and circulation by applying oxygen, obtaining intravenous access, and administering a 20-mL/kg bolus of isotonic crystalloid. This child is crying and vigorous; thus, fluid resuscitation is the current priority. During intravenous catheter placement, laboratory tests, including a complete blood cell count with differential, blood culture, and glucose, electrolyte panel, blood urea nitrogen, and creatinine measurement, are ordered.

Undifferentiated abdominal pain in a febrile child can be due to gastroenteritis, mesenteric adenitis, lower respiratory tract infection, urinary tract infection, pyelonephritis, or musculoskeletal trauma or infection. In this young child with a confusing presentation, graded compression ultrasonography was performed and revealed an 8-mm noncompressible appendix containing an appendicolith.

Analgesia should be considered in any child who presents to the ED in pain. There is an increasing body of literature supporting the use of early analgesia in children with acute abdominal pain and, in particular, those with appendicitis. Opiate administration has been shown to decrease pain scores but did not appear to impair the final diagnosis, increase time to surgical disposition, increase missed diagnosis rate, or lead to unnecessary surgical interventions.

chapter 9

Nontraumatic Orthopedic Emergencies

Kemedy K. McQuillen, MD, FAAP, FACEP
Ronald I. Paul, MD, FAAP, FACEP

Objectives

1 Discuss the epidemiology, pathophysiology, assessment, and treatment of nontraumatic pediatric orthopedic conditions.

2 Describe the assessment and treatment of a child with a limp.

3 Identify the radiographic findings for developmental dysplasia of the hip (DDH), nursemaid elbow, Legg-Calvé-Perthes (LCP) disease, slipped capital femoral epiphysis, Osgood-Schlatter disease, and acute septic arthritis.

Chapter Outline

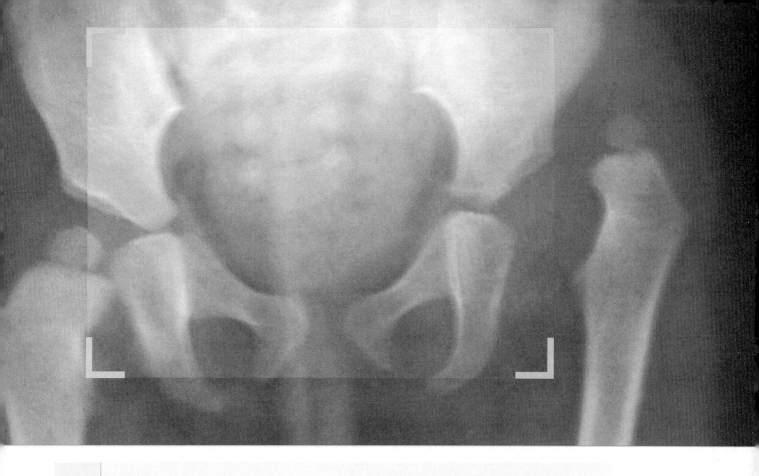

CASE SCENARIO 1

During your evaluation of a 5-week-old girl, you feel a clunk as you do the Ortolani maneuver on the left hip. You also note asymmetric skinfolds and decreased abduction. The results of the rest of the examination, including the right hip, are normal, and the child is in no distress. On questioning, the mother tells you that her daughter was born on time after an uncomplicated antenatal course. Specifically, the mother did not have multiple gestations or oligohydramnios, and the infant was born head first. The infant is breastfeeding well and gaining weight. The mother has had no problems with diaper changes, and her daughter does not appear to be in pain. After discussing your findings with the mother, you arrange for further testing and contact a specialist.

1. *What is the diagnosis?*
2. *How do you proceed in your evaluation?*
3. *What is the most likely course of treatment for this child?*

Introduction

As a result of the physiologic and anatomical differences between children and adults, pediatric patients are susceptible to orthopedic problems that do not affect the adult population.

Developmental Dysplasia of the Hip

Developmental dysplasia of the hip (DDH), formerly known as congenital dislocation of the

hip, is an abnormal formation of the hip joint occurring between organogenesis and fetal maturity.[1] It encompasses a spectrum of disease that ranges from subluxable (loose) hips to frankly dislocated hips. The origin of DDH is not entirely clear, but it might be related to intrauterine positioning, primary acetabular dysplasia, and/or ligamentous laxity.

In white neonates, the incidence of dysplasia is 1%, and the incidence of dislocated hips is 0.1%. Dysplasia is more common in Native

American populations and less common in black, Korean, and Chinese populations. There seems to be a familial predilection. Developmental dysplasia of the hip is more common in girls and most commonly unilaterally (80%). With unilateral involvement, there is a slight predilection for the left side. Associated birth factors include oligohydramnios, breech presentation, torticollis, talipes equinovarus, metatarsus adductus, and being the first born.[2] Postnatally, swaddling infants with hips and knees in extension predisposes them to hip dislocation.

Clinical Features

Developmental dysplasia of the hip might be diagnosed at birth, or despite frequent and appropriate physical examinations, it might not present until later in life.[3] Conversely, more than 50% of infants found to have unstable hips at birth will develop spontaneous hip stability within 3 to 4 days.[4]

The presentations and physical findings of DDH are as diverse as the disease itself. This variability is due to the differences in the severity of the dysplasia and the progressive changes that occur over time.

In infants up to 6 months of age, the diagnosis of DDH is based on physical examination findings and specific testing. The leg length, skinfolds, range of motion, and the results of the Barlow provocative test and the Ortolani reduction maneuver are abnormal (Table 9-1).

Skinfold asymmetry can be noted in the groin, below the buttock, and along the thighs. Skinfold asymmetry is not specific for DDH and can be found in approximately 30% of infants with normal hips. Hip range of motion is also helpful in diagnosing DDH. Asymmetries in hip flexion, abduction, and external rotation should prompt further investigation. The physical diagnostic cornerstones for diagnosing DDH in young infants are the Ortolani reduction maneuver and the Barlow provocative test. The Ortolani reduction maneuver is done in an attempt to reduce a dislocated hip back into a normal position, and the Barlow provocative test detects the subluxable or dislocatable hip. Abnormal findings include the presence of a "clunk" with the Ortolani test and any abnormal movement

between the femoral head and the acetabulum with the Barlow maneuver.

From 4 to 6 months of age, soft tissue contractures develop and the Ortolani and Barlow tests are less helpful in detecting unstable hips, whereas range of motion abnormalities become more apparent. Limited or asymmetric leg movements or difficulty with diapering might be noticed. On examination, there is limited abduction, a relative shortening of the femoral segment (Galeazzi sign), and skinfold asymmetry. In children with bilateral DDH, the diagnosis is even more difficult beyond the first few months of life because there might be no asymmetry. After contractures develop, physical findings in bilateral DDH include widening of the perineum, abduction less than 4°, and the appearance of abnormally short thigh segments.

With the onset of walking, gait asymmetry or asymmetric in-toeing or out-toeing are clues to the presence of DDH. Adduction and flexion contractures, a positive Galeazzi sign, hyperlordosis, and a waddling gait are common findings. Clinical observation will reveal a Trendelenburg sign: while standing, the patient lifts one leg up at a time, and because the gluteal muscles are weakened on the affected side, the pelvis will drop to the opposite side. With bilateral DDH, the child will present with a wide-based waddling gait.

TABLE 9-1 Ortolani and Barlow Maneuvers	
Ortolani (Reduction) Maneuver	Barlow (Provocative) Test
• Stabilize the pelvis with one hand. • With the other hand, slightly abduct the infant's hip. • With the index and long fingers over the greater trochanter, pull the thigh up to gently reduce the hip.	• Stabilize the pelvis with one hand. • Place the thumb on the inner aspect of the thigh near the lesser trochanter. • Adduct the hip. • Exert downward pressure on the thigh with the thumb, pushing it into the table.

Diagnostic Studies

Radiographs of infant hips are extremely difficult to interpret and can provide a false sense of security if they seem normal. At 3 to 6 months of age, the femoral head ossifies. Before this time, an abnormal relationship between the upper end of the femur and the acetabulum might not be apparent. In addition, in infants with unstable but located hips, radiographs show the hip in position and the instability is undetected. A better imaging test before femoral head ossification is ultrasonography.[5] Because a large percentage of infants will have abnormal sonographic evaluation in the first week of life, with many of these abnormalities resolving within a few weeks,[1,6] it is best to delay ultrasonography in children with located but possibly unstable hips until 4 to 6 weeks of age.[3,7] Children with dislocated hips should undergo ultrasonography immediately. After approximately 6 weeks, the ossific nucleus of the femoral head is detectable and radiographs are more likely to reveal abnormalities and asymmetries. A standard anteroposterior pelvis radiograph with both legs extended in neutral abduction is then sufficient for diagnosis.

Findings on radiographic evaluation can be subtle, but two features are typical for DDH: the Shenton line is displaced laterally (**Figure 9.1**), and the acetabular angle is widened. The Shenton line, an arc running from the inferior border of the femoral neck up and extending to the superior border of the obturator foramen, is used to identify displacement of the hip on an anteroposterior (AP) pelvis film. The acetabular angle is formed by the angle produced by a line drawn between two points on the acetabulum and the Hilgenreiner line (**Figure 9.2**). Angles greater than 30° are considered abnormal, and angles greater than 40° indicate dislocation (**Figure 9.3**).

Differential Diagnosis

The differential diagnosis for DDH is broad and includes trauma, infections, cerebral palsy, and congenital abnormalities.

Management

Treatment of DDH is most successful when begun early; delays in detection can lead to a significantly worse prognosis. Patients with untreated

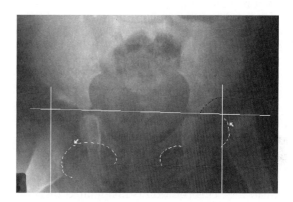

Figure 9.1 Shenton line displaced laterally in a hip with developmental dysplasia of the hip.

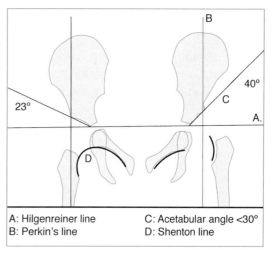

A: Hilgenreiner line	C: Acetabular angle <30°
B: Perkin's line	D: Shenton line

Figure 9.2 Acetabular angle and Hilgenreiner line.

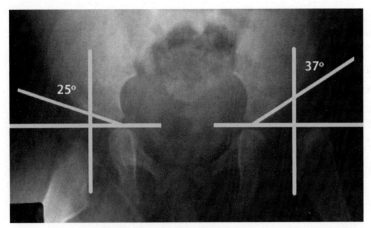

Figure 9.3 Widened acetabular angle in developmental dysplasia of the hip.

abnormal hips persisting beyond the newborn period are at risk for osteoarthritis, pain, abnormal gait, leg length discrepancy, and decreased agility. All infants who are seen in the emergency department (ED) should have their hips examined regularly until they are able to walk. Neonates who have a dislocated hip at birth should be referred to an orthopedic surgeon or pediatric orthopedic surgeon if available. When a newborn has a loose but located hip, referral can be made within 2 weeks. Children who present after the newborn period require immediate referral.

The essential goal of treatment is concentric reduction of the hip. After concentric reduction, stability must be obtained so that when the leg is allowed to move, it does not subluxate or dislocate. This position is maintained until all the dysplastic features of the bone and cartilage have resolved. The two most important complications are failure to achieve these goals and aseptic necrosis of the femoral head.

In the first 6 months of life, the Pavlik harness is the mainstay of treatment. It is a dynamic splint that allows movement while preventing hip extension or adduction. If the harness is

unsuccessful, a hip spica cast is usually the next choice. Beyond 6 months of age, a hip spica cast or fixed orthosis is required. Surgical release of contracted muscles might be required in older infants and children, with open surgical reduction if complete closed reduction is not achieved. Femoral and/or pelvic osteotomy might be necessary to reduce and stabilize dislocated hips in children older than 2 or 3 years.[8] Beyond 4 years in bilateral cases and 8 years in unilateral cases, reduction should not be attempted. The risk of aseptic necrosis and the potential for a poor result are too high.[2]

WHAT ELSE?

Differential Diagnosis of DDH

- Cerebral palsy
- Spina bifida
- Metatarsus adductus
- Internal tibial torsion
- Femoral anteversion
- Septic arthritis
- Osteomyelitis
- Trauma

THE CLASSICS

Radiographic Clues to DDH

- Sonogram showing displacement
- Shenton line displaced
- Acetabular angle greater than 30°

KEY POINTS

Management of DDH

Birth to 6 months of age:

- Infants younger than 6 weeks—ultrasonography
- Infants older than 6 weeks—plain radiography
- Orthopedic referral for closed reduction as appropriate and Pavlik harness

6 to 18 months of age:

- Plain radiography
- Orthopedic referral for closed reduction and spica cast

Older children:

- Plain radiography
- Orthopedic referral for closed reduction or leave unreduced

A father brings his 2-year-old daughter to the ED because she will not move her left arm. Earlier that day, as she was walking with her mother, she tripped and her mother grabbed her arm to prevent her from falling. Since that time she has not moved her arm and cries if anyone touches it. The father thinks she has hurt her wrist. The girl is otherwise healthy without any medical problems or allergies. She is not taking any medications. Excluding the left arm, results of the physical examination are normal. The child is holding her left arm at her side in mild flexion with the forearm pronated. Her wrist, elbow, and shoulder are nontender. She has no tenderness of any of her bones in her left upper extremity.

1. What is the diagnosis?
2. How do you treat it?
3. What is the prognosis?

Radial Head Subluxation

Radial head subluxation, commonly referred to as nursemaid elbow, is a frequent condition encountered in the ED. Classically, it occurs when there is a sudden traction on a child's arm. Simple maneuvers, such as swinging a child by the wrists or pulling the child up by the hands, are associated with radial head subluxation. Other associated histories include taking off or putting on a sweater or coat, falls, and self-induced episodes during temper tantrums. In up to one half of cases, no history of sudden traction of the arm is elicited. However, many of these infants likely had unwitnessed falls or pulls of their arms by other children. Studies have shown a higher frequency of occurrence in the left arm and a slightly higher incidence in girls compared with boys. Radial head subluxation usually occurs between 1 and 5 years of age, with an average age of approximately 2.5 years.[9–11] There are reported cases in infants younger than 6 months.[2,12] A recurrence rate has been described of up to 26%.[10]

The proposed mechanism of injury is the entrapment of the annular ligament between the radial head and capitellum.

Clinical Features

The child usually presents with the affected arm held at the side in mild flexion with the forearm pronated. Frequently, children hold their

> ## YOUR FIRST CLUE
>
> **Nursemaid Elbow**
> - History of traction to the arm or swinging of the child by the arms
> - Absence of edema or bruising of the upper extremity
> - Child holds the arm by the side with forearm flexed and pronated

wrists as they attempt to support their arms and elbows, causing parents to erroneously think the injury is at the wrist instead of the elbow. Patients can have involvement of both arms.[13] Examination of most children reveals a nontender extremity unless the forearm is supinated, which causes the child to cry and resist supination. There should be no edema or induration at the elbow. If detected, the physician should consider other diagnoses, including elbow fracture, contusion, or infection.

Differential Diagnosis

The differential diagnosis for nursemaid elbow includes trauma, infection, and tumor. If the history and physical findings are not classic, then radiographs will help distinguish these conditions from nursemaid elbow.

Diagnostic Studies

Radiographs, if obtained, can either be normal or reveal an abnormality in a line drawn through the longitudinal axis of the radius and capitellum.[14] In uninjured elbows this line should bisect the capitellum. A patient with a true radial head subluxation might return from the radiology department with a reduced subluxation because positioning for a lateral elbow radiograph sometimes provides the necessary treatment procedure even before the radiograph is taken. Overall, radiographs are not recommended before attempts at reduction, especially if there is a classic history of a pulled arm and a compatible examination result. Even without a classic history, many physicians will attempt a reduction if the examination results are compatible with radial head subluxation and then reevaluate clinically before getting a radiograph.[15]

Management

Treatment of radial head subluxation is fairly straightforward, with two different types of procedures described. The classic method of reduction involves supination of the wrist/forearm followed by flexion at the elbow (**Figure 9.4**). Studies have found this technique to be successful in 80% to 90% of cases.[10,11] An alternative technique is hyperpronation at the wrist; flexion is not required[16] (**Figure 9.5**). Although both techniques have been found to be highly successful, hyperpronation might provide a slightly higher

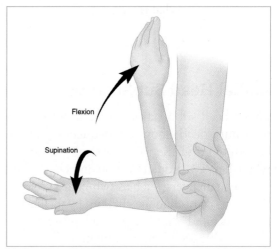

Figure 9.4 Treatment of radial head subluxation with supination and flexion.

Macias CG, Bothner J, Wiebe R. A comparison of supination/flexion to hyperpronation in the reduction of radial head subluxations. *Pediatrics.* 1998;102:10. Reprinted with permission.

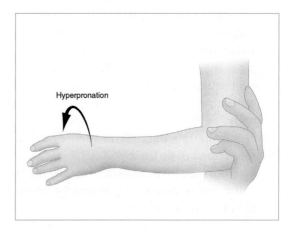

Figure 9.5 Treatment of radial head subluxation with pronation.

Macias CG, Bothner J, Wiebe R. A comparison of supination/flexion to hyperpronation in the reduction of radial head subluxations. *Pediatrics.* 1998;102:10. Reprinted with permission.

success rate, especially in the left arm.[16,17] In addition, one study suggested that it might be less painful to the patient.[17] It is helpful to know both techniques because some patients in whom one type of reduction has failed will subsequently have successful reduction when the alternative procedure is applied. In both treatment modalities, a palpable or audible click at the radial head is highly associated with a successful reduction and full use of the arm within 10 to 15 minutes. Children younger than 2 years have been associated with a slower return of use of the arm perhaps because it takes the younger child longer to realize that the arm is no longer painful. Occasionally, the subluxed elbow cannot be reduced even after several attempts. In these cases, the elbow should be splinted in 90° and referred for orthopedic follow-up. Most of these patients will have normal use of the arm at follow-up.[18]

There are no known complications of either reduction technique in patients with radial head subluxation. If attempts at reduction occur in patients with other injuries, complications can be seen, including displacement of previously nondisplaced fractures and unnecessary pain. In most cases the diagnosis is obvious and the treatment is straightforward. Once reduced, the arm should be pain free and need no specific follow-up. Guidance should be given, however, to avoid sudden traction on the arm to prevent recurrences.

The Child With a Limp

Limp can result from pain, weakness, neuromuscular abnormality, or deformity, and the differential diagnosis is extensive (Table 9-2). Determining the origin of the limp requires an understanding of the gait cycle, a thorough history and physical examination, radiographic imaging, and laboratory evaluation.

Gait is divided into the swing phase, when the limb is off the ground, and the stance phase when the limb is in a heel strike, flat foot, or push-off period. When children have pain, they develop an antalgic gait or a shortened stance phase in an attempt to shorten the time in which the limb is contact with the ground.

Determining the source of a limp begins with a thorough history and physical examination. History should elicit the presence, location, and nature of pain, as well as any factors that aggravate or alleviate the symptoms. Some children with hip conditions might experience knee pain. Other children might limp due to abdominal pain from appendicitis or a psoas abscess. If the child is unable to sit comfortably they might have a back condition. Onset and progression of symptoms can suggest a cause; gradually worsening symptoms can suggest a bone tumor, rheumatologic disorders, or a stress fracture; intermittent pain at rest or at night is seen with bone tumors[19]; and rheumatologic disorders can cause pain that is worse after a period of inactivity or first thing in the morning. Migratory pain might result from the polyarthralgias of acute rheumatic fever and gonococcal infection. An inciting trauma can suggest a fracture, sprain, strain, or contusion. Clarify associated symptoms such as fever (eg, osteomyelitis or septic arthritis), conjunctivitis (reactive arthritis), or rash (gonococcal arthritis). Excessive bruising can suggest leukemia or a hemarthrosis associated with a bleeding disorder. Ask about a recent pharyngitis (acute rheumatic fever), upper respiratory tract infection (transient synovitis), or diarrheal illness (reactive arthritis). A child who has been in areas endemic for Lyme disease should be queried about outside play, tick bites, and rashes. Sexual activity can suggest gonococcal or reactive arthritis. Fever, anorexia, weight loss, and night sweats are concerning for malignant disease.

The goal of the physical examination is to identify the type of limp and localize the pain. The child should be undressed and observed at rest in the supine and prone positions. Assessment of children while they are in the prone position allows for flexion and extension of the knee without movement of the hip and also permits for simultaneous comparison of hip rotation that can detect subtle differences in inward rotation. Hip flexion contractures that might be concealed by lumbar hyperlordosis will also be revealed in the prone position.[20] With the patient at rest, the position of comfort should be noted and symmetry, erythema, swelling, and deformity assessed. The back, abdomen, and extremities should be palpated to locate masses,

TABLE 9-2 Causes of Limp in Childhood

Cause	Specific Examples	
Infection	• Septic arthritis • Osteomyelitis • Diskitis • Appendicitis • Meningitis	• Gonococcal arthritis • Lyme disease • Psoas abscess • Myositis/pyomyositis
Inflammation	• Transient synovitis • Reactive arthritis • Acute rheumatic fever	• Juvenile idiopathic arthritis • SLE • Ankylosing spondylitis
Malignant neoplasm	• Leukemia/lymphoma • Ewing sarcoma • Osteosarcoma	• Neuroblastoma • Wilms tumor • Spinal cord tumors
Congenital abnormalities	• DDH • Clubfoot	• Limb length disparity
Neuromuscular	• Cerebral palsy • Muscular dystrophy	• Myelomeningocele • Tethered cord
Benign neoplasm	• Osteoid osteoma	• Osteoblastoma
Osteonecrosis	• Sickle cell disease	• Thalassemia
Overuse	• Stress fracture • Chondromalacia patellae • Osgood-Schlatter disease	• Sever disease • Jumper's knee • Osteochondritis dissecans
Trauma	• Soft tissue injury • Hemarthrosis	• Fracture
Developmental	• SCFE	• Legg-Calvé-Perthes

Abbreviations: DDH, developmental dysplasia of the hip; SCFE, slipped capital femoral epiphysis; SLE, systemic lupus erythematosus.

organomegaly, or areas of tenderness. Asymmetric skinfolds or limb length discrepancies should be noted. Compress the iliac wings toward each other to assess for sacroiliac joint disease. The following areas of muscle attachment to the pelvis should be palpated: the anterior superior iliac spine where the sartorius attaches, the anterior inferior iliac spine where the rectus femoris attaches, and the ischium where the hamstrings attach. Pain on resisted movement should be assessed for each of the muscles. Range of motion in each joint should be checked, with special attention paid to adjacent joints to rule out referred pain. The stance and swing phases of walking and running should be observed and any abnormal upper body posturing or frontal plane abnormalities noted. If the child is unable to walk but can crawl, he or she likely has pain in the lower leg. The physical examination should be completed with attention to the presence or absence of conjunctivitis, rash, muscle atrophy, or hypertrophy. In addition, the body habitus should be noted.

Laboratory evaluation is directed by the findings of the history and physical examination. If infection, inflammation, or malignant disease is suspected, obtain a C-reactive protein (CRP), erythrocyte sedimentation rate (ESR), and complete blood cell (CBC) count with differential. Blood cultures should be obtained in the evaluation of infection. If septic arthritis is suspected, joint fluid should be obtained for culture, Gram stain, and cell count. Other laboratory testing is listed in Table 9-3.

TABLE 9-3 Laboratory Evaluation of the Child With a Limp

Condition	Laboratory Test
Acute rheumatic fever	Throat culture, antistreptolysin-O titer, anti-deoxyribonuclease B titer
Gonococcal arthritis	Urethral, cervical, pharyngeal, and rectal cultures
Hemophilia	Coagulation profile, factor levels
Lyme disease	Lyme titer
Reactive arthritis	Urethral and stool cultures
Systemic lupus erythematosus	Antinuclear antibody, rheumatoid factor

Initial imaging studies include AP and lateral views of the area of concern. When imaging the hip, frog-leg radiograph can be performed in lieu of true lateral radiography unless there is a concern for an acute slipped capital femoral epiphysis (SCFE). In a child with an acute SCFE, the frog-leg positioning can cause worsening of the slip.[21] Children who have nonfocal examination results and cannot localize their pain should have the entire lower leg imaged. Children who have stress fractures, toddler's fractures, LCP disease, osteomyelitis, or septic arthritis can have initial radiographs that are normal. Advanced imaging might be necessary in a child with a concerning story but no symptoms detected on evaluation. Bone scintigraphy, magnetic resonance imaging (MRI), and computed tomography (CT) are all options for further imaging, although MRI has replaced bone scintigraphy in many cases because it does not expose the child to radiation and can give greater anatomical detail. Magnetic resonance imaging offers excellent visualization of joints, soft tissues, cartilage, and medullary bone, whereas CT scanning is useful in imaging cortical bone.[22] Ultrasonography of the hip can assess for the presence of hip effusions, but it cannot differentiate among sterile, purulent, or hemorrhagic fluid.[23,24] Ultrasonography is also useful in guiding hip joint aspiration.

CASE SCENARIO 3

A woman brings her 4-year-old daughter to the ED. For the past 3 weeks, the child has been intermittently limping and experiencing right leg pain. She has otherwise been well without fever, chills, or a preceding viral illness. She does not have a history of recent injury to her leg. She has never been hospitalized and is not taking any medications. On physical examination, the girl is in the 10th percentile for height and weight. Results of the physical examination are normal except for her right leg. Her legs are the same length, and she limps on the right leg. She has normal range of movement of her ankle and knee and has no bony tenderness. When you attempt to move her hip, she tenses up and whimpers. She has limited range of motion of the hip in all directions. There is no redness, swelling, or deformity of her right leg. Anteroposterior and frog-leg lateral radiographs of the pelvis show the right femoral head to be smaller than the left with a relatively widened joint space. Her CBC count and ESR are normal.

1. What is the diagnosis?
2. What is the treatment for this illness?
3. What is the prognosis?

Legg-Calvé-Perthes Disease

Legg-Calvé-Perthes (LCP) disease is a localized disorder of the hip characterized by ischemic necrosis of the femoral head, subsequent collapse, and fragmentation, followed by reossification. Although the disease was first described in the early 1900s, its causes and methods of treatment remain elusive and controversial.[25] The origin of LCP disease is thought to be a localized manifestation of a generalized disorder of the epiphyseal cartilage. This process is manifested in the femoral head because of its precarious blood supply. Vascular pathologic conditions also might be contributing to ischemic injury of the femoral head.[26]

Most cases of LCP disease occur between the ages of 4 and 9 years, although cases have been reported as early as 2 years or as late as 13 years.[27] The disease affects boys more often than girls and is found to be bilateral in 10% of cases.[25] A history of other family members with the disease has been found in approximately 10% of cases.[25] Low birth weight and growth delay have been associated with LCP disease, with some patients having a bone age that is between 1 and 3 years below chronological age.[25,27]

Clinical Features

Clinical symptoms in patients with LCP disease typically include pain and/or limp in the affected extremity; symptoms and limp tend to be worse at the end of the day. Similar to patients with slipped capital femoral epiphysis (SCFE), symptoms can be referred to the groin, thigh, or knee. Therefore, any child presenting with knee pain should have a thorough examination of the hip. A history of minor trauma frequently brings the chronic symptoms to medical attention but is not the cause of the disease. Gait disturbances can be due to pain, limb length discrepancy, or a limited range of motion at the hip. The examination should include gait, limb length measurement, and range of motion at the hip. Limited internal rotation and abduction at the hip joint is frequently found.

Diagnostic Studies

The diagnosis of LCP disease is confirmed with AP and frog-leg lateral pelvis radiographs.

Initially, the femoral head appears smaller and the articular cartilage space appears wider than the contralateral normal side. Within several months, a crescent-shaped radiolucent line can be seen on the lateral radiograph (crescent sign). This line is caused by subcortical collapse of the trabecular bone. Later, the femoral head develops a fragmented appearance and is less radiopaque (**Figure 9.6**). Reossification then takes place, but a residual deformity in the femoral epiphysis and acetabulum can persist. If standard radiographs are not conclusive, MRI and bone scintigraphy can be used to clarify the diagnosis.[28,29]

Differential Diagnosis

The differential diagnosis of LCP disease includes other entities that present with knee or hip pain in children, including septic arthritis, transient synovitis, fractures, malignancies, and SCFE. Although SCFE usually presents in older children, there is overlap of age presentations

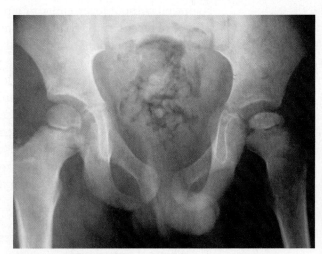

Figure 9.6 Anteroposterior radiograph of Legg-Calvé-Perthes disease.

between 10 and 13 years. Radiographs should easily distinguish these two entities. Other diagnoses can be eliminated by either history or radiographic evidence.

Management

Treatment of LCP disease is controversial.[25,30] Long-term studies of the natural history are rare, and multiple classification schemes exist, which makes it more difficult to compare treatment modalities. The disease process is self-limiting but can last for several years. The early goals of treatment are to alleviate pain and hip stiffness. The limp can persist for 2 to 4 years.[27] Non-steroidal anti-inflammatory medications and reduction of activities will help reduce pain. Occasionally, non–weight-bearing with crutches and/or braces will be necessary. A physical therapy program might improve range of motion and decrease stiffness. Long-term goals of therapy include reducing residual deformities of the femoral head and surrounding acetabulum. One approach to maintaining a spherical femoral head on reossification is femoral head containment, which requires positioning the proximal femur in abduction with braces or doing so during surgical procedures.[30] Prognosis depends primarily on age of healing, with better outcomes found in younger children, especially those whose diagnosis is made before the age of 5 years.[30] Long-term studies reveal a higher incidence of osteoarthritis and total hip replacement as patients approach their sixth and seventh decades of life.[25] These late-term complications might be dependent on the shape of the femoral head and acetabulum at the time of healing.

A mother brings her 12-year-old son to the ED after he collided with another boy while playing baseball. After the collision, which is described as minor, he started to experience left knee pain. He tells you he has been having mild, intermittent knee pain for the past 2 months but it is now worse and he cannot walk. He denies hip, ankle, or foot pain. No other injuries were sustained in the collision. On physical examination, he is in the 90th percentile for weight and 25th percentile for height. On examination, he is lying on the stretcher with his leg held in flexion with external rotation and abduction. The knee, ankle, and foot are normal. Any attempt to move his hip elicits extreme pain, and he has limited range of motion, especially with abduction and internal rotation.

1. *What is the diagnosis?*
2. *What should not have been done during the physical examination?*
3. *How do you diagnose this condition?*

Slipped Capital Femoral Epiphysis

Slipped capital femoral epiphysis (SCFE) occurs when the femoral head (epiphysis) slips posteriorly and inferiorly relative to the femoral neck (metaphysis). Although it is the most common orthopedic hip disorder in adolescence, SCFE is frequently misdiagnosed early in its course because of the variety of presenting symptoms. Delays in diagnosis can lead to a more difficult treatment course and a less favorable prognosis. Therefore, SCFE has to be considered whenever a patient presents with a limp; hip, thigh, or knee pain; or both.

Patients who have SCFE are classified as having a stable or unstable slip based on their ability to ambulate: those who can ambulate with or without crutches are classified as having stable SCFE, whereas patients with unstable SCFE are nonambulatory even with crutches.[31] The latter form is treated much more like an acute fracture of the femur across the growth plate and has a poorer prognosis due to an increased incidence of avascular necrosis of the femoral head. Most patients with SCFE are stable and therefore have a favorable prognosis.

The overall incidence of SCFE is 1 to 3 per 100,000, with a slightly higher incidence in black and Hispanic children.[32–34] Males are affected almost twice as often as females. In two-thirds of cases, children are found to be obese; it is thought that the increased weight during the early adolescent growth spurt years increases the stress across the physeal plate, which is already oriented vertically and posteriorly. The mean (SD) age for development of SCFE is 12 (1.5) years in girls and 13.5 (1.7) years in boys. There is bilateral involvement in approximately 20% of patients at presentation, and another 20% to 30% will develop involvement of the other hip within 18 months of presentation.[35] Although most cases are considered idiopathic, there are associations described with hypothyroidism, growth hormone deficiency, renal osteodystrophy, and radiation therapy. The incidence of renal and endocrine dysfunction is so low in patients with SCFE that routine testing is not recommended unless the clinical presentation is atypical or the patient presents with bilateral hip involvement.

Clinical Features

Patients with SCFE usually present with a history of intermittent limp of several weeks' duration with hip, thigh, or knee pain. Often a vague history of trauma or a fall brings attention to the limp and is the initial reason for the visit. In one study, 29% of patients had their conditions misdiagnosed at the initial visit, mostly because the main symptom was thigh pain instead of hip pain.[36] Diagnoses frequently given at the initial visit include Osgood-Schlatter disease, growing pain, thigh contusion, and muscle strain. Physical examination findings depend on the degree and chronicity of slippage. Patients with early symptoms can have an antalgic gait with discomfort in the groin, thigh, and knee. If chronic slippage has developed, discomfort of the hip is seen when the hip is rotated internally and externally. Range of motion at the hip might be decreased, particularly in abduction and internal rotation. With flexion there can be outward rotation of the hip to allow the femoral neck to clear the acetabulum. On gait evaluation, patients with stable SCFE usually have an asymmetrical outward foot progression angle. Patients with acute slippage will present with severe pain, similar to those with an acute fracture. Attempts to rotate or flex the hip are not advised because they can cause severe discomfort. The hip is typically held in a position of flexion, external rotation, and abduction. The acute slippage can disrupt circulation to the femoral head, especially the superior retinacular arteries, which supply blood flow to the outer two-thirds of the femoral head, thus increasing the risk for avascular necrosis of the femoral head.[37]

Diagnostic Studies

The diagnosis of SCFE can be confirmed with plain radiographs. Both AP and frog-leg or true lateral pelvic radiographs should be obtained (**Figure 9.7**). Early in the course, AP radiographs can appear normal because the early slippage is in the posterior direction and will be seen only on a lateral view. The first radiographic sign is physeal widening; an anteroposterior (AP) pelvic view should be obtained to compare the width of the physis between the right and left sides of the hip. In normal pelvic radiographs, the Klein line can be drawn along the anterior aspect of the neck of the femur at the base of the greater trochanter and should intersect the epiphysis (**Figure 9.8**). In patients with SCFE, an abnormal Klein line does not intersect the epiphysis as it should. With an unstable slip, radiographs show an abrupt displacement of the femoral head posterior, inferior, and medial relative to the femoral neck. These patients are in such severe pain that only one projection of the hip can be obtained, usually an AP view. In suspicious cases with normal radiographs, advanced imaging with CT, MRI, or bone scintigraphy should be obtained.[20,35]

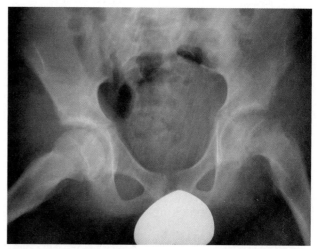

Figure 9.7 Frog-leg view of a left slipped capital femoral epiphysis.

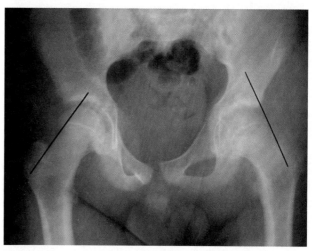

Figure 9.8 Anteroposterior radiograph of slipped capital femoral epiphysis revealing normal Klein line on the right hip, intersecting the edge of the epiphysis, and an abnormal Klein line on the left hip, missing the epiphysis.

> ## YOUR FIRST CLUE
>
> ### Signs and Symptoms of SCFE
> - Obese preadolescent or adolescent
> - Hip, thigh, groin, or knee pain
> - Limp
> - Decreased range of motion of the hip

Differential Diagnosis

The differential diagnosis includes other causes of hip and knee pain, including toxic synovitis, septic hip, LCP disease, Osgood-Schlatter disease, and other hip and knee conditions.

Management

Treatment is always surgical, so early orthopedic consultation is advised. Once their conditions are diagnosed, patients should be non–weight-bearing on the affected extremity to prevent further slippage. Initial ED management consists of bed rest, pain management, and relief of muscle spasms. Treatment of patients with stable SCFE consists of a single screw placed through the femoral neck into the epiphysis, thus eliminating the possibility of further slippage. The treatment of patients with unstable SCFE is more controversial in both the type of surgical procedure recommended and the timing of the procedure.[38]

The most common complications are avascular necrosis of the femoral head and chondrolysis. The risk of either process increases with the severity of the initial slippage.[38,39] Children with avascular necrosis can have a rapidly developing arthritis of the hip, ultimately requiring a hip replacement early in adulthood. Chondrolysis, a loss of articular cartilage, can occur in 5% to 7% of patients with SCFE and can lead to chronic pain and loss of normal hip motion. Barring the development of either complication, the child can resume running and contact sports after closure of the physis.

A woman brings her 5-year-old daughter to the ED. For the past day, the child has been limping and experiencing left leg pain. She has otherwise been well without fever. She had a mild upper respiratory tract infection 2 weeks ago. She does not have a history of recent injury to her leg. She has never been hospitalized and is not taking any medications. On physical examination, the girl has normal findings except for her left leg. Her legs are the same length, and she limps on the left leg. She has normal range of movement of her ankle and knee and has no bony tenderness. She has mild restriction of internal rotation of the left hip when compared with the right. There is no redness, swelling, or deformity of her left leg. Anteroposterior and frog-leg lateral radiographs of the pelvis are unremarkable. Her CBC count and ESR are normal.

1. *What is the diagnosis?*
2. *How is it diagnosed?*
3. *How long should her symptoms last?*

CASE SCENARIO 5

Transient Synovitis

Transient synovitis is the most common cause of hip pain in childhood.[40] It is a self-limited inflammatory condition caused by a nonpyogenic inflammatory response of the synovium. Its peak incidence is between 3 and 6 years of age. Transient synovitis of the hip is more common in boys and has a slight predilection for the right side. Less than 5% of cases are bilateral. Its onset is acute in approximately half of patients and more insidious in others, with symptoms occurring for weeks to months before medical evaluation.[41] It is most common in the hip, but can also affect the knee.

The etiology of transient synovitis is unknown. Current theories imply an association with active or recent infection, trauma, or allergic hypersensitivity. Transient synovitis of the hip can occur in up to 3% of children. Hip or groin pain is the most common initial finding, but referred pain to the medial aspect of the thigh or knee is found in 10% to 30% of patients. Affected patients either walk with a limp or, with severe pain, refuse to walk at all. The leg is held in flexion with slight abduction and external rotation. On examination, passive movement is usually pain free; however, there can be pain and a slightly decreased range of motion with extreme internal rotation or abduction. Although most children with transient synovitis tend to otherwise be well, some will have a low-grade fever and malaise.

The diagnosis of transient synovitis is one of exclusion and relies on the history and physical examination in combination with limited laboratory testing and AP and frog-leg lateral radiographs of the pelvis. Laboratory tests are used to help differentiate children with transient synovitis from those with septic arthritis. In transient synovitis, laboratory values might be normal or might reveal mild elevations in the white blood cell (WBC) count and ESR, both consistent with a nonspecific inflammatory process. One study found four predictors of septic arthritis: fever, inability to bear weight, ESR of 40 mm/h or greater, and a serum WBC greater than 12,000 cells/mm³. Patients with three of the four predictors had a 93% chance of having septic arthritis, and those who had all four had a 99% likelihood of pyarthrosis.[42] A subsequent study to validate these findings showed that patients with zero of the predictors had a 2% probability of septic arthritis, with one criterion the probability of septic arthritis was 9.5%, with two criteria it was 35%, with three criteria the probability was 73%, and in patients who had all four predictors the probability of septic arthritis was 93%.[43] However, when this algorithm was tested at another institution the presence of all four criteria predicted septic arthritis only 59% of the time.[44]

The overlap of laboratory values and historical features is too great to provide a foolproof diagnostic algorithm when differentiating transient synovitis and septic arthritis.

Although radiographs of the hip and pelvis tend to be normal in transient synovitis, they are helpful in excluding other diseases. Radiographic findings consistent with transient synovitis include medial joint space widening, an accentuated pericapsular shadow, and Waldenström sign, which is lateral displacement of the femoral epiphysis with surface flattening secondary to effusion. However, these findings are also apparent in LCP disease and, if present, mandate close follow-up or further investigation with MRI. If joint aspiration is necessary to clarify the diagnosis, ultrasonography can be used to guide hip joint aspiration. Effusions are present in 60% to 70% of cases of transient synovitis; however, they are also present in septic arthritis, osteomyelitis, acute SCFE, LCP disease, rheumatoid and infectious arthritis, malignant neoplasm, and osteoid osteoma. As such, the presence of an effusion on ultrasonography cannot be used to distinguish transient synovitis from other causes of hip pain.[45] Nuclear scintigraphy in patients with transient synovitis is helpful in differentiating transient synovitis from osteomyelitis (with or without septic arthritis), LCP disease, and SCFE. Scintigraphy can demonstrate asymmetry in uptake in the capital femoral epiphysis, with decreased uptake early in the disease and increased uptake later on. The early changes are also seen with very early LCP disease and suggest that some children with transient synovitis experience ischemia of the capital femoral epiphyses. This ischemia can be caused by an intracapsular effusion that tamponades vessels along the femoral neck. These ischemic findings have not yet been shown to have clinical significance.

Most cases of transient synovitis can be managed at home with close follow-up by the child's primary care physician. Generally, these children have a mild limp and, if treated with nonsteroidal anti-inflammatory drugs, often show improvement in symptoms. Patients with severe symptoms, fever, and an elevated ESR should be evaluated for septic arthritis. If there is any doubt about the diagnosis, immediate orthopedic consultation is necessary.

Treatment of transient synovitis includes rest and reduction of synovitis with anti-inflammatory medications. Rarely, bed rest is required. Temperatures should be monitored closely, and any fever should be reported to the physician. Children are allowed a gradual return to activity as the pain subsides, and full, unrestricted activity is permitted when the hip is completely pain free with no evidence of a limp. Although many children with transient synovitis have an effusion, aspiration of the joint is not routinely performed, and there is no strong evidence that aspiration shortens the clinical course or prevents osteonecrosis. Additional examination is recommended for all children within 12 to 24 hours and then again after 10 to 14 days if the symptoms have not resolved.

The prognosis for children with transient synovitis is excellent: approximately 75% of patients have complete resolution of pain within 2 weeks and 88% within 4 weeks. The remainder can have less intense but persistent pain for up to 8 weeks. It is recommended that children with persistent symptoms undergo ultrasonography to evaluate for the presence of an effusion: persistent joint effusion beyond 4 to 6 weeks is concerning for the subsequent development of LCP disease.[46] Relapse is infrequent and tends to occur within 6 months. In general, there are infrequent long-term sequelae of transient synovitis.

A woman brings her 2-year-old son to see you because he has a fever and has been crying. He had been well until yesterday, at which time he became cranky with frequent crying spells. Later that day he developed a fever, with a temperature of 39°C (102°F), which the mother treated with ibuprofen. His fever subsided but he continued to cry intermittently, especially during diaper changes. He has been lying around and seems to be favoring his left leg. He has no current cold symptoms, vomiting, diarrhea, or rash. He has not had any recent falls or injuries. Three weeks earlier, he had a cold that got better without any treatment. The child is healthy, has never been admitted to the hospital, and has never been seriously ill. He takes no medications and has no allergies.

As you start to examine the child, you notice that he is lying still on the bed and looks tired but not severely ill; he has no increased work of breathing, and his skin is flushed. His initial assessment findings are normal except for a heart rate of 140/min and a temperature of 39°C (102°F). On focused and detailed physical examination, you find no abnormalities in his head, eyes, ears, nose, throat, lung, abdomen, or heart. His cranial nerves are intact. Deep tendon reflexes are normal, but as you lift his left leg to check his left patellar reflex, he winces with pain. The results of the remainder of his neurologic examination are normal. On extremity examination, he has full range of motion of both upper extremities and his right lower extremity. His left foot, ankle, and knee are normal. On examination of the left hip, he cries with pain and pushes your hand away. He has limited range of motion of his left hip, especially with flexion, abduction, and external rotation. There is no redness, swelling, or warmth of the left hip.

After your examination, you discuss your concerns with the mother and order blood tests and radiographs. As you wait for results, you treat the child's pain and fever and call a consultant.

1. What is the diagnosis?
2. What tests were ordered and why?
3. Who did you consult and why?

Acute Septic Arthritis

Septic arthritis refers to microbial invasion and infection of the joint space. Bacterial pathogens are common in patients with acute septic arthritis, whereas fungal and mycobacterial pathogens tend to be associated with chronic septic arthritis. Acute septic arthritis occurs in all age groups but is more common in children. Approximately 70% of cases occur in children younger than 4 years, and the peak incidence is between 6 and 24 months of age. Boys are affected twice as frequently as girls. Predisposing factors include preceding viral infection, trauma, immunodeficiency, hemoglobinopathy, hemophilia with recurrent hemarthroses, diabetes, intravenous drug abuse, rheumatoid arthritis, and intra-articular injections or surgical procedures. Seventy-five percent of septic arthritis cases involve the joints of the lower extremity, with the knee being most commonly involved and the hip being the second most commonly involved. Other affected joints, in order of involvement, include the ankle, elbow, shoulder, and wrist. More than 90% of cases are monoarticular.

Hematogenic seeding, local spread, or traumatic or surgical infection can cause septic arthritis. In children, it most commonly results from hematogenic spread as bacteria pass into the synovial space through the highly vascular synovial membrane. The synovial membrane lacks a limiting basement membrane, which facilitates bacterial translocation. The bacteria then bind to bone and cartilage and initiate an inflammatory response that breaks down the joint by two mechanisms: directly through the effects of proteolytic enzymes and indirectly through pressure necrosis caused by accumulation of purulent synovial fluid.

The contiguous spread of infection from osteomyelitis to the joint space occurs in approximately 10% of cases and is more common in newborns and young infants. The most common bacterial causes of septic arthritis are listed in Table 9-4. In all age groups, *Staphylococcus aureus* is the most common cause of septic arthritis, and infection with community-acquired methicillin-resistant *S aureus* is becoming more common.[47] In addition to the organism listed in Table 9-4, additional causative organisms include *Neisseria gonorrhoeae* in neonates and sexually active adolescents, *Pseudomonas aeruginosa* and *Candida* species in intravenous drug abusers, *Salmonella* species in children with sickle cell disease, and gram-negative bacteria in immunosuppressed children. *Kingella kingae*, a fastidious gram-negative coccobacillus (previously classified as *Moraxella*) that colonizes the respiratory and oropharyngeal tract in children, has been implicated as a common cause of

YOUR FIRST CLUE

Signs and Symptoms of Septic Arthritis

- Irritability
- Fever
- Erythema
- Limp or refusal to walk
- Decreased range of motion of the affected limb
- Hip held in abduction and external rotation

TABLE 9-4 Septic Arthritis Pathogens and Treatment		
Age	Organism	Treatment
Birth to 2 months	Group B *Streptococcus* *Staphylococcus aureus* Gram-negative rods	Nafcillin, 50 mg/kg per dose, and gentamicin, 2.5 mg/kg per dose, or cefotaxime, 50 mg/kg per dose; add vancomycin, 10 mg/kg per dose, if MRSA is suspected or known
2 months to 3 years	*S aureus* *Haemophilus influenzae* *Streptococcus pneumoniae* *Kingella kingae*	Nafcillin, 50 mg/kg per dose, and ceftriaxone, 50 mg/kg per dose; add vancomycin, 10 mg/kg per dose, if MRSA is suspected or known
3 years to 12 years	*S aureus* *S pneumoniae* *S pyogenes*	Ampicillin/sulbactam, 50 mg/kg of ampicillin per dose, or cefuroxime, 50 mg/kg per dose; add vancomycin, 10 mg/kg per dose, if MRSA is suspected or known
>12 years	*S aureus* *S pneumoniae* *Neisseria gonorrhoeae*	Nafcillin, 50 mg/kg per dose, and ceftriaxone, 50 mg/kg per dose; add vancomycin, 10 mg/kg per dose, if MRSA is suspected or known

Abbreviation: MRSA, methicillin-resistant *Staphylococcus aureus*.

osteoarticular infections in young children. Culture- and *K kingae*–specific polymerase chain reaction was used to identify *K kingae* as the causative agent in 45% of osteoarticular infections.[48] Fortunately, *K kingae* is susceptible to a wide array of antibiotics that are usually given empirically to young children for septic arthritis.

Clinical Features

The clinical picture of septic arthritis varies with age. Infants tend to have fever, failure to feed, lethargy, pseudoparalysis of the extremity, and pain with diaper changes. Most older children have systemic symptoms of fever, malaise, poor appetite, and irritability, as well as localized symptoms of pain, with limp or refusal to walk. With septic arthritis, the onset of symptoms is more acute than seen with osteomyelitis. Physical examination reveals local erythema, warmth, and swelling. If the hip is affected, it is often held in flexion, abduction, and external rotation. Range of motion is decreased due to pain and muscle spasm, and passive joint movement is painful. In infants, joint dislocation might be observed.

Diagnostic Studies

Helpful initial laboratory studies for diagnosis of septic arthritis include a WBC count, ESR, CRP, and blood cultures. In patients with septic arthritis, the peripheral WBC count, ESR, and CRP are generally elevated, although occasionally CRP is normal, especially with *K kingae* infection.[49] A combination of history, physical examination, and laboratory test results will suggest the diagnosis and prompt an evaluation of synovial fluid. On the first day of illness,

a CRP might be more appropriate than an ESR: CRP levels increase early in infection, whereas the ESR is slower to rise. Physicians can order both CRP and ESR because they might be useful in tracking the course of the infection.

Blood cultures are positive in 20% to 50% of cases of septic arthritis.[50] Identification of the causative organism not only helps direct antibiotic treatment but also provides an organism for serum bactericidal testing when the child is switched to oral antibiotics.

Synovial fluid evaluation is the mainstay for diagnosing septic arthritis. If septic arthritis is suspected, joint aspiration should be performed without delay and the sample sent for Gram stain, aerobic and anaerobic cultures, cell count with differential, and glucose measurement. The synovial fluid of septic arthritis tends to be turbid or grossly purulent with a WBC count greater than 40,000 cells/mm³ and a predominance of polymorphonuclear cells. Synovial glucose can be low (synovial fluid/blood glucose ratio <0.5) and protein and lactate levels elevated (Table 9-5). Because of the intrinsic immunoglobulins in the synovial fluid, cultures of the fluid will be positive in only half of children with a clinical picture consistent with septic arthritis. Joint fluid should be inoculated directly into blood culture bottles to enhance identification of fastidious organisms

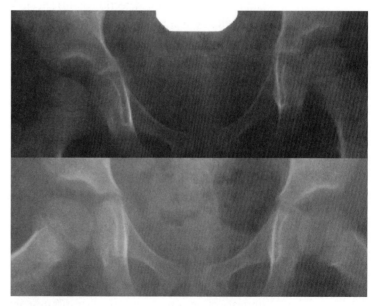

Figure 9.9 Septic arthritis of the hip with large joint effusion.

THE CLASSICS

Diagnostic Studies in Septic Arthritis

- WBC is elevated >15,000 cells/mm³ (50%)
- ESR is elevated >60 mm per hour (90% of cases)
- CRP >20 mg/L (94%)

TABLE 9-5 Synovial Fluid Findings in Different Types of Arthritis

	Character	WBC Count, cells/mm³	PMNs %	Mucin Clot	Other
Normal	Clear; yellow	<200	<10	Good	
Juvenile rheumatoid arthritis	Turbid	250–50,000	50–70	Fair to poor	50% with decreased complement
Reactive arthritis	Cloudy to turbid; can be clear	1,000–150,000	50–70	Fair to poor	Increased complement
Lyme arthritis	Turbid	500–100,000	>50	Poor	
Septic arthritis	Turbid; white-gray	10,000–250,000	>75	Poor	Low glucose and high lactate

Abbreviations: PMNs, polymorphonuclear cells; WBC, white blood cell.

such as *K kingae*.[49] Cultures might need to be incubated for a week or more.[51]

In septic arthritis, plain radiographs of the hip can be normal or, in the presence of a large joint effusion, can show periarticular soft tissue swelling, widening of the joint space, obliteration or displacement of the gluteal lines, and asymmetric fullness of the iliopsoas and obturator soft tissue planes (**Figure 9.9**). Late in the course of infection, subchondral bone erosions and narrowing of the joint space can be seen.

Ultrasonography is much more sensitive than plain radiography in the detection of hip effusion and provides direct visualization of the fluid and needle during joint aspiration. Scintigraphy can also be useful in diagnosing septic arthritis: during the "blood pool" or delayed images of the joint, symmetric uptake in the periarticular tissues on both sides of the joint is seen. Scintigraphy is diagnostic of septic arthritis earlier than other imaging techniques and is also a useful adjunct in identifying associated osteomyelitis or avascular necrosis of the femoral head. Both CT and MRI can confirm the presence of an effusion but do not differentiate septic from nonseptic arthritis.

Management

Septic arthritis requires immediate hospital admission, antibiotics, and surgical intervention. Surgical options range from needle aspiration to open surgical drainage; however, no random-

THE CLASSICS

Joint Effusions and Joint Space Widening in the Hip on Plain Radiographs

- Infants—measure from the inner border of the ramus to the top femur at the junction with the physis
- Children—measure from the teardrop on the pelvis to the femoral head; >2-mm difference between the sides with the hips in neutral position is abnormal

ized controlled trials exist that compare these two treatment approaches. Some authors recommend surgical drainage in all infants and young children with septic arthritis because needle aspiration has been shown to be inferior in this population.[52] Indications for surgical drainage in children with septic arthritis include involvement of the hip joint, the presence of large amounts of pus or debris in the joint, loculated fluid, recurrence of joint fluid after four or five aspirations, and lack of clinical improvement within 3 days of the initiation of appropriate therapy.[52–54] In joints other than the hip, the need for surgical drainage is determined on a case-by-case basis.

Empiric antibiotic therapy for septic arthritis is directed against the most likely organisms based on patient age and comorbidities (Table 9-4). Treatment can then be changed after culture results and sensitivities are known. To maximize culture results, antibiotics should not be given until a specimen of joint fluid is obtained. However, antibiotic therapy should not be delayed if arthrocentesis cannot be performed in a timely manner. Initial treatment is parenteral to ensure adequate serum concentrations of antibiotic. After the patient's clinical condition is stabilized, oral antibiotic therapy can be instituted. In general, doses two to three times those used for mild infections are sufficient. Response to therapy is measured with clinical improvement and acute phase reactants, including the ESR or CRP.

The mortality rate associated with septic arthritis has decreased to less than 1%, but the morbidity rate remains significant. Sequelae include leg length discrepancy, persistent pain, limited range of motion and ambulation, and aseptic necrosis of the femoral head. Predictors of poor outcome include infection of the hip and shoulder, adjacent osteomyelitis, a delay of 4 days or more before antibiotics and surgical intervention, and prolonged time to sterilization of synovial fluid.

KEY POINTS

Management of Septic Arthritis
- Admission
- Parenteral antibiotics
- Surgical intervention: aspiration and/or surgical drainage

A 12-year-old and her mother come to see you because the girl has been having right knee pain. It started about 1 month ago and has been getting worse. The pain is worse when she goes up or down stairs and when she plays soccer. It also hurts when she touches it. There is a small amount of swelling of the knee but no redness. She has not fallen on the knee and there are no other symptoms. On examination of the right knee, she has point tenderness at the tibial tubercle. There is full range of motion of the knee and on extension against resistance her pain is reproduced. Her ligaments are stable and there is no knee effusion.

1. What is the diagnosis?
2. Does she need a radiograph?
3. What is the treatment?

Osgood-Schlatter Disease

Osgood-Schlatter disease is generally a benign lesion of the tibial tubercle at the site of the patellar tendon insertion. It affects adolescents during growth spurts and is most commonly seen in boys 12 to 14 years old and in girls 10 to 11 years old.[55] Most cases are unilateral, but bilateral cases are not uncommon. Osgood-Schlatter disease occurs frequently in boys due to greater participation in sports. It is becoming more common in girls as they are increasingly involved in athletic activities. Common sports associated with Osgood-Schlatter disease include basketball, football, soccer, gymnastics, and ballet. During these activities, repetitive quadriceps stress contractions are applied to the patellar tendon at its insertion at the tibial tuberosity. This can result in a partial avulsion fracture through the ossification center, which subsequently leads to heterotopic bone formation at the tendon insertion site. Tibial tuberosity fuses with the tibial metaphysis at the age of 15 years in girls and 17 years in boys. The avulsed segment can fail to unite, leaving a small palpable mass.[55]

Clinical Features

Patients with Osgood-Schlatter disease present with a painful soft tissue swelling at the tibial tubercle. The area is very tender to palpation, and the pain can be reproduced by having the patient extend the knee against resistance or by squatting with the knee in full flexion. History usually reveals that running, going up and down stairs, and jumping cause increased pain.

YOUR FIRST CLUE

Signs and Symptoms of Osgood-Schlatter Disease

- History of repetitive running, jumping, or sports activity
- Swelling and pain over the tibial tubercle
- Pain over tibial tubercle with knee extension or squatting

KEY POINTS

Management of Osgood-Schlatter Disease

- Mild to moderate symptoms
  - Decrease activity; nonsteroidal anti-inflammatory agents
- Moderate to severe symptoms
  - Knee immobilizer or cylindrical cast
- Very severe cases
  - Surgical intervention (rare)

Diagnostic Studies

The diagnosis of Osgood-Schlatter disease is usually clinical. Radiographs are frequently obtained to rule out other conditions, including neoplasm, cysts, infections, stress fractures, and other musculoskeletal diseases involving the knee. Although a lateral knee radiograph might reveal a fracture through the tibial tubercle, frequently only soft tissue swelling is seen. Some patients who present with radiographic fragmentation of the tubercle will develop chronic symptoms. Those with no fragmentation are usually asymptomatic at long-term follow-up.[56]

Management

Treatment of patients with Osgood-Schlatter disease is almost always nonsurgical and depends on the extent of the presenting symptoms.[55] Patients with mild symptoms should be given nonsteroidal anti-inflammatory drugs and be advised to avoid activities that cause repeated quadriceps contraction. For many adolescents, the latter advice is frequently hard to follow. Symptoms usually improve in weeks to months. More advanced cases can be treated with a knee immobilizer (and, rarely, a cylindrical cast). Steroid injections are not indicated. Rarely, patients with unresolved lesions will require surgery directed at excision of all the intratendon ossicles and possible removal of the tibial tubercle.[57] In most patients, the condition is self-limiting and results in no long-term complications.

Summary

The approach to children with orthopedic symptoms should be based on age, history of symptoms, and physical findings. Causes of nontraumatic orthopedic conditions vary significantly with age, and a complete history and physical examination will be necessary to exclude systemic disease.

THE BOTTOM LINE

- Causes of nontraumatic orthopedic emergencies vary with patient age.
- Obtain a complete history to include character, location, quality, and time course of symptoms.
- Establish whether the condition is associated with an acute traumatic event or repetitive activity.
- Always examine the hips in any patient with knee pain.
- Radiographs might be needed to establish the diagnosis.
- Prompt orthopedic or primary care referral is necessary.

Check Your Knowledge

1. Which of the following statements regarding Legg-Calvé-Perthes (LCP) disease is correct?
   A. Can be bilateral
   B. Classically presents in toddlers
   C. Generally seen in large, obese children
   D. Has no findings on radiograph

2. Which of the following statements regarding slipped capital femoral epiphysis (SCFE) is correct?
   A. Most common in the early 20s
   B. Occurs when the femoral head slips anteriorly and superiorly relative to the femoral neck
   C. Often presents as knee pain
   D. Treated nonsurgically

3. Which of the following statements regarding transient synovitis is correct?
   A. Children tend to be well-appearing.
   B. Decision rules are reliable in diagnosing transient synovitis.
   C. The presence of an effusion on ultrasonography is diagnostic of transient synovitis.
   D. Most children are still symptomatic 8 weeks after presentation.

4. Which of the following statements regarding septic arthritis is correct?
   A. Always yields bacterial growth from the synovial fluid
   B. Most common in teenagers
   C. Most commonly caused by *Neisseria meningitidis*
   D. Treated with joint drainage and intravenous antibiotics

5. Which of the following statements regarding children with Osgood-Schlatter disease is correct?
   A. All have knee effusions
   B. Have increased pain when they squat with the knee in full flexion
   C. Require surgery for a cure
   D. Usually play a lot of video games

References

1. Marks DS, Clegg J, al-Chalabi AN. Routine ultrasound screening for neonatal hip instability: Can it abolish late-presenting congenital dislocation of the hip? *J Bone Joint Surg Br.* 1994;76:534–538.
2. Novacheck TF. Developmental dysplasia of the hip. *Pediatr Clin North Am.* 1996;43:829–848.
3. Donaldson JS, Feinstein KA. Imaging of developmental dysplasia of the hip. *Pediatr Clin North Am.* 1997;44:591–614.
4. Barlow TC. Early diagnosis and treatment of congenital dislocation of the hip. *J Bone Joint Surg Br.* 1962;44:292.
5. Boal DK, Schwenkter EP. The infant hip: Assessment with real-time ultrasound. *Radiology.* 1985;157:667–672.
6. Tionnis D, Storch K, Ulbrich H. Results of newborn screening for congenital dislocation of the hip with and without sonography and correlation of risk factors. *J Pediatr Orthop.* 1990;10:145–152.
7. Gull F, Muller D. Results of hip ultrasonographic screening in Austria. *Orthopade.* 1997;26:25–32.
8. French LM, Dietz FR. Screening for developmental dysplasia of the hip. *Am Fam Physician.* 1999;60:177–184.
9. Choung W, Heinrich SD. Acute annular ligament interposition into the radiocapitellar joint in children (nursemaid's elbow). *J Pediatr Orthop.* 1995;15:454–456.
10. Schunk JE. Radial head subluxation: Epidemiology and treatment of 87 episodes. *Ann Emerg Med.* 1990;19:1019–1023.
11. Quan L, Marcuse EK. The epidemiology and treatment of radial head subluxation. *Am J Dis Child.* 1985;139:1194–1197.
12. Newman J. "Nursemaid's elbow" in infants six months and under. *J Emerg Med.* 1985;2:403–404.
13. Foster DL. Bilateral nursemaid's elbow. *Pediatr Emerg Care.* 1991;7:128.
14. Frumkin K. Nursemaid's elbow: A radiographic demonstration. *Ann Emerg Med.* 1985;14:690–693.
15. Sacchetti A, Ramoska EE, Glascow C. Nonclassic history in children with radial head subluxations. *J Emerg Med.* 1990;8:151–153.
16. Macias CG, Bothner J, Wiebe R. A comparison of supination/flexion to hyperpronation in the reduction of radial head subluxations. *Pediatrics.* 1998;102:e10.
17. McDonald J, Whitelaw C, Goldsmith LJ. Radial head subluxation: Comparing two methods of reduction. *Acad Emerg Med.* 1999;6:715–718.

18. Jones J, Cote B. "Irreducible" nursemaid's elbow. *Am J Emerg Med.* 1995;13:491.

19. Widhe B, Widhe T. Initial symptoms and clinical features in osteosarcoma and Ewing sarcoma. *J Bone Joint Surg Am.* 2000;82:667–674.

20. Laine JC, Kaiser SP, Diab M. High risk pediatric orthopedic pitfalls. *Emerg Clin N Am.* 2010;28:85–102.

21. Loder RT. Controversies in slipped capital femoral epiphysis. *Orthop Clin North Am.* 2006;37:211–221.

22. Flynn JM, Widmann RF. The limping child: Evaluation and diagnosis. *J Am Acad Orthop Surg.* 2001;9:89–98.

23. Navarro OM, Parra DA. Pediatric musculoskeletal ultrasound. *Ultrasound Clin.* 2009;4:457–470.

24. Vieira RL, Levy JA. Bedside ultrasound to identify hip effusions in pediatric patients. *Ann Emerg Med.* 2010;55:284–289.

25. Wenger DR, Ward WT, Herring JA. Legg-Calvé-Perthes disease. *J Bone Joint Surg Am.* 1991;73:778–788.

26. Yasmin DH, Montgomery SM, Ekbom A, Nilsson OS, Behmanyar S. Legg-Calvé-Perthes disease and risks for cardiovascular diseases and blood diseases. *Pediatrics.* 2010;125:e1308–e1315.

27. Weinstein SL. Natural history and treatment outcomes of childhood hip disorders. *Clin Orthop.* 1997;344:227–242.

28. Lahdes-Vasama T, Lamminen A, Merikanto J, Marttinen E. The value of MRI in early Perthes disease: An MRI study with 2-year follow-up. *Pediatr Radiol.* 1997;27:517–522.

29. Lamer S, Dorgeret S, Khairouni A, et al. Femoral head vascularisation in Legg-Calvé-Perthes disease: Comparison of dynamic gadolinium-enhanced subtraction MRI with bone scintigraphy. *Pediatr Radiol.* 2002;32:580–585.

30. Herring JA. The treatment of Legg-Calvé-Perthes disease: A critical review of the literature. *J Bone Joint Surg Am.* 1994;76:448–458.

31. Loder R, Richards B, Shapiro P, Reznick LR, Aronson DD. Acute slipped capital femoral epiphysis: The importance of physeal stability. *J Bone Joint Surg Am.* 1993;75:1134–1140.

32. Lehmann CL, Arons RR, Loder RT, Vitale MG. The epidemiology of slipped capital femoral epiphysis: An update. *J Pediatr Orthop.* 2006;26:286–290.

33. Swiontkowski MF, Gill EA. Slipped capital femoral epiphysis. *Am Fam Physician.* 1986;33:167–171.

34. Loder RT. Slipped capital femoral epiphysis. *Am Fam Physician.* 1998;57:2135–2142.

35. Frick SL. Evaluation of the child who has hip pain. *Orthop Clin N Am.* 2006;37:133–140.

36. Ledwith CA, Fleisher GR. Slipped capital femoral epiphysis without hip pain leads to missed diagnosis. *Pediatrics.* 1992;89:660–662.

37. Maeda S, Kita A, Funayama K, Kokubun S. Vascular supply to slipped capital femoral epiphysis. *J Pediatr Orthop.* 2001;21:664–667.

38. Loder RT. Unstable slipped capital femoral epiphysis. *J Pediatr Orthop.* 2001;21:694–699.

39. Rattey T, Piehl F, Wright JG. Acute slipped capital femoral epiphysis: Review of outcomes and rates of avascular necrosis. *J Bone Joint Surg Am.* 1996;78:398–402.

40. MacEwen GD, Dehse R. The limping child. *Pediatr Rev.* 1991;12:268.

41. Haueisen DC, Weiner DS, Weiner SD. The characterization of "transient synovitis of the hip" in children. *J Pediatr Orthop.* 1986;6:11–17.

42. Kocher M, Zurakowski D, Kasser J. Differentiating between septic arthritis and transient synovitis of the hip in children: An evidence-based clinical prediction algorithm. *J Bone Joint Surg Am.* 1999;81:1662–1670.

43. Kocher M, Mandiga R, Zurakowski D, Barnewolt C, Kasser JR. Validation of a clinical prediction rule for differentiation between septic arthritis and transient synovitis of the hip in children. *J Bone Joint Surg Am.* 2004;86:1629–1635.

44. Luhmann SJ, Jones A, Schootman M, Gordon JE, Schoenecker PL, Luhmann JD. Differentiation between septic arthritis and transient synovitis of the hip in children with clinical prediction algorithms. *J Bone Joint Surg Am.* 2004;86:956–962.

45. Zamzam MM. The role of ultrasound in differentiating septic arthritis from transient synovitis of the hip in children. *J Pediatr Orthop B.* 2006;15:418–422.

46. Eggl H. Ultrasonography in the diagnosis of transient synovitis of the hip and Legg-Calvé-Perthes disease. *J Pediatr Orthop B.* 1999;8:177–180.

47. Arnold SR, Elias D, Buckingham SC, et al. Changing patterns of acute hematogenous osteomyelitis and septic arthritis. *J Pediatr Orthop.* 2006;26:703–708.

48. Chometon S, Benito Y, Chaker M, et al. Specific real-time polymerase chain reaction places Kingella kingae as the most common cause of osteoarticular infections in young children. *Pediatr Infect Dis J.* 2007;25:377–381.

49. Gutierrez K. Bone and joint infections in children. *Pediatr Clin N Am.* 2005;52:779–794.

50. Kallio MJ, Unkila-Kallio L, Aalto K, Peltola H. Serum C-reactive protein, erythrocyte sedimentation rate and white blood cell count in septic arthritis of children. *Pediatr Infect Dis J.* 1997;16:411–413.

51. Osteomyelitis/septic arthritis caused by Kingella kingae among day care attendees—Minnesota, 2003. *MMWR Morb Mortal Wkly Rep.* 2004;53:241–243.

52. Dunkle LM. Toward optimum management of serious focal infections: The model of suppurative arthritis. *Pediatr Infect Dis J.* 1989;8:195–196.

53. Green NE, Edward K. Bone and joint infections in children. *Orthop Clin North Am.* 1987;18:555–576.

54. Nade S. Acute septic arthritis in infancy and childhood. *J Bone Joint Surg Am.* 1983;65:234–241.

55. Dunn JF. Osgood-Schlatter Disease. *Am Fam Physician.* 1990;41:173–176.

56. Krause BL, Williams, JP, Catterall A, Chir M. Natural history of Osgood-Schlatter disease. *J Pediatr Orthop.* 1990;10:65–68.

57. Binazzi R, Felli L, Vaccari V, Borelli P. Surgical treatment of unresolved Osgood-Schlatter lesion. *Clin Orthop.* 1993;289:202–204.

CASE SUMMARY 1

During your evaluation of a 5-week-old girl, you feel a clunk as you do the Ortolani maneuver on the left hip. You also note asymmetric skinfolds and decreased abduction. The results of the rest of the examination, including the right hip, are normal, and the child is in no distress. On questioning, the mother tells you that her daughter was born on time after an uncomplicated antenatal course. Specifically, the mother did not have multiple gestations or oligohydramnios, and the infant was born head first. The infant is breastfeeding well and gaining weight. The mother has had no problems with diaper changes, and her daughter does not appear to be in pain. After discussing your findings with the mother, you arrange for further testing and contact a specialist.

1. *What is the diagnosis?*
2. *How do you proceed in your evaluation?*
3. *What is the most likely course of treatment for this child?*

In this case, the infant showed signs of developmental dysplasia of the hip (DDH): asymmetry of skinfolds and asymmetrical range of motion of the hip. Because she was only 5 weeks old, routine radiographs might not be helpful and you obtain immediate ultrasonography of both hips. On ultrasonography, she was found to have a normal right hip with DDH of the left hip. The infant was seen by an orthopedic surgeon within 2 days and placed in a Pavlik harness. The orthopedic surgeon instructed the parents in the use and care of the harness, as well as how to change diapers and handle the infant without disrupting the alignment of the hip. The orthopedist is confident that this infant's hip will respond to this therapy and will continue to follow her closely for the next several months.

CASE SUMMARY 2

A father brings his 2-year-old daughter to the emergency department (ED) because she will not move her left arm. Earlier that day, as she was walking with her mother, she tripped and her mother grabbed her arm to prevent her from falling. Since that time she has not moved her arm and cries if anyone touches it. The father thinks she has hurt her wrist. The girl is otherwise healthy without any medical problems or allergies. She is not taking any medications. Excluding the left arm, results of the physical examination are normal. The child is holding her left arm at her side in mild flexion with the forearm pronated. Her wrist, elbow, and shoulder are nontender. She has no tenderness of any of her bones in her left upper extremity.

1. *What is the diagnosis?*
2. *How do you treat it?*
3. *What is the prognosis?*

The girl has radial head subluxation of her left arm. You explain the injury to the father and the girl. After explaining the hyperpronation reduction technique, you proceed with the maneuver and feel a clunk under your thumb. Within 5 minutes the girl is playing and using her left arm normally. The father is told that this is a common problem in young children and it might recur but should not cause any long-term problems. You also instruct him to avoid maneuvers that put traction on the arm to minimize the risk of recurrence.

A woman brings her 4-year-old daughter to the ED. For the past 3 weeks, the child has been intermittently limping and experiencing right leg pain. She has otherwise been well without fever, chills, or a preceding viral illness. She does not have a history of recent injury to her leg. She has never been hospitalized and is not taking any medications. On physical examination, the girl is in the 10th percentile for height and weight. She has normal physical examination results except for her right leg. Her legs are the same length, and she limps on the right leg. She has normal range of movement of her ankle and knee and has no bony tenderness. When you attempt to move her hip, she tenses up and whimpers. She has limited range of motion of the hip in all directions. There is no redness, swelling, or deformity of her right leg. Anteroposterior and frog-leg lateral radiographs of the pelvis show the right femoral head to be smaller than the left with a relatively widened joint space. Her CBC count and ESR are normal.

1. *What is the diagnosis?*
2. *What is the treatment for this illness?*
3. *What is the prognosis?*

The girl has LCP disease. The mother is informed that LCP is a progressive disease with a variable prognosis. The girl is under 5 years of age, so her prognosis is better than if she had presented later in childhood. You also let the mother know that treatment modalities are quite variable. She needs to see an orthopedic surgeon who will consider her age and degree of femoral head deformity and formulate a treatment plan. The girl is sent home with an appointment to see an orthopedist in 3 days.

A mother brings her 12-year-old son to the ED after he collided with another boy while playing baseball. Following the collision, which is described as minor, he started to experience left knee pain. He tells you he has been having mild, intermittent knee pain for the past 2 months but it is now worse and he cannot walk. He denies hip, ankle, or foot pain. No other injuries were sustained in the collision. On physical examination, he is in the 90th percentile for weight and 25th percentile for height. On examination, he is lying on the stretcher with his leg held in flexion with external rotation and abduction. The knee, ankle, and foot are normal. Any attempt to move his hip elicits extreme pain and he has very limited range of motion, especially with abduction and internal rotation.

1. *What is the diagnosis?*
2. *What should not have been done during the physical examination?*
3. *How do you diagnose this condition?*

The boy has (acute or chronic) unstable SCFE. Because of the instability of the hip, manipulation during initial evaluation should be minimized. He had AP and frog-leg pelvic radiographs done that showed the slippage, and an orthopedic surgeon was consulted. He is admitted to the hospital for pain control and complete bed rest, and is scheduled for surgical stabilization.

A woman brings her 5-year-old daughter to the ED. For the past day, the child has been limping and experiencing left leg pain. She has otherwise been well without fever. She had a mild upper respiratory tract infection 2 weeks ago. She does not have a history of recent injury to her leg. She has never been hospitalized and is not taking any medications. On physical examination, the girl has normal findings except for her left leg. Her legs are the same length, and she limps on the left leg. She has normal range of movement of her ankle and knee and has no bony tenderness. She has mild restriction of internal rotation of the left hip when compared with the right. There is no redness, swelling, or deformity of her left leg. Anteroposterior and frog-leg lateral radiographs of the pelvis are unremarkable. Her CBC count and ESR are normal.

1. *What is the diagnosis?*
2. *How is it diagnosed?*
3. *How long should her symptoms last?*

The girl's WBC count, CRP level, and ESR are normal. The radiograph of her left hip shows no widening of the joint space with no bony abnormality. These findings in a child with her clinical picture are highly suggestive of transient synovitis of the hip. She was treated with nonsteroidal anti-inflammatory medications and followed up with her primary care physician. Her symptoms improved and were completely resolved within 3 weeks.

A woman brings her 2-year-old son to see you because he has a fever and has been crying. He had been well until yesterday, at which time he became cranky with frequent crying spells. Later that day he developed a fever, with a temperature of 39°C (102°F), which the mother treated with ibuprofen. His fever subsided, but he continued to cry intermittently, especially during diaper changes. He has been lying around and seems to be favoring his left leg. He has no current cold symptoms, vomiting, diarrhea, or rash. He has not had any recent falls or injuries. Three weeks earlier, he had a cold that got better without any treatment. The child is healthy, has never been admitted to the hospital, and has never been seriously ill. He takes no medications and has no allergies.

As you start to examine the child, you notice that he is lying still on the bed and looks tired but not severely ill; he has no increased work of breathing, and his skin is flushed. His initial assessment findings are normal except for a heart rate of 140/min and a temperature of 39°C (102°F). On focused and detailed physical examination, you find no abnormalities on his head, eyes, ears, nose, throat, lung, abdomen, or heart. His cranial nerves are intact. Deep tendon reflexes are normal, but as you lift his left leg to check his left patellar reflex, he winces with pain. The results of the remainder of his neurologic examination are normal. On extremity examination, he has full range of motion of both upper extremities and his right lower extremity. His left foot, ankle, and knee are normal. On examination of the left hip, he cries with pain and pushes your hand away. He has limited range of motion of his left hip, especially with flexion, abduction, and external rotation. There is no redness, swelling, or warmth of the left hip.

After your examination, you discuss your concerns with the mother and order blood tests and radiographs. As you wait for results, you treat the child's pain and fever and call a consultant.

1. *What is the diagnosis?*
2. *What tests were ordered and why?*
3. *Who did you consult and why?*

The boy's WBC count is elevated with a left shift, and his CRP level is 19. The radiograph of his left hip shows slight widening of the joint space with no bony abnormality. These findings in a child with his clinical picture are highly suggestive of septic arthritis of the hip. The consultant, an orthopedic surgeon, agrees with the clinical assessment and takes the boy to the operating room to tap his hip. The boy's synovial fluid is purulent and has a WBC count of 90,000 cells/mm³, with a preponderance of polymorphonuclear cells. On Gram stain, the synovial fluid shows WBCs and gram-positive cocci in clusters. Intravenous antibiotic therapy was started intraoperatively. His hip was surgically drained and intravenous antibiotic therapy was continued until he became afebrile and his hip pain resolved. He was then switched to oral antibiotics and discharged home. He continues to take oral antibiotics and has remained afebrile and pain free.

A 12-year-old and her mother come to see you because the girl has been having right knee pain. It started about 1 month ago and has been getting worse. The pain is worse when she goes up or down stairs and when she plays soccer. It also hurts when she touches it. There is a small amount of swelling of the knee but no redness. She has not fallen on the knee and there are no other symptoms. On examination of the right knee, she has point tenderness at the tibial tubercle. There is full range of motion of the knee and on extension against resistance her pain is reproduced. Her ligaments are stable, and there is no knee effusion.

1. *What is the diagnosis?*
2. *Does she need a radiograph?*
3. *What is the treatment?*

The girl has Osgood-Schlatter disease. It was exacerbated with daily playing during soccer season. She does not need a radiograph for this diagnosis. She was treated with nonsteroidal anti-inflammatory medications and rest (avoidance of activities causing repeated quadriceps contraction), and her symptoms resolved completely. She is advised that her symptoms might recur until her tibial tuberosity fuses at approximately 15 years of age.

chapter 10

Medical Emergencies

Jeffrey R. Avner, MD, FAAP

Ghazala Q. Sharieff, MD, FACEP, FAAEM

Objectives

1 Discuss the evaluation of an infant or child with suspected sepsis.

2 Formulate the diagnostic evaluation of a very young infant with a fever.

3 Formulate the diagnostic evaluation of an immunocompromised child with a fever.

4 Describe emergencies encountered with children with sickle cell disease.

5 Identify rashes that indicate serious illnesses.

6 Recognize signs and symptoms of genitourinary emergencies in male patients.

7 Plan management of hypertensive urgencies and emergencies.

8 Classify causes of syncope.

Chapter Outline

Introduction
Sepsis
Fever in Very Young Infants
Fever in Children
Sickle Cell Disease
Dermatologic Emergencies
Epididymitis
Balanitis/Balanoposthitis
Urinary Tract Infections—Cystitis and Pyelonephritis
Hypertension
Acute Glomerulonephritis
Nephrotic Syndrome
Syncope

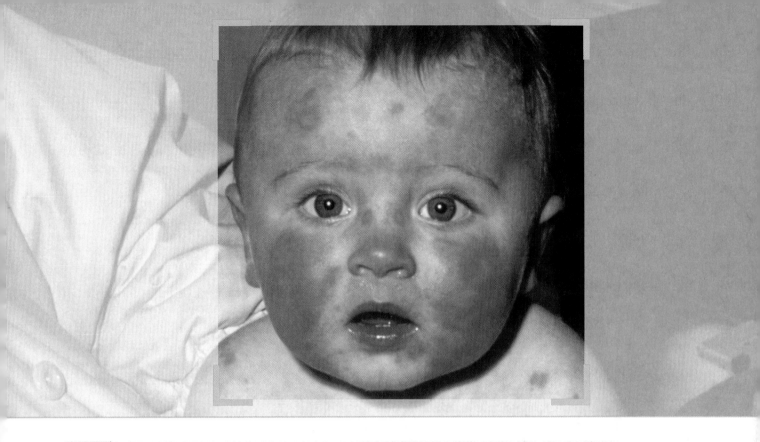

A previously healthy 15-month-old boy is brought to the emergency department with a 1-day history of fever and "not acting like himself." He was well until 3 days ago when he had symptoms of an upper respiratory tract infection. Yesterday he developed a low-grade fever that his mother treated with ibuprofen. Today he has continued fever and decreased oral intake, urine output, and activity level. He has no history of vomiting, diarrhea, cough, or rash. He is not taking any prescription medication.

On physical examination he appears tired and cranky when stimulated. His breathing is not labored, and he is pink. His respirations are 40/min, pulse is 162/min, blood pressure is 92/70 mm Hg, and temperature is 38.9°C (102°F). He has dry lips but moist mucous membranes without oral lesions. His neck is supple. The results of an examination of lungs, heart, abdomen, and extremities are unremarkable. There are a few scattered petechiae on his abdomen and lower extremities. His peripheral pulses are normal, and capillary refill time is 3 seconds.

1. *What is your general impression of this child?*
2. *What are the most likely diagnoses?*
3. *What would be your initial management strategy?*

Introduction

Most patients who present with medical emergencies have recognizable presenting signs and symptoms, allowing the physician to formulate an appropriate management plan. At the same time, the physician must be aware of those conditions that can be life threatening so that immediate care and treatment are not delayed. This chapter addresses both common and life-threatening medical emergencies.

Sepsis

The body's host defense system responds to an infectious agent with a complex cascade of cytokines and other proinflammatory mediators. This inflammatory response is mediated through the cellular and humoral immune systems, as well as the reticuloendothelial system. In certain situations, regulation limiting the extent of the inflammation is lost, leading to a massive systemic reaction that results in damage ranging from tissue and capillary injury to organ dysfunction. The term sepsis is often used to refer to a process of systemic inflammation accompanied by systemic signs, such as alteration in body temperature, tachypnea and tachycardia, leukocytosis, or leukopenia. It is also helpful to categorize sepsis into more specific clinical categories: bacteremia, systemic inflammatory response syndrome, sepsis (systemic inflammatory response syndrome response to documented infection), and septic shock (sepsis plus cardiovascular organ dysfunction).[1] Sepsis-like syndromes can also be caused by trauma, burns, neoplasms, and other conditions.

Clinical Features

The pathophysiology of bacteremia and sepsis is essentially a battle between the infecting organism and the host defense. The organism tries to multiply and invade various organ systems, whereas the host tries to contain and then eliminate the organism. If the host wins, there is complete resolution; if the organism wins, there is focal infection. The effects of this battle are the signs of inflammation, which produce characteristic clinical manifestations. Fever is usually apparent, especially early in the course of bacteremia. Hypothermia, although less common, portends a worse prognosis. As the severity of sepsis increases, so do the clinical features. Initially, there is tachycardia and an increase in cardiac output to preserve systemic blood pressure and organ perfusion. As a result of end organ vascular and tissue injury, the body generates lactic acid. Tachypnea results from increased oxygen demands and a response to metabolic acidosis. Hypoxemia can affect other organ systems, including the central nervous system (eg,

confusion, lethargy, and irritability) and the kidneys (eg, decreased urinary output). Increased capillary leak and vascular permeability cause volume depletion, increased systemic vascular resistance, and the clinical signs of decreased peripheral perfusion (ie, cold shock). On the other hand, vasodilation and warm extremities, despite the presence of inadequate organ perfusion, characterize the warm shock of sepsis.

Diagnostic Studies

The peripheral white blood cell (WBC) count in children with sepsis typically shows a leukocytosis with a left shift of the differential and increased band forms. When sepsis is overwhelming, the WBC count can be low, with or without neutropenia. Hypoglycemia is common, especially in young infants, due to limited glycogen stores but conversely can be elevated due to stress.[2] The serum bicarbonate level is usually low, consistent with metabolic acidosis that results from cellular demand exceeding the supply of necessary substrates. As tissue hypoperfusion worsens, the serum lactate level might rise, causing an elevated anion gap acidosis. Depending on the degree of metabolic acidosis and the child's respiratory reserve, a partial respiratory compensation

YOUR FIRST CLUE

Signs and Symptoms of Sepsis
- Fever
- Headache
- Fatigue
- Myalgias
- Leg pains
- Cool extremities
- Abnormal skin color (pallor or mottling)
- Arthralgias
- Lethargy, irritability, or confusion
- Rigors
- Tachypnea
- Tachycardia
- Skin signs of shock
- Petechiae/purpura

can occur. Thus, arterial blood gas analysis can demonstrate a low pH (<7.25), a base deficit, and evidence of respiratory compensation. In severe sepsis, excessive work of breathing and/or respiratory failure can exacerbate metabolic acidosis. The serum albumin, total protein, and total calcium levels might be low in sepsis; therefore, it is important to measure the ionized calcium for an accurate determination. Disseminated intravascular coagulation can cause abnormalities in coagulation studies and thrombocytopenia. Selective cultures of the blood, urine, cerebrospinal fluid (CSF), and/or stool are necessary for determining a bacterial origin. Administration of antibiotics and other supportive therapy must not be delayed for laboratory testing.

Infants who appear ill and those with respiratory findings should undergo chest radiography to evaluate for the presence of pneumonia or pulmonary edema. Abnormal heart size on a chest radiograph might suggest hypovolemia (small heart), cardiac failure (large heart), or congenital heart disease in younger infants. An electrocardiogram (ECG) is necessary if cardiac disease or dysfunction is suspected. An abdominal radiograph might show evidence of intestinal perforation (free air), small bowel obstruction (dilated small bowel loops with air-fluid levels), or intussusception (paucity of air in the right lower quadrant).

Differential Diagnosis

Many infectious and noninfectious processes can present as sepsis or sepsislike conditions. Infection is the most common cause of sepsis in children. Common bacterial causes are listed in Table 10-1.[2]

Infants with congenital cardiac lesions, especially those with left-sided outflow tract obstruction (eg, coarctation of the aorta or hypoplastic left heart syndrome), present with tachycardia, tachypnea, poor peripheral perfusion, and cold, mottled extremities and might be difficult to differentiate from infants with neonatal sepsis.[3] Depending on the type of congenital heart lesion and the duration of illness, a heart murmur or signs of congestive heart failure (eg, hepatomegaly or rales) might or might not be present. Diagnosis is supported by cardiomegaly or findings characteristic of a heart defect on chest radiograph and ECG and then is usually confirmed by echocardiography.[3] Supraventricular tachycardia is a common dysrhythmia in pediatric patients. Supraventricular tachycardia can be well tolerated in infants for 24 to 48 hours; however, prolonged tachycardia will produce signs and symptoms of heart failure. Similarly, patients with myocarditis present with ill appearance and congestive heart failure, often in the presence of fever.

TABLE 10-1 Common Bacterial Causes of Sepsis and Empiric Therapy		
Patient Group	Pathogen	Empiric Therapy
Infants <4–6 weeks	Group B *Streptococcus* Gram-negative bacilli	Ampicillin and cefotaxime OR ampicillin and gentamicin
Infants >4–6 weeks	Pneumococcus Meningococcus	Cefotaxime or ceftriaxone; add vancomycin if patient is toxic and/or if a gram-positive organism is suspected
Children	Pneumococcus Meningococcus *Staphylococcus aureus*	Cefotaxime or ceftriaxone; add vancomycin if patient is toxic and/or resistant gram-positive organism is suspected or if high staphylococcal or pneumococcal resistance
	Group A *Streptococcus*	Penicillin and clindamycin
For neutropenic patients with potential *Pseudomonas* infection, add ceftazidime or cefepime.		

Schexnayder SM. Pediatric septic shock. *Pediatr Rev.* 1999;20:303–308.[2]

Infections of the gastrointestinal (GI) tract can lead to an intra-abdominal abscess with peritonitis, bowel ischemia, or perforation of the intestinal wall. Necrotizing enterocolitis usually presents with the sudden onset of bilious vomiting, abdominal distention, lethargy, and lower GI tract bleeding. Although most common in premature infants, necrotizing enterocolitis can occasionally occur in stressed, full-term infants. Diagnosis is confirmed by the presence of pneumatosis intestinalis on abdominal radiograph, but this finding is variable. Presenting signs and symptoms of volvulus or malrotation of the GI tract include abdominal pain, distention, bilious vomiting, and possibly melena. Children with intussusception classically present with intermittent, severe, colicky abdominal pain and vomiting. As the intussusception progresses, lethargy or paradoxical irritability develops. As the bowel becomes ischemic, the initially guaiac-positive stool is mixed with blood and mucus, producing the "currant jelly" finding that occurs late in intussusception.

Congenital adrenal hyperplasia, usually caused by deficiency of the enzyme 21-hydroxylase, has abrupt symptom onset in the first couple of weeks of life with vomiting, diarrhea, lethargy, and shock. Female patients might have virilization of the external genitalia; male patients might have hyperpigmentation of the nipples and scrotum but often have no physical findings. The presence of hyponatremia, hyperkalemia, and metabolic acidosis is a vital clue suggestive of this disorder.

Many inborn errors of metabolism can present as sepsislike syndrome. After a minor stress such as a viral illness, the child becomes tachycardic, tachypneic, acidotic, and frequently hypoglycemic. Treatment is aimed at fluid resuscitation and reduction of catabolism by administration of intravenous fluids and glucose.

Management

Management of suspected sepsis begins with rapid assessment of the airway, breathing, and circulation (ABCs). High-flow oxygen should be given and intravenous or intraosseous access obtained. Aggressive cardiovascular support is critical and begins with intravenous administration of isotonic fluids (normal saline or lactated Ringer's solution) in 20-mL/kg boluses. If perfusion does not improve after repletion of the intravascular space (at least 60 mL/kg), inotropic drugs (dopamine or epinephrine [adrenaline]) might be indicated.[4,5] Under-resuscitation with fluid therapy, particularly before the addition of inotropic and vasopressor agents, has been associated with significantly increased mortality rates.[4,6] Early antibiotic therapy is essential and must not be delayed while attempting other procedures. Empiric therapy should be started based on the possible causative agent as outlined in Table 10-1.[2] In some cases of bacterial sepsis, antibiotic therapy can worsen the clinical findings through the release of endotoxins from lysed organisms. All ill-appearing children should undergo rapid bedside glucose measurement and should be given glucose intravenously if hypoglycemic. Other electrolyte abnormalities should also be addressed. (See Chapter 3 Shock, for further treatment.)

Fever in Very Young Infants

Infants younger than 2 months have immature immune responses and might not be able to contain certain infections. Although most well-appearing, febrile infants have benign, self-limited illness, those with serious bacterial illness (SBI) often have difficult-to-diagnose conditions and high morbidity rates. In fact, up to 10% of febrile infants in this age group have SBI, including bacteremia or bacterial meningitis in up to 3%.[7-13] Therefore, fever is an important symptom for identifying infants who need immediate evaluation and treatment.

> ## KEY POINTS
>
> **Management of Sepsis**
> - Provide supplemental oxygen.
> - Obtain prompt vascular access.
> - Begin fluid resuscitation.
> - Order laboratory studies and cultures.
> - Begin empiric antibiotic therapy.

Differential Diagnosis of the Septic-Appearing Infant

- Infectious diseases
  - Bacteremia/bacterial sepsis
  - Meningitis
  - Viral infections
- Cardiac disease
  - Congestive heart failure
  - Ductal-dependent lesions
  - Left-sided outflow tract obstruction
  - Myocarditis
  - Supraventricular tachycardia
- Child abuse
  - Shaken baby syndrome
- Endocrine disorders
  - Congenital adrenal hyperplasia
- GI disorders
  - Appendicitis (perforated)
  - Gastroenteritis
  - Hirschsprung enterocolitis
  - Incarcerated inguinal hernia
  - Intussusception
  - Pyloric stenosis (with dehydration)
  - Necrotizing enterocolitis
  - Volvulus
- Hematologic disorders
  - Anemia
  - Methemoglobinemia
- Metabolic disorders
  - Dehydration (hyponatremia, hypernatremia, and isotonic)
  - Hypoglycemia
  - Urea cycle defects
- Neurologic disorders
  - Infant botulism
- Genitourinary disorders
  - Obstructive uropathy
  - Posterior urethral valves
  - Pyelonephritis
- Toxins

Clinical Features

Although most febrile infants who have SBI appear ill, fever might be the first and only presenting sign. Useful clinical clues from observation include quality of the infant's cry, general activity and alertness, eye contact, reaction to stimulation, skin color, and hydration status. However, clinical impression alone is an unreliable predictor of serious infection in this age group; at this age, the ability of the infant to interact in a clear, social manner, such as with a social smile, is inconsistent. Thus, a febrile infant with SBI can present with signs of sepsis—irritability, lethargy, tachypnea, grunting, or poor peripheral perfusion—or the infant can appear well.

Diagnostic Studies

Although some differences in practice patterns exist for infants 30 to 60 days old, almost all experts agree that febrile infants younger than 28 days should undergo a complete sepsis workup, consisting of a complete blood cell (CBC) count with differential, urinalysis, and lumbar puncture (LP), with cultures of blood, urine, and CSF. A low threshold for a chest radiograph should be maintained for evaluation of any respiratory symptoms, and a stool culture should be obtained if the patient has diarrhea. The extent of the evaluation of the febrile infant 30 to 60 days old is more controversial. A conservative approach maintains the same diagnostic testing as for the infant younger than 1 month. However, some physicians withhold the LP if the infant appears well and will be either admitted to the hospital and observed or discharged with close follow-up care provided by the primary care physician. The decision to perform LP is a clinical one and should not be dependent on CBC count results, as they have little predictive value in this age group.[14] Regardless of age, if the infant is in shock or has episodes of apnea, LP should be deferred until the infant's condition is stable, and antibiotics should be administered before diagnostic studies are performed.

Differential Diagnosis

Life-threatening illness in febrile infants is usually the result of bacteremia, sepsis, or bacterial meningitis. In infants younger than 1 month, infection is usually due to organisms acquired perinatally—group B *Streptococcus*, gram-negative enteric organisms, and, historically, *Listeria monocytogenes*. Infants older than 6 weeks have a high risk of infection with community-acquired organisms, such as pneumococcus and, less commonly, *Neisseria meningitidis* and *Haemophilus influenzae* type b. Significant overlap exists for the ages of acquisition of all of these infections. Other focal bacterial infections include urinary tract infection (UTI), bacterial gastroenteritis, cellulitis (including omphalitis and mastitis), pneumonia, and otitis media.

Although bacterial infection is the primary concern because of its high morbidity rates, benign viral illness is the most common cause of fever in the well-appearing infant. During the winter months, respiratory syncytial virus can present with or without tachypnea, wheezing, and respiratory distress. Apnea and cyanosis can be the only presenting signs of respiratory syncytial virus in infants younger than 6 weeks, especially if they were born prematurely. Influenza can present with mild symptoms (eg, upper respiratory tract infection or nasal discharge) or with more severe symptoms that mimic bacterial sepsis. Furthermore, young infants are at higher risk for complications from influenza, including pneumonitis and otitis media. Aseptic meningitis from Enterovirus is common throughout the year and presents with irritability and (usually) fever. Although most cases of aseptic meningitis are generally self-limited, herpes encephalitis can be devastating.

Management

Febrile infants younger than age 60 days mandate a full or partial sepsis workup. All infants 28 days old and younger should be treated with empiric antibiotics (eg, ampicillin and cefotaxime) and admitted. As noted earlier, because of concerns of apnea and/or bradycardia in the very ill infant, LP should be deferred if the infant is in shock or experiencing apneic spells; *however, treatment with antibiotics must not be delayed.*

There are several approaches to the management of fever in well-appearing infants older than 1 month. All high-risk infants, regardless of age, should be admitted and treated with empiric antibiotics. In an effort to avoid routine hospitalization, investigators have devised criteria to identify febrile infants unlikely to have serious illness (Table 10-2). Well-appearing febrile infants 30 to 90 days old judged to be at low risk, who have no focal findings on physical examination, are not chronically ill, and are receiving close follow-up care, can be managed as outpatients. The use of empiric antibiotics as part of outpatient management for well-appearing, low-risk, 1- to 3-month-old infants is controversial.[7-13] Options are close follow-up without empiric therapy or treatment with parenteral ceftriaxone once daily until culture results are negative (usually at 48 hours). Strong consideration of performing LP should be made before any antibiotic administration in patients younger than 8 weeks.

Fever in Children

Fever in the Immunocompromised Child

Advances in care and treatment have led to high survival rates for children with cancer, human immunodeficiency virus (HIV) infection, sickle cell disease, and other immunosuppressive disorders. In many cases, treatment has moved from the inpatient to the ambulatory setting. Thus, presentation of immunocompromised children to the emergency department is common. Although fever in these children often represents benign illness (eg, upper respiratory tract infection, otitis media, or viral syndrome), the risk of SBI can be as high as 20%.[15] Therefore, fever in children who are immunosuppressed requires immediate attention.

The degree of immunosuppression varies with the child's underlying disease and can often be estimated using specific laboratory tests. In general, severe neutropenia is indicated by an

Criteria	Boston[12]	Philadelphia[11]	Rochester[13]
Age, d	28–89	29–56	0–60
Temperature, °C (°F)	>38 (100.4)	>38.2 (100.8)	>38 (100.4)
History	No immunizations or antibiotics within preceding 48 hours, not dehydrated	Not specified	Term infant, no perinatal antibiotics or underlying disease
WBC /mcL	<20,000	<15,000	5,000–15,000
Differential WBC count	Not specified	Band total to neutrophil ratio <0.2	Absolute band count <1,500/mcL
Urinalysis, WBC/hpf	<10	<10, no bacteria	<10
Chest radiograph	No infiltrate	No infiltrate	Not required
Cerebrospinal fluid, WBC/mcL	<10	<8	Not required

TABLE 10-2 Low-Risk Criteria for Well-Appearing Febrile Infants

Abbreviations: WBC, white blood cell.

absolute neutrophil count (ANC) less than 500/mcL or less than 1,000/mcL and decreasing. In addition to a low ANC, a low total lymphocyte count, in particular a low CD4 lymphocyte count, is a risk factor for SBI in children with HIV.

Clinical Features

General appearance is an important clinical feature in children who are immunosuppressed. Children with sepsis present with alteration in mental status (eg, lethargy or irritability), signs of increased work of breathing (eg, tachypnea or retractions), and decreased peripheral perfusion (eg, prolonged capillary refill, mottled extremities, or weak pulse). However, fever might be the only sign of serious illness. Although a child might appear well at presentation, the potential for acute deterioration mandates immediate evaluation.

Particular attention should be given to potential sources of bacterial invasion of the bloodstream. Many children who are immunosuppressed have indwelling intravascular catheters. Repeated use of these catheters to draw blood and administer intravenous medications increases the likelihood of colonization and bacteremia. Although catheter-related bacteremia can cause clinical signs of sepsis, catheter

infections can be more indolent, presenting with several days of low-grade fever. Other potential sources of bacteria include the respiratory tract (eg, pneumonia), GI tract (eg, stomatitis, perianal cellulitis, and typhlitis), genitourinary tract (eg, UTI), and skin (eg, cellulitis and ecthyma gangrenosum). Although bacterial infections are the most common cause of serious disease, viral infections, such as herpesvirus or cytomegalovirus, can disseminate, causing cardiovascular collapse and death. In particular, any vesicles noted on the skin should raise significant concern for herpes simplex or varicella-zoster infections.

Diagnostic Studies

A CBC count should be obtained in any child with fever who is potentially immunosuppressed, with attention to the degree of leukopenia or leukocytosis. Comparison with recent WBC counts (as well as the timing of the last chemotherapy) is particularly helpful for children undergoing chemotherapy and those children with HIV. Blood and urine cultures should be routinely obtained, although urethral catheterization should be avoided in children likely to be neutropenic (as should taking temperatures rectally). In children with indwelling intravascular catheters, an aerobic blood culture should be drawn from each catheter lumen, as well as from a peripheral site (if possible), to determine whether the catheter is the source of infection. These blood cultures should be of sufficient volume (minimum of 3 mL) to allow detection of fungi and bacterial pathogens. Specific areas of potential focal infection might require investigation with radiography, ultrasonography, or computed tomography.

Differential Diagnosis

Gram-positive bacteria account for most cases of culture-proven sepsis in oncologic patients. Children with indwelling intravenous catheters are at risk for line sepsis caused by coagulase-negative staphylococci, *Streptococcus viridans*, and *Staphylococcus aureus*. The catheter insertion site should be examined for pus, erythema, and tenderness along the catheter tract. Cellulitis, skin irritation, and abrasions can also be a source of invasion by *Staphylococcus*. Mucosal tenderness, sores, or ulcers suggest infection with *S viridans* and anaerobes, particularly in profoundly immunocompromised children (eg, acute myelogenous leukemia). Gram-negative infections with *Escherichia coli, Klebsiella, Pseudomonas aeruginosa,* and other Enterobacteriaceae are less common but often more virulent. Typhlitis, a severe form of colitis of the terminal ileum and cecum associated with chemotherapy, should be suspected in any child with neutropenia and abdominal tenderness.

In addition to these considerations, children with HIV and sickle cell disease are at high risk for sepsis due to infection with pneumococcus and *Salmonella*, which can present without antecedent illness or focus of infection on physical examination. *Pneumocystis jirovecii* pneumonia (formerly known as *P carinii* pneumonia and still referred to as PCP) can occur in young children with HIV (or who are immunocompromised) and is accompanied by tachypnea, cough, and hypoxemia.

Management

Rapid assessment and immediate management of suspected sepsis in immunocompromised children are often lifesaving. Regardless of how ill the patient appears or how high the fever is, all children should undergo complete examination, determination of CBC count with differential, and empiric antibiotic therapy. The choice of antibiotics is based on a combination of factors, including likely pathogens (ie, clinical diagnosis), previous history of sepsis, and local antibiotic resistance patterns. Children with neutropenia are treated with an antipseudomonal antibiotic, such as ceftazidime or cefepime. An aminoglycoside is usually added for patients who appear very ill or toxic. Because of concerns of increasing gram-positive resistance, empiric administration of vancomycin should be reserved for children with severe mucositis, patients at risk for resistance to monotherapy (eg, methicillin-resistant *S aureus* [MRSA] colonization or risk factors for resistant *S viridans*), and patients who present with septic shock. Regardless of the antibiotic choice, close monitoring for deterioration is essential because endotoxin release or progression of sepsis after antibiotic administration can cause cardiovascular instability.

The management of children with HIV infection is controversial. Children who are febrile but appear well and who have an ANC above 500/mcL can usually be managed as outpatients with oral or parenteral antibiotics and close followup. Ill appearance or a low ANC mandates admission and empiric parenteral antibiotic therapy. Children who are not neutropenic and those with sickle cell disease are often treated with ceftriaxone until culture results are known, often as outpatients.

KEY POINTS

Management of Immunocompromised Children With Neutropenia

- Obtain intravenous access and begin fluid resuscitation for signs of shock.

- Assess and treat respiratory distress.

- Order laboratory studies as indicated, including cultures of blood and urine.

- Begin empiric antibiotic treatment with ceftazidime or cefepime and consider the addition of gentamicin and/or vancomycin if there is suspected catheter-related infection or severe sepsis.

- Admit for inpatient care.

Fever With Petechiae

Although most types of petechiae in children are usually benign, the combination of fever and petechiae always raises the concern of invasive bacterial illness, especially due to meningococcus (*N meningitidis*).[16] In one study, meningococcus was found to be present in only approximately 2% of children with petechiae who were well enough to be treated as outpatients but in up to 20% of those treated as inpatients.[17] Furthermore, the mortality rate associated with meningococcus is as high as 20%. Discriminating the small number of patients with fever and petechiae due to bacterial sepsis from most patients with more benign conditions is a difficult but important task.[17]

Clinical Features

There is a continuum of clinical features of meningococcemia, ranging from asymptomatic to mild infection to sepsis and shock. The nonspecific prodrome can include an upper respiratory tract illness with early symptoms of fever, headache, fatigue, myalgias, and arthralgias. Common early findings include cold hands and feet, leg pain, and abnormal skin color (pallor or mottling).[18] Within hours, the child might become lethargic, tachypneic, and tachycardic, with poor peripheral perfusion. Petechiae can be present at any stage of the illness. In the more fulminant cases, petechiae progress to purpura (**Figure 10.1**).

Diagnostic Testing

Laboratory testing in all children with fever and petechiae should include CBC count, coagulation studies (prothrombin time [PT] and partial thromboplastin time [PTT]), C-reactive protein measurement, and blood culture. Because streptococcal pharyngitis can present with petechiae, a throat culture and rapid antigen testing should be considered in older children. Lumbar puncture should be performed if the child appears ill or has signs of meningitis, assuming the child is clinically stable and has normal coagulation times and platelet counts.

Differential Diagnosis

Most well-appearing children with fever and petechiae have a viral condition. In particular, influenza, Enterovirus, infectious mononucle-

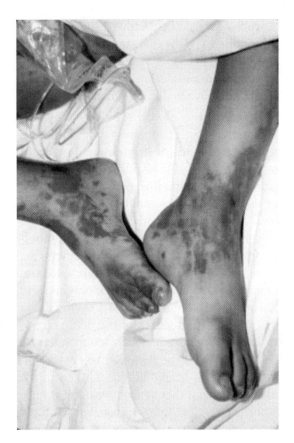

Figure 10.1 Purpura in a patient with meningococcemia.

osis, adenovirus, atypical measles, and other viral illnesses can all present with petechiae. In addition to meningococcemia, any cause of bacterial sepsis can cause petechiae, including pneumococcus, *H influenzae* type b, group *A Streptococcus, S aureus, E coli,* and *Neisseria gonorrhoeae.* Children with Rocky Mountain spotted fever (RMSF; *Rickettsia rickettsii*) are generally ill appearing and present with petechiae over the wrists and ankles accompanied by headache and myalgias. Leukemia can be suggested by an abnormal CBC count with anemia, thrombocytopenia, and either leukopenia or leukocytosis (often with blasts on the peripheral smear). Signs of heart failure or a history of acute rheumatic fever or congenital heart disease can suggest bacterial endocarditis.

One important caveat in the evaluation is the presence of petechiae above the nipple line (upper chest and face). Increases in intrathoracic pressure that accompany cough, vigorous crying, and emesis can cause petechiae in the distribution of the superior vena cava. If petechiae are restricted to this distribution with a clear origin and the child appears well, the risk of SBI is much less likely; however, it is always important to consider the child's entire clinical presentation when deciding management.[16]

Management

Children who are ill appearing or immunocompromised should undergo immediate evaluation for sepsis and be admitted for empiric parenteral antibiotic therapy. The management of well-appearing children with fever and no clear source of the petechiae is somewhat controversial.[17] Children younger than 12 months have a higher risk of invasive bacterial illness and therefore should be hospitalized and treated with empiric antibiotic therapy. Older children with normal WBC counts between 5,000/mcL and 15,000/mcL, band count less than 500/mcL, normal ANC, C-reactive protein of less than 6 mg/L, and normal PT can be observed in the emergency department for several hours and then treated as outpatients if they remain well and no new petechiae develop. Empiric treatment with parenteral antibiotics in the outpatient management of these children is varied. Children who are well appearing and have pharyngitis with a positive streptococcal antigen test result can be treated as outpatients with an antistreptococcal antibiotic.

Sickle Cell Disease

A single amino acid substitution of valine for glutamate in the β chain of the hemoglobin molecule is responsible for sickle cell disease. This disorder is most commonly seen in African, Indian, Middle Eastern, and Mediterranean populations. In the United States, approximately 0.15% of the black population carries the homozygous form of sickle cell disease, and 8% carry the hemoglobin (*HbS*) gene.

Clinical Features

Although symptoms of sickle cell disease can present in infancy, most patients do not have clinical manifestations before they are 6 months old. Sickle cells are more readily deformed than normal red blood cells, which leads to hemolysis and thrombosis within the small blood vessels, with resultant tissue ischemia and end-organ

damage. There are four classic presentations of sickle cell disease: vaso-occlusive crisis, splenic sequestration, aplastic crisis, and infection.

Vaso-occlusive Crisis

These painful crises typically involve the chest, abdomen, extremities (usually the long bones such as the tibia, femur, and humerus), and back. Infants can present with dactylitis (swelling of the hands and feet) due to occlusion of the nutrient arteries supplying the metacarpals and metatarsals (**Figure 10.2**). Triggers for all vaso-occlusive crises include infection, dehydration, high altitude, hypoxia, stress, and cold water immersion. Priapism, a result of vaso-occlusion of the corpus cavernosum, is a true emergency because sustained priapism can result in long-term impotence. Acute chest syndrome presents with a combination of cough, chest pain, tachypnea, and/or dyspnea. Although the results of initial chest radiographs can be negative, an infiltrate might develop 2 to 3 days after symptom onset (**Figure 10.3**). Between 5% and 10% of children will develop cerebral disease, such as thrombotic stroke, seizures, coma, subarachnoid hemorrhage, and cranial nerve palsies (**Figure 10.4**).

Splenic Sequestration

Splenic sequestration typically occurs in children younger than 5 years and presents with hypotension, pallor, and splenomegaly. Preceding infections with parvovirus B19, echovirus, and rhinovirus have been implicated. Reticulocyte counts are elevated, and hemoglobin levels are markedly decreased. Rapid treatment with blood transfusion (10 mL/kg of packed red

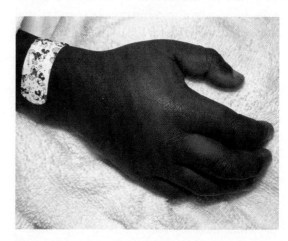

Figure 10.2 Child with dactylitis.

blood cells) is imperative. Exchange transfusion and splenectomy might also be warranted.

Aplastic Crises

Profound inhibition of erythropoiesis can result in hemoglobin levels less than 3 g/dL and inappropriately low reticulocyte counts (<3%). Possible causes include parvovirus B19, bone marrow toxic drugs, and folic acid deficiency. Treatment includes blood transfusions and supportive therapy.

Infection

Splenic infarction due to multiple episodes of splenic thrombosis usually results in splenic autoinfarction (and functional asplenia) by the age of 5 years. Therefore, in these children, infections with the encapsulated organisms (such as *Streptococcus pneumoniae, H influenzae* type b, *E coli*, and *S aureus*) can lead to overwhelming sepsis and death. Patients with sickle cell disease are also at increased risk for meningitis, bacteremia/septicemia, UTIs, bacterial pneumonia, and osteomyelitis. The most common causes of pneumonia are *S pneumoniae* and *Mycoplasma*. Fifty percent of osteomyelitis cases are caused by *Salmonella typhimurium*, with *S aureus* and *E coli* also being contributing organisms. The use of prophylactic oral penicillin for children younger than 6 years has decreased the incidence of sepsis. In addition, vaccination against *S pneumoniae* and *H*

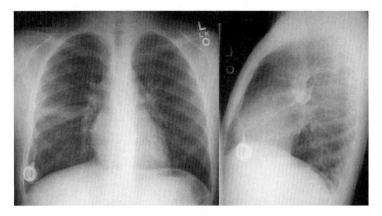

Figure 10.3 Acute chest syndrome. This 13-year-old with sickle cell disease developed cough, chest pain, and tachypnea. This chest radiograph demonstrates streaky infiltrates in his right lung.

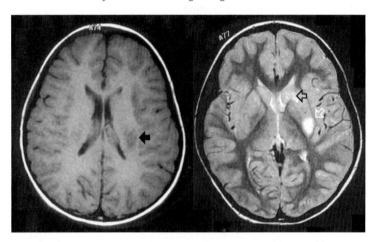

Figure 10.4 Patients with sickle cell disease are at increased risk for thrombotic strokes. This magnetic resonance image is of a 7-year-old. On the T1 image the infarct is visible in the posterior left putamen (black arrow). The T2 image is a lower cut through the center of the infarct. The infarct appears as a white lesion in the left caudate nucleus (black outlined arrow) and the left putamen (white outlined arrow). This study is read as an infarct in the left basal ganglia, the posterior limb of internal capsule, and the head of the caudate.

influenzae type b is crucial for patients with sickle cell disease because these two organisms are the most common bacterial pathogens.

Diagnostic Studies

In patients who present with sickle cell crisis, CBC and reticulocyte counts should be determined. Typical hemoglobin levels in patients with sickle cell disease range from 6 to 9 g/dL; baseline platelet counts and WBC counts are often elevated. Typical baseline reticulocyte counts range from 5% to 15%; counts lower than 3% should raise the suspicion of an aplastic crisis. Blood cultures should be obtained in patients with fever (temperature >38°C [100.4°F]).

Urinalysis and urine culture are indicated in patients with fever, dysuria, or hematuria and in young infants. Liver enzyme studies might be warranted in the evaluation of right upper quadrant pain or if cholecystitis is suspected. Chest radiographs should be obtained in patients with dyspnea, fever, chest pain, cough, or hypoxia. Other testing might include a bone scan or magnetic resonance imaging (osteomyelitis), extremity radiographs (avascular necrosis of the femoral or humeral head), or head CT or magnetic resonance imaging (transient ischemic attack or cerebral infarct).

Management

Patients who present with sickle cell crisis are typically underhydrated and are routinely treated with a fluid bolus with 10 to 20 mL/kg of normal saline solution; ongoing fluid therapy should be 1.5 times the maintenance rate. Pain control is imperative; many patients have tried oral analgesics before presenting to the emergency department and will require parenteral therapy. Morphine, hydromorphone, and ketorolac are good analgesic agents. Meperidine should be used sparingly because high doses

can lead to seizures due to accumulation of the toxic metabolite normeperidine.

Patients with hypoxemia should be given supplemental oxygen. Even without hypoxemia, supplemental oxygen can be beneficial. Patients with splenic sequestration, aplastic crisis, central nervous system syndromes, priapism, and acute chest syndrome often require a blood transfusion to decrease the concentration of circulating sickled red blood cells. Patients with severe conditions can ultimately require exchange transfusion. Patients with acute chest syndrome can splint due to pain, and therefore adequate pain control is imperative to avoid atelectasis. Empiric antibiotic therapy with a broad-spectrum cephalosporin and a macrolide is typically warranted in this condition. Patients with priapism require prompt urologic consultation; surgical intervention might be necessary if the priapism is not relieved. If outpatient pain management fails and multiple doses of parenteral medications are needed, the patient should be admitted for treatment with patient-controlled analgesia.[19]

Dermatologic Emergencies

Almost any infectious illness can present with skin manifestations, as do many systemic inflammatory conditions. In most cases, rashes are one manifestation of a benign illness. However, certain rashes can be a warning sign of a more serious disease.

Clinical Features

A thorough history and physical examination often lead to a diagnosis. Information about the child's general health, immune status, medication use, and history of chronic illness can identify risk factors for associated illness. Related signs and symptoms might include a viral prodrome, fever, mucous membrane involvement, myalgias, arthralgias, or arthritis. Progression of the rash—how the rash started, inciting agents, spread, duration, and presence of pruritus—is also important.

On physical examination, the type of primary lesion should be determined. A macule is a small, flat lesion with a different skin color. A papule is a small, elevated lesion. A vesicle is a

---

> ## KEY POINTS
>
> **Management of Sickle Cell Crisis in Infants and Children**
>
> - Assess and treat for signs of respiratory distress/failure and shock.
> - Administer oxygen to patients with hypoxia or acute chest syndrome.
> - Obtain vascular access and begin fluid resuscitation.
> - Obtain blood for CBC and reticulocyte counts and other laboratory studies as indicated.
> - Begin antibiotic therapy for documented infections.
> - Provide pain control.
> - Start transfusion as indicated.
> - Obtain prompt urologic consultation for priapism.

blister containing clear fluid; a pustule contains purulent fluid. A bulla is a large blister. The rash can be generalized, suggesting a diffuse exposure or a systemic illness, or confined to specific areas. There can be characteristic patterns, such as linear (poison ivy) or dermatomal (herpes zoster), or a characteristic appearance, such as purpura or target lesions.

Diagnostic Studies

Laboratory evaluation is based on the child's appearance and the nature and likely causes of the rash. If the child is febrile and ill appearing, CBC count, erythrocyte sedimentation rate, C-reactive protein level, and blood culture should be obtained. In addition to evaluation for possible sepsis, children with purpura and/or petechiae should undergo measurement of platelet count and coagulation studies (PT and PTT) to investigate for a bleeding disorder. The presence of multinucleated giant cells on a Tzanck smear (obtained by unroofing an intact blister)

is diagnostic for herpes simplex, varicella, and herpes zoster and can be discovered quickly. The results of a Gram stain of fluid from a lesion might be consistent with bacterial causes but are often indeterminate; viral cultures and polymerase chain reaction testing are also useful for the identification of herpes simplex, varicella, and herpes zoster.

Differential Diagnosis

The differential diagnosis of dermatologic lesions is extensive. Although many rashes are self-limited, those that are potentially life threatening or indicative of significant disease should be identified.

Maculopapular Rashes

Erythema multiforme is a hypersensitivity reaction characterized by diffuse erythematous macules with central clearing called target or iris lesions (**Figure 10.5**). Drug exposure (especially penicillins, sulfonamides, and anticonvulsants) and herpes infection are commonly identified

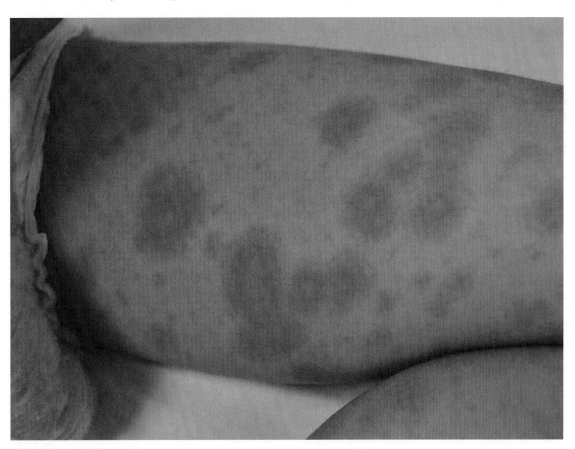

Figure 10.5 Erythema multiforme.

causes. Most cases of erythema multiforme are self-limited, but the presence of mucous membrane involvement can be a sign of Stevens-Johnson syndrome, which has a mortality rate of up to 25%. Children with Stevens-Johnson syndrome have areas of extensive mucosal necrosis accompanied by severe systemic symptoms, including ill appearance, fever, cough, vomiting, and diarrhea.

Rocky Mountain spotted fever usually begins with a maculopapular rash before progressing to petechial lesions, beginning on the wrists and ankles and spreading inward in a centripetal manner. Not all patients with RMSF exhibit the classic petechial rash (or exhibit lesions on the palms and soles). Systemic symptoms of RMSF include fever, headache, and lethargy.

Kawasaki disease is an illness characterized by fever for at least 5 days and four of the following five features: nonspecific, polymorphous, maculopapular rash; conjunctivitis; mucositis (ie, red lips and strawberry tongue); edema/swelling of the hands and feet (often with erythematous palms and soles); and adenopathy (usually a single, nontender cervical node). Coronary artery aneurysms can develop in as many as 20% of untreated children. (See Chapter 4 Cardiovascular System.)

Many viral illnesses have characteristic maculopapular rashes. In measles, the rash begins on the face and then progresses to the torso and extremities during a 3-day period, lasting 5 or 6 days before fading. Cough, coryza, conjunctivitis, and a high temperature (40°C [104°F]) accompany the rash. Erythema infectiosum (fifth disease), caused by parvovirus B19, presents with a slapped-cheek erythema or a lacy, reticulated, erythematous rash on the torso and extremities (**Figure 10.6**). Apart from the rash, symptoms are usually absent in young children, but adolescents can have mild fever and arthralgias. Transmission of this virus to pregnant women is a concern. Roseola, associated with human herpesvirus 6 infection, typically presents with 3 days of high temperatures followed by abrupt defervescence and the appearance of a diffuse, rose-colored papular rash.

Toxic shock syndrome (TSS) is an acute systemic illness characterized by fever and a diffuse macular erythematous rash with rapid

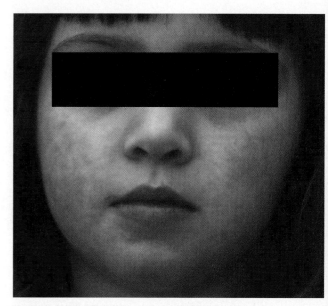

Figure 10.6 Slapped-cheek rash of erythema infectiosum.

onset of hypotension, renal failure, and multisystem organ involvement. It is caused by toxin-producing strains of either *Staphylococcus* or *Streptococcus pyogenes* (group A *Streptococcus*). Although public awareness increased in the early 1980s when TSS was associated with tampon use in menstruating women, menstrual cases currently account for approximately 50% of reported cases.[20] Risk factors for *S aureus*–mediated TSS include primary *S aureus* infection (eg, cellulitis, carbuncle, osteomyelitis, and sinusitis), postoperative wound infection, skin or mucous membrane disruption (eg, burns, influenza, and varicella), and both surgical and nonsurgical foreign-body placement (eg, catheters, tampons, and sutures). Currently, most cases of community-acquired MRSA infection do not produce the TSS toxin.[20] Streptococcal TSS in children is usually associated with varicella or a focal, invasive tissue or blood infection with group A *Streptococcus*.

Petechial and Purpuric Rashes
Purpura is the result of bleeding into the skin and, unlike most other rashes, does not blanch when pressure is applied across the skin surface. The most common causes of purpura in children are local trauma, sepsis, vasculitis, and bleeding disorder. When accompanied by fever or ill appearance, purpura, like petechiae, can be a sign of invasive bacterial illness or disseminated viral

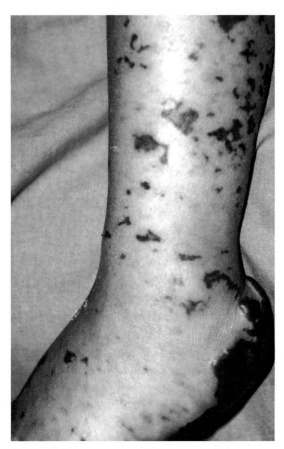

Figure 10.7 Child with meningococcemia and purpura fulminans.

although hematuria (the most common manifestation) and proteinuria are usually mild, some children might develop nephritis or nephrotic syndrome and even end-stage renal disease.

Purpura can also be a presenting sign of a bleeding disorder, such as hemophilia or von Willebrand disease. Diagnosis is based on abnormal platelet function analysis (von Willebrand disease), abnormal PTT (hemophilia and severe von Willebrand disease), and factor activity (factor VIII in hemophilia A and factor IX in hemophilia B).

Immune thrombocytopenic purpura (ITP), an immune disorder causing increased platelet destruction, is the most common cause of thrombocytopenia in children. The child appears well but has a combination of petechiae, bruising, purpura, or mucosal bleeding. All other cell lines on the CBC count are normal in ITP, whereas children with leukemia often have significant anemia and/or abnormalities with the WBC count.

illness. In particular, sepsis caused by meningococcemia (as well as other microorganisms) can lead to disseminated intravascular coagulation, resulting in diffuse areas of purpura, some evolving with central necrosis (**Figure 10.7**). Henoch-Schönlein purpura (HSP) is the most common vasculitis in children, usually occurring between the ages of 3 and 9 years. This leukocytoclastic vasculitis of the small blood vessels involves primarily the skin, GI tract, joints, and kidneys. The characteristic rash of HSP is palpable purpura located predominantly on the buttocks and lower extremities but seen in other dependent areas on infants and younger children (**Figure 10.8**). Associated symptoms include colicky abdominal pain, GI bleeding, arthritis (usually in the lower extremities), scrotal edema, and hematuria. Some children with HSP develop intussusception of the small bowel (eg, ileoileal) that cannot be identified using standard intussusception studies (eg, barium enema). Renal disease is the most concerning manifestation;

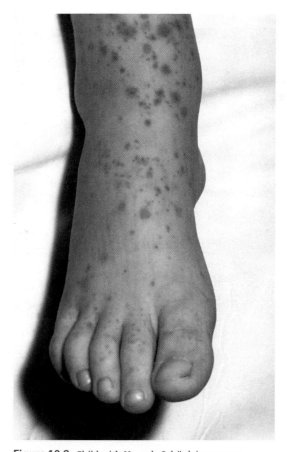

Figure 10.8 Child with Henoch-Schönlein purpura.

Vesiculobullous and Vesiculopustular Rashes

Herpes viruses are a common cause of vesicular eruptions in children. Herpes simplex virus causes gingivostomatitis, usually accompanied by fever and irritability. With varicella (chickenpox), the cutaneous lesions follow a mild prodrome of fever, sore throat, and malaise. The rash begins with scattered pruritic papules and progresses to vesicles on a red base, central umbilication, and then crusting. Smallpox has been eradicated for more than 25 years but remains a bioterrorism threat. The vesicles of smallpox are similar to varicella; however, there are key differences in their presentations. Varicella lesions occur in crops during different stages of the illness, whereas smallpox lesions appear all at the same time. Varicella usually begins on the torso and spreads to the extremities; smallpox begins on the arms, face, and legs and progresses to the torso during approximately 7 days. Scab formation occurs 4 to 7 days after the rash begins in varicella and 10 to 14 days in smallpox. Herpes zoster is a reactivation of dormant varicella that presents with pain, itching, and then grouped macular, papular, and vesicular lesions in a dermatomal distribution (**Figure 10.9**). Any herpes infection can disseminate in an immunosuppressed child and can be life threatening.

Desquamating Skin Disorders

Staphylococcal scalded skin syndrome is a severe systemic reaction to a staphylococcal toxin and occurs primarily in young children and infants. After a prodrome of fever, malaise, and possibly evidence of impetigo, a fine erythematous rash erupts on the face and neck. During the next 1 to 2 days, the rash spreads over the entire body and the skin becomes tender. At this stage, slight skin pressure can cause skin sloughing or blister formation (Nikolsky's sign) as separation occurs between layers within the epidermis. Desquamation occurs 1 to 2 weeks after the initial infection.

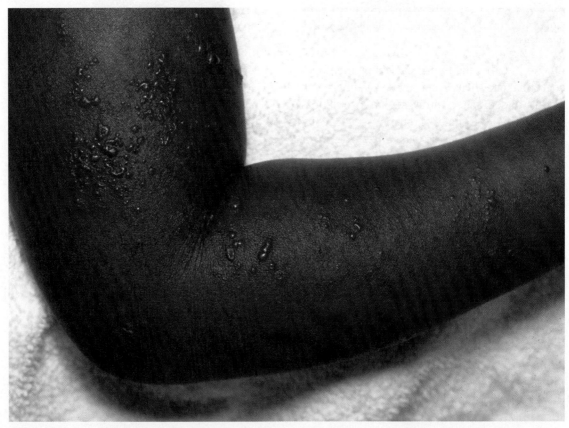

Figure 10.9 Girl with shingles (herpes zoster).

Toxic epidermal necrolysis (TEN), a hypersensitivity reaction to medications, presents with similar clinical findings as staphylococcal scalded skin syndrome. However, TEN has higher morbidity and mortality because the skin sloughing in TEN occurs at a deeper layer—the dermal-epidermal junction.

Bacterial Skin Infections/MRSA

Community-acquired MRSA infection has emerged as a frequent cause of cellulitis, furuncles, and abscess formation in previously healthy children; patients often report having a spider bite. The mainstay of MRSA abscess treatment includes incision and drainage. Culture and susceptibility results are useful for management of individual patients and to help determine the prevalence of *S aureus* susceptibility to β-lactam and non–β-lactam agents. Prevention is imperative, and all patients with suspected MRSA infection should be advised to pay strict attention to hand washing. Wounds should be kept covered, and towels, clothing, razors, and sheets should not be shared with others.

Management

Management of dermatologic emergencies is based on the underlying cause. Most viral illnesses require little more than supportive care and maintenance of the child's hydration status. Antiviral agents, such as acyclovir, can provide a benefit in healthy children with varicella or herpes gingivostomatitis. However, herpesvirus infection in neonates, children who are immunocompromised, and children with eczema herpeticum warrants hospital admission and parenteral antiviral therapy. Rashes typical of bacterial infection or sepsis should be treated with the appropriate antibiotics. Severe, diffuse skin reactions, such as TSS, staphylococcal scalded skin syndrome, TEN, or Stevens-Johnson syndrome, call for hospital admission with intensive monitoring, fluid therapy, antibiotics if appropriate, and burn care. Any patient with a presentation suggestive of measles should be rapidly isolated and reported to the public health authorities.

Appropriate therapy of abscesses is incision and drainage. (See Online Chapter 25, Office Procedures, Procedure 5.3 skin abscess drainage.) Routine use of antibiotics after incision and drainage remains controversial in clinical practice, with some experts stating that antibiotics are not warranted if there is no surrounding cellulitis and proper incision and drainage are performed. If antibiotics are used, clindamycin or trimethoprim-sulfamethoxazole is the initial drug of choice for outpatient management, depending on local sensitivities. Patients who have severe or rapidly advancing disease can be treated with intravenous vancomycin, clindamycin, or linezolid. Treatment of undifferentiated cellulitis without abscess formation in the era of MRSA presents a difficult scenario. Many physicians will treat with two antibiotics—a β-lactam (for *Streptococcus*) and an antimicrobial effective against MRSA—but recent evidence suggests that a β-lactam and close follow-up care might still be the most appropriate therapy.[21]

Early treatment of Kawasaki disease with intravenous immunoglobulin and aspirin prevents the development of coronary artery aneurysms. Children with bleeding disorders might require transfusion of blood or factor concentrates. Many cases of ITP require no therapy; however, treatment is indicated for very low platelet counts, severe mucosal bleeding, or persistent symptoms. Corticosteroids are the best treatment option for ITP. Anti-RhD immune globulin is another treatment option for children with ITP who are Rh positive. Intravenous immunoglobulin (IgG) can be used for Rh-negative patients. Children with suspected HSP should undergo urinalysis to check for hematuria and protein and, if the results are positive, measurement of blood urea nitrogen (BUN) and creatinine.

Epididymitis

Epididymitis results from inflammation of the epididymis, which is located along the posterior aspect of the testis and serves as the storage center for sperm. Bacterial infection is the most common concern, but sterile inflammation is probably much more common in younger age groups.[22] Adolescents should be evaluated for possible sexually transmitted diseases, such as *N gonorrhoeae* and *Chlamydia trachomatis*.

Clinical Features

Patients with epididymitis usually present with a unilaterally tender, edematous scrotum. The epididymis is in its normal location, posterolateral to the testes. In adolescents, a urethral discharge might be present when the epididymitis is secondary to a sexually transmitted disease. Systemic symptoms, such as nausea, vomiting, low-grade fever, and lower abdominal, scrotal, and testicular pain, can also be present. As the swelling increases, obliteration of the sulcus between the testis and epididymis occurs, making clinical differentiation from torsion extremely difficult. Relief of pain with scrotal elevation (Prehn's sign) is unreliable. In the absence of torsion, a cremasteric reflex should be present.

Diagnostic Studies

A urinalysis and urine culture should be obtained. However, a lack of pyuria does not rule out epididymitis because 20% to 50% of patients can have a normal urinalysis result. A leukocytosis can be present on a peripheral blood smear in more severe cases. Any urethral discharge should be cultured and sent for Gram stain, including studies for *N gonorrhoeae* and *C trachomatis*. Great care should be taken in relying on a clinical diagnosis because the sensitivity and specificity of physical examination findings are imperfect. Color-flow duplex Doppler sonography, or less commonly radionuclide scintigraphy, should be used to exclude testicular torsion. In epididymitis, the testis is normal and vascular flow is preserved or increased.

Differential Diagnosis

Although acute scrotal or testicular pain is often caused by a benign underlying diagnosis, the emergency physician should always be concerned about diagnoses that can cause irreversible genitourinary injury with resultant testicular loss, atrophy, or infertility. Patients who present with acute pain should be evaluated for testicular torsion, epididymitis, strangulated or incarcerated inguinal hernia, testicular rupture, or hemorrhage into a testicular mass. Other diagnoses to consider include torsion of the testicular or epididymal appendages, orchitis, HSP, idiopathic scrotal edema, varicocele, and hydrocele (Table 10-3). The diagnosis that must be excluded is testicular torsion because delay or misdiagnosis can result in testicular infarction.[23] Painless causes of scrotal or testicular swelling are listed in Table 10-4.

Management

The treatment of epididymitis in prepubertal children is controversial. Some physicians treat mild epididymitis with nonsteroidal anti-inflammatory drugs alone on the premise that the underlying cause is a sterile inflammation.[22] Children with more severe disease or a positive urinalysis (or culture) result should be treated for typical uropathogens (eg, with cefdinir). Patients with systemic symptoms and toxic effects should be treated with intravenous antibiotics (eg, ceftriaxone). In addition to antibiotic administration, pain control is imperative: scrotal elevation, placement of cold packs on the swollen area, nonsteroidal anti-inflammatory agents, or narcotics can all be helpful. If there is urethral discharge, the patient should be treated for both *N gonorrhoeae* and *C trachomatis* infection. Children should be referred for urology follow-up care to ensure that there are no contributing urologic abnormalities. If epididymitis is found to be sexually transmitted in a young child, the appropriate child protective agency should be contacted immediately and a report filed by the emergency department staff.

Balanitis/Balanoposthitis

Balanitis (inflammation of the glans) and balanoposthitis (inflammation of the glans and the foreskin) can occur in both circumcised and uncircumcised males. The primary cause of

TABLE 10-3 **Painful Causes of Scrotal or Testicular Swelling**
• Epididymitis
• Testicular torsion
• Torsion of the appendix testis
• Incarcerated strangulated hernia
• Testicular rupture
• Hemorrhage into a testicular tumor
• Hydrocele
• Varicocele

Barkin RM ed. Pediatric Emergency Medicine Concepts and Clinical Practice, 2nd ed. St. Louis, Mo: Mosby;1140. Reprinted with permission.

TABLE 10-4 **Painless Causes of Scrotal or Testicular Swelling**	
• Henoch-Schönlein purpura	• Hydrocele
	• Inguinal hernia
• Varicocele	• Testicular tumor

Barkin RM ed. Pediatric Emergency Medicine Concepts and Clinical Practice, 2nd ed. St. Louis, Mo: Mosby;1140. Reprinted with permission.

balanoposthitis is infection; however, chemical irritation, trauma, fixed drug eruption, or contact dermatitis can also be contributory.

Clinical Features

The typical organisms involved in infection-related balanoposthitis are gram-positive and gram-negative organisms that are normal flora. Group A β-hemolytic streptococci have been reported to cause balanitis.[24] *Candida albicans* can also be contributory in infants and prepubertal males, and recurrent cases should raise the suspicion of diabetes mellitus. In adolescents, sexually transmitted diseases can lead to inflammation and subsequent balanoposthitis. Physical examination can reveal penile erythema, edema, and occasionally a discharge. Systemic symptoms are unusual.

Diagnostic Studies

The diagnosis of both balanitis and balanoposthitis is clinical. In male adolescents, cultures for *N gonorrhoeae* and *C trachomatis* are warranted if the clinical presentation is suggestive of sexually transmitted disease.

Management

The mainstay of management is emphasis on adequate hygiene with gentle retraction and cleaning of the foreskin and sitz baths to promote irrigation. In patients with edema and cellulitis, a 5- to 7-day course of a first-generation cephalosporin might be required. Some physicians also treat empirically with topical antifungals, depending on the presentation. Circumcision might be required for recurrent disease.

Urinary Tract Infections— Cystitis and Pyelonephritis

Diagnosing UTIs in infants and young children can be challenging because the clinical signs are typically nonspecific (eg, fussiness, fever, or lethargy). Early diagnosis is imperative to avoid the potential complications of sepsis and renal scarring. The risk of experiencing a UTI before the age of 12 years is approximately 3% for girls and 1% for boys. Significantly, 7% of children younger than 2 years with a temperature greater than 39°C (102.2°F) without a clear source have an occult UTI.[25] Uncircumcised male newborns are significantly more likely to develop a UTI than female newborns. Beyond the newborn period, girls younger than 2 years and uncircumcised boys younger than 12 months are especially at risk of UTI.[25]

E coli is the predominant cause of UTIs in children, although *Klebsiella, Enterobacter, Proteus,* and *Enterococcus,* as well as group B *Streptococcus* in neonates are also important pathogens.

In neonates and young infants, bacteremia can occur concomitantly. The significance of UTIs, particularly pyelonephritis, is that acute infection might cause permanent scarring in a significant percentage of children. Such scarring is believed to be a risk factor for long-term renal insufficiency, hypertension, and end-stage renal disease.[26]

Clinical Features

In neonates, the signs and symptoms of UTIs are usually nonspecific and include fever, decreased oral intake, lethargy, jaundice, and irritability. Children 3 to 24 months old can additionally present with abdominal pain and vomiting. Children older than 2 years often have more recognizable symptoms: abdominal pain, dysuria, or hematuria. New bedwetting might be a sign of a UTI. Cystitis is usually associated with local symptoms, such as suprapubic tenderness and dysuria, whereas patients with pyelonephritis typically have more systemic symptoms, such as fever, costovertebral angle tenderness, and vomiting.

Diagnostic Studies

There are several methods for collecting urine samples from children. Because of the difficulty

in adequately cleansing the perineal area, the bag-collection method poses an excessive risk of contamination, with a high rate of false-positive results. Although a negative urine culture result from a bag specimen can be helpful, a positive culture result must be confirmed by urethral catheterization or suprapubic bladder aspiration.

For a clean-catch urine sample from a toilet-trained child, the parent can clean the child with soap and water before urination. A urine sample with greater than 10 WBC/hpf and a significant number of epithelial cells should be considered contaminated, and either an improved clean-catch method or catheterization must be tried. Females with a vaginal discharge or vaginal bleeding should be catheterized.

Bladder catheterization is less prone to contamination and is the method of choice for obtaining urine samples in ill- or septic-appearing infants.[27] Urethral catheterization is relatively simple and poses little risk, although it might be more difficult in uncircumcised boys or young infants. There is a minimal risk of trauma to the urethra or introduction of bacteria into the urinary tract with this technique. A No. 5 feeding tube can be used in young infants. For patients who are excessively difficult to catheterize, suprapubic aspiration is an acceptable option, particularly with the aid of bedside ultrasonography.

Nitrite and leukocyte esterase urinalysis markers have the highest combined sensitivity and specificity for infection. However, in children younger than 2 years, urinalysis alone is not considered adequate for ruling out UTIs. Ten percent to 50% of young children with positive urine culture results can have false-negative urinalysis results (bacteria without pyuria). Therefore, performing a urine culture is mandatory, regardless of the urinalysis result.[28]

Differential Diagnosis

There are several other causes of dysuria in children. Irritants, such as bubble bath or soaps, can cause a local irritation and dysuria. A retained foreign body in the vagina (such as toilet paper) can cause irritation or bacterial growth with associated dysuria and vaginal discharge. Pinworms in the genitourinary area can cause itching and scratching. Balanitis in uncircumcised males can also cause dysuria and pyuria. Unintentional injuries to the genital area can cause abrasions, lacerations, and subsequent dysuria. Sexual or physical abuse must always be considered in any young child with a history of multiple UTIs. In adolescents at risk for sexually transmitted disease, it is in the patient's best interest to actively consider urethritis (which requires a pelvic examination for cultures) rather than make a presumptive diagnosis of cystitis.

Management

Because of the risk of associated sepsis and pyelonephritis, infants younger than 2 months with a UTI are typically admitted to the hospital for empiric intravenous antibiotic therapy.[29] However, a recent multicenter study suggested that infants 29 to 60 days old who are well appearing in the emergency department and do not have a high-risk medical history (eg, prematurity of <37 weeks' gestation, genitourinary abnormalities, previous UTIs, and infections or severe systemic disease) can be managed by brief hospitalization or outpatient management with close follow-up care.[30] Follow-up is essential to ensure resolution of the infection and to obtain imaging studies to determine the presence of renal scarring, posterior urethral valves, and vesicoureteral reflux. Oral antibiotic therapy for infants with febrile UTI (ie, presumed pyelonephritis) should be administered for 10 to 14 days. Antibiotic choice includes cephalosporins, such as cefprozil, cefdinir, or cefixime, or amoxicillin-clavulanate, with cefixime receiving the most formal study.

In older children with simple cystitis, a shorter 3- to 5-day course of antibiotics, such as amoxicillin, amoxicillin-clavulanate, cephalosporins, or trimethoprim-sulfamethoxazole (or a quinolone for patients older than 18 years) should be prescribed. Attention should be paid to local resistance patterns given the marked increase in resistance noted in recent years.

Hypertension

Stage 1 hypertension is defined as a systolic and/or diastolic blood pressure higher than the 95th

percentile for sex, age, and height of the patient. Stage 2 hypertension is defined as 5 mm Hg above the 99th percentile.[31] This diagnosis requires accurately measured blood pressures for several weeks. A correct-sized cuff should be chosen (a bladder width that is 40% of the arm circumference, with a cuff width of two-thirds the length of the upper arm). A child who is in pain or agitated can have falsely elevated blood pressure readings, so additional measurements should be obtained when the patient is more comfortable.

Hypertension can develop throughout childhood in both boys and girls. Primary (essential) hypertension by definition has no underlying identifiable cause. Predisposing factors include obesity, physical inactivity, and strong family history. Secondary hypertension results from endocrinologic, cardiac, neurologic, or other factors, such as certain drugs or poisons. Children with significant hypertension usually have an underlying renal (eg, glomerulonephritis) or renovascular cause.

Clinical Features

Asymptomatic or mildly symptomatic hypertension can be discovered while measuring vital signs in children who are being evaluated for an unrelated illness. On questioning, these children might report headaches, abdominal pain, irritability, or nosebleeds. Sometimes personality changes and difficulties in school are noted.

The distinction between a hypertensive urgency and hypertensive emergency is important. Hypertensive urgencies are considered severe elevations in systolic and/or diastolic blood pressures (patients younger than 10 years—systolic blood pressure of greater than or equal to 160 mm Hg and diastolic blood pressure of greater than or equal to 105 mm Hg; patients older than 10 years—systolic blood pressure of greater than or equal to 170 mm Hg and diastolic blood pressure of greater than or equal to 110 mm Hg) without signs or symptoms of end-organ damage.

Patients with hypertensive emergencies have clinical signs of end-organ damage, such that severe elevation in blood pressure is associated with acute neurologic changes or encephalopathy, pulmonary edema, myocardial ischemia, papilledema, or severe proteinuria. An ECG might show signs of ischemic strain or ventricular hypertrophy. Chest radiographs might reveal cardiomegaly or pulmonary edema. Rapid treatment of a hypertensive emergency is crucial. However, overly aggressive treatment of the long-standing hypertension can produce relative hypotension and lead to worsening neurologic sequelae.

Pertinent historical questions include a previous history of hypertension, UTIs, hematuria, or edema (or umbilical artery catheterization in neonates). A history of joint pain or swelling, palpitations, weight loss, flushing of the skin, drug ingestion, or family history of hypertension is important. The presence of hematuria suggests the possibility of acute glomerulonephritis.

Physical examination should focus on the central nervous system and cardiovascular system. Examination of the optic fundus might reveal papilledema or hemorrhages. Signs of congestive heart failure or a difference in the upper and lower extremity blood pressures (coarctation of the aorta) should be noted. A renal cause for the hypertension is suggested by the presence of peripheral edema (nephrotic syndrome) or palpable kidneys. An abdominal bruit suggests renovascular hypertension.

Symptoms of hypertensive encephalopathy include headache, vomiting, altered mental status, vision disturbances (including blurred vision and diplopia), seizures, and stroke. Papilledema, retinal hemorrhage, and cranial nerve palsies might be found on examination. The diagnosis is confirmed when the symptoms and signs improve rapidly after the blood pressure is lowered. The differential diagnosis of hypertensive encephalopathy includes meningitis, brain tumor, intracerebral hemorrhage, stroke, and uremia.

Diagnostic Studies

In addition to a thorough history and physical examination, laboratory and radiographic studies (usually inpatient) can help determine both the cause of severe hypertension and the presence of a hypertensive emergency. Initial minimal laboratory tests include a CBC count; measurement of electrolytes, BUN, and creatinine; urinalysis; urine culture; radiography; and ECG.

Management

Initial management of severe hypertension begins with the ABCs of resuscitation. Intravenous access should be established if the patient has signs consistent with a hypertensive emergency (eg, end-organ damage by physical examination or laboratory or radiographic results). Continuous blood pressure monitoring is required (an arterial catheter is preferable in severe cases). The initial goal of therapy is to reduce the mean arterial blood pressure by 10% to 20% over several minutes to hours, depending on the nature and extent of the emergency, but usually not more than 25% during the initial 6 to 8 hours. Headache and vomiting require blood pressure control for several hours, whereas intracranial bleeding or herniation requires reduction in several minutes. To avoid overly aggressive treatment and resultant relative hypotension, medications that can be titrated by intravenous infusions are preferred.[28] Commonly used agents include the following: nitroprusside (0.3-0.5 mcg/kg/min; titrate to effect; usual dose is 3 mcg/kg/min; maximum dose is 10 mcg/kg/min), esmolol (load of 100-500 mcg/kg for 1 minute, followed by a maintenance drip of 25-100 mcg/kg per minute), nicardipine (1-3 mcg/kg/min; titrate every 15 minutes), or labetalol (0.2- to 1-mg/kg bolus [maximum dose, 20 mg] or 0.4-1 mg/kg/h [maximum dose, 3 mg/kg/h]). Admission to a pediatric intensive care unit should be arranged.

β-Blockers (esmolol and labetalol) are contraindicated in patients with decreased cardiac output and clinical signs of congestive heart failure. Oral nifedipine is contraindicated in patients with signs of end-organ damage (such as intracerebral bleeding) because of the inability to accurately control the blood pressure reduction.[28]

In patients with hypertensive urgency, an oral antihypertensive agent should be administered to prevent end-organ sequelae. Angiotensin-converting enzyme inhibitors (captopril,

0.3-0.5 mg/kg, given 2-4 times a day; maximum dose, 6 mg/kg/d) or calcium channel blockers (nifedipine, 0.25-0.5 mg/kg/d) are useful first-line agents. The child should be observed for a few hours after administration of the medication to evaluate effectiveness. The child can then be discharged home with a prescription for the agent used to lower the blood pressure with close follow-up care. However, if these medications are unsuccessful in lowering the blood pressure or reducing the symptoms, the patient should be admitted for continued monitoring and further evaluation and therapy.

Children with mildly elevated blood pressures (5-10 mm Hg above normal) unrelated to their presenting complaints require repeated blood pressure measurements before treatment for hypertension is begun. If the blood pressure is moderately elevated and the patient is asymptomatic, the patient can be discharged home for outpatient workup of the hypertension.

Acute Glomerulonephritis

The most common type of glomerulonephritis seen in the United States in children between the ages of 3 and 7 years is acute poststreptococcal glomerulonephritis (PSGN). It is a nonsuppurative complication of infection with strains of nephritogenic *Streptococcus*, which is not generally preventable by antibiotics. There is typically a delay in the onset of nephritis of approximately 8 to 14 days after pharyngitis and 14 to 21 days after a streptococcal skin infection.

Clinical Features

Thirty percent to 50% of patients present with gross hematuria or tea-colored urine. Dependent edema might also be present. Other signs and symptoms include mild to moderate hypertension (50%-90%), pallor, oliguria, nausea, fever, abdominal pain, vomiting, and headache. Less frequent but more severe presentations include pulmonary edema, congestive heart failure, and hypertensive encephalopathy.

Diagnostic Studies

The hallmark of glomerulonephritis is red blood cell casts in freshly spun urine. Hematuria, pyuria, and proteinuria are also present. Blood samples should be evaluated for elevated BUN, creatinine, potassium, and chloride levels, with low sodium, bicarbonate, and albumin levels. Hemoglobin level and platelet counts are typically normal, although dilutional anemia can be present. Cultures of the throat and skin lesions should be obtained for *Streptococcus*. Other laboratory tests to obtain include streptozyme, antistreptolysin O titers (elevated with pharyngitis), anti-DNase B (elevated with pyoderma), antihyaluronidase (elevated), and C3 complement (decreased in 90% of patients in first 2 weeks).

Differential Diagnosis

Other causes of glomerulonephritis include hereditary nephritis, lupus nephritis, IgA nephropathy, HSP nephritis, toxin-mediated nephritis (lead, hydrocarbons, and mercury), and membranoproliferative glomerulonephritis.

Management

Most patients with PSGN should be admitted and undergo nephrology consultation. Most will benefit from diuretic therapy to help control hypertension. Fluid restriction and a low-sodium/low-protein diet are indicated for patients with acute renal insufficiency. Patients with congestive heart failure should be treated with diuretics (furosemide), morphine (0.1 mg/kg), and oxygen, as well as fluid restriction. Hypertension and hypertensive encephalopathy should be treated as outlined earlier. Hyperkalemia can be treated with sodium polystyrene sulfonate (1 g/kg), bicarbonate (1 mEq/kg), calcium gluconate

---

> ## THE CLASSICS
>
> **Diagnostic Findings in Glomerulonephritis**
> - Red blood cell casts on urinalysis
> - Elevated BUN, creatinine, potassium, and chloride levels
> - Decreased sodium, bicarbonate, and albumin levels and complement factors

(100 mg/kg), or glucose and insulin (2-4 mL/kg D25 solution and 0.1 U/kg of insulin).

Nephrotic Syndrome

Hypoalbuminemia, nephrotic range proteinuria, hyperlipidemia, and peripheral edema characterize nephrotic syndrome. Primary nephrotic syndrome applies to diseases limited to the kidney. Secondary nephrotic syndrome results from systemic illnesses such as PSGN. Renal biopsy is used to categorize patients and will determine therapeutic and prognostic decisions when the presentation is not classic.

Between two and seven cases of nephrotic syndrome per 100,000 children are diagnosed each year. Boys are affected twice as often as girls, but this ratio equalizes by adulthood. Primary nephrotic syndrome occurs more commonly in children younger than 5 years, and secondary nephrotic syndrome occurs more often in older children. Of children with nephrotic syndrome, 90% have the primary disease, with 85% having minimal change nephrotic syndrome, 10% focal sclerosis, and 5% mesangial proliferation. The etiology of primary nephrotic syndrome is thought to be idiopathic, but various theories involving bacterial or viral infections, allergic reactions (eg, pollens or poison ivy), and drug ingestion (eg, heroin or mercury) have been implicated.

Clinical Features

Characteristic findings include edema, hypoalbuminemia, proteinuria, and hyperlipidemia. The onset of edema can be insidious and can initially present with only periorbital edema. As a child's weight increases from the retained fluid, parents might report that the child's pants and shoes are tight. The edema continues to progress, but the child usually does not appear ill unless large pleural effusions or ascites are present. Anorexia, nausea, and vomiting can be present as a result of edema of the intestinal wall. Hypertension, hematuria, or oliguria might also occur as the disease progresses. Acute renal failure is rare in primary nephrotic syndrome.

Children with nephrotic syndrome are at some risk for thrombosis due to hemoconcentration, thrombocytosis, hyperfibrinogenemia, and urinary loss of antithrombotic proteins, with up to 2% of nephrotic children having thromboembolic complications. Renal vein thrombosis can cause flank pain, hematuria, and worsening renal function. Children with nephrotic syndrome should not undergo punctures to deep vessels because of this risk of thrombosis. Most cases of typical nephrotic syndrome are treated with corticosteroids. Because of steroid therapy, urinary loss of opsonizing proteins, and decreased levels of immunoglobulins, children with nephrotic syndrome are at risk for bacterial infections of encapsulated organisms (S pneumoniae) and E coli.

Diagnostic Studies

Proteinuria in nephrotic syndrome is defined as more than 3.5 g/1.73 m^2/24 h or greater than 50 mg/kg/24 h (in the absence of gross hematuria). This corresponds to 3+ or 4+ on the dipstick reading. Specific gravity might be high due to the proteinuria. Microscopic hematuria might also be present. Total serum protein level usually is low at 4.5 to 5.5 g/dL, and serum albumin is less than 2 g/dL.

Hyperlipidemia can occur due to the increased serum cholesterol level. Hyponatremia can be present, but other electrolytes are usually normal. Both BUN and creatinine levels are also usually normal, and hemoglobin and hematocrit levels can be elevated due to hemoconcentration.

A chest radiograph might reveal a pleural effusion or pulmonary edema. The heart appears normal or small on chest radiograph due to intravascular hypovolemia. An abdominal radiograph might reveal ascites, and renal ultrasonography can help rule out renal abnormalities. A renal biopsy is important for diagnostic and therapeutic decisions and should be performed in children who present with atypical features: age older than 6 years, evidence of hematuria, low complement, elevated BUN level, persistent hypertension, or failure to respond to steroids.

Differential Diagnosis

Other renal diseases that cause edema include glomerulonephritis and renal failure. A vasculitis or acute thrombosis of the renal vessels must also be considered. The GI causes that produce hypoproteinemia include cirrhosis, cystic fibrosis, and protein-losing enteropathy. In addition, HSP can initially present as scrotal or lower-extremity edema.

Management

Despite the edema, children with signs of hypovolemia or shock should be resuscitated in the usual manner with a crystalloid solution or 25% albumin (possibly followed by intravenous administration of furosemide for signs of pulmonary edema). If the patient is hypertensive, treatment should be initiated as previously outlined in this chapter.

After consultation with a pediatric nephrologist, patients between 12 months and 5 years old with no gross hematuria or atypical features for primary (idiopathic) nephrotic syndrome are treated with corticosteroids (prednisone, 2 mg/kg/24 h, orally divided into doses of either two or three times a day). Relapses or steroid resistance might necessitate a second course of steroids. Diuretics, such as furosemide, might be indicated for respiratory distress or significant ascites. Salt restriction is usually required. Fluid intake should be restricted only if edema is present despite salt restriction or if the child exhibits hyponatremia due to an impaired ability to excrete excess water. The relative immunocompromised state of nephrotic children increases their risk of infection. A fever or signs of peritonitis must be aggressively evaluated. In the presence of ascites, paracentesis should be performed and fluid sent for Gram stain and culture. These children should be admitted and treated with antibiotics.

Syncope

Syncope is a sudden brief loss of consciousness associated with a decrease in muscle tone that usually results from a transient decrease in cerebral blood flow. Most cases of syncope in children are self-limited and benign.[32, 33] The incidence is more common among adolescents, but syncope can be seen at any age.

Clinical Features

By the time the child arrives in the emergency department, the episode of syncope is usually resolved. Therefore, information on most of the clinical features must be obtained from a careful history. Helpful clues are obtained from the circumstances immediately preceding the event (specific activities, environmental factors, and symptoms), the duration of the syncope, the occurrence of premonitory symptoms (eg, dizziness and vision changes), and the symptoms noted during the event (eg, tonic-clonic movements and cyanosis).

Diagnostic Studies

Because the differential diagnosis of syncope can range from benign to life-threatening causes, the initial workup is varied and patient dependent.

Differential Diagnosis

The most important aspect in the evaluation of a child with syncope is differentiating life-threatening and benign events. It is helpful to divide the causes of syncope into three clinical categories: vasovagal (neurocardiogenic), noncardiac, and cardiac.

Vasovagal

Vasovagal (neurocardiogenic) syncope is the most common type of syncope. Often there is a clearly identifiable precipitating event, such as fear, pain, exhaustion, or prolonged standing. The child might feel faint, lightheaded, sweaty, and/or short of breath. The child then briefly loses consciousness and falls forward. During the event, bradycardia usually occurs, associated with the transient hypotension. It is not uncommon for the child to experience a few brief myoclonic jerks immediately after collapsing.

After a short time, the child awakens but might report mild headache, nausea, and/or fatigue. The results of physical examination are unremarkable. Confident diagnosis is dependent on the presence of premonitory symptoms.

Noncardiac

Most noncardiac events are not episodes of true syncope but rather loss of consciousness as an associated symptom. Seizure is usually associated with tonic-clonic movements and incontinence. In contrast to vasovagal syncope episodes, seizures usually have a more prolonged postictal state, and patients do not remember the events immediately preceding the loss of consciousness. Orthostatic syncope can be the result of intercurrent viral illness, dehydration, anemia, drug ingestion, or associated medication use.

Breath-holding spells occur in young children, typically 6 months to 4 years old. The child experiences a sudden fright (such as a minor head injury) or becomes angry (as when a favorite toy is taken away), begins to cry, holds his or her breath, and then passes out, occasionally with a few myoclonic jerks of the extremities that can be easily confused with seizure activity. Breath-holding spells can be pallid (the child's face turns pale) or cyanotic (perioral or facial cyanosis). Although very concerning to the parents and other caregivers, true breath-holding spells are harmless.

Psychiatric (hysterical) syncope usually occurs in front of an audience when children faint and fall gently backward, rarely hurting themselves. Other than hypoglycemia, metabolic causes of syncope are rare. Other noncardiac causes of syncope include pregnancy, hyperventilation, subarachnoid hemorrhage, and situational syncope (venipuncture).

Cardiac

Although uncommon, cardiac causes of syncope are potentially life threatening. Therefore, every evaluation for syncope must involve careful history, physical examination, and evaluation for cardiac causes. Suggestive features include palpitations, tachycardia, chest pain, and syncope associated with exertion. Cardiac causes can be grouped into outflow obstruction (eg, myxoma or critical aortic stenosis), hypertrophic cardiomyopathy, and dysrhythmias (eg, ventricular tachycardia, prolonged QT syndrome, sick sinus syndrome, or Brugada syndrome). Other cardiovascular disorders have been linked to sudden death in young athletes, including hypertrophic cardiomyopathy, congenital coronary artery abnormalities, and commotio cordis.[34]

Management

Initial management is based on the likely diagnoses. Diagnostic testing should be patient specific but can include a serum hemoglobin level, serum glucose level, ECG, and urine pregnancy test (as appropriate). Other tests should be ordered based on history and physical examination findings. If cardiac syncope is suspected, ECG, chest radiograph, troponin measurement, and cardiology consultation should be obtained. Inpatient monitoring, echocardiography, and Holter monitoring might be needed. Evaluation for noncardiac causes might also include electroencephalography and a urine toxicology screening.

KEY POINTS

Management of Syncope

- Complete a thorough history and physical examination.
- Consider obtaining blood for serum hemoglobin and serum glucose measurement.
- Perform an ECG.
- Perform a urine pregnancy test (as appropriate).
- Obtain a cardiology consultation for all children with suspected cardiac syncope.

CHAPTER REVIEW

Check Your Knowledge

1. Which of the following pathogens has been associated with aplastic crises in sickle cell disease?
   A. *Escherichia coli*
   B. *Klebsiella*
   C. Parvovirus B19
   D. *Salmonella typhimurium*

2. Which of the following finding is the best in distinguishing epididymitis from testicular torsion?
   A. Abnormal results on urinalysis in epididymitis
   B. Absence of cremasteric reflex in testicular torsion
   C. Normal or increased vascular flow on Doppler ultrasonography in epididymitis
   D. Normal testicular orientation for epididymitis

3. An 8-month-old boy is brought to the emergency department for evaluation of fever, vomiting, and listlessness. On examination, he is lethargic with a temperature of 39°C (103°F), a weak pulse of 160/min, a respiratory rate of 44/min, and cool, mottled extremities with a capillary refill time of 6 seconds. After evaluation of airway, breathing, and circulation, which of the following is the next step in management?
   A. Administer normal saline bolus intravenously; if the white blood cell (WBC) count is elevated, give parenteral antibiotics.
   B. Attempt to give a rehydration solution orally.
   C. Obtain a blood culture and administer normal saline bolus and antibiotics intravenously.
   D. Obtain a blood culture, attempt lumbar puncture (LP), and then give parenteral antibiotics.

4. A 13-year-old girl is brought to the emergency department on a hot summer morning after she passed out in church. According to bystanders, she was standing when she fainted. By the time the ambulance arrived, she was awake. She has no significant medical history, and the results of her physical examination are normal. Which of the following is the most likely explanation for this event?
   A. Breath-holding spell
   B. Dysrhythmia
   C. Seizure
   D. Vasovagal syncope

References

1. Annane D, Bellissant E, Cavaillon JM. Septic shock. *The Lancet*. 2005;365:63–78.
2. Schexnayder SM. Pediatric septic shock. *Pediatr Rev*. 1999;20:303–308.
3. Pickert CB, Moss MM, Fiser DH. Differentiation of systemic infection and congenital obstructive left heart disease in the very young infant. *Pediatr Emerg Care*. 1998;14:263–267.
4. Carcillo JA, Davis AL, Zaritsky A. Role of early fluid resuscitation in pediatric septic shock. *JAMA*. 1991;266:1242–1245.
5. Ceneviva G, Paschall A, Maffei F, Carcillo JA. Hemodynamic support in fluid-refractory pediatric septic shock. *Pediatrics*. 1998;102:e19.
6. Han YY, Carcillo JA, Dragotta MA, et al. Early reversal of pediatric-neonatal septic shock by community physicians is associated with improved outcome. *Pediatrics*. 2003;112:793–799.
7. Baker MD, Avner JR. The febrile infant: What's new? *Clin Pediatr Emerg Med*. 2008;9:213–220.
8. Pantell RH, Newman TB, Bernzweig J, et al. Management and outcomes of care of fever in early infancy. *JAMA*. 2004;291:1203–1212.
9. ACEP Clinical Policies Committee. Clinical policy for children younger than three years presenting to the emergency department with fever. *Ann Emerg Med*. 2003;42:530–545.
10. Goldman RD, Scolnik D, Chauvin-Kimoff L, et al. Practice variations in the treatment of febrile infants among pediatric emergency physicians. *Pediatrics*. 2009;124:439–445.
11. Baker MD, Bell LM, Avner JR. Outpatient management without antibiotics of fever in selected infants. *N Engl J Med*. 1993;329:1437–1441.
12. Baskin MN, O'Rourke EJ, Fleisher GR. Outpatient treatment of febrile infants 28 to 89 days of age with intramuscular administration of ceftriaxone. *J Pediatr*. 1992;120:22–27.
13. Jaskiewicz JA, McCarthy CA, Richardson AC, et al. Febrile infants at low risk for serious bacterial infection—an appraisal of the Rochester Criteria and implications for management. *Pediatrics*. 1994;94:390–396.

14. Bonsu BK, Harper MB. Utility of the peripheral blood white blood cell count for identifying sick young infants who need lumbar puncture. *Ann Emerg Med.* 2003;41:206–214.

15. Dayan PS, Pan SS, Chamberlain JM. Fever in the immunocompromised host. *Clin Pediatr Emerg Med.* 2000;1:138–149.

16. Klinkhammer MD, Colletti JE. Pediatric myth: Fever and petechiae. *CJEM.* 2008;10:479–482.

17. DiGiulio GA. Fever and petechiae: No time for a rash decision. *Clin Pediatr Emerg Med.* 2000;1:132–137.

18. Thompson MJ, Ninis N, Perera R, et al. Clinical recognition of meningococcal disease in children and adolescents. *The Lancet.* 2006;367:397–403.

19. Givens T. Sickle cell disease. In: Baren J, Rothrock S, Brennan J, et al, eds. *Pediatric Emergency Medicine.* Philadelphia, PA: Saunders; 2008:898–904.

20. American Academy of Pediatrics. Staphylococcal infection. In: Pickering LK, ed. *2009 Red Book: Report of the Committee on Infectious Diseases.* 28th ed. Elk Grove Village, IL: American Academy of Pediatrics; 2009:601–607.

21. Elliott DJ, Zaoutis TE, Troxel AB, Loh A, Keren R. Empiric antimicrobial therapy for pediatric skin and soft-tissue infections in the era of methicillin-resistant *Staphylococcus aureus. Pediatrics.* 2009;123:e959–e966.

22. Somekh E, Gorenstein A, Serour F. Acute epididymitis in boys: evidence of a post-infectious etiology. *J Urol.* 2004;171:391–394.

23. Kadish H. Pediatric surgical emergencies: the tender scrotum. *Clin Pediatr Emerg Med.* 2002;3:5–6.

24. Orden B, Martinez R, Lopez de los Mozos A, Franco A. Balanitis caused by group A beta-hemolytic streptococci. *Pediatr Infect Dis J.* 1996;15:920–921.

25. Shaikh N, Morone NE, Bost JE, Farrell MH. Prevalence of urinary tract infection in childhood: a meta-analysis. *Pediatr Infect Dis J.* 2008;27:302–308.

26. Shaikh N, Ewing AL, Bhatnagar S, Hoberman A. Risk of renal scarring in children with a first urinary tract infection: A systematic review. *Pediatrics.* 2010;126:1084–1091.

27. American Academy of Pediatrics, Committee on Quality Improvement, Subcommittee on Urinary Tract Infection. Practice parameter: The diagnosis, treatment, and evaluation of the initial urinary tract infection in febrile infants and young children. *Pediatrics.* 1999;103:843–852.

28. McCollough M, Sharieff G. Renal and genitourinary tract disorders. In: Marx J, Hockberger R, Walls R, eds. *Rosen's Emergency Medicine Concepts and Clinical Practice.* 7th ed. St Louis, MO: Mosby; 2010:2200–2217.

29. Chang SL, Shortliffe LD. Pediatric urinary tract infections. *Pediatr Clin North Am.* 2006;53:379–400, vi.

30. Schnadower D, Kuppermann N, Macias CG, et al. Febrile infants with urinary tract infections at very low risk for adverse events and bacteremia. *Pediatrics.* 2010;126:1074–1083.

31. National High Blood Pressure Education Program Working Group on High Blood Pressure in Children and Adolescents. The fourth report on the diagnosis and treatment of high blood pressure in children and adolescents. *Pediatrics.* 2004;114;555–576.

32. Willis J. Syncope. *Pediatr Rev.* 2000;21:201–204.

33. Zhang Q, Du J, Wang C, Du Z, Wang L, Tang C. The diagnostic protocol in children and adolescents with syncope: A multi-centre prospective study. *Acta Paediatr.* 2009;98:879–884.

34. Maron BJ. Sudden death in young athletes. *N Engl J Med.* 2003;349:1064–1075.

A previously healthy, 15-month-old boy is brought to the emergency department with a 1-day history of fever and "not acting like himself." He was well until 3 days ago, when he had symptoms of an upper respiratory tract infection. Yesterday he developed a low-grade fever that his mother treated with ibuprofen. Today he has continued fever and decreased oral intake, urine output, and activity level. He has no history of vomiting, diarrhea, cough, or rash. He is not taking any prescription medication.

On physical examination he appears tired and cranky when stimulated. His breathing is not labored, and he is pink. His respirations are 40/min, pulse is 162/min, blood pressure is 92/70 mm Hg, and temperature is 38.9°C (102°F). He has dry lips but moist mucous membranes without oral lesions. His neck is supple. The results of an examination of lungs, heart, abdomen, and extremities are unremarkable. There are a few scattered petechiae on his abdomen and lower extremities. His peripheral pulses are normal, and capillary refill time is 3 seconds.

1. *What is your general impression of this child?*
2. *What are the most likely diagnoses?*
3. *What would be your initial management strategy?*

On presentation, the child is ill-appearing, febrile, tachycardic, and tachypneic, with physical examination results remarkable for scattered petechiae on the abdomen and lower extremities. The primary concern is whether this child is in shock. The tachycardia and slightly delayed capillary refill with a normal peripheral pulse and blood pressure are consistent with compensated shock. Because the child is febrile and has a history of an upper respiratory tract illness with no history of excessive fluid loss, the most likely cause of the shock is sepsis. Any ill-appearing child with fever and petechiae should be assumed to have a serious bacterial illness, most likely meningococcemia. Although patients with many other conditions, such as viral infection (eg, influenza, Enterovirus, infectious mononucleosis, and adenovirus), group A *Streptococcus* infection, or Rocky Mountain spotted fever, can present with fever and petechiae, meningococcal infection is rapidly progressive and life threatening. Initial management begins with 100% oxygen by a nonrebreather mask. As this case developed, continuous pulse oximetry showed an oxygen saturation of 98% with the oxygen therapy. Intravenous access was established, and a blood sample was tested for complete blood cell count, serum electrolytes levels, coagulation times, and blood culture. Rapid bedside glucose determination was 120 mg/dL. An intravenous bolus of normal saline was given in response to evidence of compensated shock. Because the child was tachypneic and had signs of shock, LP was deferred and intravenous antibiotics were administered immediately. The child was admitted to a monitored inpatient unit.

Initial laboratory tests revealed the following: WBC count, 21,000/mcL with 25% band; serum bicarbonate, 11 mEq/L; prothrombin time, 15 seconds; and partial thromboplastin time, 28 seconds. During the next several hours he became more obtunded, developed purpura, had increasing respiratory distress, and had labile blood pressure. He was intubated and intravenous pressors were initiated. His blood culture yielded *N meningitidis*.

chapter 11

Neonatal Emergencies

Chris Colby, MD, FAAP
William Carey, MD, FAAP

Objectives

1 Describe the resuscitation of the newborn.

2 Prepare for transport of the newborn from the emergency department.

Chapter Outline

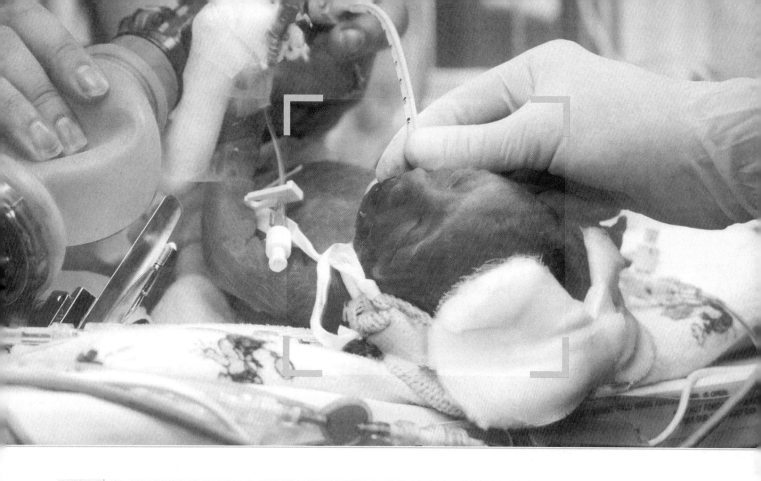

CASE SCENARIO 1

A 25-year-old pregnant woman arrives in your emergency department with frequent uterine contractions every 1 to 2 minutes. She is diaphoretic and anxious yet conversational between contractions but has rapid, pursed-lip respirations during contractions. Vital signs reveal a respiration rate of 20/min, a heart rate of 130/min, a blood pressure of 120/75 mm Hg, and a temperature of 38°C (100.4°F).

1. *What three questions should the patient be asked to predict the need for resuscitation of the newly born?*
2. *What steps should be taken to prepare for the resuscitation of this infant?*

Introduction

The newborn presents unique challenges to health care professionals not familiar with the distinct physiologic characteristics encountered in the neonatal period. This population can present with unique disease processes. The anatomical and physiologic characteristics of the neonate require special consideration during resuscitation and ongoing care.

Historically, the neonatal age group extends from the time of birth to 28 days. The focus of this chapter is the resuscitation of the newborn and preparation of the newborn for transport.

The chapter begins with a review of resuscitation principles, highlighting the differences in neonatal physiologic characteristics that can make resuscitation preparation and procedures unique. In the second part of the chapter, care of the newborn beyond the immediate evaluation and resuscitation period is discussed.

Resuscitation of the Newborn

Approximately 10% of newborns require some assistance to begin breathing at birth. Less than 1% of newborns will require extensive resuscitation to survive. Most newborns will make the transition to extrauterine life with little or no difficulties.[1] Although the percentage of newborns requiring resuscitation is low, the number of births is large; thus, those providing health care in an environment where an expectant mother might deliver must be familiar with the processes required for successful resuscitation.

Preparation for Delivery

Resuscitation-Oriented History

Before the ultimate delivery of the newborn, it is useful to obtain a limited obstetrical history to help you anticipate the requirements of the resuscitation (Table 11-1). Questions that should be asked during the history are as follows:

1. How many newborns are going to be delivered? If multiple newborns are expected, preparation for each infant must be made, including setting up multiple resuscitation areas, each stocked with appropriate equipment, and establishing a resuscitation team for each newborn.

2. How far along in pregnancy are you? If the mother states that she is about to deliver a premature infant and time permits, serious consideration should be given to notify available resources (a neonatal resuscitation team) if available at your hospital. If the mother is going to deliver a newborn at the margin of viability, immediate consultation with a local neonatologist will be helpful. The potential complexity of the resuscitation of the neonate increases with decreasing gestational age, and decisions about viability are often difficult and require neonatal expertise.

3. What color is the amniotic fluid? Green color of the amniotic fluid signifies the passage of meconium in utero. Meconium-stained amniotic fluid is observed in approximately 12% of all deliveries. Risk factors for passage of in utero meconium include small for gestational age, postmature infants, and those with

umbilical cord complications.[2] Despite the common observation of meconium staining of the amniotic fluid, meconium aspiration syndrome can occur as infrequently as in 4% of newborns born through meconium-stained amniotic fluid.[3] Recognition of meconium-stained amniotic fluid will guide your initial steps of resuscitation.

TABLE 11-1 Brief Resuscitation History

Question	Implication
How many newborns are you going to deliver?	More than one newborn will require additional equipment and staff.
How far along in pregnancy are you?	If the newborn is premature, consider calling for neonatal expertise.
What color is your amniotic fluid?	If meconium is present, follow resuscitation guidelines accordingly.

Anticipation

The obstetric history and fetal heart monitoring can lend valuable information as you prepare for the resuscitation of the newborn. Once the three key questions for planning for neonatal resuscitation have been asked, if time permits, further history can be valuable. Significant anatomical abnormalities on prenatal ultrasonography can help you anticipate the level of resuscitation that will be required. Some anatomical malformations identified on prenatal ultrasonography include congenital heart disease, spina bifida, gastroschisis, omphalocele, and congenital diaphragmatic hernia. If there is concern about the infant having a major malformation, consultation with a local neonatologist is advised. The well-being of the fetus as reflected by fetal heart rate monitoring can also guide your level of concern and preparation. A fetus who is exhibiting significant late decelerations might have hypoxemia and acidosis that will need to be addressed once delivered. Maternal well-being is also important to consider. A mother with diabetes is at increased risk for delivering an infant who is large for his or her gestational age who is at risk for hypoglycemia. A mother who is febrile, has a tender uterus and/or foul smelling discharge, and has a fetus who is tachycardic will likely deliver an infant who will need to be evaluated and treated for suspected neonatal sepsis. If narcotics are given to the laboring mother for analgesia during delivery, the infant will be at risk of respiratory depression.

Preparation of Equipment

Gathering and preparing the necessary equipment before delivery will facilitate a successful resuscitation (Table 11-2).

Environment

The first thing to identify is where the newborn will be placed once delivery has occurred. Ideally, this would be on a radiant warmer that provides the newborn with an exogenous source of heat. More commonly, the newborn can be placed on an examining table or crib sufficient for evaluation and resuscitation, ensuring that the wet newborn is kept warm and does not fall. Temperature maintenance can be facilitated with warm blankets and dry towels and warming the temperature of the room if possible, particularly if the newborn is anticipated to be preterm.

Efforts to evaluate and resuscitate the newborn in close proximity to an oxygen source and suction will enhance the ability to provide optimal care. Additional equipment that might be necessary includes a blended oxygen source with the ability to provide oxygen concentrations from room air to 100% and an oxygen saturation monitor with a probe that should be placed on the newborn's right wrist or hand to measure the oxygen saturation of preductal blood.

Airway Management

If there is evidence of airway obstruction or positive pressure ventilation is required, it will be necessary to clear the airway. Equipment that can be used includes a bulb syringe or wall suction device and a number of commercially available suction catheters appropriately sized for the newborn's mouth and upper airway. If the newborn requires positive pressure ventilation (PPV), an appropriately sized face mask connected to a device capable of delivering PPV will be needed. These devices include an infant-sized self-inflating bag, a flow inflating bag, or mechanical resuscitator or ventilator. If the newborn requires endotracheal intubation, appropriately sized laryngoscope blades and endotracheal tubes will be needed. For the newborn with difficult airway access, a laryngeal mask airway can offer airway support if bag-mask ventilation is ineffective and endotracheal intubation is difficult. The smallest size of laryngeal mask airway devices currently available restricts their use primarily to infants greater than approximately 2.0 kg.

An exhaled carbon dioxide detector is recommended to confirm appropriate placement of an endotracheal tube. The endotracheal tube should be secured in place at the correct depth of insertion. A special consideration is the need for a meconium aspirator for the infant who requires airway clearance beyond the vocal cords.

TABLE 11-2 Equipment for Neonatal Resuscitation

Environment
- Radiant warmer, crib, examination table
- Heat source, blankets, towels
- Increase room temperature if feasible

Oxygen administration and monitoring
- Source for adjustable blended oxygen (room air to 100%)
- Oxygen saturation monitoring
- Neonatal oxygen saturation probe to place on right wrist or hand

Airway management
- Suction source (bulb suction, suction catheters)
- Appropriately sized facial masks for bag-mask ventilation
- Source for positive pressure ventilation (self-inflating bag, flow inflating bag, T-piece Resuscitator or ventilator)
- Appropriately sized laryngoscope blade (00, 0, 1 Miller blade)
- Appropriately sized endotracheal tubes (2.5, 3.0, 3.5, 4.0)
- Laryngeal mask airway
- Exhaled carbon dioxide detector or monitor
- Tape
- Stethoscope

Healthy Newborn

The term gestation newborn who has good muscle tone and activity level and is breathing spontaneously should receive routine care. Universal suctioning of the newborn's mouth once delivered is no longer considered mandatory.[4] It is recommended that suctioning immediately after birth should be reserved for newborns who have obvious obstruction to spontaneous breathing or require ventilatory support with positive pressure. Newborns are born wet and will experience heat loss rapidly in the absence of a heat source. For the vigorous, well-appearing infant, this could be prevented by allowing the infant, once dried off, to be held by the mother skin to skin. Ongoing evaluation of risk factors (potential infection, stable blood glucose) should be pursued. Stimulating a newborn can include slapping or flicking of the soles of the feet or gentle rubbing of the newborn's back, trunk, or extremities during the drying process. Delayed cord clamping for longer than 30 seconds is reasonable for those term and preterm infants who do not require resuscitation.[4a]

The Newborn Requiring Assessment and Intervention

The premature newborn or term newborn who has poor respiratory effort or decreased tone should have a comprehensive evaluation of clinical stability. This newborn should be brought to the area that you prepared for neonatal evaluation

Immediate Care of the Newborn

Primary Assessment

Most newborns transition to extrauterine life without significant distress. Once born, all newborns require an assessment of risk for requiring resuscitation. The primary assessment of a newborn includes an evaluation of the infant's respiratory effort and muscle tone (**Figure 11.1** and Table 11-3).

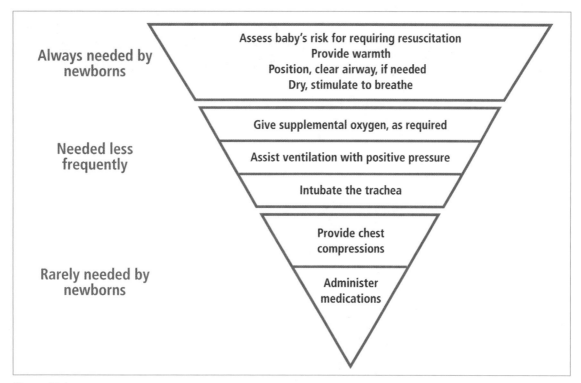

Figure 11.1 The neonatal resuscitation pyramid lists practices when caring for any infant and practices that are only needed in the context of resuscitation.

Kattwinkel J, ed. *Textbook of Neonatal Resuscitation, 6th ed.* Elk Grove Village, IL: American Academy of Pediatrics and American Heart Association; 2011: 3. Reprinted with permission.

TABLE 11-3 **Critical Assessment of the Newborn Immediately After Delivery**
1. Term gestation?
2. Breathing or crying?
3. Good tone?

and resuscitation. During transfer, it is essential to support the newborn's head. There must be careful placement and attention to the position of the head and neck. The correct position of the newborn's head and neck is slight extension in the "sniffing" position. Hyperextension or flexion of the neck should be avoided (**Figure 11.2**).

The initial evaluation of the newborn should include an assessment of the newborn's respiratory effort, muscle tone, and heart rate. If there is decreased respiratory effort (gasping, apnea) or if the heart rate is less than 100/min, the newborn should have the airway cleared and positive pressure ventilation initiated. If an infant has labored breathing or persistent cyanosis, the airway should be positioned and cleared, and supplementary oxygen given as needed.

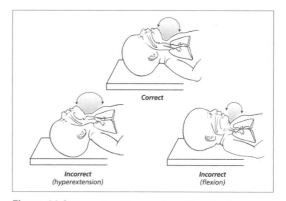

Figure 11.2 Correct and incorrect positions for the newborn's head.

Kattwinkel J, ed. *Textbook of Neonatal Resuscitation, 6th ed.* Elk Grove Village, IL: American Academy of Pediatrics and American Heart Association; 2011: 41. Reprinted with permission.

During these interventions, if respiratory support or supplemental oxygen is considered necessary, a team member should place a pulse oximetry probe on the newborn's right hand or wrist to enhance monitoring oxygen saturation and heart rate. Application of an oxygen saturation probe can take up to 2 minutes and might not function well during poor cardiac output. Direct auscultation of the precordium or palpation of the heart rate by gently squeezing the base of the umbilicus can also provide additional heart rate data (Table 11-4).

The Neonatal Resuscitation Algorithm–2015 Update serves as a useful tool for further assessment of the newborn (**Figure 11.3**).

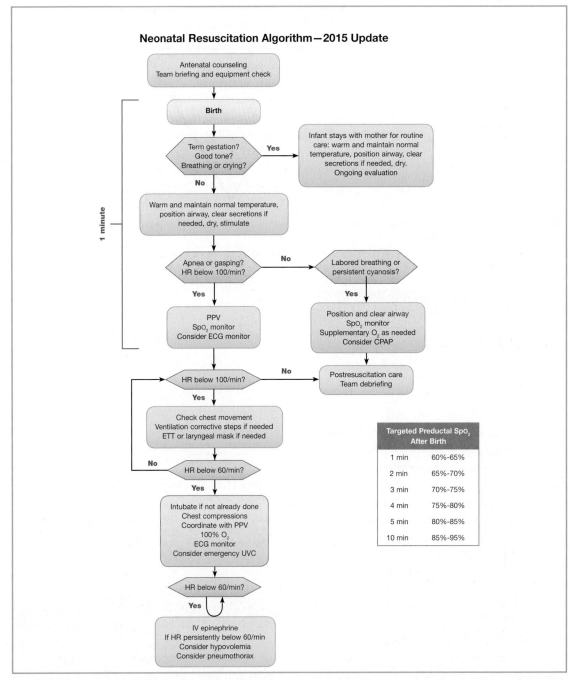

Figure 11.3 The Neonatal Resuscitation Algorithm–2015 Update.

Reprinted with permission. *Circulation.* 2015; 132:S543-S560. © 2015 American Heart Association, Inc.

Oxygenation Assessment

Included in the *Textbook of Neonatal Resuscitation* 6th edition resuscitation algorithm is a table that indicates the target preductal (right hand) oxygen saturation in newborns. The uncompromised term newborn will transition from fetal circulation to extrauterine circulation during the first 10 minutes of life. It is normal for the uncompromised newborn to have an oxygen saturation in the range of 60% to 70% in the first minute of life. During this transition in circulation, using patient color as an assessment of the newborn's well-being is unreliable.

There is a growing body of literature that supports the harmful effect of either insufficient or excessive oxygen delivery to the newborn. To properly assess the need for supplemental oxygen or whether the resuscitation of the newborn will involve the administration of supplemental oxygen or PPV, an oxygen saturation probe should be placed on the right wrist or surface of the right palm.

It is recommended that the saturation of newborns being resuscitated at birth be targeted at the mean preductal saturations demonstrated by healthy term newborns after vaginal birth at sea level. Achievement of such targets can best be achieved by administering an adjustable blend of oxygen and air titrated to established preductal normal values. If blended oxygen is not available, resuscitation should begin with air (21% oxygen) for term infants. For preterm infants (<35 wk), resuscitation should be initiated with low oxygen concentration (21 to 30% oxygen) titrated to achieve preductal oxygen saturation.[4a] If oximetry is not available, the concentration of oxygen should be adjusted to achieve relief of cyanosis and correction of bradycardia. Bradycardia will generally require PPV and will not improve with supplemental oxygen alone (Table 11-5).

Positive Pressure Ventilation

If the infant requires resuscitation beyond warming, drying, stimulation, and clearance of the airway, the algorithm suggests application of PPV. Effective PPV requires the selection and placement of the appropriately sized facial mask (**Figure 11.4**).

The primary indicator of effective PPV resuscitation is improvement in heart rate. If no improvement in heart rate is observed

TABLE 11-5 Indications for Oxygen Saturation Monitoring
1. Resuscitation is anticipated based on risk factors (eg, prematurity).
2. PPV is administered for more than a few breaths.
3. Cyanosis is persistent.
4. Supplemental oxygen is administered.

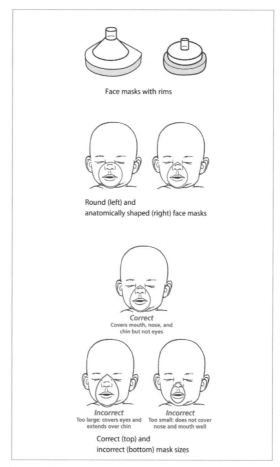

Figure 11.4 Correct and incorrect mask sizes and placement.

Kattwinkel J, ed. *Textbook of Neonatal Resuscitation*, 6th ed. Elk Grove Village, IL: American Academy of Pediatrics and American Heart Association; 2011: 88. Reprinted with permission.

during positive pressure, assessment of chest rise is recommended. The initial peak inspiratory pressure is variable. Some newborns will experience an improvement in heart rate and chest rise with peak inspiratory pressures of 20 cm H_2O, whereas other compromised apneic term newborns can require up to 40 cm H_2O to establish effective ventilation. The initial assisted ventilation rate recommended for newborns is between 40 and 60/min. For preterm infants, the use of 5 cm H_2O PEEP is suggested when PPV is needed.

Troubleshooting Ineffective PPV

Despite application of a facial mask and positive pressure assisted ventilation, the newborn might not respond to this intervention. It is important to remember a number of factors that can contribute to ineffective ventilation (no improvement in heart rate or chest rise) (Table 11-6).

TABLE 11-6 Troubleshooting Ineffective Ventilation

1. Is the mask appropriately sized and positioned correctly?
2. Is there a tight seal between the mask and face?
3. Is there airway obstruction?
4. Is the head positioned slightly hyperextended?
5. Is adequate pressure being delivered?
6. Does the self-inflating bag have a PEEP valve?

Laryngeal Mask Airway

A laryngeal mask airway (LMA) has been shown to be effective for assisted ventilation of newborns who weigh more than 2 kg or are delivered at 34 weeks' gestation or later.[5–7] The appropriately sized device in this population is a size 1 neonatal. Laryngeal mask airways have not been studied for the use during the resuscitation of the newborn delivered through meconium-stained amniotic fluid or for the administration of medications into the trachea. However, there are indications for the use of LMA in this population:

- Congenital anomalies involving the mouth, lip, or palate resulting in difficulties in obtaining a proper seal with face mask ventilation (eg, cleft lip or palate).
- Anomalies of the mouth, tongue, pharynx, or neck where there is difficulty visualizing the larynx with a laryngoscope (eg, cystic hygroma of neck or Beckwith-Wiedemann syndrome and macroglossia).
- A very small mandible or relatively large tongue (eg, Robin sequence).
- PPV provided by bag and mask is ineffective and attempts at intubation are not feasible or are unsuccessful.

Endotracheal Tube Placement

Endotracheal intubation might be indicated during neonatal resuscitation. Indications for endotracheal intubation are included in the NRP resuscitation algorithm. In addition, if the newborn requires prolonged mask ventilation or was born nonvigorous through thick meconium, endotracheal intubation is recommended. Meconium should be suctioned from the trachea, using an endotracheal tube and meconium aspirator, if the newborn is meconium stained, is nonvigorous, or has a persistent bradycardia.

Selecting the appropriately sized endotracheal tube is essential for successful and safe insertion. The proper tube size and insertion depth are dependent on the newborn's birth weight and gestational age (Table 11-7).

TABLE 11-7 Endotracheal Tube Size for Infants of Various Weights and Gestational Ages

Weight (grams)	Gestational Age (weeks)	Tube Size (Inside Diameter mm)
<1,000	<28	2.5
1,000–2,000	28–34	3.0
2,000–3,000	34–38	3.5
>3,000	>38	3.5–4.0

Kattwinkel J, ed. *Textbook of Neonatal Resuscitation 6th ed.* Elk Grove Village, IL: American Academy of Pediatrics and American Heart Association; 2011: 165. Reprinted with permission.

Similar to assisted PPV with mask and bag, an improvement in heart rate is the best indicator that the endotracheal tube is in the proper position and effective ventilation is occurring. Tracheal intubation is best confirmed with exhaled carbon dioxide detection. Cyclical rise of condensation in the endotracheal tube, chest rise, and auscultation of symmetric breath sounds are also helpful signs.

Intubation of the newborn can be a high-acuity, low-frequency event at certain locations. If the practitioner is unfamiliar with the unique challenges of intubating a newborn, airway backup should be called for, and effort should certainly be focused on providing effective PPV with face mask and device instead of spending time unsuccessfully placing an endotracheal tube. Placement of an LMA can be helpful in larger newborns.

Chest Compressions

If the heart rate remains below 60/min despite adequate PPV, chest compressions are recommended. It is important to reinforce that before initiation of chest compressions, practitioners should ensure that assisted ventilation is being delivered optimally. The preferred technique in the newborn for delivery of higher peak systolic pressures and coronary perfusion pressure is the two-thumb technique. This technique involves encircling the newborn's torso with both hands. The thumbs are placed on the sternum and the fingers are placed under the infant's back, supporting the spine. The thumbs can be placed side by side or, on a small infant, one over the other (**Figure 11.5**).

Compressions and ventilations should be coordinated to avoid simultaneous delivery. The chest should be permitted to fully reexpand during relaxation. There should be a 3:1 ratio of compressions to ventilations with 90 compressions and 30 breaths to achieve approximately 120 events per minute to maximize ventilation at an achievable rate. It is recommended that 3:1 be used for neonatal resuscitation, but rescuers should consider using higher ratios (15:2) when the arrest is believed to be of cardiac origin.

Medications

Epinephrine (Adrenaline)

There are indications within the NRP algorithm for the administration of epinephrine (adrenaline). It is important to remember that most cases of bradycardia in the newborn are secondary to inadequate lung inflation or hypoxemia. If these interventions are ineffective at improving the heart rate, administration of epinephrine (adrenaline) might be warranted.

The preferred route of administration of epinephrine (adrenaline) is intravenous. If it appears that the infant might need epinephrine (adrenaline), the practitioner should obtain venous access, usually by cannulating the umbilical vein. If administration of epinephrine (adrenaline) is indicated before obtaining venous access, an endotracheal dose can be administered. The dose of endotracheal epinephrine (adrenaline) of 0.05 to 0.1 mg/kg is recommended. This is a higher dose than had previously been recommended and remains higher than the recommended intravenous dose. Once venous access has been obtained, epinephrine (adrenaline) can be given with a recommended dose of 0.01 to 0.03 mg/kg per dose. The concentration of epinephrine (adrenaline) for either route should be 1:10,000 (0.1 mg/mL).

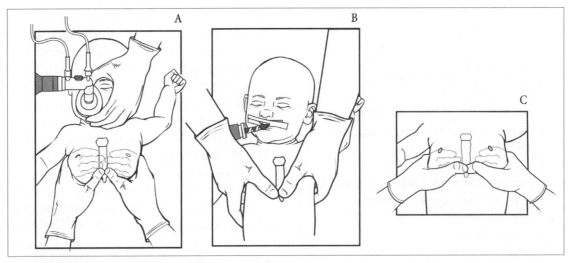

Figure 11.5 Thumb technique of chest compressions administered from the bottom (A), from the top (B), and for small chests, with thumbs overlapped (C).

Kattwinkel J, ed. *Textbook of Neonatal Resuscitation, 6th ed.* Elk Grove Village, IL: American Academy of Pediatrics and American Heart Association; 2011: 139. Reprinted with permission.

Volume Expansion

If the newborn has not responded to other resuscitation efforts or if the patient is hypotensive with poor perfusion, volume expansion with normal saline or blood can be considered. The starting dose is 10 mL/kg and can be repeated.

Special Considerations

Meconium-Stained Amniotic Fluid

Passage of meconium while in utero can contribute to meconium aspiration syndrome with dark, viscous material aspirated into the terminal airspaces. The approach to the newborn delivered through meconium-stained amniotic fluid has evolved over time. The current recommendation is that if a newborn is delivered through meconium-stained amniotic fluid and has poor tone and respiratory effort at birth, the initial steps of resuscitation should occur under the radiant warmer. If the heart rate is less than 100 bpm or the infant is not breathing, positive pressure ventilation should be initiated. Routine intubation for tracheal suctioning is not recommended.[4a]

Induced Hypothermia

Several trials of hypothermia of newborns of 36 weeks' gestation and later with moderate to severe hypoxic ischemic encephalopathy revealed that the newborns who were cooled within the first 6 hours of life had significantly less death and neurodevelopmental disability at 18-month follow-up.[8-10] If a newborn requires extensive resuscitation and has low Apgar scores during resuscitation, prompt consultation with a local tertiary care neonatal intensive care unit would be appropriate to decide whether hypothermia treatment should be initiated.

Discontinuing Resuscitative Efforts

In a newborn with an Apgar score of 0 after 10 minutes of resuscitation and no detectable heart rate, it may be reasonable to stop assisted ventilation; however, the decision to continue resuscitation efforts beyond 10 minutes should take into consideration factors such as the presumed cause of the arrest, the gestation of the newborn, the presence or absence of complications, the potential role of therapeutic hypothermia, and the parents' consent and request for continued resuscitation.[4a]

Preparing the Newborn for Transfer From the Emergency Department

Once the primary assessment and resuscitation of a newborn have been stabilized in the emergency department, steps must be taken to maintain the infant's stability before and during transfer to an appropriate nursery. Whether the newborn is healthy and full term or exhibits symptoms and signs warranting intensive care, one must consider the basic needs of a newborn for an appropriate degree of warmth and an adequate delivery of glucose and fluids. For infants who require resuscitation or who show signs of instability after delivery, infectious disease should be suspected and treated expeditiously. Jaundice can be identified at birth or in a days-old newborn who presents for evaluation in the emergency department, so familiarity with basic principles of management is essential. Umbilical vascular catheter placement and thoracostomy drainage of a pneumothorax are sometimes required in the treatment of the critically ill newborn.

Temperature

Although there is no consensus for what temperature should be considered "normal" for a newborn infant, there are published ranges that practitioners can use to guide their postresuscitation care of the newborn in the emergency department. The American Academy of Pediatrics recommends that an axillary temperature of 36.5° to 37.4°C (97.7° to 99.3°F) should be obtained to safely discharge an infant home,[11] so this range could be considered a safe and acceptable range to target when preparing a newborn for transfer. Measurement of the temperature in the central axilla with the arm held to the infant's side allows for rapid and easy measurement of the temperature without the risks associated with rectal measurements.

Maintaining the temperature of a well, term, or near-term newborn consists of replacing the wet linens used during the resuscitation with warmed, dry linens. Swaddling the newborn from the level of the shoulders down protects the newborn from heat loss while keeping the face free of obstructions. An appropriately sized cap can be placed over the head to limit heat loss. For those newborns who require frequent assessment and intervention, continuous visible assessment of the skin must be countered with any of several measures to limit heat loss. Careful attention to drying the exposed newborn will limit evaporative heat loss. Increasing the ambient temperature of the newborn resuscitation room and limiting drafts will minimize convective heat loss. Periodic replacement of cold linens with warmed linens can prevent some degree of conductive heat loss, and a radiant source of heat can mitigate radiant heat loss as well.

Glucose

The energy needs of a newborn reflect a balance between energy expenditure and energy stores on which the infant can draw. Factors that increase energy expenditure (eg, thermogenesis in response to cold stress, increased metabolic rate in the setting of sepsis) and certain characteristics of the newborn (eg, small for gestational age, prematurity) can be present in a newborn delivered in the emergency department, so it is essential for emergency personnel to identify and manage these problems appropriately. Providing intravenous dextrose is often sufficient to overcome the deficits present in a newborn, so a basic knowledge of neonatal glucose needs is helpful in preparing for these emergencies.

Glucose is the principal energy source for the fetus and newborn, with most neonates consuming glucose at a rate of 4 to 8 mg/kg per minute.[12] In neonates, most of circulating glucose is consumed by the brain, so prompt provision of exogenous glucose is essential to optimize a newborn's chance for normal neurodevelopment. For any newborn that requires an advanced level of care, placement of a peripheral intravenous catheter should be followed by the administration of dextrose sufficient to meet the typical needs of a newborn. For example, a simple 10% dextrose solution run at 4 mL/kg per hour would provide a dextrose infusion rate of approximately 7 mg/kg per minute. Fluids can be titrated to maintain a blood glucose level in the normal range. If the newborn is noted to be hypoglycemic, a bolus of 2 mL/kg of 10% dextrose is indicated, and an increase in the basal glucose delivery should be considered. A repeat blood glucose measurement should be obtained with accompanying interventions until the newborn's glucose level is normal.

Fluids

The fluid and electrolyte requirements of the newborn are different from those of older infants, children, and adults. At the time of birth, the newborn possesses a store of excess extracellular fluid, which during the first few days of life is excreted in an isotonic diuresis. Thus, the provision of dextrose-containing fluids must be tempered by the need to promote the negative fluid and electrolyte balance that is a normal aspect of transitional newborn physiologic characteristics. Unlike fluids provided to older infants and children, the maintenance intravenous fluid provided to most newborns should not contain sodium chloride—a simple solution of 10% dextrose would be most appropriate via a peripheral vein. If a peripheral intravenous catheter is the only site available for fluid administration, the rate of 10% dextrose infusion can be increased incrementally or the dextrose concentration could be increased up to 12.5%, a safe upper limit for peripheral veins. Fluids containing higher concentrations of dextrose must be administered into a central vein, preferably via an umbilical venous catheter.

Hypotension in the newborn is rarely due to hypovolemia, and there is little evidence to suggest that bolus volume infusion is an effective treatment for hypotension in newborns who require resuscitation.[13] However, bolus infusions of 10 mL/kg of normal saline can be used cautiously, depending on a practitioner's clinical assessment and the newborn's diagnosis. For example, one might expect considerable volume loss in a newborn with gastroschisis, in which case supplemental volume infusions could be used to treat suspected hypovolemia. For more careful assessment of volume status, central venous pressures can be transduced through an umbilical venous catheter, although this information should be interpreted with the assistance of an expert in neonatal care.

Infection

Newborns of any gestational age are at high risk for infectious diseases due to pathogens acquired in utero, during the delivery process, or later in the neonatal period. There are risk factors that increase the likelihood of infection in the newborn (eg, prematurity, maternal infection), and these can be elucidated from the maternal medical and obstetric history and newborn physical examination. Acute infectious disease in the newborn most often is caused by bacterial pathogens, the identity of which can be suspected based on the timing of presentation. Perinatal viral infections also can present acutely in the newborn, so these less common but aggressive pathogens must be considered.

Early-onset bacterial sepsis is generally considered to occur during the first 3 days of life. Term infants account for most cases, but the likelihood of infection is greater in premature infants. Gram-negative bacteria now account for most early-onset infections, although the gram-positive group B *Streptococcus* remains another common pathogen. These infections can present in a florid manner with circulatory, respiratory, and neurologic signs, but many newborns present initially with limited, nonspecific symptoms (eg, lethargy or intermittent apnea). As a consequence, careful review of the maternal history and critical assessment of the neonate in the emergency department is essential to prevent undiagnosed and untreated early-onset sepsis. Any risk factor or sign of infection should prompt the physician to order a complete blood cell count with differential white blood cell count, blood culture, and lumbar puncture with cerebrospinal fluid differential cell count, chemical analyses, and culture. Radiography of the chest should be ordered to assess for pneumonia. Parenteral antibiotic therapy with ampicillin and gentamicin should be instituted without delay and, when indicated, can precede the blood culture if obtaining an adequate blood sample proves difficult.

Late-onset bacterial sepsis occurs beyond the third day of life and most often is caused by gram-negative rods and group B *Streptococcus*. These infections are more likely to present with variable symptoms, but a fulminant presentation can be seen as well. The diagnostic workup includes the above laboratory and radiographic studies but, in addition, urine samples should be obtained for analysis and culture. In late-onset bacterial disease in particular, the urinary tract can be the primary site of bacterial infection or it can be secondarily infected after hematogenous spread of the pathogen. In either case, the pathogen and its antibiotic sensitivity profile can be identified rapidly from the urine. Collection of the urine sample should occur under sterile conditions via urethral catheterization or suprapubic aspiration and not by bag collection (because of the possibility of contamination). As with early-onset sepsis, ampicillin and gentamicin are appropriate for empiric antibiotic coverage.

Perinatal or congenital viral infections can present with profound circulatory, respiratory, and neurologic compromise in the newborn. Although these are most often acquired in utero or during parturition, affected neonates typically do not present until late in the first week of life. Although several viruses are known pathogens in neonates, herpes simplex virus (HSV) merits special consideration in this chapter. Neonates with systemic HSV are by far most likely to have acquired their infection during delivery from a mother with a primary HSV outbreak. As a consequence, there might be no history of prior maternal HSV infection, or the mother might report that vesicles were identified at the time of delivery. Systemic HSV in the neonate must be considered based on the timing and mode of presentation (common signs include fever, seizures, and cardiorespiratory compromise). The virus can be detected in many bodily fluids, including blood, urine, and cerebrospinal fluid, and culture of conjunctivae, nasopharynx, and rectum can yield virus as well. Prompt provision of parenteral acyclovir is essential in suspected cases and, as is the case with antibacterial agents, initiation of therapy should not be delayed in the event that diagnostic samples have been difficult to obtain. To prevent spread of the virus to health care workers in the emergency department, contact isolation should be instituted in cases of suspected disseminated HSV infection.

Jaundice

Approximately half of all term neonates are jaundiced to some degree during the first week of life. Most of these neonates are well, with levels of unconjugated bilirubin that pose no threat to their neurodevelopment. Nevertheless, any neonate presenting to the emergency department for evaluation of jaundice must be carefully assessed by history, physical examination, and laboratory studies to ensure that pathologic jaundice is not present.

Historical findings that would suggest that a neonate is at risk for unsafe levels of unconjugated bilirubin include excessive weight loss or inadequate weight gain since the time birth, poor feeding per parental report, and limited urine or stool output. A physical examination revealing signs of dehydration or infection, pallor (suggesting hemolysis), or depressed sensorium should prompt the clinician to suspect that an infant's jaundice can be pathologic and not an incidental finding. More so than historical or physical examination findings, however, laboratory evaluation is of critical importance in assessing jaundice in the neonate.

Laboratory testing of the jaundiced neonate must include both total and direct serum bilirubin levels. Although it is the unconjugated (indirect) form of bilirubin that is associated with bilirubin encephalopathy or kernicterus, it is important to exclude hepatobiliary causes of jaundice by assessing the conjugated (direct) fraction of serum bilirubin. The American Academy of Pediatrics has established guidelines for managing total serum bilirubin levels in term and near-term neonates, and this tool is valuable when deciding whether or when a neonate must be seen again by a clinician or whether inpatient hospitalization would be required for phototherapy and additional laboratory studies (**Figure 11.6**).[14] Unless this information is already available to the emergency department clinician, the blood type of both the mother and neonate should be determined and a direct antiglobulin (Coombs) test performed on the neonate's blood. This information, coupled with the neonate's hematocrit, can provide evidence that hemolysis is contributing to the jaundice. In such cases, consultation with a local expert in neonatal care is recommended.

Umbilical Vascular Catheter Placement

Placement of umbilical vascular catheters can be indicated in the treatment of a newborn who presents to the emergency department in critical condition. Although knowledge of these procedures is essential for emergency department clinicians, it is recommended that clinicians seek consultation with a local neonatologist or an in-hospital pediatrician before performing these procedures if time permits.

The umbilical vasculature is composed of one vein and two arteries. The vein can be identified by its thin wall and larger diameter, whereas the arteries are small, thick-walled vessels, which most often are tightly constricted on inspection. Catheterization of the umbilical vein permits access to the central venous system, with the tip of the catheter coursing through the portal sinus, ductus venous, and inferior vena cava to its ideal location in the right atrium. A catheter placed in the umbilical artery would pass through the internal iliac artery from which the umbilical artery originates before it ultimately is located in the descending aorta. Either of two locations of the umbilical artery catheter tip would be appropriate: between the sixth and ninth thoracic vertebrae (a "high line") or between the third and fourth lumbar vertebrae (a "low line") (**Figure 11.7**).

Although the above information is helpful in identifying what is ideal for umbilical vessel catheter placement, it is much more likely that an emergency department clinician would need to obtain emergency vascular access for the administration of fluids or medications. In the event that peripheral venous access cannot be obtained, the umbilical vein can be rapidly and safely catheterized by a skilled clinician. After sterilizing the base of the umbilical cord

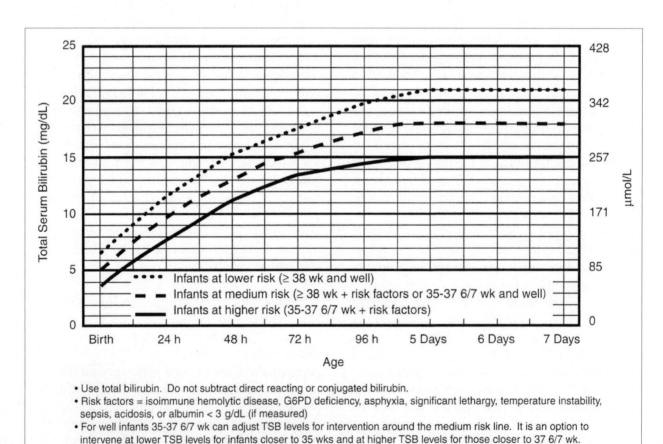

- Use total bilirubin. Do not subtract direct reacting or conjugated bilirubin.
- Risk factors = isoimmune hemolytic disease, G6PD deficiency, asphyxia, significant lethargy, temperature instability, sepsis, acidosis, or albumin < 3 g/dL (if measured)
- For well infants 35-37 6/7 wk can adjust TSB levels for intervention around the medium risk line. It is an option to intervene at lower TSB levels for infants closer to 35 wks and at higher TSB levels for those closer to 37 6/7 wk.
- It is an option to provide conventional phototherapy in hospital or at home at TSB levels 2-3 mg/dL (35-50mmol/L) below those shown but home phototherapy should not be used in any infant with risk factors.

Figure 11.7 Management of hyperbilirubinemia in the newborn.

Reproduced with permission from *Pediatrics*, Volume 114, Page 297, Copyright 2004 by the American Academy of Pediatrics.

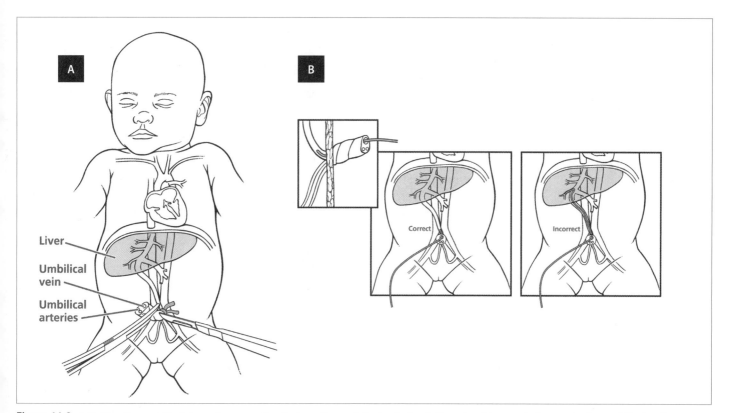

Figure 11.8 A. Cutting the umbilical stump in preparation for inserting umbilical catheter. B. Correct and incorrect placement of an umbilical catheter.

Kattwinkel J, ed. *Textbook of Neonatal Resuscitation, 6th ed.* Elk Grove Village, IL: American Academy of Pediatrics and American Heart Association; 2011: 215-216. Reprinted with permission.

or stump and the surrounding skin, a sterile tie should be firmly tightened around the base of the cord. The cord stump should be cut horizontally with a scalpel, with careful attention to avoid lacerating the skin at the base of the cord, to expose the umbilical vessels. Once the umbilical vein is visualized, a saline-flushed catheter of appropriate size can be inserted just a few centimeters below the cut surface of the cord until blood return is documented on drawing back on the syringe. With the catheter in place, maintenance or bolus fluids and emergency medications can be safely administered. The catheter should be secured to the non-skin portion of the umbilical cord (known as Wharton jelly) with a suture as soon as is permissible.

Thoracostomy Drainage of a Pneumothorax

Pneumothorax is a known complication of neonatal resuscitation and can be due to anatomical or physiologic characteristics of the neonate or the manner in which resuscitation is conducted. When small in volume, pneumothoraces might not result in any symptoms or signs of respiratory distress but instead might appear as an incidental finding on a chest radiograph. Larger pneumothoraces will result in tachypnea, retractions and nasal flaring in the newborn, diminished breath sounds on the affected side, and hypoxemia. Tension pneumothorax will present with more severe hypoxia and severe cardiovascular comprise with a shift of the heart sounds and trachea to the contralateral side. Suspected pneumothorax can be confirmed by chest radiography if the patient is stable.

When significant respiratory distress is thought to be due to pneumothorax, immediate evacuation of the air in the pleural space is essential. The affected side can be determined immediately by transillumination and clinical assessment. Needle aspiration of a pneumothorax can be performed quickly using a small-bore (18- or 20-gauge) percutaneous catheter. The newborn should be turned on the side so that the side of the pneumothorax is up. After the fourth intercostal space has been located at the anterior axillary line, the skin can be sterilized and the needle inserted just superior to the fourth rib. Once the catheter has been inserted into the pleural space the needle can be removed. The catheter should then be connected to a stopcock and 20-mL syringe. Gentle aspiration of air into the syringe should be performed. If the syringe has been pulled back completely and there is evidence of further air in the pleural space, the stopcock can be turned off to the patient and the air can be expelled through the side port of the stopcock. Continue aspiration until there is resistance to aspiration. At this point the needle should be removed from the chest and a follow-up chest radiograph should be obtained (**Figure 11.8**).

If needle decompression does not completely remove the intrapleural air and symptoms persist or if it is suspected on clinical grounds that the pneumothorax would persist despite needle decompression, a thoracostomy tube can be inserted at the fifth intercostal space at the anterior axillary line (just lateral to the nipple). A thoracostomy tube of appropriate size can be inserted just over the sixth rib, after which the tube can be advanced toward the anterior aspect of the chest to an appropriate depth. After securing the tube in place, it should be connected to a suction device set to maintain negative 10-cm H_2O pressure. As above, a chest radiograph should be obtained to check the position of the tube and the status of the pneumothorax.

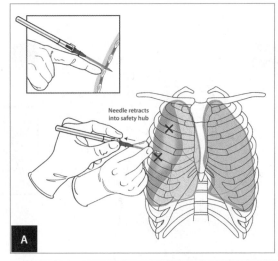

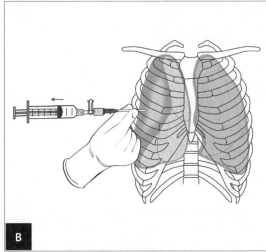

Figure 11.9 A. Locations for percutaneous aspiration of intrapleural air from the chest. Note that the needle enters just above the rib, so as to avoid the artery lying just under the rib above. B. Insertion of a percutaneous catheter for drainage of a pneumothorax or pleural fluid (see text). The needle can be placed at either of the "X" marks shown in part A but should always be perpendicular to the chest surface. Note that the needle present in part A has been removed and only the catheter remains in the pleural space.

Kattwinkel J, ed. *Textbook of Neonatal Resuscitation, 6th ed.* Elk Grove Village, IL: American Academy of Pediatrics and American Heart Association; 2011: 244. Reprinted with permission.

Preparing for Transfer

Neonatal emergencies present in a variety ways. In some cases there is time to discuss an infant's care with a local pediatrician or neonatologist, whereas in others the emergency department clinician must respond rapidly and rely on his or her own expertise. As soon as it is feasible, a health care professional with a detailed knowledge of the newborn's history and emergency department course should contact the on-call pediatric specialist to whom the newborn is likely to be referred. Even in emergency settings, it is of critical importance to provide complete and accurate information to the accepting physician so that the best advice and guidance can be provided to the emergency department staff and to the team who can transport the newborn to an intensive care nursery.

Check Your Knowledge

1. The three most important vital sings to monitor during neonatal resuscitation include:
   A. color, tone, and respiratory effort.
   B. central cyanosis, temperature, and heart rate.
   C. heart rate, respirations, and oxygenation saturation.
   D. cry, grimace, and blood pressure.

2. The recommended placement of a pulse oximetry probe in a newborn is:
   A. right hand.
   B. left hand.
   C. right foot.
   D. left foot.

3. In an apneic and bradycardic newborn being resuscitated, the most immediate (earliest) indicator of effective positive pressure ventilation is:
   A. an improvement in color.
   B. the infant beings to cry.
   C. a rise in blood pressure.
   D. an improvement in heart rate.

4. Chest compressions in a newborn should:
   A. be initiated if the heart rate is below 100.
   B. be coordinated with ventilation.
   C. be given gently to prevent fracturing the fragile sternum.
   D. be applied with a rate of 180 events per minute.

5. Epinephrine (adrenaline) during a newborn resuscitation:
   A. can be given through venous access only.
   B. can be given through an endotracheal tube only.
   C. can be given through venous access or an endotracheal tube using the same dosing ranges.
   D. can be given through venous access or an endotracheal tube using different dosing ranges.

6. Which of the following measures can help a newborn infant maintain a normal temperature?
   A. Swaddling the infant from the shoulders down and placing a cap over the scalp
   B. Increasing the ambient temperature of the room in which the infant is being resuscitated
   C. Using a radiant heat source
   D. All of the above

7. Which of the following statements regarding the initial fluid management of the newborn infant is false?
   A. Adding sodium to the initial maintenance fluids prevents hypotension.
   B. Ten percent dextrose infused at 4 mL/kg per hour should provide a sufficient supply of glucose to most newborns.
   C. If a newborn is hypoglycemic, it would be appropriate to provide a 2-mL/kg bolus infusion of 10% dextrose.
   D. None of the above

8. Which of the following statements regarding neonatal infection is false?
   A. Gram-negative bacilli are common causes of early- and late-onset sepsis.
   B. Viral infection should be considered when a newborn presents with signs of sepsis.
   C. Collection of urine by a bag placed over the perineum is the preferred method of urine collection for culture.
   D. All are correct.

9. Risk factors for indirect hyperbilirubinemia include which of the following?
   A. Parental report of poor feeding
   B. Suboptimal weight gain since discharge from birth hospital
   C. Parental report of decreased urine and/or stool output
   D. All of the above

10. Which of the following statements regarding umbilical catheter placement is true?

A. The umbilical cord contains two umbilical veins and one umbilical artery.

B. Catheterization of the umbilical vessels can be performed rapidly and safely in an emergency.

C. The exact location of an emergently placed umbilical venous catheter must be confirmed by radiography before it can be used for fluid or medication administration.

D. All are true.

References

1. Kattwinkel J. *Textbook of Neonatal Resuscitation.* 5th ed. Elk Grove, IL: American Academy of Pediatrics and American Heart Association; 2006:1–2.
2. Gregory G, Gooding CA, Phibbs RH, Tooley WH. Meconium aspiration in infants: A prospective study. *J Pediatr.* 1974;85:848–852.
3. Wiswell TE, Bent RC. Meconium staining and the meconium aspiration syndrome: Unresolved issues. *Pediatr Clin North Am.* 1993;40:955–81.
4. Kattwinkel J. *Textbook of Neonatal Resuscitation.* 6th ed. Elk Grove, IL: American Academy of Pediatrics and American Heart Association; 2010.
4a. Wyckoff MH, Aziz K, Escobedo MB, et al. Part 13: Neonatal resuscitation: 2015 American Heart Association Guidelines Update for Cardiopulmonary Resuscitation and Emergency Cardiovascular Care. *Circulation.* 2015;132(suppl2):5543–5560.
5. Singh R, Mohan CVR. Controlled trial to evaluate the use of LMA for neonatal *Resuscitation. J Anaesthesiol Clin Pharmacol.* 2005;21:303–306.
6. Trevisanuto D, Micaglio M, Pitton M, Magarotto M, Piva D, Zanardo V. Laryngeal mask airway: Is the management of neonates requiring positive pressure ventilation at birth changing? *Resuscitation.* 2004;62:151–157.
7. Gandini D, Brimacombe JR. Neonatal resuscitation with the laryngeal mask airway in normal and low birth weight infants. *Anesth Analg.* 1999;89:642–643.
8. Gluckman PD, Wyatt JS, Azzopardi D, et al. Selective head cooling with mild systemic hypothermia after neonatal encephalopathy: Multicentre randomised trial. *The Lancet.* 2005;365:663–670.
9. Shankaran S, Laptook AR, Ehrenkranz RA, et al. Whole-body hypothermia for neonates with hypoxic-ischemic encephalopathy. *N Engl J Med.* 2005;353:1574–1584.
10. Azzopardi AD, Strohm B, Edwards AD, et al. Moderate hypothermia to treat perinatal asphyxial encephalopathy. *N Engl J Med.* 2009;361:1349–1358.
11. American Academy of *Pediatrics.* Committee on Fetus and Newborn. Hospital stay for healthy term newborns. *Pediatrics.* 2010;125:405–409.
12. Ogata ES. Carbohydrate metabolism in the fetus and neonate and altered neonatal glucoregulation. *Pediatr Clin North Am.* 1986;33:25–45.
13. Wyckoff MH, Perlman JM, Laptook AR. Use of volume expansion during delivery room resuscitation in near-term and term infants. *Pediatrics.* 2005;115:950–955.
14. American Academy of Pediatrics, Subcommittee on Hyperbilirubinemia. Management of hyperbilirubinemia in the newborn infant 35 or more weeks of gestation. *Pediatrics.* 2004;114:297–316.

CHAPTER REVIEW

A 25-year-old pregnant woman arrives in your emergency department with frequent uterine contractions every 1 to 2 minutes. She is diaphoretic and anxious yet conversational between contractions but has rapid, pursed-lip respirations during contractions. Vital signs reveal a respiration rate of 20/min, a heart rate of 130/min, a blood pressure of 120/75 mm Hg, and a temperature of 38°C (100.4°F).

1. *What three questions should the patient be asked to predict the need for resuscitation of the newly born?*
2. *What steps should be taken to prepare for the resuscitation of this infant?*

To prepare for an imminent delivery, it is necessary to obtain a limited obstetric history to identify the following:

- How many newborns will be delivered
- The gestational age of the newborn(s) to be delivered
- Whether meconium is present in the amniotic fluid

The initial evaluation of the newborn should include an assessment of the following in the newborn:

- Respiratory effort
- Heart rate
- Muscle tone

CASE SUMMARY 1 CONT.

For newborns exhibiting poor respiratory effort or bradycardia (heart rate <100/min), resuscitative efforts should progress in the following sequence until clinical improvement is achieved:

- Clear the airway and stimulate the newborn.
- Place an oxygen saturation probe to the right hand or wrist.
- For spontaneously breathing newborns, provide supplemental oxygen using a blended air source, if available.
- For newborns exhibiting poor respiratory effort or apnea, provide positive pressure ventilation via a properly sized face mask.
- Endotracheal intubation should be confirmed by detection of exhaled carbon dioxide.
- Persistent bradycardia (heart rate <60/min) should be treated with chest compressions using the two-thumb technique.
- Epinephrine may be used to treat persistent bradycardia, with higher doses being required if administered via the endotracheal tube.

chapter 12

Procedural Sedation and Analgesia

Alfred Sacchetti, MD, FACEP
Teena Cortese, PharmD

Objectives

1 Identify clinical circumstances in which procedural sedation or analgesia might be indicated in the care of children.

2 Provide a pharmacologic basis for pediatric procedural sedation and analgesia (PSA).

3 Provide the basis for the development of safe and effective PSA practices.

Chapter Outline

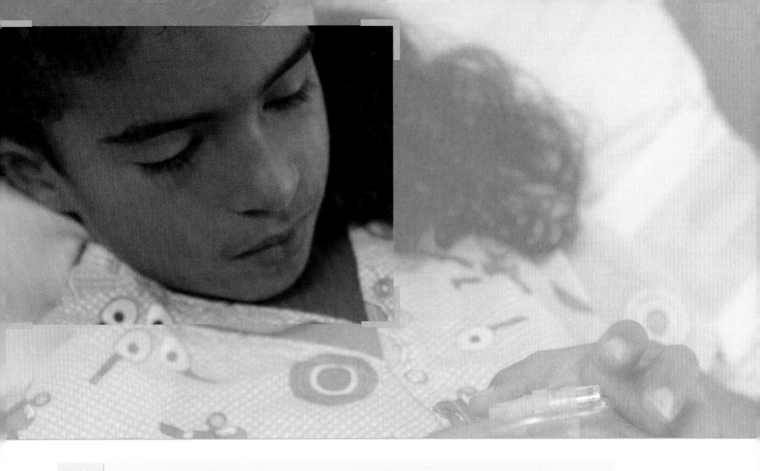

An 18-month-old boy is brought to the emergency department (ED) after a witnessed generalized tonic clonic seizure. He sustained a closed head injury and a 4-cm forehead laceration when he struck a low coffee table. His mother, who witnessed the event, notes that he has a ventriculoperitoneal shunt and a history of hydrocephalus. He was drowsy for a few minutes after the initial injury. On awakening, he cried briefly but has been abnormally quiet and withdrawn since the event. He has vomited three times and is irritable in his mother's arms. The child has no other signs of injuries. After a discussion with the patient's neurologist, it is determined that magnetic resonance imaging (MRI) would be the optimal diagnostic study to evaluate his seizure and head trauma.

1. *What are the procedural sedation options for this child for an MRI scan and laceration repair?*
2. *Can a single agent be used for both procedures?*

CASE SCENARIO 1

Introduction

Pediatric PSA has evolved greatly in the past few decades. Advances in the management of painful or anxiety-provoking procedures in children have come from not just anesthesiology but also fields as diverse as emergency medicine, pediatric dentistry, and critical care. This section will present the latest developments in the delivery of PSA to children and their applications in the varied environments in which children are treated.

Because procedural sedation overlaps so many different fields, multiple definitions exist to describe it. One of the most clinically applicable definitions of procedural sedation is the technique of administering sedatives or dissociative agents with or without analgesics to induce a state that allows the patient to tolerate unpleasant procedures while maintaining stable vital signs, an independent airway, and adequate spontaneous respirations.[1-3] The Joint Commission further distinguishes levels of sedation depending on the patient's awareness and ability to respond to stimuli. Table 12-1 lists the most recent definitions proposed by the Joint Commission.[4]

Indications

Generally accepted guidelines defining objective indications for the use of procedural sedation do not currently exist.[2] The decision to add procedural sedation to the care of a child is a combination of individual physician preference, clinical skills, practice environment, parental preference, and the procedure to be performed. In some circumstances, physicians can elect to use local anesthetics, regional blocks, and/or simple physical restraint as alternatives to procedural sedation. Even for common procedures, such as a lumbar puncture, there is no agreement on best practice options. Some physicians will routinely sedate young children for this procedure, whereas others use physical restraint with or without local anesthesia. Most physicians base their decision to use procedural sedation on whether the performance of a single major procedure, such as a complex laceration repair or fracture reduction, requires minimal movement for an optimal outcome or would be unacceptably traumatic without sedation. However, in some circumstances the combined stress of multiple minor procedures can meet or exceed that produced by a single major procedure.[5] The decision to use procedural sedation must also take into consideration the practice environment and experience of the operator performing the procedure. An experienced physician might be able to incise and treat a local abscess while the patient is under local anesthesia in minutes in a toddler, whereas a resident in training might take much longer to perform the same procedure under the direction of a supervising attending physician. It is unfair to both the patient and the resident in training to ask that any procedure be learned on a struggling, frightened, and uncomfortable child, and procedural sedation should be more liberally performed in teaching environments.[5]

Children exhibit extreme variability in their individual responsiveness to medications and their tolerance of procedures, and it is not always possible to predict in advance the degree of seda-

TABLE 12-1 Joint Commission Sedation Level Definitions	
Minimal sedation (anxiolysis)	A drug-induced state during which patients respond normally to verbal commands. Although cognitive function might be impaired, ventilatory and cardiovascular functions are unaffected.
Moderate sedation/analgesia ("conscious sedation")	A drug-induced depression of consciousness during which patients respond purposefully to verbal commands, either alone or accompanied by light tactile stimulation. No interventions are required to maintain a patient's airway, and spontaneous ventilation is adequate. Cardiovascular function is usually maintained.
Deep sedation/analgesia	A drug-induced depression of consciousness during which patients cannot be easily aroused but respond purposefully after repeated or painful stimulation. The ability to independently maintain ventilatory function might be impaired. Patients might require assistance in maintaining a patent airway, and spontaneous ventilation might be inadequate. Cardiovascular function is usually maintained.

Joint Commission Resources. *Comprehensive Accreditation Manual for Hospitals (CAMH)*. Oakbrook Terrace, IL: Joint Commission on Accreditation of Healthcare Organizations; 2005:PC–41–42, definitions 1–3.

tion required—or achieved—in a given case.[1,6] In some cases, a child might be predicted to need only moderate sedation, but the procedure might actually evolve to require deep sedation and analgesia. Alternatively, in other children, moderate sedation or analgesia might be adequate, but deep sedation or analgesia might be inadvertently attained because of variations in responsiveness to the sedative agents. As a result, operational definitions describing the intended purpose of PSA are more useful in helping physicians approach the treatment of any given child. From a practice perspective, sedation and analgesia requirements can be grouped into five clinical scenarios: (1) simple analgesia, (2) anxiolysis, (3) procedural sedation for painless intervention,

(4) procedural sedation for painful intervention, and (5) extended sedation. These scenarios are specifically defined in Table 12-2 along with clinical examples of each.

Regardless of the purpose of the sedation or the intended level of sedation, it is important that adequate PSA be provided. Inadequate sedation leading to patient agitation has been associated with an increase in complications in children.[7]

Preparation and Monitoring

Preparation for analgesia, anxiolysis, or PSA begins with patient assessment. Although some variation can be expected, all pediatric pain management or sedation needs must be examined in the context of their clinical scenario. A focused

TABLE 12-2 **Procedural Sedation and Analgesia Clinical Scenarios**		
Clinical Scenario	Definition	Examples
Simple analgesia	Relief of pain without production of an altered mental state. Sedation might be a secondary effect of medications administered for this purpose.	Administration of an opioid to a patient with an undisplaced extremity fracture or abdominal pain.
Anxiolysis	A state of decreased apprehension concerning a particular situation; there is no change in patient's level of awareness.	Benzodiazepine administration to an adolescent after severe emotional traumatic event.
Procedural sedation for painless intervention	A technique of administering sedatives, analgesics, and/or dissociative agents to induce a state that allows the patient to tolerate unpleasant procedures while maintaining function.	Barbiturate use to permit a computed tomography (CT) scan in a toddler after seizure.
Procedural sedation for painful intervention	Intended to result in a depressed level of consciousness but to allow the patient to maintain airway control independently and continuously.	Ketamine administration to a child for debridement of burns.
Extended sedation	Intentional depression of a patient's sense of awareness of surroundings to permit cooperation with ongoing care. Loss of protective airway reflexes and respiratory drive might be an intended consequence of such care in patients in whom ventilatory management has been assumed.	Barbiturate or benzodiazepine infusion to facilitate ventilator management in a head injury patient.

history and physical examination are part of the initial evaluation and should include specific questions concerning preexisting conditions, medication allergies or reactions, last oral intake, and previous sedation or analgesic experiences. A good mnemonic that covers all the salient historical points in a child undergoing procedural sedation is AMPLE, which represents:

- Allergies
- Medications
- Previous procedures and past medical history
- Last meal
- Events before procedure

A formal American Society of Anesthesiologists (ASA) classification is often applied to potential candidates to help guide their treatment. A structured, presedation assessment focusing on the airway and preexisting medical conditions has been shown to reduce complications.[8] Table 12-3 contains the ASA categorization scheme. As a general rule, ASA class I and II patients can be safely treated by nonanesthesiologists, whereas ASA class IV and V children are best treated in conjunction with an anesthesiologist or subspecialty consultant when possible. ASA class III patients can be treated by emergency physicians, intensivists, and other qualified physicians. Input from an anesthesiologist can be useful for medically complex patients and those with a potentially difficult airway. In emergent circumstances, it might be

necessary to begin treatment immediately, regardless of the ASA classification, while awaiting consultant input.[8]

TABLE 12-3 American Society of Anesthesiologists Physical Status Classification	
Class I	Normal, healthy patient
Class II	Patient with mild systemic disease
Class III	Patient with severe systemic disease
Class IV	Patient with severe systemic disease that is a constant life threat
Class V	Moribund patient who is not expected to survive without the procedure
E	Emergency procedure

The ASA physiologic status classifications are not purely objective and are open to some individual interpretation. A patient with well-controlled asthma might be considered ASA class II, whereas a patient with poorly controlled asthma might be considered class III. Patients with diseases of two systems (eg, diabetes and asthma) might be considered to be in class III even if each condition was relatively well controlled. Some physicians believe that patients with certain congenital problems, such as Down syndrome and some skeletal dysplasias, should be class III because of the multiple anomalies associated with these conditions.

Questions concerning last meals and recent activities might be appropriate for ED patients but might not be needed in intensive care unit (ICU) patients. ASA consensus-based fasting guidelines extrapolated from patients undergoing general anesthesia are often inappropriately applied to ED patients undergoing procedural sedation.[9] Pulmonary aspiration in the context of properly conducted ED procedural sedation is exceedingly unlikely, and recent oral intake is not a contraindication; this is particularly true for pediatric patients who are ASA classes I and II.[8-10] However, individual risk should always be weighed against the benefit of urgent sedation.[9] Knowledge of nothing by mouth status might influence whether a physician delays a nonemergent procedure and might influence the choice of the sedative agent (eg, ketamine, which maintains intact airway reflexes, versus propofol, which does not). For patients who are sedated who have recently eaten, an E (for emergency) code can be applied to the ASA status. Additional preparation includes determination of medications and routes of administration and initiation of appropriate patient monitoring. If intravenous medications are to be used, some form of vascular access must be established. Supplemental oxygen and suction capabilities along with respiratory and cardiovascular monitoring equipment should be readily available in every area in which PSA is to be performed.

Explanation of the planned sedation or analgesia to the child and caregiver should be reviewed during medical preparations. Assurance that a child's pain will be addressed or his anxiety managed is extremely comforting to both patient and family.

The degree to which a child's respiratory or cardiovascular status is continuously monitored is scenario specific and depends on what is intended. Children receiving simple analgesics or anxiolytics will generally not require any ongoing monitoring beyond the initial, and possibly a repeat, set of vital signs. Patients undergoing procedural sedation will require more intensive monitoring. At the very least, continuous pulse oximetry with audible tone (pitch) change indicator should be maintained on any child with an intentionally depressed level of awareness. In addition, continuous cardiac monitoring (with blood pressure) should be considered routine on all patients receiving procedural sedation.[11] Table 12-4 contains descriptions of the various monitoring techniques used for procedural sedation.

Pulse oximetry detects only arterial hypoxemia, a late finding in children who are hypoventilating or experiencing airway obstruction. The use of bedside capnography in children undergoing procedural sedation is increasingly common. Elevation of end tidal carbon dioxide levels or loss of a capnometry waveform (or a sharp

TABLE 12-4 Various Monitoring Techniques Used for Procedural Sedation	
Monitoring	Description
Bedside monitoring	Continuous monitoring and correlation between patient appearance and electronic monitoring.
Cardiac monitor	Continuous presentation of heart rate and rhythm. Will detect bradycardia indicative of significant hypoxia or tachycardia indicative of pain in iatrogenically paralyzed patient.
Pulse oximetry	Continuous presentation of oxygen saturation and heart rate. Will detect decrease in oxygen saturation or resultant bradycardia or tachycardia.
Capnometry	Continuous presentation of exhaled carbon dioxide tension. Will detect increase in carbon dioxide blood levels with hypoventilation or absence of respiratory waveform if apnea or airway obstruction develops. May detect respiratory depression before development of hypoxia.
Noninvasive blood pressure monitoring	Interval measurement of blood pressure. Will detect hypotension secondary to medication administration.
Cerebral infrared oximetry (experimental)	Monitors cerebral oxygen saturation. May detect decrease in brain oxygen saturation even in the face of normal capnometry and pulse oximetry.

decrease in exhaled carbon dioxide) is an earlier warning sign of respiratory depression or an airway obstruction.[12,13] Whether transient changes in exhaled carbon dioxide represent clinically significant hypoventilation is unclear, and the role of routine capnometry in low-risk patients who are being directly observed at the bedside has not been established. Direct observation of a child's breathing by an experienced physician, nurse, or respiratory therapist should help identify those individuals at risk for respiratory depression.[14] In procedures such as an MRI scan in which patients are not continuously visible, the use of capnometry will allow early detection of obstruction (absent waveform) before oxygen desaturation and its consequences occur. Continuous capnometry should be considered in patients sensitive to both carbon dioxide tension and oxygen saturation, such as those with elevated intracranial pressure (ICP) or certain cardiac lesions.

One concern that frequently arises is whether a physician can manage a child's sedation while simultaneously performing a procedure. This question was addressed specifically in a report from the Procedural Sedation in the Community Emergency Department (ProSCED) registry. In that report, physicians supervising procedural sedation for another physician performing a procedure had the same complication rates as single physicians both supervising the sedation and performing the procedure.[14] However, in all of these cases the patients were monitored by experienced ED nurses. The exact composition of the team providing care to a child undergoing procedural sedation should be determined individually for each institution and for each patient.

Monitoring initiated on a child must be continued beyond the time required to perform the procedure. For painful activities, such as fracture reductions or burn debridement, the observed level of sedation might increase significantly after the painful stimulus of the procedure is removed.

Specified disposition criteria should be established for children undergoing procedural sedation. As a general rule, children must return to their baseline respiratory status before consideration for discharge. Airway reflexes must also be present unless already altered by some preexisting condition. Both the level of consciousness and voluntary motor control should be observed to be spontaneously improving, although both of these might not return completely to baseline for some time if certain longer-acting agents are used.[15] Parents should be warned of this possibility and instructed not to allow children to engage in unsupervised play or high-risk activities that require coordination until all residuals of the treatment medications have dissipated.

Pain Assessment

The ability to provide pain relief to a patient is complicated by the lack of any effective objective means of assessing a patient's level of discomfort. Verbal scales and visual analog tools are useful in research studies of pain control in patients of all ages. Whether these measurement devices are more effective than an experienced physician has not been proven. General emergency physicians tend to use more local anesthetics and postprocedure narcotics than pediatricians for children undergoing the same procedures.[16] In very young children, a purely observational scoring system can alert a physician to otherwise unrecognized cues that a nonverbal child is in pain.[8] Use of interactive scoring systems, such as numerical scales or a faces pictorial, might not be perfectly accurate, but it does force the treating health care professionals to recognize that a child's pain needs to be assessed. **Figures 12.1A**, **12.1B**, and **12.1C** contain examples of three age-related scoring systems.

The selection of any single pain scoring system is not as important as the consistent application of some form of repeated patient assessment. Toddlers and small children in particular might be hesitant or developmentally unable to verbalize their discomfort, and mechanisms should be in place to specifically offer these patients pain medication. In communicative children, the regular offer of additional analgesia might be even more effective than using clinical judgment or a scoring system to determine when pain medications are needed.

Not every child undergoing a procedure or study will require some form of sedation. Cooperation can sometimes be elicited by engagement or distraction for brief diagnostic studies, such as simple head computed tomography

FLACC Observation Scale for Infants and Small Children			
Category	Scoring		
	0	1	2
Face	No particular expression or smile	Occasional grimace or frown, withdrawn disinterested	Frequent to constant quivering chin, clenched jaw
Legs	Normal position or relaxed	Uneasy, restless, tense	Kicking, or legs drawn up
Activity	Lying quietly, normal position, moves easily	Squirming, shifting back and forth, tense	Arched, rigid, or jerking
Cry	No cry (awake or asleep)	Moans or whimpers; occasional complaint	Crying steadily, screams or sobs, frequent complaints
Consolability	Content, relaxed	Reassured by occasional touching, hugging, or being talked to, distracted	Difficult to console or comfort
FLACC: F-Face, L-Legs, A-Activity, C-Cry, C-Consolability			

Figure 12.1A Pain assessment scale.

Merkel SI, Voepel-Lewis T, Shayevitz JR, Malviya S. The FLACC: a behavioral scale for scoring postoperative pain in young children. *Pediatr Nurs.* 1997;23:293–297.

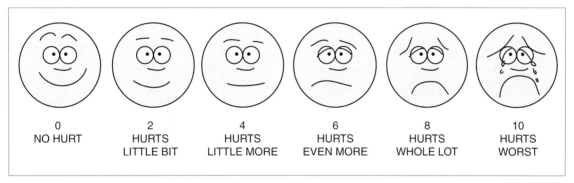

Figure 12.1B FACES scale for children older than 3 years.

From Hockenberry MJ, Wilson D. *Wong's essentials of pediatric nursing.* ed 8. St. Louis, 2009, Mosby. Used with permission. Copyright Mosby.

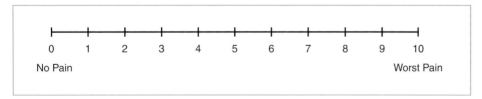

Figure 12.1C Linear scale for older children and adolescents.

(CT) scans. Briefly painful procedures, such as the reduction of a subluxed radial head, might be more appropriately performed without sedation if completed quickly and efficiently. The decision to proceed without pharmacologic assistance is determined by clinical experience and anticipated duration of the procedure. However, the ability to successfully complete a procedure does not preclude the use of some form of PSA. Just because a lumbar puncture can be completed in one attempt by an experienced physician does not imply that the child should not receive local anesthesia or procedural sedation.

For children with altered mental states, communicative handicaps, or central nervous system (CNS) injuries, it might be difficult to determine if appropriate procedural sedation is being provided during a painful procedure (although the FLACC scale in Figure 12.1A does not rely on patient self-reporting). In these patients, parents might be sensitive in recognizing discomfort or agitation that might otherwise by unrecognized by health care professionals unfamiliar with the patient.

Management

Principles of Analgesia and Sedation

The determination of the need for analgesia or sedation is determined by the physicians immediately caring for a child with parental input. Regardless of the cause of a patient's pain, waiting for an examination by a consultant or the results of a diagnostic study is never an indication to withhold analgesics. Published studies contradict the notion that the judicious use of opioid analgesics masks the important physical findings in any symptom complex, including children with abdominal pain, head injuries, extremity injuries, or headaches.[7,17,18] As with adults, the administration of opioid analgesics does not interfere with their ability to provide consent for any surgical procedure in older adolescents.

If the need for some form of analgesia or sedation is established, then a determination must be made as to the optimum approach for that particular child. Available options on the best technique, route of administration, medications, monitoring, follow-up, and personal preferences must all be considered. Every procedural sedation should be approached with the realization that any given child might require or experience substantially deeper sedation than expected and that the personnel and equipment required for any degree of sedation will need to be present at the bedside.

If a pharmacologic approach is selected for a child, the route of administration of the medication must be determined. Oral administration of pain medications is convenient and well tolerated in patients of all ages. Medications given in this manner can be liquids, pills, and even gelatin cubes. Transmucosal delivery routes include intranasal, transbuccal, and rectal, which allow administration of traditionally parenteral medicines, such as fentanyl or midazolam, that would otherwise require placement of an intravenous catheter.

Both the oral and transmucosal routes have the advantage of ease of administration regardless of the vehicle for the medications.

The primary disadvantage of these routes is the difficulty in titrating dosages to a specific effect and might not be appropriate for procedural sedation in an ED. Because of variability in the absorption of medications given via these routes, the time to onset and peak effect can never be determined exactly. Physicians treating such patients might be uncertain whether a lack of visible effect is the result of a delay in absorption or an inadequate dose. This might not be an issue for children treated with simple analgesia or anxiolysis but can be a major obstacle for those undergoing procedural sedation. If the transmucosal route is selected, it should only be used with medications demonstrating a predictable response with a single dose. Transdermal medications can also be given, although they are generally used for long-term analgesia or provision of local anesthesia (such as topical lidocaine [lignocaine] anesthetic cream).[19]

Parenteral administration of drugs provides a more rapid onset with more predictable outcomes. The major disadvantage of these approaches is that they require some form of a painful injection. For intramuscular and subcutaneous medications, a separate injection is required for each administration, making these routes less desirable for procedures requiring multiple doses or titration.[2,8] Intravenously administered medications require an initial puncture, but all subsequent doses can be delivered painlessly. The minimal time delays between administration of a drug and observed effect allows for much easier titration with this route.

Regardless of the route of administration, every physician must be knowledgeable of the time to peak effect for the medication selected. When titrating to a specific clinical response, it is important to allow enough time to elapse for a drug to take effect before delivering any additional doses or adding a second medication. If an additional dose is administered too quickly, drug stacking occurs and can lead to an inadvertent overdose. The rate of administering additional doses is also affected by the degree of agitation of the patient or amount of pain present before initiation of the procedure.[20]

Many drugs demonstrate an inverse age-dosing relation with higher doses per weight necessary in infants and toddlers. Ketamine, remifentanil, and propofol demonstrate this effect.[21]

Patient controlled analgesia is an option for most children older than 3 years.[22] Most of these systems use intravenously administered opioid analgesics delivered through an infusion pump. The pumps are programmed to allow the children to self-administer pain medications as needed while using lockout features to prevent unintentional delivery of excessive amounts. These devices have been used in acute care settings and are ideal for children with exacerbations of recurrent painful conditions.

Inhalation of nitrous oxide, long used in the dental suite, is finding increased use in the acute care medical setting. The onset time is virtually immediate, making titration of response straightforward. Delivery mechanisms and fixed gas concentrations are the primary limiting factors to the use of this agent. Older children can use self-delivery systems that use demand valves to shut off flow when the appropriate level of sedation is achieved. Younger children receive inhaled nitrous oxide through a fixed delivery system that must be controlled by an attending physician.[23,24]

Because of the imaginative and curious nature of children, they are also good candidates for nonpharmacologic techniques. In newborns, nonnutritive sucking or pacifier use can reduce the distress associated with heel blood sampling and circumcision.[25,26] Distraction techniques using visual or audio cues (such as bubble blowers, pinwheels, or music) have proven effective in diverting children's attention from brief painful procedures or extended nonpainful diagnostic studies.[8,27,28] The presence of child life specialists has been shown to reduce pain and anxiety in children by both direct intervention and education of the medical staff.[8]

Medications Used in Analgesia and Sedation

There is no single ideal agent for pediatric pain control, anxiety management, or procedural sedation. The best medication for a given patient will be determined by the clinical scenario, child's age, clinical condition, and the personal preferences and experience of the physician providing the care, as well as the preferences of the patient and caregivers. What is universal is that a sound knowledge of the pharmacology of sedation or analgesia agents is essential to their safe and effective use. Table 12-5 summarizes medications used in pediatric sedation and analgesia.

Acetaminophen (Paracetamol)

Acetaminophen (paracetamol) is an analgesic with both antipyretic and mild analgesic actions. It has an excellent safety profile and is frequently combined with opioid analgesics for mild to moderate pain.

Nonsteroidal Anti-Inflammatory Drugs

Nonsteroidal anti-inflammatory drugs (NSAIDs) possess both antipyretic and analgesic actions. NSAIDs produce their effect through enzyme inhibition in the prostaglandin synthesis pathways. As a result, these drugs are particularly effective with prostaglandin-mediated pain, such as biliary or renal colic, dysmenorrhea, and inflammatory arthritis. They have also proven effective in the treatment of mild to moderate pain associated with musculoskeletal injuries and surgery. NSAIDs also decrease blood flow to the gastric mucosa, which might produce gastritis or ulcers with long-term use. Gastritis or ulcers are generally not a concern with short-term use in children with no underlying gastrointestinal problems. NSAIDs have an antiplatelet effect, which might result in bleeding and bruising in some types of injuries.

Ibuprofen is the prototypical NSAID. As a single agent, it is effective for mild pain but can be combined with opioid analgesics for more severe pain.[29] Ketorolac is no more potent than ibuprofen or other orally administered NSAIDs but has the option for parenteral administration. Compared with opioid analgesics, there is a delay in onset of its analgesic effect even with parenteral use, and the drug is not easily titratable. Ketorolac is also commonly used in conjunction with opioid analgesics for sickle cell crisis and postoperative pain.[30,31]

TABLE 12-5 **Medications**

Medication	Dose, mg/kg	Route	Max Unit Dose, mg	Duration	Interval between redosing when titrating to effect	Precautions
Acetaminophen (paracetamol)	10–15	Oral/rectal	1,000	4 h		
Ibuprofen	5–10	Oral	800	6 h		
Ketorolac	0.5	IM/IV	30 mg IV 60 mg IM	4–6 h		
Morphine	0.1	IM/IV	10	3–4 h	30 min IM 15 min IV	Histamine release Respiratory depression
Fentanyl	0.001 0.005–0.015 0.0015	IV Transmucosal Intranasal	0.05 400 mcg 100 mcg	0.5–1 h 0.5–1 h	10 min IV	Rigid chest Vomiting Decrease dose in infants
Remifentanil	0.15 mcg/kg/min (10 mcg/kg/h) infusions	IV	0.2 mcg/kg/min 12 mcg/kg/h	5 min	2 min	Respiratory depression
Meperidine	1–1.8	IM/IV	100 IM	3–4 h	30 min IM 10 min IV	Reduce dose for IV administration Toxic metabolites Seizure, irritability
Hydromorphone	0.01	IM/IV	2	3–4 h	30 min IM 10 min IV	
Hydrocodone	0.2	Oral	10	4–6 h		Combined with acetaminophen (paracetamol)
Codeine	1	Oral	60	4–6 h		GI upset, vomiting Combined with acetaminophen (paracetamol)
Pentobarbital	2–5 4	IV IM	200	0.5–1.5 h	See text IV 20 min IM	Titrate IV Avoid all barbiturates in children with porphyria
Methohexital	0.5–1 18–25	IV Rectal	100	20–60 min	5 min IV	Respiratory depression Avoid all barbiturates in children with porphyria

TABLE 12-5 **Medications, continued**

Medication	Dose, mg/kg	Route	Max Unit Dose, mg	Duration	Interval between redosing when titrating to effect	Precautions
Thiopental	2.5–5 25	IV Rectal	300	20–60 min	5 min IV	Respiratory depression Avoid all barbiturates in children with porphyria
Midazolam	0.05-0.2 0.3-0.7	IM/IV Oral		1–2 h	10 min IV	Respiratory depression Agitation with low doses
Chloral hydrate	50–100	Oral/rectal	1,000	6–24 h		Avoid in liver disease
Propofol	0.5–1 1–6 mg/kg/h	IV bolus Infusion	100	6–10 min	5 min IV	Respiratory depression
Etomidate	0.1–0.23	IV bolus	20	15–20 min	10 min IV	Myoclonic jerks
Ketamine	1–2 4	IV IM		0.5–2 h 1–2 h	5 min IV 20 min IM	Airway secretions
Naloxone	0.005–0.01 (partial reversal) 0.1 (total reversal)	IM/IV	2	20 min		Opiate antagonist
Flumazenil	0.01	IV	0.2	30 min		Avoid in patients with seizure disorder
Lidocaine (lignocaine)		Infiltrated	4.5 mg/kg	30–120 min		
Lidocaine (lignocaine) with epinephrine (adrenaline)		Infiltrated	7 mg/kg	1 h		
Bupivacaine		Infiltrated	2.5 mg/kg	2–8 h		

Abbreviations: IM, intramuscular; IV, intravenous.

Opioid Analgesics

Opioids produce pain relief through stimulation of multiple receptors in the peripheral nervous system and CNS. All of the clinically used opioid analgesics stimulate each of the receptors to some degree, although preferential activity of different receptor types exists among various drugs. Most of the variability in the observed actions of different drugs results from their receptor binding behavior and their metabolism and ability to cross into the CNS.

Opioid analgesics produce some degree of sedation, and although not the primary purpose, this effect can be used to some advantage in patients with both pain and anxiety. All of the opioids can produce dose-related respiratory depression, which is more prominent in neonates and young children. Hypoxia and hypercarbia can result from depressed ventilation, and in children with sensitive conditions these changes can result in elevation of ICP or pulmonary or cardiac shunting. Hypotension as a result of both peripheral vasodilation and myocardial depression is another potential systemic physiologic effect of this group of agents. Many of the opioids also release histamine, and transient urticaria or flushing can occur, which can be confused with allergy. All opioids have the potential to induce nausea. Although concomitant administration of an antiemetic has not been shown to prevent this effect in controlled trials, many physicians find that once nausea occurs, antiemetics might be helpful.

Morphine is the classic opioid analgesic. It is a potent pure agonist with excellent analgesic properties. Morphine can be administered orally, intramuscularly, subcutaneously, intravenously, intra-articularly, epidurally, and intrathecally. When delivered intravenously, its actions are easily titrated. Morphine is unusual in that it is better absorbed subcutaneously than intramuscularly, which allows for use of a much smaller and less painful needle for delivery. Hydromorphone is a more potent semisynthetic opioid (approximately five to eight times that of morphine) with excellent analgesic properties. Its pharmacology is similar to that of morphine, and it is frequently preferred for patient controlled analgesia programs.

Meperidine is a synthetic opioid agonist in a different structural class than morphine, albeit with similar analgesic properties. Meperidine is frequently described as producing more euphoria than morphine, resulting in its elimination from many pain protocols in conditions requiring long-term or long-term intermittent pain management, such as sick cell disease. One of the major disadvantages of meperidine is that one of its principle metabolites, normeperidine, can accumulate with repeated dosing of this drug, resulting in neuroexcitatory symptoms, CNS stimulation, dysphoria, and seizures. Normeperidine can interact adversely with certain monoamine oxidase inhibitors and should be avoided in any patients taking this class of drugs.

Fentanyl is an extremely potent, relatively short-acting synthetic opioid analgesic. Unlike other agents that are dosed as milligrams per kilogram, fentanyl is dosed in micrograms per kilogram. It has few histamine-releasing effects and a minimal effect on the cardiovascular system, making it suitable for patients with hypotension or cardiac disease. Fentanyl's increased potency extends to its sedative and respiratory depressant actions as well, with a much greater apnea risk than morphine. One characteristic unique to high-potency opioids, such as fentanyl, is chest wall rigidity, which occurs if it is administered too rapidly or at high dosages. Fentanyl also tends to induce more nausea and vomiting in children, particularly when administered as a transbuccal lollipop. The onset of action of fentanyl is rapid, with a correspondingly short duration of action of approximately 20 minutes. These clinical characteristics make it more appropriate for procedural sedation than simple analgesia. When used in this manner, it is commonly (and carefully) combined with a pure sedative.[2] Fentanyl is also finding increasing use as an intranasal agent. When administered as an intranasal spray (by an atomizer), fentanyl is able to provide rapid, narcotic analgesia without the necessity of placing an intravenous catheter.[32]

Alfentanil, sufentanil, and remifentanil are synthetic relatives of fentanyl with different potencies that can be used for pediatric PSA.[33] Remifentanil is a relatively new synthetic opioid that demonstrates equal potency to fentanyl but with a much shorter duration of action. Remifentanil's half-life of only 5 minutes makes it an ideal agent for short painful procedures. Remifentanil has a significant potential for respiratory depression, and apnea has been reported in up to 50% of children during procedural sedation.[34-38] Remifentanil is metabolized by red blood cell esterases, making it a good option for patients with hepatic or renal problems.

Because of its short duration of action, remifentanil is best administered as a continuous infusion of 0.15 mcg/kg per minute (10 mcg/kg per hour). A bolus of 1 mcg/kg can be administered 1 minute before the procedure if the physician thinks a deeper degree of sedation is required. Remifentanil infusions are also effective for sedation of children receiving ventilatory support. One interesting observation about remifentanil is that it appears to be ineffective in children who are anxious before the start of the procedure. In these children, a low dose of pure sedative, such as lorazepam, or a barbiturate will be required.

Codeine is a low-potency opioid agent. It is most commonly given orally in combination with acetaminophen (paracetamol) for mild to moderate pain. However, studies suggest that the combination of codeine and acetaminophen (paracetamol) might be no more effective than ibuprofen alone, while demonstrating a greater incidence of adverse effects.[39] Gastrointestinal discomfort, nausea, and vomiting are well-recognized adverse effects of this drug.

Like codeine, hydrocodone and oxycodone are orally available opioid agonists used primarily in combination with acetaminophen (paracetamol) or ibuprofen to treat moderate to severe pain. These are clearly superior to codeine, with greater potency and fewer gastrointestinal adverse effects.

Opioid Antagonists

Because all the opioid medications act through a specific opioid receptor site, their actions might be reversed through blockade of those receptors. Naloxone, the traditional opioid antagonist that physicians have the most experience with, rapidly reverses the respiratory and cardiovascular depressant effects of any opioid agent. The half-life of naloxone is approximately 60 minutes, which is shorter than the duration of action of many opioid drugs. Because of this, any patient administered this agent must be observed well beyond this time frame to be certain an unwitnessed relapse of respiratory depression does not occur.

Barbiturates

As a class, the barbiturates are the model sedative-hypnotic agents. They produce their effects through neuronal γ-aminobutyric acid (GABA) receptors. The GABA receptor is the CNS's primary neuroinhibitor. Barbiturates operate through this same mechanism, and their differences in clinical characteristics are reflective of chemical differences in lipid solubility, CNS penetration, and metabolism. Because their CNS actions are relatively nonspecific, in addition to their sedative-hypnotic properties, barbiturates can also depress respirations, resulting in hypoxia and hypercarbia. Barbiturates can also induce hypotension through both myocardial and peripheral vascular effects. The neuroinhibitory actions of these drugs are cerebroprotective and can interrupt seizure activity, reduce cerebral metabolism, and lower elevated ICP, generally resulting in cerebroprotection. Barbiturates are also metabolically active compounds that induce liver enzymes, which affects the pharmacokinetics of many other drugs. Although barbiturates have no analgesic effects, if a deep enough state of sedation is induced, brief painful procedures can be performed without excessive distress.

Pentobarbital is a short-acting sedative hypnotic typically used for painless diagnostic procedures. The recommended protocol for pentobarbital use involves titrated intravenous bolus doses. Once a patient is appropriately monitored for respiratory depression, a loading dose of 2.5 mg/kg is administered intravenously. If the child is not sleeping within 1 to 2 minutes, a dose of 1.25 mg/kg is administered, followed another 2 minutes later by a dose of 1.25 mg/kg if a final dose is needed. In general, the second or third doses are rarely required. Children older than 12 years are more difficult to sedate with this protocol, although this might only represent the fact that children of this age who require sedation are more likely to have significant underlying neurodevelopmental problems that require additional agents. In direct comparisons with other pure sedatives, pentobarbital is consistently shown to be equipotent or superior for painless diagnostic studies.[40,41]

Methohexital is a rapid-acting, short duration, potent barbiturate, with an action profile almost identical to thiopental.[42] Administered intravenously, it is generally used as an induction agent for general anesthesia, although its use has been described for ED procedural sedation. In children, methohexital is commonly used as a rectal preparation for sedation in painless diagnostic studies. Administered in this manner, it acts rapidly and consistently with a reasonable safety profile with proper monitoring for respiratory depression, which can occur in 3% to 10% of patients.[43,44]

Benzodiazepines

As a family of drugs, the benzodiazepines parallel the barbiturates. Benzodiazepines also activate the GABA receptor, and, as would be expected, the clinical actions of this class of drugs include sedation, hypnosis, respiratory depression, and anticonvulsant activity. Cardiovascular depression is not as prominent as with barbiturates. Benzodiazepines also appear to be more variable in their dose response effects in children than both opioids and barbiturates.[45] As a result, their visible effects are less predictable, and it is possible to produce paradoxical disinhibition and even agitation with recommended doses.

Midazolam is a short-acting, rapid-onset benzodiazepine sedative used for painless diagnostic studies or in combination with opioids for painful procedures. This drug can be administered orally, intranasally, intravenously, and intramuscularly if necessary. The recommended dose range for midazolam is broad, and paradoxical reactions are well documented. The treatment of a child who becomes agitated after receiving this medication is additional medication until sedation is achieved.[45,46] Midazolam is also a potent amnestic and can be useful as a single agent for some procedures, such as sexual assault examinations.

Diazepam is similar to midazolam in its actions, with a slightly longer time to onset and a longer duration of action. Lorazepam is a longer-acting benzodiazepine sedative hypnotic whose primary use is seizure control and anxiolysis.

Benzodiazepine Antagonists

Like the opioids, the action of benzodiazepines can be reversed with an antagonist. Flumazenil competitively inhibits all of the actions of benzodiazepines and will effectively reverse sedation, respiratory depression, and hypotension. However, flumazenil will also antagonize the anticonvulsant properties of benzodiazepines and should be used with extreme caution in children with underlying seizure disorders treated with benzodiazepines.

Other Sedatives and Analgesics

Propofol is an ultrashort-acting sedative hypnotic with an extremely rapid onset. A modified phenol, propofol's exact mechanism of action is unclear, although some suspect both a direct membrane effect and a GABA receptor action. Used for both rapid sequence intubations and procedural sedation, propofol has an immediate onset with duration of action of 6 to 8 minutes. The speed of onset is related to propofol's high lipid solubility, which allows it to easily penetrate the highly lipophilic CNS. For procedural sedation in children, propofol is generally titrated beginning with a 0.5- to 1.0-mg/kg bolus, repeated slowly to the desired level of sedation. For more prolonged sedation, a continuous infusion is required. Like the barbiturate induction agents, propofol will induce apnea if injected rapidly or in too large a dose. Hypotension secondary to peripheral vasodilation is another well-described effect that is easily reversed with saline boluses. Reports of a fatal propofol infusion syndrome have been described in patients taking high doses of propofol for extended periods (>4 mg/kg per hour for more than 48 hours), but it is generally not an issue in the acute care setting. Propofol is a potent skeletal muscle relaxant that makes it particularly valuable for reduction of large joint dislocations. Propofol also possesses antiemetic properties.

The lipid-like nature of propofol requires that it be suspended as an emulsion. Some of the generic preparations of propofol have a high sulfite concentration in their suspensions, which can induce bronchospasm in susceptible asthmatic patients. Propofol's sedative effects make it useful for both painful and nonpainful procedures, whereas its short duration of action minimizes postprocedure monitoring times.[38,46–50] In the ProSCED registry, propofol was one of the safest drugs for procedural sedation in children.[51]

Fospropofol is a phosphorylated prodrug version of propofol. Initial studies with the drug resulted in problems with the determination of the actual pharmacokinetics of propofol release from the prodrug, so the specifics of its pharmacodynamics have not been clearly determined. Unlike propofol, fospropofol is water soluble and in clinical studies to date has been reported to produce less pain at the injection site along with less respiratory depression. Currently, there are no pediatric dosing recommendations for this drug.[52]

Etomidate is another anesthesia induction agent that has found use in procedural sedation in children. Used to provide both analgesia and sedation, etomidate is useful for brief painful procedures. Etomidate has the potential to induce myotonic jerks, making it unsuitable for diagnostic procedures that require a motionless patient. Etomidate also produces nausea and vomiting in some patients. Use of etomidate has been documented to produce adrenal suppression, the clinical significance of which is the subject of considerable debate.[53–55] Considering the concerns over the use of etomidate in critically ill children, an alternative sedation agent should be considered in this group of patients when possible.

Chloral hydrate is a pure oral sedative hypnotic. Chloral hydrate produces consistent sedation at a dose of 50 to 75 mg/kg and has been commonly used for painless diagnostic studies. The major disadvantage of this medication for ED and outpatient use is its prolonged duration of action, which can last 2 to 24 hours. The unreliable effect, inability to titrate chloral hydrate, and potential for inadvertent deep sedation make this a less than ideal sedative agent in the acute care setting.[56]

Ketamine is the only dissociative procedural sedation agent. Ketamine produces its effect through inhibition of the N-methyl-D-aspartate receptor, the CNS binding site for the excitatory neurotransmitter glutamic acid. By disrupting communication between the cortical and limbic systems, ketamine induces a trance-like dissociative state that has been described as follows: "Someone is doing something painful to my body, but I'm separated from my body right now, so I don't notice it." Patients are not sedated in the traditional sense but tolerate both painful procedures and painless diagnostic studies well. Unlike any of the other agents, ketamine is a mild sympathomimetic, which produces an increase in both heart rate and systolic blood pressure. It was believed that ketamine produced elevations in intraocular pressure and ICP; however, more recent studies have documented that ketamine actually can reduce ICP and preserve cerebral perfusion pressure.[57] Ketamine also produces an endogenous release of epinephrine (adrenaline), which is responsible for its bronchodilatory effects.

Ketamine also differs from other sedative hypnotics or opioids in that it does not blunt the ventilatory response to carbon dioxide and therefore is less likely to produce respiratory depression; however, apnea can occur if large doses are given or if it is pushed too rapidly.[58] Ketamine can produce excessive salivation, which can contribute to the increased incidence of coughing and risk of laryngospasm. Some physicians pretreat their patients with either atropine or glycopyrrolate before administration of ketamine to prevent hypersalivation, although recent studies have demonstrated that this is likely unnecessary.[58] Some physicians believe that ketamine should be used with caution in patients with oral disease or upper respiratory tract infections in whom the risk of laryngospasm is greatest.[21,59–64] However, this has recently been refuted in a large meta-analysis.[58]

Even though its effect on the lower airway muscles is one of relaxation, ketamine causes an exaggeration of upper airway reflexes, leading to an increased incidence of coughing and risk of laryngospasm (0.3%).[58] This effect is rare but is more common with large intravenous boluses (>1 mg/kg) given rapidly or with intramuscular administration.[65] If this occurs, the patient can be supported by suctioning, supplemental oxygen, and assisted ventilation, if necessary. There are reports that laryngospasm can be relieved by applying bilateral pressure at the base of the skull just anterior to the mastoid process above the condyle from the mandible (**Figure 12.2**).[66–68]

Ketamine is associated with a number of other less serious adverse effects. It can produce agitated emergence reactions in 2% to 17% of patients.[69] The concomitant administration of benzodiazepines with ketamine has been recommended to reduce the incidence of emergence agitation, but well-controlled ED studies have shown no significant reduction in agitation with benzodiazepine use.[62,63,69] Vomiting also occurs in a few patients given ketamine and is usually brief and self-limited.[69] Ketamine can have the greatest margin of dosing safety of all procedural sedation medications. Patients administered 10 times the intended dose experienced no significant long-term adverse outcomes.[64] Despite such a large therapeutic index, patients given ketamine require preparation and vigilance equal to that afforded patients given other sedatives or analgesics because serious respiratory events are still possible.[58,64]

Dexmedetomidine is another sedative agent with a unique mechanism of action. Unlike other sedative analgesic agents, which work through the GABA receptor, dexmedetomidine is an α_2-adrenoreceptor agonist. Like the GABA agonists, dexmedetomidine produces sedative-hypnotic effects but without the respiratory depression found in these other agents. Dexmedetomidine is administered as a continuous infusion and has proven effective for prolonged sedation in critical care unit patients, particularly in postcardiac surgery patients, and for extended radiology procedures and for children with neurodevelopmental problems.[70]

Droperidol is a butyrophenone used in the pharmacologic control of acutely psychiatrically agitated patients. Useful for both psychotic conditions and alcohol-induced delirium in older adolescents, droperidol has also been combined with fentanyl to produce general anesthesia. Droperidol produces rapid somnolence, although patients are easily aroused and exhibit no significant respiratory depression. Recently, the Food and Drug Administration issued what is termed a black box warning for cases of arrhythmias thought to be due to prolongation of the QT interval produced by droperidol administered as an antiemetic after general anesthesia. The emergency medicine and pediatric implications of this warning are unclear, and the significance of the warning itself has been questioned. A study of adolescents administered droperidol for acute agitation found no evidence of any cardiac arrhythmias, even in the presence of multiple illicit drugs of abuse. Currently, there is no effective alternative sedative agent that exhibits droperidol's agitation control without significant respiratory compromise. When droperidol is used, it is recommended to also provide cardiac monitoring in light of the liability risk engendered by the Food and Drug Administration warning.[71,72]

Diphenhydramine is a common antihistamine with sedative-hypnotic effects. Available as an over-the-counter sleep aid and antihistamine, it can also be administered to children to provide cooperation for control during painless diagnostic studies. Diphenhydramine is particularly effective in children who are already exhausted from extensive crying. Hydroxyzine, another histamine$_1$-receptor antagonist, has been used effectively in combination with chloral hydrate for sedation for dental procedures in children.

Nitrous oxide, a potent analgesic, is an inhalation agent available for use as a fixed nitrous oxide–oxygen mixture. Nitrous oxide produces

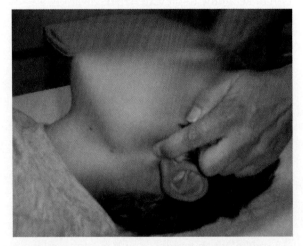

Figure 12.2 Procedure to relieve laryngospasm during ketamine sedation.

a linear dose-related sedative-hypnotic effect. It has a rapid onset and offset of action and is excreted unmetabolized from the lungs. The minimum recognized effective mixture is 30% nitrous oxide and 70% oxygen, although to be truly effective, a 50% concentration of nitrous oxide or higher is probably required; a 70% nitrous oxide concentration is even more effective, and few adverse events (other than vomiting) have been observed.[73] Nitrous oxide is best used alone or as an adjunct with local anesthetics for short, painful procedures. Care should be taken when combining nitrous oxide with other sedative analgesic agents.[9] Because the gas readily diffuses into any body cavity, it should not be used in patients with a bowel obstruction or pneumothorax.[74]

High concentrations of sucrose can provide analgesia as measured by less crying or fewer actions suggestive of pain in neonates and children up to the age of 6 weeks when administered 1 to 3 minutes or more before a procedure.[9,25,26,75] However, a more recent study has questioned this.[76] Generally 1 to 2 mL of a 25% to 30% sucrose solution are used and supplemented with nonnutritive sucking. The proposed mechanism of sucrose's effect is thought to be through enkephalin release.

Local Anesthetics

The two local anesthetics commonly used in the management of acute painful conditions in children are lidocaine (lignocaine) and bupivacaine. These agents inhibit nerve conduction through blockade of sodium channels in the axons of sensory nerves. These agents can be infiltrated directly into a wound or injected around a peripheral nerve to produce a nerve block. In all instances, care must be taken to avoid excessive dosing of either lidocaine (lignocaine) or bupivacaine. In the setting of excess dosing, neuroexcitatory effects, such as agitation, seizures, and even death, can result.

The pain of infiltration of local anesthetics can be reduced through buffering of these agents. Adjusting the pH closer to 7.4 allows more rapid absorption of the anesthetic into the myelinated axon fibers and decreases the pain on injection. Buffering can be accomplished by creation of an approximate 10:1 lidocaine (lignocaine) to bicarbonate (8.4%) ratio solution. For a fresh 30-mL bottle of lidocaine (lignocaine), this would require removing 3 mL of solution and replacing it with 3 mL of sodium bicarbonate solution. Other procedures shown to reduce the pain of injection include warming of solutions, use of small gauge needles (27 or 30 g), slow infiltration (as opposed to rapid infiltration), and pretreatment with topical anesthesia.

Lidocaine (lignocaine) is an amide anesthetic with a rapid onset of action and a duration of 30 to 120 minutes. A more prolonged effect results when the drug is combined with epinephrine (adrenaline) to produce localized vasoconstriction. The maximum recommended dose of this drug is 4.5 mg/kg (0.45 mL/kg of 1% solution) when used alone and 7 mg/kg (0.7 mL/kg of 1% solution) when combined with epinephrine (adrenaline) for subcutaneous infiltration. Lidocaine (lignocaine) solutions containing epinephrine (adrenaline) have always been described as causing potential tissue damage when injected near end arteries, such as in fingers, the penis, and the nose. This risk is actually minimal; however, infiltration will likely result in a noticeably prolonged vasoconstricted (white) area so patients should be advised of this ahead of time.

Bupivacaine is another amide anesthetic with a slightly slower onset of action but a duration of action of 2 to 6 hours. The safe dose of bupivacaine is up to 2.5 mg/kg (1 mL/kg of a 0.25% solution) for subcutaneous infiltration or nerve block.

Tetracaine is generally used in combination with lidocaine (lignocaine) and epinephrine (adrenaline) as a topical wound anesthetic preparation. Commonly referred to as LET (lidocaine [lignocaine], epinephrine [adrenaline], and tetracaine) or LAT, this solution produces good wound anesthesia without the need for infiltration with a needle.[8] To correctly use topical anesthetics for local lacerations, a cotton ball is completely saturated with the LET solution. A gauze pad should not be used for this purpose because the gauze is designed to hold onto solutions rather than release them into the tissue. The edges of the laceration are pulled apart, and the cotton ball is placed directly into the wound and loosely taped in place with a single piece of tape. If the solution is not dripping out of the wound, an inadequate amount of solution is being applied and is a common reason for failure.

Topical anesthetic agents can also be used in patients before painful percutaneous procedures or as an alternative to local anesthetic infiltration.[8] The thinner stratum corneum in children permits greater penetration of topical anesthetic agents to the underlying nerve endings, producing effective elimination of pain sensation in the skin for intravenous insertions, central port access, or lumbar punctures. Most topical preparations contain some mixture of local anesthetics, such as lidocaine (lignocaine), prilocaine, or tetracaine (amethocaine), and are available in ready-to-apply creams. Topical agents are best applied 60 minutes before the percutaneous procedure, although some anesthesia can be present at 30 minutes. Attempts to shorten the time to anesthesia by heating the area, stripping with tape, or adding nitroglycerin preparations have met with mixed success.[77–80]

Medication Selections

The choice of which agent to use again depends on the child's medical history, the clinical scenario, and physician preference. Providing physicians with the widest possible selection of agents permits the greatest opportunity to select the medication or medication combination most appropriate for any given child.

For simple analgesia, the use of acetaminophen (paracetamol), ibuprofen, or a combination of either with an oral opioid is appropriate. For more severe painful conditions, an intranasal or parenteral opioid analgesic is commonly used. Anxiety can be managed with an oral or parenteral benzodiazepine.

Painful procedures can be managed with a high-potency opioid analgesic, ketamine, etomidate, propofol, or an opioid sedative combination. Fentanyl and remifentanil have been combined successfully with midazolam or propofol for such procedures. When combining opioid analgesics and sedatives, not only are their effects enhanced but their risks of respiratory depression are enhanced as well. Because of this, the initial doses of both agents should be reduced, and they should be titrated more carefully. As a general rule with such combinations, the opioid is administered first and titrated to pain relief, followed after a few minutes by the sedative. Another drug combination that has been described for painful procedures is propofol and ketamine. Administered as a combination of 0.5 mg/kg of ketamine and 0.5 to 1 mg/kg of propofol, this regimen provides effective procedural sedation with potentially shorter recovery times than full-dose ketamine.[81,82] Nitrous oxide has also been used for many of these less painful procedures. Procedural pain associated with angiography or the repair of complex lacerations can be frequently managed with a pure sedative and a local or topical anesthetic.

Although the use of multiple sedative and analgesic agents has advantages, it also makes the drug administration process more complex. Administering multiple drugs (calculating volumes, drawing up from vials, and administering the drug) increases the potential for medication errors, complications, and distraction. A single agent administered with an automated smart infusion pump minimizes error risk and distraction. For painless diagnostic studies, pure sedatives, potent opioids, ketamine, and etomidate have all been used.

The specifics of the individual case help to determine which agent within a group of agents can be used. Drugs such as the barbiturates or propofol, which lower cerebral metabolism and ICP, might be selected for a child with possibly elevated ICP, whereas hypovolemic children should be treated with a drug that will help support blood pressure, such as ketamine or etomidate. In addition, sedation regimens that might result in hypercarbia due to hypoventilation should be used cautiously. Proper monitoring is required in patients who might have intracranial hypertension because these patients might lack normal autoregulation of cerebral blood flow and might experience great increases in ICP, which can worsen cerebral perfusion.

The presence of so many different options for pediatric procedural sedation makes it difficult to identify a universally superior drug or combination. Some possible medication options for different clinical scenarios are presented in Table 12-6. In a study of sedation preferences for posttraumatic head CT scans, more than 20 different regimens were described.[83] Depending on the study examined, virtually all of the agents listed in Table 12-6 have been reported to be "the most effective agent" for a given condition. In the ProSCED registry almost all of these drugs have been applied to procedural sedation cases outside research studies. For this reason, it is important for any physician to be as knowledgeable as possible about all the analgesic and sedation options available.[84–86]

Children With Special Health Care Needs

Children with special health care needs require analgesia and sedation for problems common to all children and conditions related to their underlying diagnosis. The fact that many of these children are already taking medications sometimes simplifies or complicates the selection of a sedation or analgesia agent. Use of a drug within a class of agents already taken by a child can minimize the risk of unexpected responses or drug interactions. For example, a child taking phenobarbital along with other medications is probably best sedated with pentobarbital or methohexital for a CT scan or MRI. If an analgesic or sedative class of agents is not among the medications a child is taking, then one must be selected, taking into account the child's unique physiologic features.[87,88]

In children with cardiac problems, a palliative procedure might have been performed using a shunt or some form of mixing communication between the pulmonary and systemic circulations. In these children, a balance must be maintained between the resistance in the two circulations. Analgesic or sedative agents that decrease peripheral vascular resistance can direct blood flow from the pulmonary to systemic circulations, resulting in cyanosis. In these instances, a relatively neutral agent, such as fentanyl or ketamine, might be the best choice, although carefully titrated propofol and etomidate have been safely used in these conditions.[89] Ketamine has also proven safe and effective in patients with pulmonary hypertension.[90]

Children with intracranial lesions can receive any number of agents, although care should be taken to prevent cerebral vasodilation secondary to either hypoxia or hypercarbia. Children who are developmentally delayed are at greater risk for airway obstruction when sedated for diagnostic studies than other children.[91] Children with endocrine problems, particularly those with adrenal problems and those with alterations in cellular immunity, should probably not be treated with etomidate because of its adrenal suppressive effects. Barbiturates should be avoided in children with porphyria, whereas chloral hydrate should not be used in patients with liver failure.

Complications and Disposition

Complications can and do occur with pediatric analgesia and sedation.[92] Overwhelmingly, most of these complications are related to inadequate patient monitoring or airway difficulties, multiple medications with synergistic effects on ventilation and airway patency, and procedural sedation conducted in inappropriately equipped facilities, which have all been noted to increase the risk of an adverse outcome in sedated children.[51,84] Problems are uncommon in children sedated in EDs, ICUs, properly attended radiology suites, or correctly staffed endoscopy units.[56,93–96]

Brief periods of hypoxia are not a problem in a sedated child when recognized and treated promptly. In most instances, repositioning of the head, lifting of the jaw, or administration of supplemental oxygen is all that is required to treat this problem. Brief bag-mask ventilation might be required in more severe cases. Reversal agents are rarely indicated because apnea that results from procedural sedation is generally short-lived and often temporally related to excessively rapid drug administration.

Hypoxia can be fatal if it is unrecognized and/or uncorrected. Continuous pulse oximetry during procedural sedation by personnel trained to recognize and react to airway obstruction and/or hypoxia will minimize this problem. Immediate access to physicians skilled at pediatric airway management with the proper equipment immediately available at the bedside is also important in any facility contemplating pediatric procedural sedation.

TABLE 12-6 Potential Sedation Options

Scenario	Options	
Extremity injury (minor)	Oral opioid Acetaminophen (paracetamol) or ibuprofen with or without an opioid	
Extremity injury (major)	Parenteral or oral opioid Patient controlled analgesia Regional anesthesia Ketamine	Propofol Etomidate Nitrous oxide
Small area burn	Oral opioid Acetaminophen (paracetamol) or ibuprofen with or without an opioid IM opioid Local anesthetic infiltration Topical anesthetic (LET)	
Large area burn	IV opioid Regional anesthesia Patient controlled analgesia	Ketamine Remifentanil
Multiple minor injuries	Parenteral opioid Acetaminophen (paracetamol) or ibuprofen with or without an opioid Distraction Hypnosis Oral opioid	
Multiple trauma	IV opioid Ketamine Etomidate	Patient controlled analgesia Fentanyl Remifentanil
Joint dislocation	Propofol Nitrous oxide IV opioid/sedative Diazepam Etomidate Intra-articular lidocaine (lignocaine) Remifentanil	
Vaso-occlusive painful crisis (mild)	Acetaminophen (paracetamol) / opioid combinations (PO) May be combined with ibuprofen (PO)	
Vaso-occlusive painful crisis (severe)	Morphine (IV) Hydromorphone (IV) Patient-controlled analgesia	Opioid should be combined with: Ibuprofen (PO) Ketorolac (IV)
Abdominal pain	Parenteral opioids Ketorolac (for biliary/renal colic) Patient controlled analgesia	
Pelvic pain (nonpregnant)	Parenteral opioids Oral NSAIDs Ketorolac	

TABLE 12-6 **Potential Sedation Options,** continued

Scenario	Options	
Pregnant nonobstetric painful condition	Oral opioid Acetaminophen (paracetamol) and opioid IM/SQ opioid Distraction Regional anesthesia	
Toothache	Oral opioid Acetaminophen (paracetamol) or ibuprofen with or without an opioid Hypnosis Local anesthesia	
Laceration in cooperative child	Lidocaine (lignocaine) Bupivacaine LET	
Laceration in uncooperative child	Oral midazolam and local anesthetic or LET Fentanyl and midazolam Propofol and local anesthetic Ketamine and local anesthetic	
Lumbar puncture	Propofol Ketamine Fentanyl and midazolam Pentobarbital Local anesthesia	
CT/ MRI	Pentobarbital Propofol Fentanyl or remifentanil Methohexital IV/PR	Midazolam Diphenhydramine Chloral hydrate Ketamine
Outpatient painless diagnostic study	Midazolam PO Chloral hydrate Pentobarbital PO Diphenhydramine Sleep deprivation	
Sepsis workup	Oral Sucrose Ketamine IM Nitrous oxide Transmucosal opioid IM/SQ opioid	
Multiple minor procedures	Ketamine IM Nitrous oxide Transmucosal opioid IM/SQ opioid	

Abbreviations: CT, computed tomography; IM, intramuscular; IV, intravenous; LET, lidocaine (lignocaine), epinephrine (adrenaline), and tetracaine; MRI, magnetic resonance imaging; NSAIDs, nonsteroidal anti-inflammatory drugs; PO, oral; PR, per rectum; SQ, subcutaneous.

Because hypoxia can be a sign (albeit late) of hypoventilation, some authors have suggested that administration of prophylactic supplemental oxygen to a sedated child could delay the early detection of this problem. In these cases, the fear is that more extreme hypoventilation, carbon dioxide retention, and respiratory acidosis will occur before hypoxia appears if a child is routinely given oxygen during procedural sedation. To date, there is no evidence supporting or refuting this concept. Close clinical observation of the patient permits detection of airway obstruction and/or significant hypoventilation before a decrease in oxygenation occurs. Oxygen supplementation provides a margin of safety and a longer time to correct the problem. In instances in which close clinical monitoring is not possible, such as during MRI, combining capnography with pulse oximetry serves to detect airway obstruction through loss of carbon dioxide waveform at an earlier time, often before desaturation, and can provide an additional margin of safety.

In outpatient facilities, a sedative should not be administered until the child is present in the facility and under the observation of competent staff. By the same token, children should not be discharged until respiratory status and protective airway reflexes have returned to baseline.

Deaths have occurred in sedated children in car seats during transport home from outpatient diagnostic sites. Physicians asked to arrange outpatient procedures that require sedation should only allow the procedures to be performed in sites with the capabilities to monitor and safely treat sedated children.

Putting It All Together

The successful delivery of procedural sedation or analgesia to a child is more than simply a knowledge of pharmacology and a working pulse oximeter. The entire treatment team, including nurses, technicians, aids, and physicians, must all have an understanding of the entire clinical scenario and how the PSA fits into the care of the particular patient. A formal presentation of all the potential PSA protocols for all the combinations of different agents and clinical scenarios is beyond the scope of this text. Even Table 12-6 barely touches the multitude of options used in clinical practice. Table 12-7 is a protocol of how a PSA agent such as propofol might be applied in a clinical setting. The safe application of such a protocol will hinge on the unit's education, pretreatment, monitoring, and credentialing practices.

TABLE 12-7 Propofol Administration Protocol Example

Clinical indication	• Extended sedation for painless or painful procedures
Intended sedation level	• Deep sedation
Anticipated agent and route	• Propofol intravenous
Specific precautions	• Hypotension • Egg allergy, soy allergy • Asthma
Supervising physician	• Credentialed for use of propofol
Location	• Approved unit for use of propofol sedation

Preparation	• History and physical examination to be performed in compliance with hospital's preprocedure assessment protocols and to include at the least:
	  - Direct inspection of mouth and posterior pharynx
	  - Assessment of lungs and respiratory capabilities
	  - Recent vital signs
	  - Cardiac monitor, continuous pulse oximetry with continuous audible tone (pitch) change indicator, intermittent blood pressure
	  - Immediate access to suction, airway rescue equipment, oxygen
	  - Normal saline infusion
	  - Oxygen by nasal prongs or mask (see section describing oxygen use)
	  - Optional pretreatment of vein with lidocaine (lignocaine)*

Medications delivery	• Propofol bolus 0.5–1 mg/kg over 0.5–2 minutes, repeated until sedation level is achieved, followed by propofol infusion at 3–6 mg/kg per hour • Inadequate sedation: rebolus 0.5–1 mg/kg, repeated until sedation level is achieved, followed by optional infusion increase of 1 mg/kg per hour
Postprocedure care	• Terminate infusion • Continue monitoring until return to baseline physical examination (6–10 min)

* To reduce the pain of propofol bolus infusion, some physicians pretreat the vein. Intravenous infusion is stopped, and the vein is occluded with a finger 1 to 2 cm proximal to catheter tip. Slow infusion of 0.5 to 1 mL of 1% lidocaine (lignocaine) without epinephrine (adrenaline), not to exceed 1 mg/kg (0.1 mL/kg). Hold finger occlusion in place for 2 minutes.

CHAPTER REVIEW

Check Your Knowledge

1. What would be the American Society of Anesthesiologists (ASA) classification in a 7-year-old child with occasional asthma relieved with as needed albuterol (salbutamol) metered-dose inhaler puffs?
   A. Class I
   B. Class II
   C. Class III
   D. Class IV

2. Selection of an agent for procedural sedation in an infant is determined by which of the following:
   A. Age of child
   B. Indication for procedural sedation
   C. Painful or painless procedure
   D. All of the above
   E. None of the above

3. A stable, 3-year-old, ASA class I child has severe abdominal pain and is scheduled for an abdominal computed tomographic (CT) scan in 2 hours. He is administered 0.1 mg/kg of morphine sulfate subcutaneously. What monitoring is appropriate for this child?
   A. Continuous pulse oximetry
   B. End tidal capnography
   C. Initial and repeat vital signs
   D. Pulse oximetry and cardiac monitoring

4. Which agent does not produce respiratory depression?
   A. Ketamine
   B. Methohexital
   C. Propofol
   D. Thiopental

5. Discharge criteria after procedural sedation include:
   A. return to baseline ambulation status.
   B. return to baseline level of alertness.
   C. return to baseline respiratory status.
   D. two hours of observation after conclusion of procedure.

6. Which agent should not be used in a hypotensive trauma patient?
   A. Etomidate
   B. Ketamine
   C. Midazolam
   D. Propofol

7. What is the maximum volume of 1% lidocaine (lignocaine) with epinephrine (adrenaline) that can be safely given as a subcutaneous infiltration in a 20-kg child?
   A. 14 mL
   B. 20 mL
   C. 27 mL
   D. 38 mL

8. Which of the following are effects that can be experienced with ketamine?
   A. Dissociative state
   B. Excessive salivation
   C. Laryngospasm
   D. Sympathomimetic effects and bronchodilation
   E. All of the above

9. Which sedative agent has the longest duration of action?
   A. Chloral hydrate
   B. Midazolam
   C. Morphine
   D. Pentobarbital
   E. Propofol

References

1. Godwin SA, Caro DA, Wolf SJ, et al; American College of Emergency Physicians. Clinical Policies Subcommittee on Procedural Sedation and Analgesia. Clinical policy: Procedural sedation and analgesia in the emergency department. *Ann Emerg Med*. 2005;45:177–196.

2. Sacchetti A, Schafermeyer R, Geradi M, et al. Pediatric analgesia and sedation. *Ann Emerg Med*. 1994;23:237–250.

3. American College of Emergency Physicians. The use of pediatric sedation and analgesia. www.acep.org/practres.aspx?LinkIdentifi er=id&rid=32884&fid=2144&Mo=No&taxid=117952. Accessed October 10, 2010.

4. Joint Commission Resources. *Comprehensive Accreditation Manual for Hospitals (CAMH)*. Oakbrook Terrace, Il: Joint Commission on Accreditation of Healthcare Organizations; 2002:TX-15, definitions 1–3.

5. Sacchetti A, Baren J, Carraccio C. Total procedural requirements as indication for emergency department sedation. *Pediatr Emerg Care*. 2010;26:209–211.

6. Dial S, Silver P, Bock K, Sagy M. Pediatric sedation for procedures titrated to a desired degree of immobility results in unpredictable depth of sedation. *Pediatr Emerg Care*. 2001;17:414–420.

7. Lightdale JR, Valim C, Mahoney LB, Wong S, DiNardo J, Goldmann DA. Agitation during procedural sedation and analgesia in children. *Clin Pediatr*. 2010;4:35–42.

8. Zempsky WT, Cravero JP, American Academy of Pediatrics Committee on Pediatric Emergency Medicine, Section on Anesthesiology and Pain Medicine. Relief of pain and anxiety in pediatric patient in emergency medical systems. *Pediatrics*. 2004;114:1348–1356.

9. Mace SE, Brown LA, Francis L, et al., EMSC Panel (Writing Committee) on Critical Issues in the Sedation of Pediatric Patients in the Emergency Department. Clinical policy: Critical issues in the sedation of pediatric patients in the emergency department. *Ann Emerg Med*. 2008;51:378–399.

10. Agrawal D, Manzi SF, Gupta R, Krauss B. Preprocedural fasting state and adverse events in children undergoing procedural sedation and analgesia in a pediatric emergency department. *Ann Emerg Med*. 2003;42:636–646.

11. Krauss B, Green SM. Sedation and analgesia for procedures in children. *N Engl J Med*. 2000;342:938–944.

12. Deitch K, Miner J, Chudnofsky CR, Dominici P, Latta D. Does end tidal CO2 monitoring during emergency department procedural sedation and analgesia with propofol decrease the incidence of hypoxic events? A randomized, controlled trial. *Ann Emerg Med*. 2010;55:258–264.

13. Padmanabhan P, Berkenbosch JW, Lorenz D, Pierce MC. Evaluation of cerebral oxygenation during procedural sedation in children using near infrared spectroscopy. *Ann Emerg Med*. 2009;54:205–213.

14. Hogan K, Sacchetti A, Aman L, Opiela D. The safety of single-physician procedural sedation in the emergency department. *Emerg Med J*. 2006;23:922–923.

15. D'Agostino J, Terndrup TE. Chloral hydrate versus midazolam for sedation of children for neuroimaging: A randomized clinical trial. *Pediatr Emerg Care*. 2000;16:1–4.

16. Quinn M, Carraccio C, Sacchetti A. Pain, punctures, and pediatricians. *Pediatr Emerg Care*. 1993;9:12–14.

17. Kim MK, Strait RT, Sato TT, Hennes HM. A randomized clinical trial of analgesia in children with acute abdominal pain. *Acad Emerg Med*. 2002;9:281–287.

18. Sharwood LN, Babl FE. The efficacy and effect of opioid analgesia in undifferentiated abdominal pain in children: a Review of four studies. *Paediatr Anaesth*. 2009;19:445–451.

19. Zernikow B, Michel E, Anderson B. Transdermal fentanyl in childhood and adolescence: A comprehensive literature review. *J Pain*. 2007;8:187–207.

20. Luten R, Broselow J. Doses and Dosing Intervals for Procedural Sedation eBroselow-Luten, The Artemis Project. 2010.

21. Dallimore D, Herd DW, Short T, Anderson BJ. Dosing ketamine for pediatric procedural sedation in the emergency department. *Pediatr Emerg Care*. 2008;24:529–533.

22. Nelson KL, Yaster M, Kost-Byerly S, Monitto CL. A national survey of American Pediatric Anesthesiologists: Patient-controlled analgesia and other intravenous opioid therapies in pediatric acute pain management. *Anesth Analg*. 2010;110:754–760.

23. Zier JL, Tarrago R, Liu M. Level of sedation with nitrous oxide for pediatric medical procedures. *Anesth Analg*. 2010;110:1399–1405.

24. Annequin D, Carbajal R, Chauvin P, Gall O, Tourniaire B, Murat I. Fixed 50% nitrous oxide oxygen mixture for painful procedures: A French survey. *Pediatrics*. 2000;105:E47.

25. Stevens B, Ohlsson A. Sucrose for analgesia in newborn infants undergoing painful procedures. *Cochrane Database Syst Rev*. 2001;4:CD001069.

26. Carbajal R, Chauvet X, Couderc S, Olivier-Martin M. Randomised trial of analgesic effects of sucrose, glucose and pacifiers in term neonates. *BMJ*. 1999;319:1393–1397.

27. Baghdadi ZD. Evaluation of audio analgesia for restorative care in children treated using electronic dental anesthesia. *J Clin Pediatr Dent*. 2000;25:9–12.

28. Rusy LM, Weisman SJ. Complementary therapies for acute pediatric pain management. *Pediatr Clin North Am*. 2000;47: 589–599.

29. Tobias JD. Weak analgesics and nonsteroidal anti-inflammatory agents in the management of children with acute pain. *Pediatr Clin North Am*. 2000;47:527–543.

30. Lieh-Lai MW, Kauffman RE, Uy HG, Danjin M, Simpson PM. A randomized comparison of ketorolac tromethamine and morphine for postoperative analgesia in critically ill children. *Crit Care Med*. 1999;27:2786–2791.

31. Beiter JL Jr, Simon HK, Chambliss CR, Adamkiewicz T, Sullivan K. Intravenous ketorolac in the emergency department management of sickle cell pain and predictors of its effectiveness. *Arch Pediatr Adolesc Med*. 2001;155:496–500.

32. Borland M, Jacobs I, King B, O'Brien D. A randomized controlled trial comparing intranasal fentanyl to intravenous morphine for managing acute pain in children in the emergency department. *Ann Emerg Med*. 2007;49:335–440.

33. Bates BA, Schutzman SA, Fleisher GR. A comparison of intranasal sufentanil and midazolam to intramuscular meperidine, promethazine, and chlorpromazine for conscious sedation in children. *Ann Emerg Med*. 1994;24:646–651.

34. Keidan I, Berkenstadt H, Sidi A, Perel A. Propofol/remifentanil versus propofol alone for bone marrow aspiration in paediatric haemato-oncological patients. *Paediatr Anaesth*. 2001;11:297–301.

35. Sammartino M, Garra R, Sbaraglia F, De Riso M, Continolo N. Remifentanil in children. *Paediatr Anaesth*. 2010;20:246–255.

36. Litman RS. Conscious sedation with remifentanil during painful medical procedures. *J Pain Symptom Manage*. 2000;19:468–471.

37. Beers R, Camporesi E. Remifentanil update: Clinical science and utility. *CNS Drugs*. 2004;18:1085–1104.

38. Duce D, Glaisyer H, Sury M. An evaluation of propofol combined with remifentanil: A new intravenous anaesthetic technique for short painful procedures in children. *Paediatr Anaesth.* 2000;10:689–690.

39. Drendel AL, Gorelick MH, Weisman SJ, Lyon R, Brousseau DC, Kim MK. A randomized clinical trial of ibuprofen versus acetaminophen with codeine for acute pediatric arm fracture pain. *Ann Emerg Med.* 2009;54:553–560.

40. Greenberg SB, Adams RC, Aspinall CL. Initial experience with intravenous pentobarbital sedation for children undergoing MRI at a tertiary care pediatric hospital: The learning curve. *Pediatr Radiol.* 2000;30:689–691.

41. Moro-Sutherland D, Algern JT, Penelope TL, Kozinetz A, Shook, J. Comparison of intravenous midazolam with pentobarbital for sedation for heat computed tomography imaging. *Acad Emerg Med.* 2000;7:1370–1375.

42. Beekman RP, Hoorntje TM, Beek FJ, Kuijten RH. Sedation for children undergoing magnetic resonance imaging: Efficacy and safety of rectal thiopental. *Eur J Pediatr.* 1996;155:820–822.

43. Pomeranz ES, Chudnofsky CR, Deegan TJ, Lozon MM, Mitchiner JC, Weber J. Rectal methohexital sedation for computed tomography imaging of stable pediatric emergency department patients. *Pediatrics.* 2000;105:1110–1114.

44. Sedik H. Use of intravenous methohexital as a sedative in pediatric emergency departments. *Arch Pediatr Adolesc Med.* 2001;155:665–668.

45. Karian VE, Burrows PE, Zurakowski D, Connor L, Mason KP. Sedation for pediatric radiological procedures: Analysis of potential causes of sedation failure and paradoxical reactions. *Pediatr Radiol.* 1999;29:869–873.

46. Havel CJ, Strati RT, Hennes H. A clinical trial of propofol vs. midazolam for procedural sedation in a pediatric emergency department. *Acad Emerg Med.* 1999;6:989–997.

47. Golden S. Combination propofol-ketamine anaesthesia in sick neonates. *Paediatr Anaesth.* 2001;11:119–122.

48. Jayabose S, Levendoglu-Tugal O, Giamelli J, et al. Intravenous anesthesia with propofol for painful procedures in children with cancer. *Am J Pediatr Hematol Oncol.* 2001;23:290–293.

49. Skokan EG, Pribble C, Bassett KE, Nelson DS. Use of propofol sedation in a pediatric emergency department: Prospective study. *Clin Pediatr.* 2001;40:663–671.

50. Cannon ML, Glazier SS, Bauman LA. Metabolic acidosis, rhabdomyolysis, and cardiovascular collapse after prolonged propofol infusion. *J Neurosurg.* 2001;95:925–926.

51. Sacchetti A, Stander E, Ferguson N, Maniar G, Valko P. Pediatric Procedural Sedation in the Community Emergency Department: Results from the ProSCED registry. *Pediatr Emerg Care.* 2007;23:218–222.

52. Garnock-Jones KP, Scott LJ. Fospropofol. *Drugs.* 2010;70:469–477.

53. Dickinson R, Singer A, Carrion W. Etomidate for pediatric sedation prior to fracture reduction. *Acad Emerg Med.* 2001;8:74–77.

54. Walls RM, Murphy MF. Clinical controversies: Etomidate as an induction agent for endotracheal intubation in patients with sepsis: Continue to use etomidate for intubation of patients with septic shock. *Ann Emerg Med.* 2008;52:13–14.

55. Sacchetti A. Etomidate: Not worth the risk in septic patients. *Ann Emerg Med.* 2008;52:14–16.

56. Hoffman GM, Nowakowski R, Troshynski TJ, Berens RJ, Weisman SJ. Risk reduction in pediatric procedural sedation by application of an American Academy of Pediatrics/American Society of Anesthesiologists process model. *Pediatrics.* 2002;109:236–243.

57. Bar-Joseph G, Guilburd Y, Tamir A, Guilburd JN. Effectiveness of ketamine in decreasing intracranial pressure in children with intracranial hypertension. *J Neurosurg Pediatr.* 2009;4:40–46.

58. Green SM, Roback MG, Krauss B, et al. Predictors of airway and respiratory adverse events with ketamine sedation in the emergency department: An individual-patient data meta-analysis of 8,282 children. *Ann Emerg Med.* 2009;54:158–168.

59. Green SM, Rothrock SG, Harris T, Hopkins GA, Garrett W, Sherwin T. Intravenous ketamine for pediatric sedation in the emergency department: Safety profile with 156 cases. *Acad Emerg Med.* 1998;5:971–976.

60. Green SM, Denmark TK, Cline J, Roghair C, Abd Allah S, Rothrock SG. Ketamine sedation for pediatric critical care procedures. *Pediatr Emerg Care.* 2001;17:244–248.

61. Green SM, Kupperman N, Rothrock SG, Hummel CB, Ho M. Predictors of adverse events with intramuscular ketamine sedation in children. *Ann Emerg Med.* 2000;35:35–42.

62. Sherwin TS, Green SM, Khan A, Chapman DS, Dannenberg B. Does adjunctive midazolam reduce recovery agitation after ketamine sedation for pediatric procedures? A randomized double-blind placebo controlled trial. *Ann Emerg Med.* 2000;35:229–238.

63. Wathen JE, Roback MG, Mackenzie T, Bothner JP. Does midazolam alter the clinical effects of intravenous ketamine sedation in children? A double-blind, randomized, controlled, emergency department trial. *Ann Emerg Med.* 2000;36:579–588.

64. Green SM, Clark R, Hostetler MA, Cohen M, Carlson D, Rothrock SG. Inadvertent ketamine overdose in children: Clinical manifestations and outcome. *Ann Emerg Med.* 1999;34:492–497.

65. Melendez E, Bachur R. Serious adverse events during procedural sedation with ketamine. *Pediatr Emerg Care.* 2009;25:325–328.

66. Kino A, Hirata S, Mishima S. The use of "laryngospasm notch" in two patients whose oxygen saturations dropped after tracheal extubation [in Japanese]. *Masui.* 2009;58:1430–1432.

67. Soares RR, Heyden EG. Treatment of laryngeal spasm in pediatric anesthesia by retroauricular digital pressure: Case report. *Rev Bras Anesthesiol.* 2008;58(6):631-6.

68. Larson CP Jr. Laryngospasm—the best treatment. *Anesthesiology.* 1998;89:1293–1294.

69. Green SM, Roback MG, Krauss B, et al. Predictors of emesis and recovery agitation with emergency department ketamine sedation: An individual-patient data meta-analysis of 8,282 children. *Ann Emerg Med.* 2009;54:171–180.

70. Lubisch N, Roskos R, Berkenbosch JW. Dexmedetomidine for procedural sedation in children with autism and other behavior disorders. *Pediatr Neurol.* 2009;41:88–94.

71. Horowitz BZ, Bizovi K, Moreno R. Droperidol-behind the black box warning. *Acad Emerg Med.* 2002;9:615–617.

72. Szwak K, Sacchetti A. Droperidol use in pediatric emergency department patients. *Pediatr Emerg Care.* 2010;26:248–250.

73. Babl FE, Oakley E, Seaman C, Barnett P, Sharwood LN. High-concentration nitrous oxide for procedural sedation in children: Adverse events and depth of sedation. *Pediatrics.* 2008;121:e528–e532.

74. Luhmann JD, Kennedy RM, Porter FL, Miller JP, Jaffe DM. A randomized clinical trial of continuous flow nitrous oxide and midazolam for sedation of young children during laceration repair. *Ann Emerg Med.* 2001;37:20-27.

75. Mace SE, Barata IA, Cravero JP, et al. American College of Emergency Physicians. Clinical policy: Evidence-based approach to pharmacologic agents used in pediatric sedation and analgesia in the emergency department. *Ann Emerg Med.* 2004;44:342-377.

76. Slater R. Cornelissen L, Fabrizi L, et al. Oral sucrose as an analgesic drug for procedural pain in newborn infants: A randomized controlled trial. *The Lancet.* 2010;376:1225-1232.

77. Kleiber C, Sorenson M, Whiteside K, Gronstal BA, Tannous R. Topical anesthetics for intravenous insertion in children: A randomized equivalency study. *Pediatrics.* 2002;110:758-761.

78. Chen BK, Cunningham BB. Topical anesthetics in children: Agents and techniques that equally comfort patients, parents, and clinicians. *Curr Opin Pediatr.* 2001;13:324-330.

79. Liu DR, Kirchner HL, Petrack EM. Does using heat with eutectic mixture of local anesthetic cream shorten analgesic onset time? A randomized, placebo-controlled trial. *Ann Emerg Med.* 2003;42:27-33.

80. Soltesz S, Dittrich K, Teschendorf P, Fuss I, Molter G. Topical anesthesia before vascular access in children: Comparison of a warmth-producing lidocaine-tetracaine patch with a lidocaine-prilocaine patch [in German]. *Anaesthesist.* 2010;59:519-523.

81. Andolfatto G, Willman E. A prospective case series of pediatric procedural sedation and analgesia in the emergency department using single-syringe ketamine-propofol combination (ketofol). *Acad Emerg Med.* 2010;17:194-201.

82. Sharieff GQ, Trocinski DR, Kanegaye JT, Fisher B, Harley JR. Ketamine-propofol combination sedation for fracture reduction in the pediatric emergency department. *Pediatr Emerg Care.* 2007;23:881-884.

83. Conners GP, Sacks WK, Leahey NF. Variations in sedating uncooperative, stable children for post-traumatic head CT. *Pediatr Emerg Care.* 1999;15:241-244.

84. Sacchetti A, Senula G, Strickland J, Dubin R. Procedural sedation in the community emergency department: Initial results of the ProSCED registry. *Acad Emerg Med.* 2007;14:41-46.

85. Sacchetti A, Harris RH, Packard D. Emergency department procedural sedation formularies. *Am J Emerg Med.* 2005;23:569-570.

86. Sacchetti A, Stander E, Ferguson N, Maniar G, Valko P. Pediatric Procedural Sedation in the Community Emergency Department: Results from the ProSCED registry. *Pediatr Emerg Care.* 2007;23:218-222.

87. Sacchetti A, Turco T, Carraccio C, Hasher W, Cho D, Gerardi M. Procedural sedation for children with special health care needs. *Pediatr Emerg Care.* 2003;19:231-239.

88. Sacchetti AD, Gerardi M. Procedural sedation for patients with special health needs. In: Krauss B, Brustowicz RB, eds. *Pediatric Procedural Sedation and Analgesia.* Baltimore, MD: Lippincott Williams & Wilkins; 1999:189-199.

89. Gozal D, Rein AJ, Nir A, Gozal Y. Propofol does not modify the hemodynamic status of children with intracardiac shunts undergoing cardiac catheterization. *Pediatr Cardiol.* 2001;22:488-490.

90. Williams GD, Maan H, Ramamoorthy C, et al. Perioperative complications in children with pulmonary hypertension undergoing general anesthesia with ketamine. *Paediatr Anaesth.* 2010;20:28-37.

91. Elwood T, Hansen LD, Seely JM. Oropharyngeal airway diameter during sedation in children with and without developmental delay. *J Clin Anesth.* 2001;13:482-485.

92. Pena BM, Krauss B. Adverse events of procedural sedation and analgesia in a pediatric emergency department. *Ann Emerg Med.* 1999;34:483-491.

93. Cote CJ, Karl HW, Notterman DA, Weinberg JA, McCloskey C. Adverse sedation events in pediatrics: Analysis of medications used for sedation. *Pediatrics.* 2000;106:633-644.

94. Blike G, Cvravero J, Nelson E. Same patients, same critical events-different systems of care, different outcomes: Description of a human factors approach aimed at improving the efficacy and safety of sedation/analgesia care. *Qual Manag Health Care.* 2001;10:17-36.

95. Cote CJ, Notterman DA, Karl HW, Weinberg JA, McCloskey C. Adverse sedation events in pediatrics: A critical incident analysis of contributing factors. *Pediatrics.* 2000;105:805-814.

96. Cravero JP, Beach ML, Blike GT, Gallagher SM, Hertzog JH; Pediatric Sedation Research Consortium. The incidence and nature of adverse events during pediatric sedation/anesthesia with propofol for procedures outside the operating room: A report from the Pediatric Sedation Research Consortium. *Anesth Analg.* 2009;108:795-804.

An 18-month-old boy is brought to the emergency department after a witnessed generalized tonic clonic seizure. He sustained a closed head injury and a 4-cm forehead laceration when he struck a low coffee table. His mother, who witnessed the event, notes that he has a ventriculoperitoneal shunt and a history of hydrocephalus. He was drowsy for a few minutes after the initial injury. On awakening, he cried briefly but has been abnormally quiet and withdrawn since the event. He has vomited three times and is irritable in his mother's arms. The child has no other signs of injuries. After a discussion with the patient's neurologist, it is determined that magnetic resonance imaging (MRI) would be the optimal diagnostic study to evaluate his seizure and had trauma.

1. *What are the procedural sedation options for this child for an MRI scan and laceration repair?*
2. *Can a single agent be used for both procedures?*

This case presents a unique challenge because both a painless procedure and a painful procedure must be addressed. Multiple options can be considered for the procedural sedation of this patient. Oral agents, such as diphenhydramine, oral pentobarbital, or even chloral hydrate, would not provide sufficient sedation for either procedure. The possibility of increased intracranial pressure (ICP) makes

CASE SUMMARY 1 CONT.

fentanyl a lower-priority choice because it can induce vomiting itself, which would further elevate the ICP. A pure sedative with ICP-lowering characteristics would be appropriate for computed tomography (CT) cooperation but would not permit repair of the laceration alone. If CT was chosen, because of its short scanning time, a shorter-acting and milder sedative could be used, or perhaps no sedative is necessary. Because MRI has been chosen, the scan time is much longer and the noise level is high. Deep sedation is likely necessary to complete the MRI scan. Combining such a sedative with local anesthesia of the wound might help. An option that is likely to succeed is to apply LET (lidocaine [lignocaine], epinephrine [adrenaline], and tetracaine) to the wound and sedate the child with propofol for the MRI scan. This approach would permit the LET to take effect during the MRI procedure, whereas enough residual sedation would remain after the MRI scan (or the propofol infusion rate could be decreased but not stopped) to facilitate repair of the laceration.

chapter 13

Children With Special Health Care Needs: The Technologically Dependent Child

Terry A. Adirim, MD, MPH, FAAP

Objectives

1 Explain how children with special health care needs differ from healthy children with regard to vital signs, size, and developmental level.

2 Describe the types of emergencies that medical personnel might encounter in children with special health care needs.

3 Discuss the management of various technologies used for children with special health care needs, including tracheostomy tubes, home mechanical ventilators, central venous catheters, feeding tubes, ventriculoperitoneal (VP) shunts, vagal nerve stimulators, and intrathecal baclofen pumps.

Chapter Outline

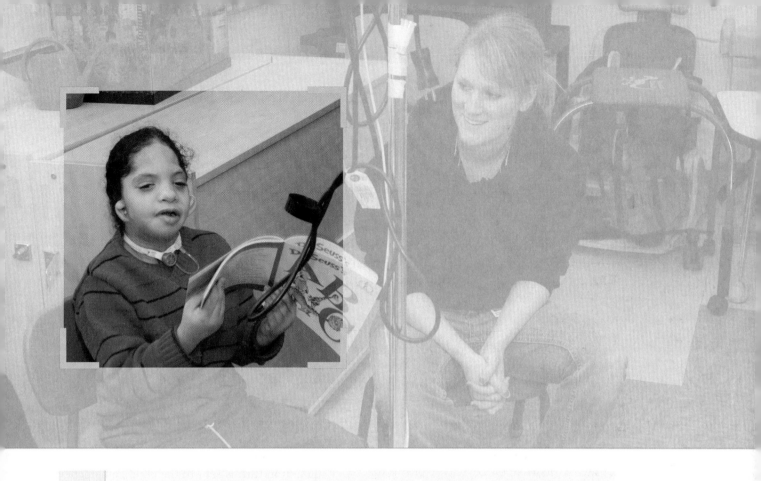

A 3-year-old boy with a mitochondrial myopathy is brought to the emergency department (ED) with a 1-day history of difficulty breathing. The boy's condition was diagnosed when he was 1 year of age, when it was noted that he had muscle weakness and frequent respiratory infections. He had a tracheostomy tube placed and home mechanical ventilation was initiated at the age of 18 months for impending respiratory failure due to severe muscle weakness. He also has a gastrostomy tube, which is reportedly functioning without a problem. Yesterday, his home health care nurse noted that he was producing more than usual secretions, which are now yellow (as opposed to clear), and he required more frequent suctioning. This morning, his mother noted that he had a temperature of 38.4°C (101.2°F), his pulse oximetry reading at home was 92%, and his baseline reading is above 95% on 0.25 L/min of oxygen. He receives ventilation mostly at night while asleep and has periods during the day while awake off the ventilator. Today, his mother kept him on the ventilator at his baseline settings for the trip to the hospital. On examination, the boy is sleepy but arousable and there are subcostal and intercostal retractions. His color is pink. His ventilator rate is set at 20 to support each breath (volume support). His respiratory rate is 40/min, heart rate is 160/min, and blood pressure is 90/60 mm Hg. Temperature in the ED is noted to be 39°C (102.2°F), and pulse oximetry is 90% on 1 L/min of oxygen. Lung examination reveals crackles on the right side of the child's chest. Capillary refill is less than 2 seconds, and the extremities are well perfused.

1. What is your initial assessment of this child's presentation?
2. How do you manage this presentation? Where do you start?
3. What issues do you need to consider?

Introduction

An estimated 34% of all ED visits involve children and adolescents. More than half of these visits are medically related, and a subset of these patients comprises children with special health care needs (CSHCN).[1,2] Children who have a variety of chronic health and behavioral conditions that are potentially disabling are considered CSHCN. A subset of these children are technology assisted and therefore depend on medical devices to support bodily functions.[3] Children who have or are at increased risk for a chronic physical, developmental, behavioral, or emotional condition and who also require health and related services of a type or amount beyond that required by children generally are considered CSHCN.[4] On the basis of this definition, it is estimated that more than 12 million, or 18%, of children in the United States have special health care needs.[5] One study at a tertiary care pediatric ED found that almost a quarter of their visits were by CSHCN. Not unexpectedly, they found that these children tended to be sicker, that they were 33 times more likely to need intensive care unit admission, and that more than half of these children needed the consultation of a subspecialty service.[1] Therefore, this population is a significant user of health care resources.[6–8]

Most parents and caregivers of CSHCN have specialized training in the care of their children. They are well versed in the care of their children's technology and medical conditions. They often carry detailed care plans that are developed with teams of specialists. However, because these children are vulnerable to serious and recurrent complications, they frequently need access to emergency care for the management of their conditions. Although most caregivers are adept at handling many of their children's emergencies, they still seek help for a variety of reasons, including the need for respite, equipment malfunction, an overwhelming medical problem, and the need for help with transport to the child's home hospital.

During these emergencies, the emergency health care professional does not have time to read often lengthy medical records. One example of a program that provides information to medical care personnel is the American Academy of Pediatrics and American College of Emergency Physicians Emergency Preparedness for Children with Special Health Care Needs Program.[9] This is an emergency notification program designed to provide specific information to medical caregivers about the special needs child. An emergency information form (EIF), downloadable at www.aap.org and www.acep.org, is completed by the child's primary care physician and/or family and is carried with the child (**Figure 13.1**). The child can also be enrolled in the MedicAlert program. MedicAlert personnel enter the information from the EIF into a database accessible to health care personnel in an emergency. Other programs, such as EMS Outreach from the Children's National Medical Center in Washington, DC, serve a similar function but are focused on the out-of-hospital environment. Enrollees in this program complete a medical information form that caregivers carry with them, and this information in turn is sent to the child's emergency medical service jurisdiction so that the personnel dispatched in an emergency are aware that the child has special health care needs.[10]

Medical personnel should be aware that CSHCN differ from well children in a variety of ways. They can be neurologically impaired and therefore developmentally delayed. Their growth might be impaired, so they might be smaller than other children of the same age. Also, depending on a child's condition, vital signs at rest might also be different and thus change management strategies. Medical personnel cannot rely on ages and weight-based norms and should either ask caregivers for this information or use length-based tapes when estimating weight and determining fluid and medication management. Developmentally delayed children might not be able to respond in the manner expected for age. Baseline vital signs can be altered, especially in children with cardiac conditions or on mechanical ventilators. For example, a child with complex congenital heart disease might have a baseline pulse oximetry reading of 85%. Some CSHCN have sensorineural deficits, such as blindness and deafness. Medical care personnel caring for special children should be sensitive to these

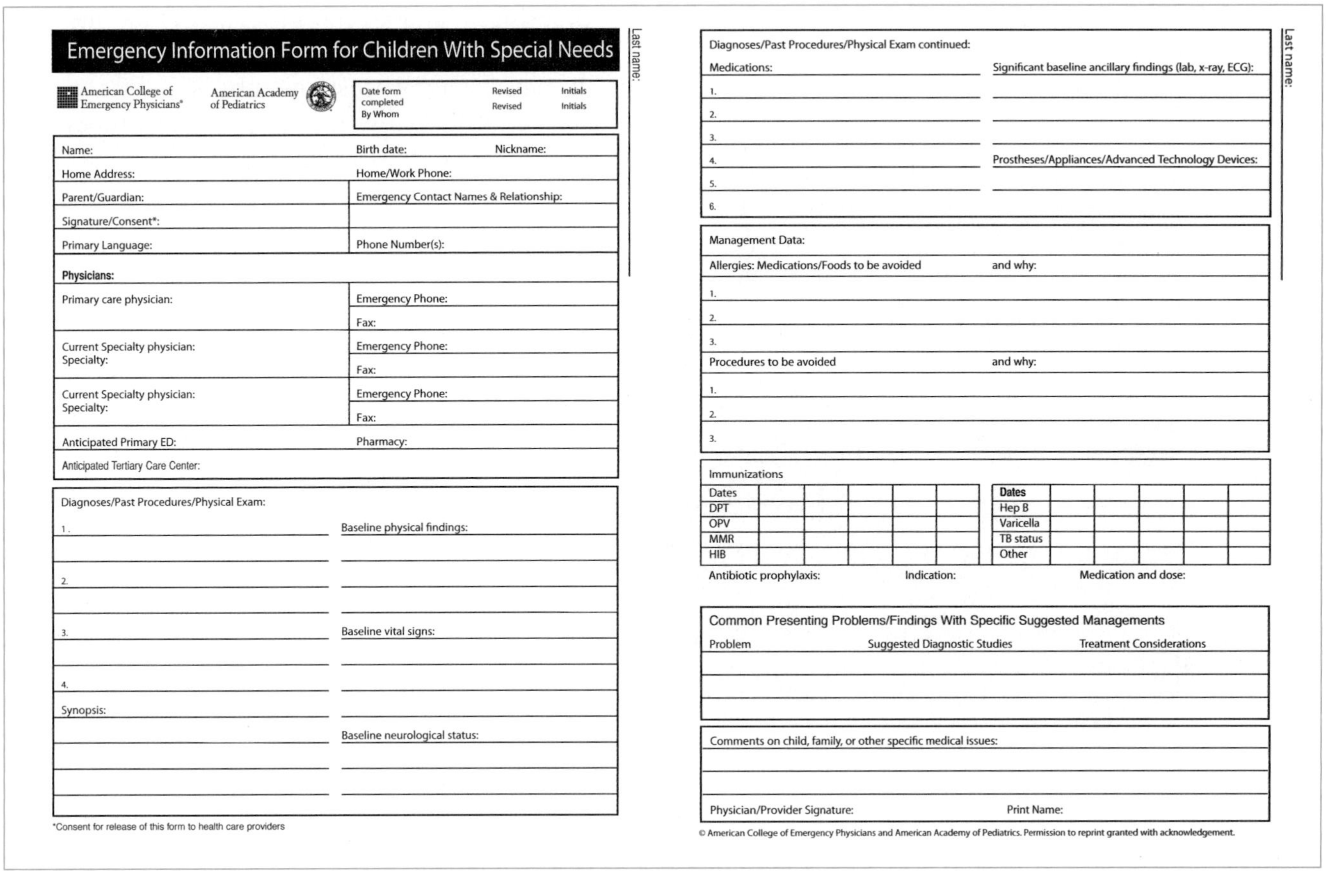

Emergency Information Form for Children With Special Needs

American College of Emergency Physicians® — American Academy of Pediatrics

Date form completed By Whom | Revised Initials | Revised Initials

Last name:

Name:	Birth date: Nickname:
Home Address:	Home/Work Phone:
Parent/Guardian:	Emergency Contact Names & Relationship:
Signature/Consent*:	
Primary Language:	Phone Number(s):
Physicians:	
Primary care physician:	Emergency Phone:
	Fax:
Current Specialty physician: Specialty:	Emergency Phone:
	Fax:
Current Specialty physician: Specialty:	Emergency Phone:
	Fax:
Anticipated Primary ED:	Pharmacy:
Anticipated Tertiary Care Center:	

Diagnoses/Past Procedures/Physical Exam:	
1.	Baseline physical findings:
2.	
3.	Baseline vital signs:
4.	
Synopsis:	Baseline neurological status:

*Consent for release of this form to health care providers

Diagnoses/Past Procedures/Physical Exam continued:	
Medications:	Significant baseline ancillary findings (lab, x-ray, ECG):
1.	
2.	
3.	
4.	Prostheses/Appliances/Advanced Technology Devices:
5.	
6.	

Management Data:	
Allergies: Medications/Foods to be avoided	and why:
1.	
2.	
3.	
Procedures to be avoided	and why:
1.	
2.	
3.	

Immunizations

Dates						Dates					
DPT						Hep B					
OPV						Varicella					
MMR						TB status					
HIB						Other					

Antibiotic prophylaxis: Indication: Medication and dose:

Common Presenting Problems/Findings With Specific Suggested Managements

Problem	Suggested Diagnostic Studies	Treatment Considerations

Comments on child, family, or other specific medical issues:

Physician/Provider Signature: Print Name:

© American College of Emergency Physicians and American Academy of Pediatrics. Permission to reprint granted with acknowledgement.

Figure 13.1 Emergency information form for children with special needs.

situations. In addition, many of these children have latex allergies, so latex-free equipment should be used when caring for CSHCN.

This chapter focuses on technology-dependent children. The more common technologies used in CSHCN will be discussed. These technologies include tracheostomy care and home mechanical ventilation, feeding tubes, central venous catheters, dialysis shunts, peritoneal dialysis catheters, VP shunts, vagal nerve stimulators (VNSs), and baclofen pumps.

Tracheostomies and Home Ventilation

Tracheostomy Tubes

A tracheostomy is a surgical opening in the anterior aspect of the neck (stoma) through the trachea that is meant to bypass the upper airway. A tracheostomy tube is placed in the stoma to facilitate mechanical ventilation, provide a bypass of the upper airway, or improve pulmonary toilet. Tracheostomy tubes allow for long-term management of the airway and for respiratory support of breathing. There are several conditions for which a child might need a tracheostomy. The most common conditions include but are not limited to tracheal stenosis, tracheomalacia, certain craniofacial anomalies, bronchopulmonary dysplasia, muscular dystrophy, spinal cord injury, and traumatic brain injury.

Tracheostomy tubes are used by most children and adolescents with tracheostomies. The tube keeps the stoma patent and can be attached to a mechanical ventilator (**Figure 13.2**). Tracheostomy tubes come in various sizes. There are several manufacturers, so there are variations in the way that they are sized and marked. Brands include Shiley, Bivona, Holinger, Portex, and Berdeen. They range in size from 00 for newborns to 7.0 for older adolescents.[10] The inner

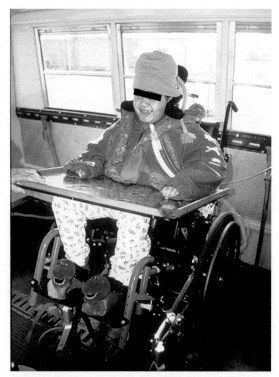

Figure 13.2 A child with a tracheostomy tube might require continuous support of ventilation with a portable ventilator.

choosing an endotracheal tube (ETT) for oral intubation or use through the stoma. The inner diameter of a tracheostomy tube is the size to choose for ETT insertion. Tracheostomy tubes also come in various lengths. Neonatal tubes are shorter than pediatric tubes, although the inner diameters might be the same.[11]

There are several types of tracheostomy tubes and attachments. Types include single cannula tubes, double cannula tubes, cuffed tubes, and fenestrated tubes (**Figure 13.4**).[3] Neonates, infants, and young children use single cannula tracheostomy tubes (**Figure 13.5**). As a child's trachea gets larger, a double cannula tube should be used. It contains an outer tube that stays in the stoma and an inner tube that is removable for cleaning and pulmonary toilet. Tracheostomy tubes for older children and adolescents often have an inflatable cuff to keep the tube in place and to prevent air leaks. Fenestrated tubes have a hole in the cephalic portion of the tube that redirects air into the upper airway, allowing the child to speak and breathe through the nose and mouth. This is facilitated by a decannulation plug attached to the opening of the tube.

Attachments to the tracheostomy tube include a tracheostomy nose, a tracheostomy collar, and a speaker valve. A tracheostomy nose is placed over the external opening of the tracheostomy tube of a child who is not receiving mechanical ventilation to provide air filtration and humidification. A tracheostomy collar is used to

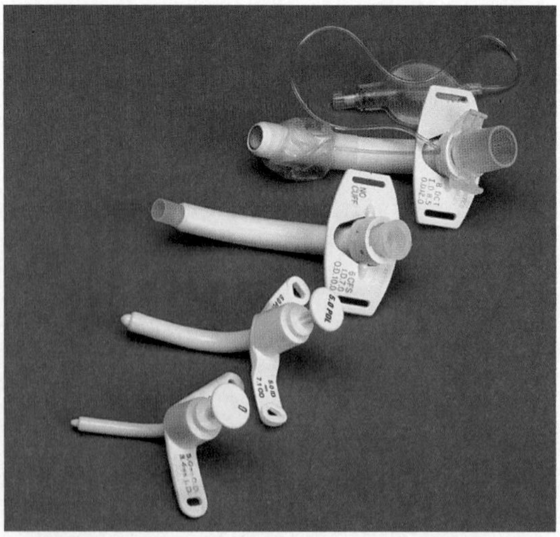

and outer diameter ranges are provided so that comparisons among brands can be made. They range from 2.5 mm for infants to 10.0 mm for adolescents and adults. Typically, the sizes are marked on the packaging and on the flange, or wings, of each tube (**Figure 13.3**). This information is also important for emergency personnel when replacing a tracheostomy tube or when

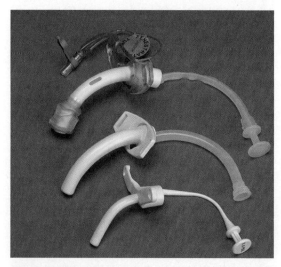

Figure 13.3 Tracheostomy tube sizes are marked on the flange, or wings.

Figure 13.4 Fenestrated, double lumen, and single lumen tracheostomy tubes (top to bottom).

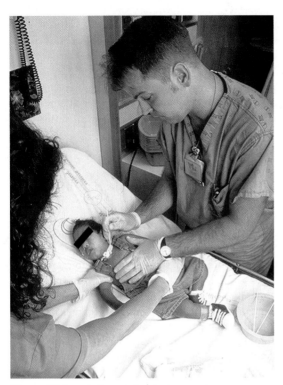

Figure 13.5 An infant with a single cannula tracheostomy tube in place.

provide humidified air or supplemental oxygen to the patient who is not receiving mechanical ventilation. A speaker valve is an attachment that redirects airflow through the upper airway to facilitate speech.

Tracheostomy Emergencies

There are many reasons a child with a tracheostomy tube can become sick, including an exacerbation of an underlying pulmonary disease. Signs and symptoms of respiratory distress include nasal flaring, retractions, increased respiratory rate, decreased breath sounds, decreased oxygen saturation, cyanosis, wheezing, rales, and increased secretions. Other causes can include a mucous plug of the tracheostomy tube or equipment failure.

The treatment approach to the child with a tracheostomy tube should begin as with any other child, with a history and attention to the ABCs (airway, breathing, circulation). Sudden onset of respiratory distress can lead one to predict a mucous plug or equipment failure as opposed to a pulmonary infection, in which fever and a more progressive onset of deterioration

of respiratory status would be expected. Assessment of the airway should include inspection of the tracheostomy tube for patency. Next, breathing is assessed by observation and auscultation of the chest. Finally, circulation is assessed by assessing color, perfusion, pulses, and auscultation of the heart sounds.

For the child with a tracheostomy tube and a pulmonary exacerbation, infection and reactive airway disease are the most likely causes. Short-term treatment would include administration of a bronchodilator nebulizer treatment through the tracheostomy tube or inline with the ventilator in a child receiving mechanical ventilation. If the child has a fever, infection should be considered and proper tracheostomy cultures and antibiotic coverage provided. Chest radiography should also be considered. Hospital admission is determined by a combination of factors, including age, medical history, severity of illness, and diagnosis. Medical personnel should consider transporting a medically complex child, if appropriate, to his or her home hospital under the advice of the physicians who know the child best.

For the child with sudden onset of respiratory distress, suctioning the tracheostomy tube can be helpful. If suctioning two to three times does not relieve the obstruction or respiratory distress, then the medical personnel should consider changing the tracheostomy tube because a thick mucous plug might be obstructing airflow through the tube. See Table 13-1 for the steps for emergency tracheostomy tube change. As with any procedure, the medical personnel should be prepared and have the appropriate supplies available (Table 13-2). If the ED or ambulance service does not have all of the supplies needed, parents and other caregivers often have them.

Home Mechanical Ventilation

Many children with tracheostomy tubes also receive mechanical ventilation. Indications for mechanical ventilation include severe lung disease and abnormal respiratory drive either from central causes or secondary to paralysis. Some children are dependent on ventilators 24 hours a day, some while asleep, and some for part of the day.

TABLE 13-1 Steps for an Emergency Tracheostomy Tube Change

1. Prepare a replacement tracheostomy tube of the same size. Ask parents for one if you do not have one.

2. For cuffed tracheostomy tubes, deflate the balloon by connecting a syringe to the valve on the pilot balloon. Draw air out until the pilot balloon collapses. Cutting the pilot balloon will not deflate the cuff.

3. If the child has a double cannula tracheostomy tube, remove the inner cannula. If removal of the inner cannula fails to clear the airway, the outer cannula should then be removed.

4. Cut the cloth or Velcro ties that hold the tracheostomy tube in place.

5. Remove the tube using a slow outward motion.

6. Gently insert the same size tracheostomy tube with the obturator in place. Point the curve of the tube downward. Never force the tube. The tube can be lubricated with a water-soluble gel or by dipping it into normal saline before insertion.

7. Securely hold the flange (wings) while removing the obturator, ventilate, assess tube placement, and ensure proper placement. Then secure tube with tracheostomy ties (or Velcro strap).

8. If the tube cannot be inserted easily, withdraw it and attempt to pass a smaller tracheostomy tube if available.

9. If insertion of a smaller tracheostomy tube fails or a smaller tube is not available, then attempt to insert an ETT into the stoma no more than 2.5 to 5 cm (1 to 2 in) into the opening. Select an ETT with an inner diameter that is equal to or smaller than the inner diameter of the last tracheostomy tube attempted. Aim downward when inserting an ETT into the stoma. If the ETT has a cuff, inflate it after checking proper placement. Note that this is only a temporizing measure until definitive treatment can be sought. An ETT in the stoma is not stable.

10. If there is no improvement in the child's clinical condition, attempt oral endotracheal intubation if this child does not have a preexisting upper airway obstruction. Bag-mask ventilation can also be attempted if there is no preexisting upper airway obstruction. If this is not possible, then attempt to ventilate by placing a manual resuscitator (bag-mask) directly over the stoma while covering the mouth and nose.

Adirim TA, Smith EL, Singh T. *Special Children's Outreach and Prehospital Education.* Sudbury, MA: Jones and Bartlett; 2006. Reprinted with permission.

Two types of ventilators are used: pressure-cycled ventilators and volume ventilators. Pressure-cycled ventilators tend to be used in infants. They are set to deliver a given pressure with each breath. Volume ventilators give a tidal volume with each breath. There are two common modes of ventilations: control modes and support modes. Control modes (also called assist control mode) deliver a set breath and the size and duration are determined by the physician and can be based on pressure or volume. Patients will get a full breath regardless of how much effort they are making. Support modes (eg, continuous positive airway pressure, bilevel positive airway pressure, pressure support volume support, and synchronized intermittent mechanical ventilation) give patients what they need above and beyond their own effort. These ventilator settings are for patients who can initiate their own breaths and serve to augment the child's own breath.

There are five types of ventilator alarms. They include low pressure/apnea, low power, high pressure, setting error, and power switchover. The causes of a low pressure alarm include a loose or disconnected circuit, a leak in the

---

YOUR FIRST CLUE

Recognizing Illness in a Child With Special Health Care Needs

- Parent or caregiver says "something is different"
- Increased work of breathing
- Need for increased oxygen
- Fever
- Change in level of functioning
- Altered level of consciousness

TABLE 13-2 Supplies Needed for Tracheostomy Tube Change

- Same size tracheostomy tube that is "ready to go" (with ties in place)
- One size smaller tracheostomy tube
- Various sized endotracheal tubes
- Laryngoscope
- Suction catheters (6.0F, 8.0F, 10.0F)
- Normal saline for suctioning (premeasured ampules, "bullets," or vials, if available)
- Towel for shoulder roll
- Sterile gloves and face mask
- Scissors
- Oxygen and suction
- Bag-mask resuscitator with appropriately sized face masks
- Water-soluble lubricating gel
- Nebulizer setup

Adirim TA, Smith EL, Singh T. *Special Children's Outreach and Prehospital Education.* Sudbury, MA: Jones and Bartlett; 2006. Reprinted with permission.

YOUR FIRST CLUE

Troubleshooting a Home Mechanical Ventilator Alarm

- Low pressure/apnea: check for loose circuits or air leak around tracheostomy tube.
- Low power: plug into an electrical outlet or the device will fail.
- High pressure: indicates obstruction in the circuit or the patient has bronchospasm; relieve tube obstruction and/or begin bronchodilator therapy.
- Setting error: indicates failure of the ventilator setup; remove the patient from the ventilator and begin ventilation with manual resuscitator.
- Power switchover: check to see whether the battery is charged; if not, connect the ventilator to an electrical outlet.

circuit, and a leak around the tracheostomy site. All circuits should be checked to ensure they are connected; if they are, the tracheostomy tube should be checked for leaks. The low power alarm means that the internal battery is nearly spent and the ventilator should be plugged into an electrical outlet. A high pressure alarm indicates an obstructed circuit or that the patient is having bronchospasm. The obstruction should be cleared or a bronchodilator administered or both. A setting error signifies that a setting might have been improperly adjusted. Under these circumstances the patient should receive manual ventilation until the ventilator can be set properly. Any time the ventilator switches from AC power to battery, an alarm will sound. Under these circumstances, the battery should be checked to ensure it is powering the unit and the "alarm silent" button pressed.[10]

A ventilator-dependent child is at risk for airway and breathing emergencies. Possible causes of respiratory distress in a ventilator-dependent child include airway obstruction (eg, an obstructed tracheostomy tube), an obstruction or leak in the ventilator tubing, problems with the oxygen supply, equipment failure involving the ventilator, and an acute medical condition. If a ventilator-dependent child is found to be in respiratory distress and the cause is not easily determined, then the child should be taken off the ventilator and given manual ventilation with a bag-mask ventilator. Manual ventilation can help determine whether the problem is equipment failure or a medical condition.

Feeding Tubes and Gastrostomy Tubes

Feeding tubes and gastrostomy tubes are placed in children who need long-term nutritional supplementation or who cannot consume food by mouth. There are many conditions that necessitate placement of an artificial feeding tube. Some of these include severe developmental delay and/or cerebral palsy (CP), coma, short bowel syndrome, neuromuscular disorders, swallowing difficulties, burns to mouth and esophagus, failure to thrive, and chronic diseases that affect nutrition, such as cystic fibrosis.

A feeding tube is a long catheter usually inserted through the nose or mouth of the child into the stomach or jejunum. The terms used for these tubes includes nasogastric, orogastric, nasojejunal, and orojejunal.

Emergency Treatment of CSHCN With Tracheostomy Receiving Home Ventilation

- Remove the child from the mechanical ventilator.
- Begin ventilation with a manual resuscitator.
- Evaluate the tracheostomy tube for obstruction (see Chapter 25, Office Procedures).
- Suction the tracheostomy tube.
- If obstruction is not relieved by suctioning, remove and replace the tracheostomy tube.
- Initiate treatment for respiratory distress as with other respiratory emergencies.

Gastrostomy tubes go directly into the stomach from a site on the abdomen (**Figure 13.6**). Most gastrostomy tubes are inserted surgically or endoscopically by gastroenterologists, surgeons, or radiologists, either at the bedside or in an outpatient procedure area by using a procedure called percutaneous endoscopic gastrostomy. There are several types of low-profile gastrostomy tubes in use, including the Button and Mic-Key.

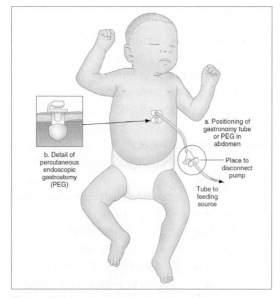

Figure 13.6 Gastrostomy tube.

A jejunostomy tube is often placed in children with gastroesophageal reflux. The tube is placed in the stomach and then passed through the duodenum into the jejunum.

Feeding and Gastrostomy Tube Emergencies

There are many potential feeding and gastrostomy tube emergencies. The most common complication with a feeding tube is displacement, which can lead to aspiration of fluid. A gastrostomy tube can become completely displaced or leak gastric contents, or the tube can become obstructed. When treating a child who has one or more of these problems with a feeding or gastrostomy tube, assessment of respiratory and hydration status is important, especially in those children who are totally dependent on their feeding tubes for hydration and nutrition. Physicians should ask about medications and whether any doses were missed.

Management

If the child has a feeding tube that has been displaced, physicians should ask if it ends in the stomach or jejunum. A nasogastric or orogastric tube can be replaced with a tube of the same size and length of the old catheter. The depth of insertion is estimated by measuring the catheter along its intended path: from the nose or mouth, down the esophagus, and into the stomach. The centimeter marking at this length should be noted. Then the tube should be lubricated and gently inserted to this mark. The tube location should be confirmed by instilling 10 to 30 mL of air into the tube while listening over the stomach for any sound of air. If air is heard, the tube is in the proper position and should be taped in place. If air is not heard or the child is not crying, the tube should be removed and the procedure repeated.

A nasojejunal or orojejunal tube is often a specially weighted tube that requires insertion under fluoroscopic guidance, so the appropriate specialist must be called for its insertion.

If a child has leaking around the gastrostomy tube or jejunostomy tube, the cause should be determined. Some possible causes of leakage include balloon deflation, coughing, constipation, bowel obstruction, and seizures. Addressing the cause might solve the problem. Consultation with the subspecialty service that manages the child's tube might be necessary.

An obstructed tube can be cleared with either a proteolytic enzyme solution or Coca-Cola. If these methods are unsuccessful, it should be replaced. Gastrostomy tubes that have been displaced should be replaced as soon as possible so that the stoma does not constrict and make replacement much more difficult. Jejunostomy tube placement is more problematic because, after placing a tube in the stomach, passing the tube to the jejunum is usually done under fluoroscopy by a radiologist familiar with this procedure. When replacing a gastrostomy tube, the medical personnel should determine when the tube was first inserted. For tubes in use for less than 3 months, consultation with the person or institution that performed the procedure is necessary because the track might not be fully formed and insertion by medical personnel not adept at replacing these tubes might create a false track.

When performing the reinsertion procedure, the physician should use a similar size and type of gastrostomy tube. The different types of tubes include Mic-Key tubes or Buttons. Parents often have an extra tube with them, but if not and the ED does not have gastrostomy tubes, a Foley catheter can be used to temporarily keep the stoma open until definitive placement can occur. Patients should not be discharged home without placement of a definitive gastrostomy tube. Discussion with the subspecialty service managing the tube is important for further advice. See Table 13-3 for a description of the gastrostomy tube insertion procedure. If there is a delay in gastrostomy tube replacement, assessment of hydration is important. For the child who cannot take fluids or medications orally, intravenous hydration should be considered.

TABLE 13-3 Steps for Gastrostomy Tube Insertion
1. Have same size gastrostomy tube and one size smaller available.
2. Check the balloon for leaks by placing in 3 to 5 mL of water. Deflate balloon before insertion.
3. Lubricate tip with water-soluble gel.
4. Insert gastrostomy tube into stoma.
5. If the tube will not pass through the stoma after two to three attempts, the procedure should be attempted with one size smaller tube. Repeat balloon check and lubrication.
6. If the smaller tube will not pass, then attempt to dilate the stoma as follows: 1) Have three sizes smaller Foley or other catheters available.   2) Insert the smallest size, lubricated catheter into the stoma. Repeat with larger catheters in a stepwise manner until the appropriate size catheter is able to pass through the stoma.   3) Pass the appropriate size gastrostomy tube into the stoma.
7. Instruct patient and family to follow up with the medical professional who regularly manages the tube. If insertion of tube is not successful, the child needs to be transferred for definitive care.

Adirim TA, Smith EL, Singh T. *Special Children's Outreach and Prehospital Education.* Sudbury, MA: Jones and Bartlett; 2006. Reprinted with permission.

A 6-year-old girl with acute lymphocytic leukemia presents to the ED with a history of fever. Her mother states that she last had chemotherapy 3 days before this ED visit. She was fine until this morning, when she stated that she was not feeling well. Her mother took her temperature orally and found that it was 38.2°C (100.8°F). The girl's oncologist advised that the child be taken to the ED. The mother denies that the child has a sore throat, vomiting, diarrhea, or contact with anyone who was ill. Her mother states that the child has a Broviac venous catheter.

On examination, the child is alert, has no labored breathing, but is somewhat pale. Her vital signs are as follows: respiratory rate, 22/min; pulse, 120/min; blood pressure, 90/50 mm Hg; and temperature, 38.6°C (101.5°F) orally. Her mucous membranes appear moist but pale. She has alopecia and is anicteric. The results of her head and neck examination are otherwise normal. Her lungs are clear to auscultation, and her heart examination reveals a soft systolic ejection murmur at the left sternal border. Her Broviac catheter site appears clean and dry, and the catheter is intact. Her abdomen is soft, and there are no masses or hepatosplenomegaly. Her extremities are warm and well perfused.

1. What is your initial assessment of this child's presentation?
2. What historical factors affect your diagnostic workup and management?
3. How do you treat this child?

Central Venous Catheters

Central venous catheters are used to deliver medications, blood products, and nutrition directly into a central vein. Blood samples can also be drawn from these lines. There are many circumstances under which a child would need a central venous catheter. These circumstances include cancer and the need for chemotherapy, sickle cell disease and the need for frequent transfusions, infections and the need for long-term antibiotic therapy, and various conditions in which nutritional supplementation is needed, such as in short bowel syndrome.

There are three types of catheters. Peripherally inserted central venous catheters are long catheters inserted into the cephalic vein via the antecubital fossa. The catheter is advanced into the subclavian vein. These tubes are placed in children who need temporary venous access for antibiotic therapy. Some potential complications include easy dislodgement because they are not sutured in place, infection (but less of a risk than with other central catheters), and obstruction.

Tunneled central venous catheters are placed surgically. They are inserted directly into a central vein, most commonly the subclavian, cephalic, or jugular. There are three common types: Broviac, Hickman, and Groshong. The first two are most commonly used in children. The distal ends rest outside the chest and can have one to three ports. Implanted vascular access ports (Port-A-Cath, PAS Port, and Med-A-Ports) are also common in children. The insertion sites and method are the same as for the tunneled central venous catheters. The distal end of the catheter consists of a reservoir that is covered with a self-healing rubber septum. This reservoir rests subcutaneously, and a special needle is needed to access this catheter.[12]

Management

The advantages of the implanted vascular ports are that they only need to be flushed with heparin once a month and after each access as opposed to daily heparin flushes. Another benefit is that they are hidden and might be more acceptable to older children when body image is more of an issue. See Table 13-4 for how to access Broviac and Hickman catheters and Table 13-5 for how to access Port-A-Caths.[13]

TABLE 13-4 How to Access Broviac and Hickman Catheters

1. Prepare equipment.

2. Use sterile technique.

3. Clamp catheter at least 7.6 cm (3 in) from cap. Either use the patient's clamp or a clamp without teeth.

4. Put sterile towel under the catheter.

5. Remove cap at end of catheter and attach 10-mL syringe filled with sterile normal saline.

6. Unclamp catheter and slowly inject 3 to 5 mL of saline into the catheter.

7. Aspirate back into the syringe to check for blood return.

8. If resistance is met to instillation of saline or no blood returns, reclamp catheter and reposition either the catheter or the patient and try the procedure again.

9. If blood return is achieved, inject the remaining sterile saline into the catheter and reclamp and remove the syringe. Intravenous tubing can then be attached to the catheter. Be sure to purge the line of any air bubbles before infusing fluid.

10. If blood needs to be drawn before fluids are infused, withdraw 8 to 9 mL of blood, reclamp the catheter, and discard the syringe. Attach an empty 10-mL syringe and remove needed blood for diagnostic tests, then return to step 9.

11. After completion of procedure, inject 3 to 5 mL of heparin into catheter, replace cap, and apply dressing.

Fuchs SM. Accessing indwelling central lines. In: King C, Henretig FM, eds. *Textbook of Pediatric Emergency Procedures, 2nd ed.* Philadelphia, PA: Wolters Kluwer Health/LippincottWilliams & Wilkins;2008:738-747. Reprinted with permission.

TABLE 13-5 Accessing Totally Implanted Catheters (Port-A-Caths)

1. In a nonemergency, a topical anesthetic cream should be placed over the site 30 to 60 minutes before skin puncture, and covered with a dressing.

2. Prepare equipment.

3. If a topical anesthetic cream was used, remove dressing and wipe cream away.

4. Perform procedure under sterile conditions; wearing sterile gloves.

5. Palpate reservoir. Wash overlying area with povidone-iodine or other sterile cleanser, then alcohol.

6. Attach a 10-mL syringe filled with sterile saline to T-connector tubing and flush saline through tubing.

7. Attach extension tubing to Huber needle and flush needle with saline to remove air. Clamp the extension tubing.

8. Put on new pair of sterile gloves.

9. Locate center of septum and stabilize reservoir between thumb and index finger. Slowly but firmly insert needle through septum to back of reservoir.

10. Unclamp extension tubing and slowly instill 2 mL of saline.

11. If resistance is met, do not force. Reclamp.

12. If resistance is not met, infuse 3 mL more saline into port.

13. Aspirate fluid back into syringe and check for blood return. If blood is needed for diagnostic purposes, then attach an empty 10-mL syringe to extension tubing and withdraw 8 to 9 mL of blood, reclamp catheter, and discard the syringe. Draw blood into a new syringe.

14. Attach a 10-mL syringe with saline and slowly inject into reservoir and reclamp extension tubing. Tape needle in place, maintaining it at a right angle to septum.

Fuchs SM. Accessing indwelling central lines. In: King C, Henretig FM, eds. *Textbook of Pediatric Emergency Procedures, 2nd ed.* Philadelphia, PA: Wolters Kluwer Health/LippincottWilliams & Wilkins;2008:738-747. Reprinted with permission.

Central Venous Catheter Emergencies

There are several circumstances under which a child with a central catheter will present for emergency treatment. These include damage to the catheter, air embolus, catheter dislodgement, and fever. Damaged catheters should be clamped proximal to the break with a hemostat. If the catheter is dislodged, apply direct pressure at the entry site to prevent or stop bleeding. This is a potentially life-threatening emergency. The child should be brought to a facility that can repair or replace the catheter. Air emboli or blood clot in the tubing can cause sudden onset of respiratory distress, chest pain, and altered mental status. If an embolus is suspected in a child with a central catheter, the medical personnel should first treat the patient, with attention to the ABCs. The catheter should be clamped; the child should be placed on the left side and given oxygen. Peripheral intravenous placement should be considered. Hyperbaric therapy should be considered for a significant air embolus.

Fever is a common problem in children with central catheters and should be considered an emergency. The central catheter is a foreign body that can act as a direct conduit for microorganisms from the outside world into the child's system. This is especially problematic in immunocompromised children, such as those undergoing treatment for cancer, because these children can easily develop sepsis.

Management

Treatment of children with central catheters and fever should include evaluation of ABCs, obtaining blood samples for complete blood cell (CBC) count and cultures from the central catheter and a peripheral vein, and starting broad-spectrum antibiotics until culture results are known. Obtain other cultures of urine, joint fluid, or cerebrospinal fluid (CSF) as indicated. If the child with a central catheter and fever is not immune suppressed and appears well, then the physician can consider discharging the child home. However, if the child with a central catheter and fever is neutropenic (absolute neutrophil count <500/mcL), the child should be admitted to the hospital for intravenous antibiotics pending blood culture results.

Dialysis Shunts and Peritoneal Dialysis Catheters

Approximately 150 cases of chronic renal failure per million persons are diagnosed in the United States each year. Most of these cases are in the adult population[10] because end-stage renal disease is not a common pediatric problem. Fewer than 15 per million children develop chronic renal failure. In fact, less than 1% of all hemodialysis patients are children. Children tend to be treated more often with transplantation and therefore might need hemodialysis or peritoneal dialysis only temporarily.

Dialysis Shunts

Hemodialysis is performed several times a week; therefore, permanent vascular access is important. A child might have a synthetic graft or arteriovenous fistulae created surgically. These sites should not be accessed outside the dialysis laboratory except in extreme emergency situations. These grafts and fistulae are susceptible to multiple complications. Some of these include graft degeneration, stenosis of the graft or fistulae, vascular aneurysm, fistula rupture, thrombosis, and infection. All of these complications should be managed by the child's nephrologist and surgeon. Until definitive care can be undertaken by appropriate specialists, management of the symptoms resulting from complications is important. Some of these children manifest signs and symptoms of volume overload and metabolic derangements, and these should be addressed in the emergency setting. Hyperkalemia is the most immediately life-threatening and should be promptly diagnosed and treated.[14] Children with dialysis shunts and fever should have blood samples drawn and empiric antibiotic therapy started pending culture results.

Peritoneal Dialysis Catheters

Peritoneal dialysis catheters tend to be more common in children than dialysis vascular shunts because peritoneal dialysis is a temporary form of managing end-stage renal disease that can be accomplished at home. A peritoneal dialysis catheter is a foreign body that provides a portal of entry for microorganisms from the external environment and therefore subjects patients to the risks of infection, most notably peritonitis.[14] This is considered a life-threatening emergency. The signs and symptoms of peritonitis include fever, abdominal pain, distended abdomen, and rebound tenderness. In immunocompromised children, signs of sepsis and/or peritonitis can be subtle.

Management

The dialysate (fluid from the peritoneal cavity) should be sent for culture, and antibiotics should be infused into the peritoneal cavity by personnel comfortable with this procedure.[15] The decision regarding systemic antibiotic treatment should be made after assessing the child's appearance and looking for signs and symptoms of sepsis. Treatment should be undertaken with consultation from the child's nephrologist.

Ventriculoperitoneal Shunts

Ventriculoperitoneal shunts are catheters inserted into the ventricles within the brain then threaded under the skin from the skull to the peritoneum, where excess CSF is drained (**Figure 13.7**).[16] In some cases, the distal end of the shunt is placed in the pleural space between the chest wall and the lung (also called a VP shunt) or in the right atrium of the heart (ventriculoatrial [VA] shunt). Both of these locations allow CSF to drain, but each can result in unique complications. There are many medical conditions in which a VP or VA shunt is necessary. The most common is hydrocephalus, where there is a blockage in the CSF circulation system. The lateral ventricles enlarge with nonabsorbed CSF, causing an increase in intracranial pressure. Hydrocephalus is found in formerly premature infants who sustain an intraventricular bleed in the neonatal period and also in children with brain tumors, spina bifida, myelomeningocele, and posttraumatic injury. These children should be assumed to have latex allergies and the necessary precautions taken.

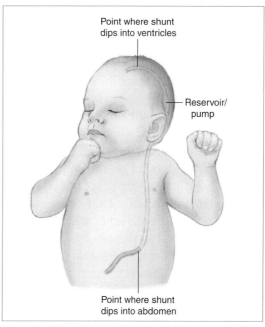

Figure 13.7 A ventriculoperitoneal shunt directs cerebrospinal fluid from the ventricles to the abdomen or, more rarely, the heart.

YOUR FIRST CLUE

Signs and Symptoms of Peritonitis in a Dialyzed Patient

- Child receiving peritoneal dialysis
- Fever
- Abdominal pain
- Distended abdomen
- Rebound tenderness
- Elevated white blood cell count in blood and peritoneal fluid

Shunt Emergencies

A child with a VP shunt is at higher risk of developing an infection of the shunt within the first 3 months postoperatively. Symptoms include fever, ill appearance, erythema over the shunt site and/or tubing, tenderness over the tubing, abdominal pain and tenderness, vomiting, and altered mental status. If a VP shunt infection is suspected, management should include assessment of the ABCs and obtaining diagnostic laboratory work. A CSF sample should be drawn from the shunt by a neurosurgeon and sent for a CBC count and culture. Broad-spectrum antibiotics should be administered pending the results of the CBC count and culture. Neurosurgeons should manage all shunt infections.

Peritonitis is another complication of VP shunts. The tip of the shunt empties into the peritoneal cavity, and a foreign body can serve as a nidus for infection. Signs and symptoms include fever, vomiting, abdominal pain and tenderness, and abdominal distention. A pseudocyst can cause symptoms similar to peritonitis, except a fever is not usually present. Management should be similar to that for VP shunt infections and should include diagnostic laboratory work, broad-spectrum antibiotics, and consultation with the neurosurgeon. Although infections of VP and VA shunts will not result in peritonitis, infection of the CSF can lead to pleural effusions and bacteremia, respectively.

The most common complication of a VP shunt is obstruction or malfunction. These can occur if there is an increase in protein in the CSF, causing a blockage in the tubing, or if there is a mechanical disruption in the shunt tubing, which can cause a buildup of CSF in the ventricles, and therefore an increase in intracranial pressure. Signs and symptoms include headache, nausea, vomiting, irritability, altered mental status, ataxia, change in vital signs, and, in infants, a bulging fontanelle. Late signs include those of the Cushing triad: bradycardia, irregular respirations, and hypertension. Initial management should include assessment and management of the ABCs, oxygen supplementation, raising the child's head to 30°, bag-mask ventilation and preparation for intubation if there are signs of increased intracranial pressure, obtaining intravenous access, and

contacting a neurosurgeon as soon as possible. If the patient is stable, an imaging study of the ventricles (computed tomography or magnetic resonance imaging) and shunt series radiographs (head, chest, and abdomen) should be obtained as needed. The definitive treatment for VP shunt malfunction is surgical shunt revision. Occasionally, the shunt tubing will break, kink, knot, or migrate to the scrotum. Every child with a VP shunt and signs of obstruction must be examined and radiographs obtained to rule out these complications.

THE CLASSICS

Radiographic Findings of Shunt Obstruction or Malfunction

- Enlarged ventricles (computed tomography or magnetic resonance imaging)
- Disconnected shunt (shunt series)
- Pseudocyst (ultrasonography)

Vagal Nerve Stimulators

Vagal nerve stimulators (VNS) are devices implanted under the skin that emit short bursts of electrical energy into the brain via the vagus nerve to prevent seizures. These devices are typically considered in children older than 12 years when other treatments fail. Intractable epilepsy affects approximately 20% to 30% of patients with seizures. Newer antiepileptic drugs and surgical procedures decrease seizure frequency in a significant number of patients. However, up to 10% of children will continue to have disabling seizures. For these patients, VNSs are used for better seizure control.[17]

The VNS is an implantable device that looks like a pacemaker. It is implanted by a neurosurgeon just under the skin in the chest. In the small number of children who have had a VNS placed, most have seen a reduction in seizure frequency of 50%. How the VNS works on the brain is not known. The vagus nerve is a peripheral nerve that leads directly to the brain, and it is there that the VNS has an effect.[18]

The VNS is programmed to provide baseline intermittent stimulation of the left vagus nerve. Although the VNS system delivers stimulation automatically in regular pulses all the time, the external magnet device can be used to deliver extra electronic stimulation between cycles. The patient or caretaker activates the device by placing a handheld magnet over the device implanted in the chest.[18] Patients who can sense that they will experience a seizure can activate the VNS themselves by passing the magnet over the device. Health care personnel who encounter a seizing patient with a VNS should assist the caregiver with its activation or seek advice from specialty consultants. Children with VNS devices should otherwise be treated as other seizing patients with careful attention to the ABCs. The magnet can also be used to stop the stimulation by holding the magnet over the device. There are times that the patient might want to shut the stimulation off. Some of these include when eating if the stimulation causes problems with swallowing and when the speaking or singing publicly because the stimulation can change one's voice.

Adverse effects of VNS therapy include hoarseness and discomfort in the throat. Patients might experience a change in voice quality during stimulation.

Treating Patients With VNSs

Children with intractable seizures might benefit from having a VNS implanted. Most children eventually improve. However, the device can stop working or might only decrease the frequency of seizures. Any child with a VNS who presents with a seizure should be treated like any child without a VNS device: with attention to the ABCs. Most children with a VNS will also be taking antiepileptic medication, and therefore those drug blood levels (when available) should be measured in a child with increased "breakthrough" seizure activity. Under these circumstances, the device should be checked to make sure it is functioning properly and medication levels adjusted under the guidance of the child's neurologist.

Intrathecal Baclofen Pump

Some children with cerebral palsy (CP) are treated with baclofen pumps inserted directly into the thecal sac surrounding the spinal cord. The device pumps baclofen directly into this space via continuous infusion. Baclofen operates by binding to receptors in the spinal cord, which leads to inhibition of spinal reflexes. Children with CP who previously could not ambulate often can after these pumps are placed.

Complications include overdose when the pump is filled incorrectly or programming is inaccurate. Overdose can lead to respiratory depression and death. Some less serious adverse effects of the medication include drowsiness, dizziness, hypotension, headache, and nausea.

Baclofen Pump Emergencies

When treating a comatose child with CP who has a baclofen pump, the physician must maintain the child's ABCs until the pump is urgently stopped with a specialized device. If this device is not readily available, then emptying the reservoir with a 22-gauge needle is an alternative treatment. This can be done by locating the pump in the abdominal wall and inserting the needle in the center of it.

Another complication is medication withdrawal due to pump failure, which is usually the result of tube obstruction or faulty pump programming. Symptoms of withdrawal include increased spasticity, tachycardia, blood pressure changes, severe hyperthermia, and rhabdomyolysis, possibly progressing to multisystem failure and death.[19]

THE BOTTOM LINE

- The initial priorities are the same; follow the ABCs.
- Ask parents and/or caregivers about the child's baseline or look for an EIF.
- Use parents and/or caregivers assistance.
- Obtain an accurate weight; do not depend on age-appropriate norms.
- Learn about the technology devices used by dependent children.

Check Your Knowledge

1. What should be your first step in treating a child with a tracheostomy tube, respiratory distress, and increased secretions?
   A. Assess color
   B. Auscultate chest
   C. Provide nebulized bronchodilator therapy
   D. Remove tracheostomy tube
   E. Suction tracheostomy tube

2. For the child with a tracheostomy tube, what is the most likely cause of a pulmonary exacerbation?
   A. Reflux of stomach contents into the lungs
   B. Mass in the lungs
   C. Tracheostomy tube dislodges
   D. Infection or reactive airway disease

3. What are the two types of mechanical ventilators?
   A. Control and support
   B. Intermittent and continuous
   C. Pressure and volume
   D. Continuous and synchronized

4. If a gastrostomy tube is clogged, which of the following can be used to clear it?
   A. Coca-Cola
   B. Ginger ale
   C. Hydrogen peroxide
   D. Pancrelipase
   E. Additional pressure

5. What is the most common complication of gastrostomy tubes?
   A. Slip into the small intestine
   B. Dislodge and need to be replaced
   C. Break
   D. Infection

6. All of the following statements regarding a central venous catheter are correct except:
   A. commonly used tunneled central venous catheters in children include Broviac and Hickman; the distal ends rests outside the chest and can have one to three ports.
   B. implanted central vascular access ports have a distal end of the catheter, which consists of a reservoir covered with a self-healing rubber septum.
   C. tunneled central venous catheters are inserted surgically into a central vein, most commonly the subclavian, cephalic, or jugular.
   D. a regular needle can be used to access an implanted port.

7. Which of the following would be the most critical and worrisome sign or symptom of a shunt obstruction?
   A. Bulging fontanelle
   B. Cushing triad
   C. Headache
   D. Nausea
   E. Vomiting

8. A seizing patient with a vagal nerve stimulator (VNS) presents to your emergency department. How should this patient initially be treated?
   A. Turn off the VNS
   B. Assess and manage airway, breathing, and circulation
   C. Administer fast-acting antiepileptic medication rectally
   D. Draw a blood sample and measure the child's antiepileptic medication level
   E. Administer an antiepileptic medication intravenously

9. A 12-year-old boy with a history of cerebral palsy presents to the emergency department with somnolence, hypoventilation, and hypotension. His mother states that 1 hour before presentation, the home health care nurse refilled his pump with baclofen. What is your first action?
   A. Draw blood for baclofen levels
   B. Turn off the pump with the wand
   C. Assess and manage his airway, breathing, and circulation
   D. Call the neurosurgeon to remove the pump
   E. Insert a 22-gauge needle and syringe into the pump's reservoir to remove the baclofen

10. Children with special health care needs:
    A. might be smaller than the average child their chronological age.
    B. might have vital signs that are out of the normal range for children their age.
    C. might be taking multiple medications.
    D. might have parents who can manage their technology.
    E. all of the above.

References

1. Reynolds S, Desguin B, Uyeda A, Davis AT. Children with chronic conditions in a pediatric emergency department. *Pediatr Emerg Care.* 1996;12:166–168.

2. Weiss HB, Mathers LJ, Forjuoh SN, Kinnane JM. *Children and Adolescent Emergency Department Visit Databook.* Pittsburgh, PA: Center for Violence and Injury Control, Allegheny University of the Health Sciences; 1997.

3. Foltin GL, Tunik MG, Cooper A, et al, eds. *Teaching Resource for Instructors in Prehospital Pediatrics.* BLS Version 2.0. New York, NY: Center for Pediatric Emergency Medicine; 1998.

4. McPherson M, Arango P, Fox H, et al. Commentaries: A new definition of children with special health care needs. *Pediatrics.* 1998;102:137–140.

5. Newacheck, PW, Strickland B, Shonkoff JP, et al. An epidemiologic profile of children with special health care needs. *Pediatrics.* 1998;102:117–121.

6. Weller WE, Minkowitz CS, Anderson GF. Utilization of medical and health related services among school-age children and adolescents with special health care needs (1994 National Health Interview Survey on Disability [NHIS-D] Baseline Data). *Pediatrics.* 2003;112(3 pt 1):593–603.

7. Williams TV, Schone EM, Archibald ND, Thompson JW. A national assessment of children with special health care needs: Prevalence of special needs and use of health care services among children in the military health system. *Pediatrics.* 2004;114:384–393.

8. Mayer ML, Skinner AC, Slifkin RT; National Survey of Children With Special Health Care Needs. Unmet need for routine and specialty care: Data from the National Survey of Children With Special Health Care Needs. *Pediatrics.* 2004;113:e109–e115. www.Pediatrics.org/cgi/content/full/113/2/e109. Accessed April 11, 2011.

9. American Academy of Pediatrics Committee on Pediatric Emergency Medicine and Council on Clinical information Technology, Physicians, Pediatric Emergency Medicine Committee. Policy Statement—Emergency Information Forms and Emergency Preparedness for Children With Special Health Care Needs. *Pediatrics.* 2010;125:829–837. http://Pediatrics.aappublications.org/cgi/content/abstract/peds.2010-0186v1. Accessed April 11, 2011.

10. Adirim TA, Smith EL, Singh T. *Special Children's Outreach and Prehospital Education.* Sudbury, MA: Jones and Bartlett; 2006.

11. Kallis JM. Replacement of a tracheostomy cannula. In: King C, Henretig FM, eds. *Textbook of Pediatric Emergency Procedures*–2nd ed. Philadelphia, PA: Wolters Kluwer Health/LippincottWilliams & Wilkins;2008:792–798.

12. Foltin GL, Tunik MG, Cooper A, et al, eds. *Paramedic TRIPP.* Version 1.0. New York, NY: Center for Pediatric Emergency Medicine; 2002.

13. Fuchs SM. Accessing indwelling central lines. In: King C, Henretig FM, eds. *Textbook of Pediatric Emergency Procedures*–2nd ed. Philadelphia, PA: Wolters Kluwer Health/LippincottWilliams & Wilkins;2008:738–747.

14. Krause RS. Dialysis complications of chronic renal failure. In: Howes DS, Talavera F, Sinert RH, Schraga ED, eds. *Medicine.* http://www.emedicine.com/ emerg/topic501.htm. Accessed April 15, 2011.

15. National Kidney Foundation. K/DOQI clinical practice guidelines for vascular access, 2000. *Am J Kidney Dis.* 2001:37(suppl 1):S137–S181.

16. Dieckmann RA, ed. *Pediatric Education for Prehospital Professionals*, 2nd ed. Sudbury, MA: American Academy of Pediatrics/Jones & Bartlett Publishers; 2006: 221–222.

17. Patwardhan R, Strong B, Bebin ME, Mathisen J, Grabb PA. Efficacy of vagal nerve stimulation in children with medically refractory epilepsy. *Neurosurgery.* 2000;47:1353–1358.

18. Epilepsy Foundation. Vagus Nerve Stimulation Therapy. http://www.epilepsyfoundation.org/answerplace/Medical/treatment/vns/. Accessed April 11, 2011.

19. Shirley K, Kothare S, Piatt J, Adirim TA. Baclofen overdose by intrathecal pump. *Pediatr Emerg Care.* 2006;22:258.

A 3-year-old boy with a mitochondrial myopathy is brought to the emergency department (ED) with a 1-day history of difficulty breathing. The boy's condition was diagnosed when he was 1 year of age, when it was noted that he had muscle weakness and frequent respiratory infections. He had a tracheostomy tube placed and home mechanical ventilation was initiated at the age of 18 months for impending respiratory failure due to severe muscle weakness. He also has a gastrostomy tube, which is reportedly functioning without a problem. Yesterday, his home health care nurse noted that he was producing more than usual secretions, which are now yellow (as opposed to clear), and he required more frequent suctioning. This morning, his mother noted that he had a temperature of 38.4°C (101.2°F), his pulse oximetry reading at home was 92%, and his baseline reading is above 95% on 0.25 L/min of oxygen. He receives ventilation mostly at night while asleep and has periods during the day while awake off the ventilator. Today, his mother kept him on the ventilator at his baseline settings for the trip to the hospital. On examination, the boy is sleepy but arousable, and there are subcostal and intercostal retractions. His color is pink. His ventilator rate is set at 20 to support each breath (volume support). His respiratory rate is 40/min, heart rate is 160/min, and blood pressure is 90/60 mm Hg. Temperature in the ED is noted to be 39°C (102.2°F), and pulse oximetry is 90% on 1 L of oxygen. Lung examination reveals crackles on the right side of the child's chest. Capillary refill is less than 2 seconds, and the extremities are well perfused.

1. *What is your initial assessment of this child's presentation?*
2. *How do you manage this presentation? Where do you start?*
3. *What issues do you need to consider?*

The initial assessment of this child reveals that he is in respiratory distress. He has an increased oxygen requirement and on lung examination is noted to have retractions, crackles in the right lung fields, and an elevated respiratory rate despite receiving mechanical ventilation. By history and examination, this child has a fever and increased tracheal secretions. The most likely diagnosis is infection.

The initial management priorities should mirror those of any other child. First, the airway should be assessed and cleared of obstruction. The tracheostomy tube should be suctioned both for therapeutic and diagnostic reasons. Sending a tracheal aspiration culture for Gram stain and culture and virus respiratory panel could be useful diagnostically and direct antibiotic management. Next, the physician should initiate treatment to improve this child's breathing. Suggested therapies could include administration of additional oxygen to maintain saturations above 94%, increase in the mechanical ventilatory support, and bronchodilator nebulizer treatment to help clear the airway of the copious secretions. Serial clinical examinations are valuable, and arterial blood gas measurements can provide useful information. The physician should next prescribe antibiotics for this child. The physician should choose a broad-spectrum antibiotic until the tracheal Gram stain and culture results are available. This child will require admission to a pediatric critical care unit, and if this type of unit is not available, this child will need to be transported by an advanced life support unit to a tertiary care center capable of caring for this child.

The following issues should be considered. This child has a chronic neuromuscular disease that has affected his ability to breathe. Children with neuromuscular disorders who are receiving mechanical ventilation are susceptible to pulmonary exacerbations of their lungs and pulmonary infections. They have a low respiratory reserve, and even seemingly simple viral infections can be serious. This child is dependent on an artificial airway that can become obstructed, so careful attention to pulmonary toilet is important. As is the case with this child, children with neuromuscular disorders often have multiple medical problems and multiple technologies. In this child, fever and respiratory distress could also be caused by other infections, such as sepsis or meningitis. A careful history and examination can help the physician determine the precise cause of his distress.

There are other issues to consider in the treatment of special needs children. These children's clinical status can deteriorate much quicker than in healthy children. Communication with the home hospital early in the child's course can be helpful to physicians in community hospitals.

A 6-year-old girl with acute lymphocytic leukemia presents to the ED with a history of fever. Her mother states that she last had chemotherapy 3 days before this ED visit. She was fine until this morning when, she stated that she was not feeling well. Her mother took her temperature orally and found that it was 38.2°C (100.8°F). The mother called the pediatric oncologist, who advised that she take the child to the ED. The mother denies that the child has a sore throat, vomiting, diarrhea, or contact with anyone who was ill. Her mother states that the child has a Broviac venous catheter.

On examination, the child is alert, has no labored breathing, but is somewhat pale. Her vital signs are as follows: respirations, 22/min; pulse, 120/min; blood pressure, 90/50 mm Hg; and temperature, 38.6°C (101.5°F) orally. Her mucous membranes appear moist but pale. She has alopecia and is anicteric. The results of her head and neck examination are otherwise normal. Her lungs are clear to auscultation, and her heart examination reveals a soft systolic ejection murmur at the left sternal border. Her Broviac catheter site appears clean and dry and the catheter is intact. Her abdomen is soft, and there are no masses or hepatosplenomegaly. Her extremities are warm and well perfused.

1. What is your initial assessment of this child's presentation?
2. What historical factors affect your diagnostic workup and management?
3. How do you treat this child?

This is a well-appearing child with fever. Her airway, breathing, and circulation are stable. Her mother confirms that she has been pale since her leukemia diagnosis. However, this is a child who is at risk for developing serious infections, such as sepsis, and so this child's respiratory and circulatory status can change rapidly.

It is important to consider that this child is undergoing treatment for leukemia. Depending on the phase of treatment, this child is at risk for neutropenia (absolute neutrophil count <500/mcL). Children with neutropenia are at risk for serious infections. In addition, this child has a central catheter, which also places her at risk for serious infection. Therefore, any child with a central venous catheter and/or neutropenia who presents with fever needs to be evaluated for serious infection and treated with broad-spectrum antibiotics until culture results are known. This child's appearance should not deter the workup.

A blood sample should be drawn from her Broviac and sent to the laboratory for a complete blood cell count and bacterial cultures. The physician should consider sending fungal cultures in the severely immunocompromised child. If this child appears well and is not neutropenic, then the physician can consider giving a dose of antibiotics through the Broviac and discharging the child home with close follow-up by the oncologist. If this child is found to be neutropenic, then the child should be admitted for an inpatient stay for antibiotic therapy until culture results are known.

Check Your Knowledge Answers

Chapter 1: Pediatric Assessment

1.C, Heart rate. Although heart rate is important, it is not a part of the Pediatric Assessment Triangle. The components of the Pediatric Assessment Triangle include appearance, work of breathing, and circulation to the skin.

2.A, Appearance and circulation. Abnormalities in appearance and work of breathing would indicate respiratory distress. Abnormalities in circulation alone could indicate compensated shock, as would occur with diarrhea. However, the combination of abnormalities in appearance and circulation to skin could indicate decompensated shock, as could occur with severe gastroenteritis or a multisystem blunt injury.

3.D, Work of breathing. Work of breathing is not an indicator of compensated or decompensated shock. A child in shock might not interact normally with his or her environment due to poor brain perfusion. Quality of pulses is a good measure of peripheral circulation and shock. Effortless tachypnea and hyperpnea occur in shock as a way of compensating for metabolic acidosis.

4.C, Offer distractions. A 6 to 12-month-old infant is socially interactive, yet has stranger and separation anxiety. Keeping the infant with the parent, getting down to the infant's level, and offering a distraction such as a penlight, will make the assessment easier. In addition, working from toe to head will not be as threatening to the child.

Chapter 2: The Pediatric Airway in Health and Disease

1.A, High-risk groups for severe bronchiolitis include infants with congenital heart disease and bronchopulmonary dysplasia. Respiratory syncytial virus (RSV) is the most common pathogen causing bronchiolitis. Initial RSV infections are usually more symptomatic. Most children have been infected with RSV by their second birthday. Infants with congenital heart disease and chronic lung disease are at increased risk for severe disease. Corticosteroids can reduce duration of symptoms but have not been shown to reduce admission rates.

2.B, Humidified oxygen. In a child with moderate to severe croup, racemic epinephrine (adrenaline) or L-epinephrine (Berkeley L-adrenaline) and dexamethasone have shown benefit in outcomes and should be administered early in the treatment course. Humidified oxygen has a theoretical benefit, but randomized trials have not shown improvement in patient outcomes.

3.A, Bronchoscopy is the "gold standard" for diagnosis and treatment of foreign body aspiration. Bronchoscopy is nearly 100% successful in the diagnosis and treatment of airway foreign body. The most commonly aspirated items are food items, with peanuts being the most common. The results of physical examination are often normal in these patients and should not lower the index of suspicion for foreign body aspiration. The most common sites of obstruction are in the lower airways. Plain radiographs are normal in approximately one-quarter of children with airway foreign body. Most foreign bodies are not radio–opaque.

4.C, Infants and children are more likely to experience oxygen desaturation. Infants and young children are more susceptible to air swallowing and emesis due to crying, diaphragmatic breathing, and a short esophagus. Infants are more likely to develop bradycardia and oxygen desaturation and have increased rates of oxygen consumption, lower lung compliance, and diminished functional residual capacity. Rapid sequence intubation for critically ill infants is a common procedure that is well tolerated.

Chapter 3: Shock

1.A, Give the patient oxygen, obtain vascular access, and fluid resuscitate up to 60 mL/kg. The key to treatment of septic shock is rapid initiation of fluid resuscitation and identification and treatment of infection; the key to reducing morbidity and mortality is to rapidly restore euvolemia. Initiation of antibiotics is important, but early fluid resuscitation to restore perfusion to vital organs is paramount.

2.D, All of the above. Distributive shock occurs when systemic vascular resistance falls and blood pressure decreases despite attempts made to increase cardiac output. There are multiple causes of distributive shock: anaphylactic shock, neurogenic shock, and septic shock.

3.A, Dopamine. Dopamine is currently the inotrope of choice for treatment of fluid resistant septic shock in children. In this scenario additional fluid boluses could be given, but treatment with dopamine should be initiated. Norepinephrine (noradrenaline) is used in warm shock (more common in adult patients) and is a profound vasoconstrictor. Vasopressin has not been well studied in children, and milrinone and nitric oxide are used in catecholamine-resistant cases of septic shock.

4.B, Increase systemic vascular resistance. The primary problem is a loss of sympathetic tone. Use of a vasopressor such as norepinephrine (noradrenaline) or dopamine temporarily to increase systemic vascular resistance and improve perfusion to an already injured cord can be of greater efficacy than fluid resuscitation.

5.C, Systemic inflammatory response syndrome in children requires abnormal leukocyte count or fever. Unlike in adults, systemic inflammatory response syndrome in children requires the presence of at least two of the following four criteria, one of which must be abnormal temperature or leukocyte count: core temperature of higher than 38.5°C (101.3°F) or lower than 36°C (96.8°F); tachycardia, defined as a mean heart rate greater than 2 SDs above normal for age OR for children younger than 1 year old; bradycardia (unexplained by other factors and that persists for more than 30 minutes); mean respiratory rate greater than 2 SDs above normal for age or mechanical ventilation for an acute process not related to underlying neuromuscular disease or the receipt of general anesthesia; leukocyte count elevated or depressed for age (not secondary to chemotherapy-induced leukopenia) or more than 10% immature neutrophils.

6.B, Epinephrine (adrenaline). Epinephrine (adrenaline) is the drug of choice for fluid refractory—dopamine-resistant shock. Delivery through a central catheter is preferred, and an umbilical venous catheter can be used. Albumin infusions have not been shown to be superior to normal saline in these cases; adenosine infusions can be used in cases of cold shock with evidence of right ventricular dysfunction, as can nitric oxide in cases of persistent pulmonary hypertension of the newborn.

7.D, In patients with suspected adrenal insufficiency. If a child is at risk for absolute adrenal insufficiency or adrenal pituitary axis failure (eg, purpura fulminans and congenital adrenal hyperplasia) and remains in shock despite norepinephrine (noradrenaline) or epinephrine (adrenaline) infusion, stress-dose steroids should be given. Hydrocortisone (1–2 mg/kg per day for stress dosing to 50 mg/kg per day for shock dosing) can be given in a continual infusion or intermittent boluses. Steroids should not be routinely given to all patients in septic shock. Hydrocortisone can also prevent hypotension in very low birth weight neonates.

8.A, Up to 40% of cardiac output might be required to support the work of breathing, and this can be unloaded by ventilation, diverting flow to vital organs. Mechanical ventilation decreases the work of breathing. It also increases intrathoracic pressure, which reduces left ventricular afterload that might be beneficial in patients with low carbon monoxide levels and high systemic vascular resistance; mild hyperventilation can also be used to compensate for the metabolic acidosis, and it facilitates temperature control and reduces oxygen consumption.

Chapter 4: Cardiovascular System

1.B, Ductus arteriosus. The ductus arteriosus closes in response to the decrease in pulmonary artery pressure and the reversal of flow through the ductus that begins the closure process. Because the newborn no longer requires flow through the ductus, it is a perinatal developmental change that results in increased flow through an infant's lungs ("right side").

2.B, Tetralogy of Fallot. The cyanotic congenital heart lesions are the five T's (transposition of the great vessels, tetralogy of Fallot, truncus arteriosus, tricuspid atresia, and total anomalous pulmonary venous return) and severe aortic stenosis and hypoplastic left heart. Ventricular septal defect is the most common structural congenital heart condition (noncyanotic unless associated with other cardiac malformations).

3.D, Prostaglandin E_1. Prostaglandin E_1 will help reverse closure of the ductus arteriosus when the congestive heart failure is secondary to the need for the shunt. It can be a lifesaving maneuver until the definitive surgical correction or extracorporeal membrane oxygenation is performed.

4.C, Erythema marginatum. The major criteria for acute rheumatic fever include arthritis, carditis, chorea, erythema marginatum (rash), and subcutaneous nodules.

5.B, Transposition of the great arteries. In tetralogy of Fallot, pulmonic valve stenosis reduces pulmonary blood flow. In Ebstein anomaly and hypoplastic right heart defects, there is reduced blood flow through the lungs. Reduced pulmonary blood flow on chest radiograph makes the lung fields look darker (hypoperfused). In transposition of the great arteries, the left ventricle is pumping blood into the pulmonary circulation which results in increased pulmonary vascularity on a chest radiograph.

6.B, Coronary artery aneurysms. Nearly all children with Kawasaki disease have fever. Abdominal pain is not a specific feature of Kawasaki disease. Dysrhythmias could result from myocarditis but are uncommon in Kawasaki disease. Fifteen percent to 20% of patients with untreated Kawasaki disease develop coronary artery aneurysms that pose risk of thrombosis and coronary artery narrowing. Early treatment with intravenous gamma globulin substantially reduces the risk of coronary artery aneurysms.

7.A, Pulmonary edema. Infants with noncyanotic congenital heart disease lesions develop congestive heart failure and subsequent pulmonary edema.

The goals of treatment are to avoid this. Right to left shunting occurs in cyanotic congenital heart disease. Most noncyanotic congenital heart disease involving shunting goes from left to right. Peripheral vasoconstriction occurs with hypovolemia and is not specific for noncyanotic congenital heart disease. Early onset coronary artery disease would not occur in infants and is not specific for noncyanotic congenital heart disease.

8.D, Soft abdomen. Poor feeding, vomiting, tachypnea, and hepatomegaly are all signs or symptoms of congestive heart failure. A soft abdomen is in patients without congestive heart failure and is not associated with an increased likelihood of congestive heart failure.

Chapter 5: Central Nervous System

1.C, Serum glucose. Many perfumes contain significant quantities of alcohol and can therefore cause hypoglycemia. A bedside glucose test is indicated. The other laboratory studies will not provide any additional information. The only other test that might be useful is a blood alcohol level.

2.D, Mild hyperventilation. Mild hyperventilation causes immediate vasoconstriction of blood vessels and thus can lower intracranial pressure. Although steroids are helpful with mass lesions, they do not act quickly. Midline positioning of the neck facilitates venous drainage and is simply a preventive measure. Hyperoxygenation has not been shown to lower intracranial pressure.

3.A, Acute renal failure. Bacterial meningitis has been associated with syndrome of inappropriate secretion of antidiuretic hormone, seizures, and subdural effusions. Clinicians must be wary of these potential complications. No association between bacterial meningitis and acute renal failure has been described.

4.C, Temperature greater than 40°C (104°F). Criteria needed to classify a seizure as a simple febrile one include age between 6 months and 5 years, generalized seizure lasting less than 15 minutes, and no neurologic deficit on evaluation. The seizure must be associated with a fever, but no specific fever threshold is defined.

Chapter 6: Trauma

1.C, Most commonly due to respiratory failure and shock. Secondary brain injury refers to a further insult to the traumatically injured brain as a result of an ongoing physiologic abnormality. The most common causes of secondary brain injury are failure to recognize and treat respiratory failure and shock. The consequences of secondary brain injury are similar to primary brain injury, and the degree of secondary brain injury is temporally related to the time when appropriate resuscitation is instituted rather than a specific time frame such as 6 hours. Because children have an exaggerated cerebrovascular response to injury compared with adults, secondary brain injury is a preeminent cause of morbidity and mortality.

2.D, Oral tracheal intubation using sedation and paralysis after preoxygenation (i.e., rapid sequence intubation). The clinical description describes a significant burn injury potential to the airways. Securing the airway with an endotracheal tube early is essential. Nasal-tracheal intubation is more difficult than oral tracheal intubation performed under rapid sequence intubation. A surgical airway is complication prone and is not necessary in most instances because the airway can be secured orally by rapid sequence intubation.

3.C, 35 mm Hg. The ideal level of ventilation is approximately 35 mm Hg. This provides effective ventilation and allows rescue hyperventilation if required. Pa_{CO_2} levels below 25 mm Hg induce ischemia from inappropriate vasospasm in the face of attenuated autoregulation. Levels above 40 mm Hg will result in vasodilatation and increase in intracranial pressure. Recent reports suggest that hyperventilation effectively treats increased intracranial hypertension; however, it can induce ischemia in areas of injured neurons, the so-called penumbra of injury.

4.A, Intraosseous needle infusion. Intraosseous infusion access can be established reliably in less than 30 seconds. Saphenous venous cutdown, internal jugular central venous access, and femoral vein central venous access will all take much longer. Nasogastric tube insertion can be used for enteral fluid replacement, but this will be slower and is not sufficient for a hypovolemic hypotensive patient.

5.E, All of the above. Only the surgeon can make the decision to operate or observe. Any child with a suspicion of intraabdominal injury must be evaluated by an appropriately trained and credentialed surgeon.

Chapter 7: Child Maltreatment

1.D, All of the above. All of the scenarios presented should raise concern that the injury was intentionally inflicted. Often a child with a major injury presents with a history of some minor mishap or the child's injuries are attributed to a young sibling who is incapable of inducing the trauma. Alternatively, the child is alleged to have sustained the injury doing some activity that the child is developmentally incapable of doing. In each of these cases, the health care professional must be concerned that the child has incurred inflicted trauma.

2.A, Abusive head injury. Head injuries remain the major cause of death from inflicted trauma. Hemorrhage, cerebral edema, and diffuse axonal injury are the physiologic changes responsible for the fatal outcome.

3.C, Skeletal dysplasia. Infants with environmental failure to thrive have growth impairment related to impaired nurturing (impaired mother-infant relationship and interactions) and disturbed social skills manifested by findings such as a watchful, wary gaze, and poor eye contact. The presence of skeletal dysplasia suggests a potential medical origin for growth impairment.

4.B, Mother who administers ipecac to her healthy child and complains about intractable vomiting. Münchausen syndrome by proxy occurs when a parent lies about, fabricates, or induces illness in a child. Administration of ipecac to induce vomiting represents Münchausen syndrome by proxy. Parental refusal to provide lifesaving health care can represent a form of medical neglect. The use of complementary and/or alternative medicines is widely practiced and, in some cases, provides some benefits.

Chapter 8: Nontraumatic Surgical Emergencies

1.C, Necrotizing enterocolitis. The only listed condition typically associated with both rectal bleeding and abdominal distention is necrotizing enterocolitis.

2.C, Nuclear medicine scan. Pneumatosis intestinalis and intrahepatic air can be seen on film radiographs. Sonographic visualization of portal circulation air bubbles is typical of necrotizing enterocolitis. Magnetic resonance imaging and computed tomography are also capable of visualizing pneumatosis intestinalis and intrahepatic air.

3.D, Midgut volvulus. Midgut volvulus is the most serious acute complication. If the midgut volvulus is not surgically relieved soon, an extensive bowel infarction results.

4.D, Roughly half of patients with appendicitis present in a nontypical manner. Younger children, such as infants, are even more likely to present with nonspecific symptoms and signs of appendicitis. Ultrasonography is dependent on the skill of the individual performing the procedure but can be highly accurate in experienced hands. Discharge sheets for any patient with abdominal pain should outline signs and symptoms that are of concern and require further evaluation.

Chapter 9: Nontraumatic Orthopedic Emergencies

1.A, Can be bilateral. Legg-Calvé-Perthes disease is bilateral in up to 10% of children. It affects children between 4 and 9 years old and tends to affect smaller children. There are multiple radiographic findings, depending on the stage of disease.

2.C, Often presents as knee pain. Slipped capital femoral epiphysis can present as hip, thigh, groin, or knee pain. The physician must examine the hips of any child presenting with knee pain because hip pain can be referred to the knee. The femoral head slips posteriorly and inferiorly relative to the femoral neck. Slipped capital femoral epiphysis presents in the early teen years and is treated surgically.

3.A, Children tend to be well appearing. With septic arthritis, they appear to be more ill appearing. Decision rules and prediction rules are helpful but are conflicting and not considered to be reliable enough. The presence of an effusion on ultrasonography is diagnostic of an effusion, but it does not indicate whether the effusion is septic or sterile. Most children with septic arthritis are symptomatic for long periods, whereas children with transient synovitis recover much sooner.

4.D, Treated with joint drainage and intravenous antibiotics. Septic arthritis most commonly presents in children younger than 4 years. Pathogens vary by age, but *Neisseria meningitidis* is not a common cause. Synovial cultures are positive in approximately 50% of cases.

5.B, Have increased pain when they squat with the knee in full flexion. Children with Osgood-Schlatter disease can reproduce the pain while squatting with knees in full flexion. They tend to be physically active in sports that require repeated contraction of the quadriceps. There is swelling over the tibial tubercle but no knee effusion.

Chapter 10: Medical Emergencies

1.C, Parvovirus B19. Parvovirus B19 has been associated with aplastic crises in patients with sickle cell disease. Encapsulated organisms are a common source of infection due to the relative asplenia seen in sickle cell patients. *Salmonella* can lead to osteomyelitis.

2.C, Normal or increased vascular flow on Doppler ultrasonography in epididymitis. With a painful and swollen scrotum, normal or increased vascular flow identified on Doppler ultrasonography rules out testicular torsion reliably. Increased flow in the area is suggestive of epididymitis. Urinalysis in epididymitis is often normal. Cremasteric reflex and testicular orientation findings can suggest one or the other but are not nearly as reliable as Doppler ultrasonography.

3.C, Obtain a blood culture and administer normal saline bolus and antibiotics intravenously. Lethargy, tachycardia, tachypnea, and poor peripheral perfusion are classic signs of shock. The cause of shock in this child is most likely hypovolemic (history of vomiting) or septic (febrile). After evaluation of airway, breathing, and circulation, the next priority is to treat for suspected hypovolemia (with a normal saline bolus intravenously) and sepsis (with antibiotics intravenously). If possible, it is helpful to obtain a blood culture before antibiotic therapy. The lumbar puncture should be deferred until the child is clinically stable.

4.D, Vasovagal syncope. This child most likely had vasovagal syncope as a result of prolonged standing on a hot summer day. There were no associated symptoms, and the results of the physical examination were unremarkable. A seizure is usually associated with tonic-clonic movements and incontinence and might have a postictal state. Although dysrhythmia is a possibility, the lack of warning signs (palpitations, tachycardia, chest pain), quick recovery, and normal examination results make it an unlikely cause. Breath-holding spells are usually seen in children younger than 4 years and have a clear history.

Chapter 11: Neonatal Emergencies

1.C, Heart rate, respirations, and oxygen saturation. One could argue that oxygen saturation is not a classic vital sign, but it has become a vital sign in resuscitation. Color, tone, and respiratory effort are not vital signs. Central cyanosis, temperature, and heart rate are useful measures, but temperature is not a useful immediate indicator or resuscitation status. Cry, grimace, and blood pressure are useful, but the first two are not vital signs, and these are not as useful as heart rate, respirations, and oxygen saturation.

2.A, Right hand. It is best to monitor oxygenation from a pre-ductus site. The lower extremities and the left hand are post-ductal and could be low with right-to-left shunting through the ductus arteriosus. A difference in the two sites is helpful in subsequent evaluation; however, for initial evaluation and resuscitation purposes, the right hand (pre-ductal site) is the most valuable.

3.D, An improvement in heart rate. With effective ventilation, all should improve, but an improvement in heart rate is a nearly immediate sign of improvement suggesting effective ventilation.

4.B, Chest compressions should be coordinated with ventilations to avoid simultaneous delivery. Chest compressions should be initiated if the heart rate is below 60/min with insufficient circulation. A fracture of the sternum is unlikely if chest compressions are given correctly. The compression rate should be approximately 90 compressions per minute, with 30 breaths coordinated every 3 compressions.

5.D, Can be given through venous access or an endotracheal tube using different dosing ranges. The preferred route of epinephrine (adrenaline) administration is intravenously at 0.01 to 0.03 mg/kg. The endotracheal dose of epinephrine (adrenaline) is 0.05 to 0.1 mg/kg.

6.D, All of the above are means to maintain a normal temperature in a newborn infant.

7.A, Adding sodium to the initial maintenance fluids prevents hypotension. This is a false statement and the correct answer. Unlike fluids provided to older infants and children, the maintenance intravenous fluid provided to most newborns should not contain sodium chloride. A total of 4 mL/kg/h of 10% dextrose is sufficient to supply the glucose to most newborns. For newborn hypoglycemia, a glucose bolus of 2 mL/kg of 10% dextrose is appropriate, followed by a glucose infusion.

8.C, Collection of urine by a bag placed over the perineum is the preferred method of urine collection for culture. This statement is false and is the correct answer. The preferred method is urine collected via urinary catheter. Gram-negative bacilli are common causes of early and late onset sepsis. Viral infection can mimic sepsis.

9.D, All of the above. All of these are risk factors for indirect hyperbilirubinemia.

10.B, Catheterization of the umbilical vessels can be performed rapidly and safely in an emergency. The vein is more easily cannulated in an emergency than the artery. The umbilical cord contains two umbilical arteries and one umbilical vein. If following the umbilical venous catheterization procedure properly, it can be used for fluid and/or medication administration before radiographic confirmation in an emergency.

Chapter 12: Procedural Sedation and Analgesia

1.B, Class II. Patients with mild systemic disease are categorized as class II. Class I patients are normal healthy patients. Class III patients are patients with severe systemic disease.

2.D, All of the above. All of these factors apply to the choice of medications selected for use in an individual child requiring sedation and/or analgesia. Some medications are appropriate for certain aged children, whereas others are not; painful procedures may require a medication with analgesic qualities, whereas a painless procedure would not; and finally, the indication for sedation can alter the priority choices for medications.

3.C, Initial and repeat vital signs. In the case of simple analgesia, continuous monitoring is not needed, provided the amount of medication administered is within the normal dose range. If additional doses of medication are needed above that expected for this child, then some form of monitoring might be indicated.

4.A, Ketamine. Methohexital, thiopental, and propofol all can cause respiratory depression. Of the listed agents, in appropriate doses, ketamine is the least likely to cause respiratory depression. All patients receiving any of these agents should undergo, at a minimum, cardiorespiratory and pulse oximetry monitoring.

5.C, Return to baseline respiratory status. At the very least, a child must demonstrate baseline respiratory activity before discharge can be considered. Some children will have some residual sleepiness or lack of coordination after procedural sedation, but this is not a contraindication to discharge. No set time frame can be used for any child for procedural sedation discharge. Some agents have durations of action of less than 10 minutes, whereas others are longer than 2 hours.

6.D, Propofol. Propofol is a potent vasodilator and can produce hypotension even in patients with normal intravascular volume.

7.A, 14-mL, A total of 7 mg/kg (0.7 mL/kg of 1%) of lidocaine (lignocaine) with epinephrine (adrenaline) is the recommended maximum for safely infiltrating wounds. Because 1% lidocaine (lignocaine) with epinephrine (adrenaline) contains 10 mg/mL, the 140 mg maximum is contained in 14 mL of solution.

8.E, All of the above. All of the above are correct. Other effects of ketamine include analgesia, emergence anxiety reactions, and vomiting.

9.A, Chloral hydrate. Chloral hydrate has the longest duration.

Chapter 13: Children With Special Health Care Needs: The Technologically Dependent Child

1.E, Suction tracheostomy tube. Assessment and management of the ABCs (airway, breathing, and circulation) include first attention to the equipment, such as the tracheostomy tube (e.g., suctioning to remove a mucous plug) and the ventilator (ensuring that all connections are intact and settings are correct). Then assess breathing (auscultate chest) and then circulation (assess color). Using a nebulized bronchodilator might be useful if the child is noted to be wheezing, but this should be done after confirming that the tracheostomy tube is clear. Removing the tracheostomy tube might be necessary if it is believed to have a plug that cannot be removed or if it is not in the trachea, in which case, it would have to be replaced immediately or the patient would have to be orally intubated with a laryngoscope if an airway or positive pressure ventilation is needed.

2.C, Tracheostomy tube dislodges. The other conditions listed are possible but would have a more gradual onset. A tracheostomy tube is at risk of dislodging at any time and will result in immediate respiratory difficulty.

3.C, Pressure and volume. The former uses pressure settings (inspiratory pressure and expiratory pressure), whereas the latter uses volume settings (tidal volume). The other answer options are different ventilator parameters as well, but they do not define the types of ventilators. In other words, a volume ventilator can be continuous or triggered by the patient's self inspiration, with a backup support rate.

4.A, Coca-Cola. Obstructed gastrostomy tubes can be cleared with either a proteolytic enzyme solution or Coca-Cola. Forcing fluid under higher pressure through the tube does not work. If the tube cannot be cleared by these means, it should be replaced. Hydrogen peroxide and pancrelipase do not work. Although ginger ale is a carbonated beverage as well, it has not been demonstrate to be effective.

5.B, Dislodge and need to be replaced. This can occur because the retention balloon has developed a leak, but it is unlikely that the tube itself will break. It would be very difficult for a gastrostomy tube to enter the small intestine because most of them are very short. Infection is possible, but uncommon.

6.D, A regular needle can be used to access an implanted port. This is the only choice that is not true. Tunneled central venous catheters are placed surgically. They are inserted directly into a central vein, most commonly the subclavian, cephalic, or jugular. There are three common types: Broviac, Hickman, and Groshong. The first two are most common in children. The distal ends rest outside the chest and can have one to three ports. Implanted vascular access ports (Port-A-Cath, PAS Port, and Med-A-Ports) are also common in children. The insertion sites and method are the same as for the tunneled central venous catheters. The distal end of the catheter consists of a reservoir covered with a self-healing rubber septum. This reservoir rests subcutaneously, and a special (Huber) needle is needed to access this catheter.

7.B, Cushing triad. Although signs and symptoms of a shunt obstruction include headache, nausea, vomiting, irritability, altered mental status, ataxia, change in vital signs, and a bulging fontanel in an infant. Late and very worrisome signs include those of the Cushing triad: bradycardia, irregular respirations, and hypertension.

8.B, Assess and manage airway, breathing, and circulation (ABCs). A child with a vagal nerve stimulator presenting with a seizure should be treated like a child without a vagal nerve stimulator, with attention to the ABCs first; then antiepileptic medication can be given, by any route. Because most of these children will be taking an antiepileptic medication, drawing a blood sample to measure the blood level (when available) is helpful, but this is done after the ABCs are assessed and managed. If the child is having breakthrough seizures, the vagal nerve stimulator should also be checked.

9.C, Assess and manage his airway, breathing, and circulation. After the ABCs are secure, then the baclofen pump can be turned off, or the reservoir can be emptied with a 22-gauge needle and syringe.

10.E, All of the above are correct.

Index

Venous thromboembolism
  management, 118
  obstructive shock, 117
Ventilators, mechanical. *See* mechanical ventilation
Ventricular septal defects, 136
Ventricular tachycardia (with pulse), 154
Ventriculoperitoneal shunts
  described, 489, 489f
  emergencies, 490
Versed. *See* midazolam
Vesiculobullous and vesiculopustular rashes, 408, 408f
Viral meningitis
  causes, 180–181
  clinical features, 181
  diagnostic studies, 181–182
  differential diagnosis, 182
  febrile seizures, 188
  management, 182–183
  signs and symptoms, 181
Vital signs, age-specific, and shock, 105–106, 106t
Vocal cords, infant and adult comparison of, 40t
Volume ventilators, 482
Volvulus, midgut. *See* malrotation and midgut volvulus
Von Willebrand disease, 407

W

Warm shock
  catecholamine-resistant shock, 113
  septic
    defined, 106
    management, 110f
West Nile virus, 180, 181
Western equine encephalitis virus, 180, 181
Wheezing, 19t
Wolff-Parkinson-White syndrome, 150, 151f, 154
Work of breathing
  abnormal audible airway sounds, 9, 11, 12t
  PAT and trauma, 208, 209f
  Pediatric Assessment Triangle, 9, 11–14, 12f, 12t, 13f
  techniques to assess, 13–14
  visual signs, 11–13, 12f, 12t, 13f
"Worrisome" appearance, 8, 8f
Wound care, initial, for burns, 251, 253, 253t

Z

Zidovudine
  sexual abuse, 281t
  sexual assault, 287t

Chapter 1
Opener © NorthGeorgiaMedia/ShutterStock, Inc.; 01.03 Courtesy of Dena Brownstein, MD.

Chapter 2
Opener © SURABKY/ShutterStock, Inc.; 02.19 © Visuals Unlimited; 02.22 Virginia Commonwealth University, Department of Radiology http://radiology.vcu.edu/09-11-02.htm.

Chapter 3
Opener © Craig Jackson/In the Dark Photography.

Chapter 4
Opener © Patrick Olear / PhotoEdit, Inc.

Chapter 6
Opener © Deborah Silver, The Stuart News/AP Photos.

Chapter 7
Opener Courtesy of Moose Jaw Police Service.

Chapter 8
Opener Courtesy of Ron Dieckman.

Chapter 9
Opener © Medical-on-Line/Alamy Images.

Chapter 10
Opener © Dr. H.C. Robinson/Photo Researchers, Inc.; 10.07 © Dr. Ken Greer/Visuals Unlimited; 10.08 © Mediscan/Visuals Unlimited; 10.09 © Mediscan/Visuals Unlimited.

Chapter 11
Opener © Eddie Lawrence/Photo Researchers, Inc.

Chapter 12
Opener © Keith Brofsky/Stockbyte/Thinkstock.

Chapter 13
Opener © Ellen B. Senisi/Photo Researchers, Inc.

Unless otherwise indicated, all photographs and illustrations are under copyright of Jones & Bartlett Learning, courtesy of Maryland Institute for Emergency Medical Services Systems, or the American Academy of Pediatrics.

Some images in this book feature models. These models do not necessarily endorse, represent, or participate in the activities represented in the images.